Current Perspectives in Hepatology

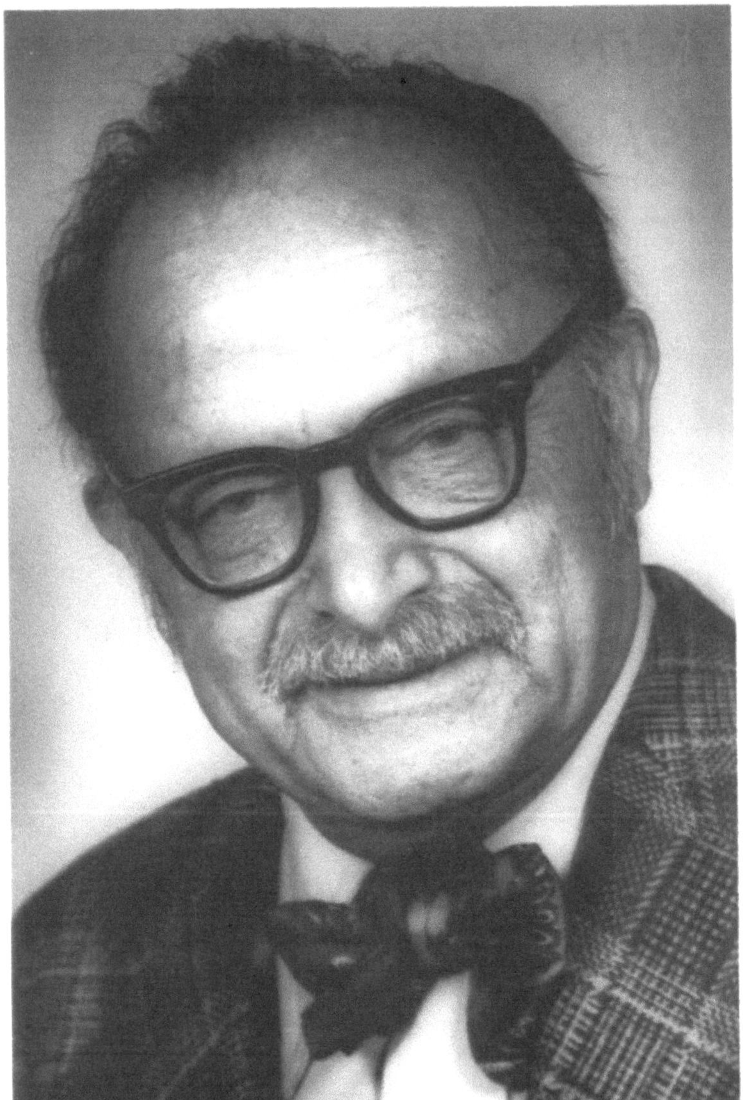

Hyman J. Zimmerman

Current Perspectives in Hepatology

Festschrift for Hyman J. Zimmerman, M.D.

Edited by

Leonard B. Seeff, M.D.

Chief, Division of Gastroenterology/Hepatology
Veterans Administration Medical Center
and Professor of Medicine
Georgetown University School of Medicine
Washington, D.C.

and

James H. Lewis, M.D., F.A.C.P., F.A.C.G.

Associate Professor of Medicine
Division of Gastroenterology
Georgetown University School of Medicine
Washington, D.C.

Plenum Medical Book Company • New York and London

Library of Congress Cataloging in Publication Data

Current perspectives in hepatology.
Includes bibliographies and index.
1. Liver—Diseases. 2. Zimmerman, Hyman J., 1914- . I. Seeff, Leonard B. II. Lewis, James H. III. Zimmerman, Hyman J., 1914- . [DNLM: 1. Liver Diseases. WI 700 C976]
RC845.C885 1989 616.3′62 88-32481
ISBN-13:978-1-4684-7043-7 e-ISBN-13:978-1-4684-7041-3
DOI: 10.1007/978-1-4684-7041-3

233 Spring Street, New York, N.Y. 10013

Plenum Medical Book Company is an imprint of Plenum Publishing Corporation

This book is dedicated
to our wives, Adele and Stephanie,
to our children,
and to the memory of the late Dr. Harry Seeff

Contributors

Charles O. Abernathy, Ph.D. • Health Effects Branch (WH-550D), Office of Drinking Water, U.S. Environmental Protection Agency, Washington, D.C. 20460

Firas H. Al-Kawas, M.D. • Associate Professor of Medicine, Georgetown University School of Medicine, Division of Gastroenterology/Hepatology/Nutrition, Veterans Administration Medical Center, Washington, D.C. 20422

Harvey J. Alter, M.D. • Chief, Department of Transfusion Medicine, Warren G. Magnuson Clinical Center, National Institutes of Health, Bethesda, Maryland 20892

Colin E. Atterbury, M.D. • Professor of Medicine, The Liver Center, Department of Internal Medicine, Yale University School of Medicine; Hepatic Hemodynamic Laboratory, Veterans Administration Medical Center, West Haven, Connecticut 06516

William F. Balistreri, M.D. • Dorothy M.M. Kersten Professor of Pediatrics, Director, Division of Pediatric Gastroenterology and Nutrition, Children's Hospital Medical Center, Cincinnati, Ohio 45229

Stanley B. Benjamin, M.D. • Associate Professor of Medicine, Chief, Division of Gastroenterology, Georgetown University School of Medicine, Washington, D.C. 20007

Martin Black, M.D. • Professor of Medicine and Pharmacology, Chief, Liver Unit, Temple University School of Medicine, Philadelphia, Pennsylvania 19140

Chao H. Chan, M.D. • Director, Gastroenterology Division, University of Arkansas for Medical Sciences; John L. McClellan Memorial Veterans Administration Medical Center, Little Rock, Arkansas 72205

Harold O. Conn, M.D. • Professor of Medicine, Yale University School of Medicine; Liver Disease Unit, Veterans Administration Medical Center, West Haven, Connecticut 06516

Stephen M. Feinstone, M.D. • Medical Officer, Laboratory of Infectious Diseases, National Institute of Allergy and Infectious Diseases, National Institutes of Health, Bethesda, Maryland 20892

Michael A. Gerber, M.D. • Department of Pathology, Tulane University School of Medicine, New Orleans, Louisiana 70112

Zachary D. Goodman, M.D., Ph.D. • Department of Hepatic Pathology, Armed Forces Institute of Pathology, Washington, D.C. 20306

Norman D. Grace, M.D. • Associate Professor of Medicine, Tufts University School of Medicine; Chief of Gastroenterology, Gastroenterology Service, The Faulkner Hospital, Boston, Massachusetts 02130

Roberto J. Groszmann, M.D. • Professor of Medicine, The Liver Center, Department of Internal Medicine, Yale University School of Medicine; Hepatic Hemodynamic Laboratory, Veterans Administration Medical Center, West Haven, Connecticut 06516

Ian D. Gust, M.D. • Professor of Clinical Virology, MacFarlane Burnet Centre for Medical Research, Fairfield Hospital, Melbourne, Australia 3078

R. Hallak, M.D. • Professor of Medicine, Yale University School of Medicine; Liver Disease Unit, Veterans Administration Medical Center, West Haven, Connecticut 06516

Jay H. Hoofnagle, M.D. • Clinical Director, Liver Diseases Section, Digestive Diseases Branch, National Institute of Diabetes and Digestive and Kidney Diseases, National Institutes of Health, Bethesda, Maryland 20892

Kamal G. Ishak, M.D., Ph.D. • Chairman, Department of Hepatic Pathology, Armed Forces Institute of Pathology, Washington, D.C. 20306-6000

Marshall M. Kaplan, M.D. • Professor of Medicine, Division of Gastroenterology, Tufts University School of Medicine, Chief, New England Medical Center Hospitals, Boston, Massachusetts 02111

Raymond S. Koff, M.D. • Chairman, Department of Medicine, Framingham Union Hospital, Framingham, Massachusetts 01701; Chief, Hepatology Section, Boston University School of Medicine, Boston, Massachusetts 02118

Jay H. Lefkowitch, M.D. • Associate Professor of Pathology, Department of Pathology, College of Physicians and Surgeons, Columbia University, New York, New York 10032

James H. Lewis, M.D. • Associate Professor of Medicine, Georgetown University School of Medicine; Division of Gastroenterology, Georgetown University Hospital, Washington, D.C. 20007

Roderick N. M. MacSween, M.D. • Titular Professor and Honorary Consultant Pathologist, Department of Pathology, University of Glasgow and Western Infirmary, Glasgow G11 6NT, Scotland, United Kingdom

Willis C. Maddrey, M.D. • Magee Professor and Chairman, Department of Medicine, Jefferson Medical College, Philadelphia, Pennsylvania 19107

Rodney S. Markin, M.D., Ph.D. • Department of Pathology and Microbiology, University of Nebraska Medical Center, Omaha, Nebraska 68105

Florabel G. Mullick, M.D. • Associate Chairman, Department of Environmental and Drug-Induced Pathology, Armed Forces Institute of Pathology, Washington, D.C. 20306

Lionel Rabin, M.D • Associate Chairman, Hepatic Pathology, Armed Forces Institute of Pathology, Washington, D.C. 20306-6000

Donald B. Rolfes, M.D. • Department of Pathology, Holy Cross Hospital, Silver Spring, Maryland 20910

Peter J. Scheuer, M.D. • Professor of Histopathology, Royal Free Hospital and School of Medicine, London NW3 2QG, England

Eugene R. Schiff, M.D. • Chief, Division of Hepatology, University of Miami School of Medicine; Chief, Hepatology Section, Veterans Administration Medical Center, Miami, Florida 33125

Leonard B. Seeff, M.D. • Professor of Medicine, Georgetown University; Chief, Gastroenterology/Hepatology/Nutrition, Veterans Administration Medical Center, Washington, D.C. 20007

J. Thomas Stocker, M.D. • Office of the Deputy Director, Armed Forces Institute of Pathology, Washington, D.C. 20306-6000

Riccardo Utili, M.D. • Clinic of Tropical and Subtropical Diseases, First Medical School, University of Naples, I-800135 Naples, Italy

Rowen K. Zetterman, M.D. • Chief, Section of Digestive Diseases and Nutrition, Department of Internal Medicine, University of Nebraska Medical Center; Veterans Administration Medical Center, Omaha, Nebraska 68105

Preface

In the spring of 1987, nearly 350 individuals gathered in a hotel in Bethesda, Maryland, just outside of Washington, D.C., to participate in a two-day medical symposium devoted to the topic of liver diseases. A small minority of this group had been attracted by what promised to be an outstanding Continuing Medical Education course. The remainder, however, although obviously interested in the content of the symposium, had come primarily to honor a man who, over the years, had profoundly touched them, personally or professionally, for the course had been conceived as a tribute to an exceptional man of medicine, a man with remarkable scholarly and personal attributes: Hyman J. Zimmerman.

Dr. Zimmerman, referred to affectionately by all as Hy, was born in 1914 in Rochester, New York, the city in which he received both his early schooling and his undergraduate education. In the late 1930s, he moved to Palo Alto to begin his medical education at Stanford University, from which he graduated cum laude in 1942, having spent an additional year acquiring a masters degree in bacteriology. Almost immediately thereafter, he entered military service, and as World War II was in progress, was assigned to duty in France. Soon after his arrival, he was made chief of an Army field hospital. A major medical problem plaguing U.S. troops at the time was viral hepatitis, which resulted in a deluge of patients admitted to his hospital. While nearly overwhelmed by the extensive numbers of hospitalized patients, he was intrigued by the varying aspects of the illness and undertook an in-depth analysis of the disease. This led to the publication, in 1947, of a now classic paper entitled: "Infectious Hepatitis: Clinical and Laboratory Features of 295 Cases."* As a consequence, his then widely varied medical interests narrowed to that of liver disease and the subsequent course of his medical career was set.

Following his discharge from the Army, Hy became aware of the efforts being made to affiliate selected Veterans Administration hospitals with local medical schools, and he surmised that this vast and far-flung hospital chain would begin to play a profoundly important role in graduate medical education and research. Accordingly, with his keen interest in both of these areas of medicine, he elected to enter the VA medical system. Thus a relationship was initiated that endures to the present, and which has brought great distinction to both.

Within two years of joining the VA medical system, Hy was invited to be the first Chief of Medicine at the Veterans Administration Hospital in Omaha, Nebraska. Indeed, he continued to hold this position until his retirement from active academic service almost 30 years later, serving as Chief of Medicine at VA hospitals in Chicago, Boston, and Washington, D.C. Even now he remains affiliated and honored as one of only a handful of VA Distinguished Physicians. During these various sojourns, Hy also served on the highest academic rungs of faculties of several medical

*_Am. J. Med. Sci._ **213**:395–409, 1947.

schools, including the Chicago Medical School where he was the Chairman of the Department of Medicine, the University of Nebraska, and Boston and George Washington universities.

Hy's contributions during these times, as administrator, researcher, and educator, raised him to the highest levels of prominence. He has, over the years, created several superb departments of medicine that have spawned and nurtured numerous outstanding physicians in all subspecialty areas. Particularly impressive has been his unusually varied and extensive attention to research in liver disease, as is apparent from a review of his voluminous bibliography, which consists of well over 300 publications. It is the field of hepatotoxicity, however, that has represented his greatest area of research interest and contribution; indeed, he has made it almost his own domain. His book, *Hepatotoxicity: The Adverse Effects of Drugs and Other Chemicals on the Liver,* now moving to its second edition, is widely and quite simply regarded as the premier reference source for students, clinicians, and scientists of all disciplines.

More than his academic accomplishments, Hy's primary appeal has always been the great regard in which he is held as a teacher and his extraordinary personal attraction. Teaching sessions conducted by him, both from the podium and at the bedside, are imbued with vitality, excitement, and erudition, making him a favorite invitee locally, nationally, and internationally, as well as a frequent honoree at numerous named lectureships. To top it all off, these achievements are accomplished by a man of uncommon charm, consideration, generosity, and compassion. Indeed, few academicians are as deeply admired and even loved as is Hy Zimmerman, a fact that prompted the American Association for the Study of Liver Diseases to bestow upon him their Distinguished Achievement Award in 1986. Little wonder then that his students, peers, and numerous friends felt compelled to organize and participate in a festschrift in his honor. The results of that symposium are represented by the contents of this book.

A final word regarding the format of the conference and of the book. One of Hy's enduring interests and strengths is that of clinicopathologic correlations of liver disease. Over the years, he has worked closely with several prominent hepatopathologists to initiate a number of highly-instructive, well-attended clinical–pathology teaching sessions. His most recent collaborator in these ventures is Dr. Kamal G. Ishak, Chairman of the Hepatic Pathology Branch of the Armed Forces Institute of Pathology, Washington, D.C., and himself a man of distinguished personal and academic stature. For more than 20 years, these two outstanding scientists have conducted a highly regarded liver pathology session at the Armed Forces Institute of Pathology, which culminated in the creation and establishment of an annual clinical–pathology course of the highest caliber. The success of these annual meetings served as the model for the festschrift and as the format of this book. An invitation to participate was extended to a number of Hy's ex-students, fellows, and friends, who are all recognized authorities in the field of hepatology or hepatopathology. While not designed to be an encyclopedic review of hepatology, each author was assigned a topic of particular expertise or relevance that touched upon Hy's vast contributions to the study of liver diseases in the process. Their efforts provide the reader with the opportunity to review many current aspects of liver disease in the unique manner of a clinical discussion followed by a pathologic correlation in what we hope and trust will be an everlasting tribute to Hy Zimmerman.

Leonard B. Seeff
James H. Lewis

Washington, D.C.

Foreword

The Four Symbols of Hy

How does one describe Hy Zimmerman? My starting point will be four symbols associated with Hy: the tennis racquet, the bow tie, the filing cabinets, and the Mustang convertible.

I remember vividly my participation in Hy's return to tennis. He and I were matched against Tom Chalmers and Dan Wright. During the first point, Hy planted himself in the center of the court on the spot formed by the confluence of the service and the midlines. From this position, he could reach almost half of the balls on our side. Only the reality that I was covering both extreme sides of the court disturbed this apparent equity. Hy would stroke, or if you will, wave at balls even beyond his reach. At times, his motions seemed to precede our opponents strokes; indeed, as if he were, in the manner of Toscanini, directing their efforts. In the epiphanal moment, just prior to my collapse, I gained an insight into one of Hy's sustaining attributes: the self-subordinating collegiality by which he stimulates and encourages colleagues of all levels to recognize and achieve their full potential.

The meaning of the bow tie remains obscure. I have consulted experts including an authoritative text, "Sexual Symbolism in Male Haberdashery," by Lauren, Steinem, and the Brothers Brooks. The latter state, and I quote, "That discarding the traditional four-in-hand is a classical symptom of the phallus rejection syndrome. However, the inexperienced clinician is advised to rule out both tie-in-soup disease and the tie-fly anomaly." Lacking access to the requisite laboratory studies, we must leave this issue unresolved. My personal preference is to interpret this Hy-tie finding as an index of his commitment to traditional values and the maintenance of vanishing skills. I will accept a recent alternative diagnosis that was proposed by a visiting fellow from Russia. In that country, apparently, the bow tie is considered to be symptomatic of an uncontrollable urge to be either a Christmas gift or the Easter Bunny.

As most of you know, Hy's capacity for information retrieval is awesome and the mechanism that underlies this process is monstrous. The origin is a desk buried under reprints—it is so chaotic that in 1970 a VAMC administrator assistant asked the search committee "How can you pick a chief with such a messy desk?" The destination in this process is the ever-increasing collection of unmarked and unmatched filing cabinets, which provides, I think, for Dr. Ishak and Dr. Zimmerman a model for a locally infiltrating lesion. But in any event, these two, the reprints and the files, are connected by an elaborate coding system.

Who among us does not remember Hy sitting through a lecture while scrawling obscure numbers on the sheaf of reprints on his lap. Despite attempts by nubile agents of several foreign powers, the secret of the code remains unbreeched. However, recent investigations, based on the sequence of winners at Pimlico, offer some possibility of solution. Of course, the process of coding

Excerpted from remarks made during an awards dinner ceremony in honor of Dr. Zimmerman April 27, 1987.

kept Hy awake during the lectures. When he became chief of the service, custom dictated that he move to the front row and propriety mandated that he forego the reprints. The predictable outcome was apparent sleep, which I found particularly frightening when some of you were our guest lecturers. I contrived to sit next to him to wiggle and jostle constantly, thereby reducing the possibility that our hero would fall from his chair and roll inexorably to the podium. My efforts were unnecessary since at the end of the lecture, each speaker was rewarded with insightful comments or questions from a refreshed host. Today, in brashness nurtured by our feeling of common affection for Hy, I will reveal the truth. Each of you received the same inquiries and comments. The lesson I believe is unmistakable—eternal vigilance may be the price of liberty, but has no essential role in the lecture hall.

I can only imagine what Hy feels when he slides behind the wheel of his Mustang convertible—suave, sophisticated, dashing, debonair; like Snoopy in search of the Red Baron. To ride with him is to experience the exhilaration of the unknown, the quest of the scientist. Will we make it in one piece? Are you supposed to look at the guy in the back seat when you talk to him? Can you really make a U-turn on a one-way street? Why is the guy in blue interested in us? And, finally, has he paid his insurance premiums? Recently, I was astonished to find that the color of the noble vehicle was changed from green to red. Had the Lone Ranger exchanged Silver for Black Beauty? No. It is the same trusty steed. The cacophony of the motor and the slope of the chassis were unmistakable. We, the Hy watchers, are still debating the meaning of the change. Is this a clever attempt to confuse the now-knowledgeable constabulary? Has he always harbored the dream of being Hyman the Fireman? Or is it possible that the little engine that could, is now signaling that it cannot?* Nevertheless, this transmutation is favorable, albeit temporizing. To Hy's wife, Kitty, I say someday, you who have tolerated so much, will have to redecorate the living room around the remains of the Z-mobile; but at least that day has been delayed.*

Having already compromised my vows of levity and brevity, let me end with some intentionally serious comments. This dinner arose only from a desire to celebrate Hy. We are here to enjoy ourselves and we frolic in the friendship that derives from our common fellowship and our shared commitments. Hy is the cement of these relationships and no institution intervenes; which brings me to my last question, how has he accomplished this without the imprimatur of institutional authority? I think a partial answer is found in John Henry Newman's definition of a university. He states, "A university exists and has ever consisted in demand and supply, in wants which it alone can satisfy and which it does satisfy, in the communication of knowledge and the relationship and bond which exists between the teacher and the taught. It's constituting animating principle is the model attraction of one class of persons to another . . ." I would note the emotional, moral, and intellectual components of this bond. Our presence this evening attests to their reality and I think in this context, much becomes clear. We are, in fact, members of the Hyman J. Zimmerman alumni association; the faculty and students of a unique college.

James D. Finkelstein, M.D.
Chief, Medical Service
Veterans Administration Medical Center
Professor of Medicine
School of Medicine
George Washington University
Washington, D.C. 20422

*His children had it refurbished and repainted on its 20th anniversary.

*Dr. Finkelstein was prescient in his remarks as the "Z-mobile" did meet an untimely end; but, good fortune was shining on the driver, who was not seriously injured. A blue T-bird sedan has taken its place.

Contents

I

Viral Hepatitis

1

Hepatitis A Infection: Clinical Aspects

Stephen M. Feinstone and Ian D. Gust

1. INTRODUCTION

The development of specific diagnostic tests first for hepatitis B virus (HBV) infections and then hepatitis A virus (HAV) infections has enabled clinicians to determine accurately the cause of hepatitis in their patients. Although non-A, non-B (NANB) hepatitis remains a diagnosis of exclusion and may be caused by more than one agent, the ability to make specific etiologic diagnoses has allowed us to study these diseases in some detail to define their clinical spectrum and epidemiology.

Hepatitis A is an acute viral illness that exhibits a wide range of symptomatology, from the common occurrence of infection without detectable disease to the very rare case of fulminant hepatitis, coma, and death. Most of the factors that determine the clinical expression of disease are unknown, and it is probably a combination of host and viral factors.

2. INCUBATION PERIOD

The incubation period—defined as the time from exposure to the virus to first expression of clinical illness—can often be established because many outbreaks of hepatitis A are point source, and the time of exposure can be determined. As early symptoms of hepatitis A are often vague, the onset of dark urine that often causes the patient to seek medical attention is frequently used as the first clinical indication of disease. In recent serologically confirmed outbreaks of hepatitis A, the incubation periods could be accurately determined. Seven of 10 members of a family who consumed partially cooked mussels collected off a pier close to where untreated sewage was being discharged from a barge developed hepatitis 29–40 days later, with a median of 34 days.[1] In a larger outbreak of hepatitis A that occurred among naval recruits in San Diego who were infected by eating salad prepared by an infected food handler, the incubation period ranged from 21 to 42 days.

Titration experiments of HAV in marmosets show that the incubation period is related to the viral dose. When the monkeys were inoculated intravenously, the incubation period increased about 1 week for each $\log_{10}$ reduction in the dose of the inoculum. The shortest incubation period

Stephen M. Feinstone • Laboratory of Infectious Diseases, National Institute of Allergy and Infectious Diseases, National Institutes of Health, Bethesda, Maryland 20892. *Ian D. Gust* • MacFarlane Burnet Centre for Medical Research, Fairfield Hospital, Melbourne, Australia 3078.

observed was only 1 week after the inoculation of 10^8 infectious doses; the longest was 7 weeks after one infectious dose[2] (Fig. 1).

3. CLINICAL FEATURES

While the clinical expression of HAV infection may vary widely, the single most important determinant yet identified that affects the severity of illness is age. More than 90% of infections in children under 5 years of age may be silent, but the proportion of symptomatic infections increases with age. In the Greenland epidemic of 1970–1974, the frequency of clinically recognizable hepatitis increased from 1% in children under 1 year of age to 24% in 15-year-old children.[3] Similar low rates of clinical expression have been noted among children involved in day-care center outbreaks of hepatitis in the United States[4]; however, adults infected in these outbreaks usually become jaundiced.

In 1969, many members of the Holy Cross University football team as well as several members of the coaching staff developed hepatitis A from drinking contaminated water.[5] Ninety members of the team developed symptoms of hepatitis or transient elevation of alanine aminotransferase levels in their sera; 32 of these members were jaundiced. When sera from these patients were studied with specific serologic tests, only those who were jaundiced could be shown to have been infected with HAV.[6]

Death due to HAV infections has been well documented, but it is a very rare event. Case fatality rates have usually been based on hospitalized patients and although rates of 1/1000 have often been reported, the rate should be much lower because of large numbers of asymptomatic and nonhospitalized symptomatic patients. In the largest hospital-based series of hepatitis A reported, of 2174 patients with serologically confirmed hepatitis A, three died (0.14%).[7] Surprisingly, two of these deaths occurred in patients under 20 years of age, when heptatitis A is usually thought to be a benign disease. Both patients were known to have previously been in good health and had no known predisposing factors that could account for their severe illness. The mean time from the onset of dark urine to encephalopathy in these three patients was 7 days, and from encephalopathy to death was 6 days. Thus, hepatic necrosis can occur very rapidly in hepatitis A.

It is not known what host or viral factors contribute to the severity of illness. Animal experiments do not seem to implicate viral dose as the major factor in determining severity of illness. If an animal receives only one infectious dose of HAV, it usually will develop hepatitis of essentially the same severity as an animal inoculated with 10^6 infectious doses; however, we do know that HAV strains can be developed in the laboratory that are infectious but that have a sharply reduced virulence.[8,9] Such strains developed by multiple in vitro cell culture passages are being studied as

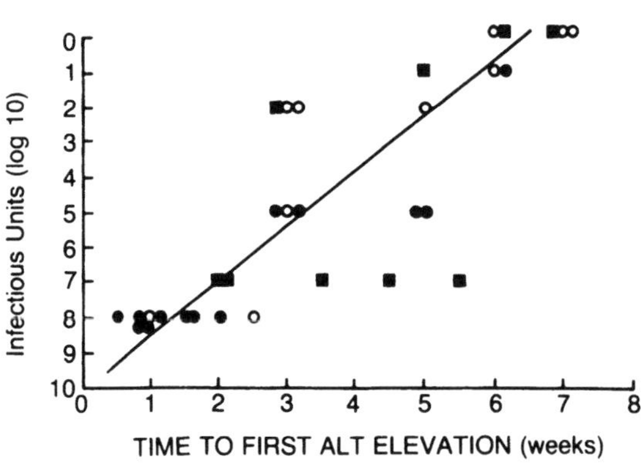

Figure 1. Inverse relationship between dose of HAV and incubation period in marmosets and chimpanzees measured from the time of intravenous inoculation to the first elevation of isocitrate dehydrogenase or alanine aminotransferase. (From ref. 2.)

live viral vaccine candidates. It is possible that viral strains with a wide range of virulence characteristics exist in nature.

In symptomatic cases of hepatitis A, patients often describe a prodromal illness of several days to 1 week or more in duration. This illness usually consists of increasing fatigue, malaise, loss of appetite, as well as nausea and vomiting; however, these symptoms are usually not severe enough to cause the patient to seek medical attention or even stay home from work. About three-fourths of patients have low-grade fever, and about 70% have headache. A variety of other symptoms have been reported, but it is not known which of these are specifically associated with HAV infections. Nausea and vomiting are commonly associated with HAV infections. Nausea and vomiting are commonly associated with hepatitis A, and inflammation of the gastric and duodenal mucosa has been reported in the older literature.[10,11] We do not know whether this is a direct result of infection by HAV or a secondary response to the hepatic disease.

Bilirubinuria followed within a few days by pale or clay-colored feces and yellow discoloration of the sclera, skin, and mucous membranes are often the first objective signs of hepatitis recognized by the patient. The return of color to the stools usually occurs within 2 or 3 weeks after the onset of illness and is a good sign of resolution of the disease. Some patients develop pruritus severe enough to require antipruritics. This symptom is frequently an indication of the cholestatic hepatitis that is occasionally associated with hepatitis A.[12]

Physical findings in patients with acute hepatitis A include the obvious jaundice, an enlarged firm tender liver, a palpable spleen in up to 15% of patients, and the possible appearance of spider naevi on the trunk.

4. NATURAL HISTORY

Hepatitis A is an acute or subacute infectious disease. Although we have recently heard of anecdotal and single cases of chronic hepatitis A, these must be thoroughly proved before they can be accepted. In general, infections by HAV never become chronic or cause chronic liver disease. No chronic carrier state of HAV is known to exist. In addition, reinfection after recovery from HAV infection is not recognized. In most cases, physical findings and laboratory tests have declined to near normal within 3 weeks of the onset of illness. Occasionally, patients have prolonged elevated serum enzyme levels, but these always resolve.[13] The cause of the prolonged abnormal liver-function tests is unclear. We have frequently observed by immunofluorescence the persistence of hepatitis A antigen in the livers of marmosets for up to 6 months after the original infection.[14] These animals all had acute infections and disease but also had recovered completely with normal liver-function tests and biopsies and had developed high levels of serum antibodies. We do not know whether the antigen observed represents complete infectious virus or only viral antigen. Since no serial biopsy material is available from humans with hepatitis A, we do not know how long viral antigen persists in humans or whether persistent antigen in the liver is associated with the prolonged enzyme elevations in some patients following acute hepatitis A.

Cholestatic hepatitis has been reported as an occasional complication of HAV infections. Gordon et al.[13] described six cases in detail. These cases showed peak serum bilirubin levels of 12–29 mg/dl, with jaundice lasting 12–18 weeks; however, ALT levels were <500 IU/liter during the icteric phase. Liver biopsies revealed centrilobular cholestasis and portal inflammation. Although the prognosis in these cases is universally favorable, Schiff has recommended a short course of rapidly tapered corticosteroids to reduce symptoms and hasten resolution.[15] The pathogenesis of this cholestatic disease is unknown.

Relapsing disease has also been reported following acute hepatitis A; recently, these cases were serologically confirmed.[16–19] Bamber et al.[16] reported three relapses among 88 patients with acute hepatitis A admitted to hospital in London, and Gruer et al.[17] reported five patients with acute hepatitis A who were readmitted with a relapse 7–10 weeks later. Chiriaco et al.[18] reported 23 children admitted to the hospital in Padua, Italy, with well-documented acute hepatitis A. All these patients had specific serologic evidence of HAV infections and no evidence of HBV, Epstein–Barr virus (EBV), or cytomegalovirus (CMV) infections. Symptoms and jaundice resolved in all these patients within 5–30 days, and ALT levels fell to normal. Each of these 23 children showed a second rise in transaminase levels to 210–2365 IU/liter (mean 710) 15–90 days (mean 31 days) later. Only four of these 23 children were icteric during the second episode, and in all 23 cases, the disease eventually resolved completely. They had no evidence of HBV, EBV, or CMV infections during the second episode.

Sjögren et al.[19] recently reported relapses in 17 of 256 patients (6.6%) with acute hepatitis A in Argentina. These patients developed ALT elevations 30–90 days after resolution of the initial episode. Serial stool samples were obtained from seven of these patients during the relapse, and evidence was found for HAV in samples from four patients by immune electron microscopy (IEM), radioimmunoassay (RIA), and molecular hybridization using a hepatitis A-cloned complementary DNA (cDNA) probe. In this case, it appears that the relapse was associated with excretion of HAV. It cannot be determined from this study whether (1) excretion of HAV ever stopped, (2) this was a relapse or reactivation of the original infection, or (3) these cases were due to a second infection with HAV. Since all these patients had high levels of serum antibody (presumably neutralizing antibody) before the relapse, all these possibilities are difficult to explain. While the mechanism of relapse has not been elucidated, it is crucial to recognize that all these cases eventually resolved without third episodes or any chronic sequelae.

5. MODE OF INFECTION

The epidemiology of hepatitis A indicates that it is spread primarily through the fecal–oral route. The virus infects the liver and is excreted through the bile into the feces. It is not known how much if any fecal HAV comes from replication within the gut; however, it is known that during the early stage of the hepatic infection, HAV can also be found in the blood.[20,21] The viremia probably ends soon after the appearance of serum antibody or at about the time of the clinical expression of illness; however, serum specimens collected soon after the onset of clinical disease that contain detectable antibody have also been shown to be infectious.[22] Therefore, even though a chronic viremic carrier state of HAV does not exist, there remains the possibility that an asymptomatic person who was incubating HAV could transmit HAV through donated blood. Francis et al.,[23] in 1946, reported a case of hepatitis of short incubation period in the recipient of a unit of blood collected 11 days before the onset of jaundice in the donor; a similar case was reported by Harden et al.[24] 1955. While these cases may have been hepatitis A, they cannot be confirmed because of the lack of specific serologic tests. This was best pointed out when an epidemic of hepatitis in a transplantation center that was associated with contaminated platelets was originally thought to be hepatitis A.[25] When specific tests were applied to these patients, it was found that the epidemic was not due to HAV but to NANB hepatitis.[26] Nevertheless, several well-documented cases of hepatitis A have been reported following transfusion of whole blood, packed red blood cells (RBC), and fresh-frozen plasma.[27–31] While it is clear that HAV can be transmitted by blood transfusion, studies on multiply transfused patients show that they do not have an increased prevalence of anti-HAV; therefore, since transfusion-associated hepatitis A must be quite rare, screening of blood supplies for HAV is not required.

Recently, an interesting outbreak of hepatitis A occurred in several cancer treatment centers around the United States (I. Weissfuss, personal communication). Several patients in a multicenter trial who were being treated with an experimental therapy consisting of interleukin-2 (IL-2) and lymphokine-activated killer (LAK) cells developed hepatitis A. The problem was first noted in August 1986, when one patient in the study, and the spouse of another patient being treated at the same center, developed hepatitis A. An epidemiologic investigation was begun by the Centers for

Disease Control (CDC). At least 30 HAV infections have been serologically confirmed, with at least two cases at each of the six centers. In addition, at least three cases occurred among household contacts of the patients receiving LAK cells.

No local factors could account for the distribution of cases. The medium used to produce the LAK cells was prepared centrally and distributed to all the centers. This tissue culture medium was supplemented with pooled human serum obtained from paid donors by a single supplier. All sera were tested for hepatitis B surface antigen (HBsAg) and anti-HIV, filtered, heated to 50°C for 30 min, pooled to produce bulk lots, and diluted to 20% in tissue culture (TC) medium. Seven batches of media were suspected to have transmitted HAV; five containing serum from a lot termed week 22 bulk lot and the other two media lots containing serum from week 31 bulk lot. Although these two lots were prepared nearly 2 months apart and did not share the same sera, 20 donors contributed to both lots.

The investigation demonstrated that the serum was the only possible source of the HAV. However, it remains surprising that pools of sera containing high levels of antibody to HAV that was also washed off the cells before they were injected back into the patient could have caused these infections, suggesting amplification in the LAK cells. This possibility is being investigated.

6. LABORATORY FEATURES OF HEPATITIS A

Liver-function tests, specifically serum levels of alanine aminotransferase (ALT) and aspartate aminotransferase (AST), that measure hepatic injury are highly sensitive means of detecting hepatitis; however, they are not specific for hepatitis type A. While some patients infected with HAV do not have elevated ALT or AST levels, many asymptomatic patients do have abnormal enzyme levels that are only detectable if blood specimens are collected. In icteric infections, serum levels of these enzymes may reach 20,000 IU/liter or even higher. Very high ALT levels may indicate severe hepatitis but are not necessarily a bad prognostic sign and may not even correlate with the patient's symptomatology. Occasional patients have ALT/AST levels persistently elevated for up to 6 months following infection, but eventual resolution is the rule.

Alkaline phosphatase may be mildly elevated in hepatitis A, and when cholestasis complicates HAV infection, the alkaline phosphatase levels are usually very high.

Giles and colleagues[32] found that children at the Willowbrook School inoculated with the MS-1 strain of HAV developed elevated levels of serum IgM within a few days of the onset of illness, which returned to normal within 4 or 5 weeks. Elevated immunoglobulin M (IgM) levels in hepatitis A have been confirmed by others in naturally acquired infections.[33,34] In a series at Fairfield Hospital in Melbourne, Australia, the mean IgM level in the first serum drawn after admission of hepatitis A patients was 443 mg/dl, compared with 270 mg/dl for hepatitis B patients, 197 mg/dl in NANB hepatitis patients, and 148 mg/dl in controls.[35] This IgM response is polyclonal, and most of the IgM elevation cannot be accounted for by the rise in specific IgM class antibody to HAV.

Many other laboratory abnormalities may be noted in HAV infection, none of which is specific. There is usually a mild lymphocytosis, and occasional atypical mononuclear cells are observed. Reductions in serum albumin and clotting factor levels are usually seen only in fulminant hepatitis.

7. SPECIFIC DIAGNOSTIC TESTS FOR HEPATITIS A

Hepatitis A virus was first detected by the technique of IEM,[36,37] a serologic technique that can be used to measure either antigen or antibody (Fig. 2). For detection of antibodies in a standard homogenate containing a known number of HAV particles, the particles are reacted with specific

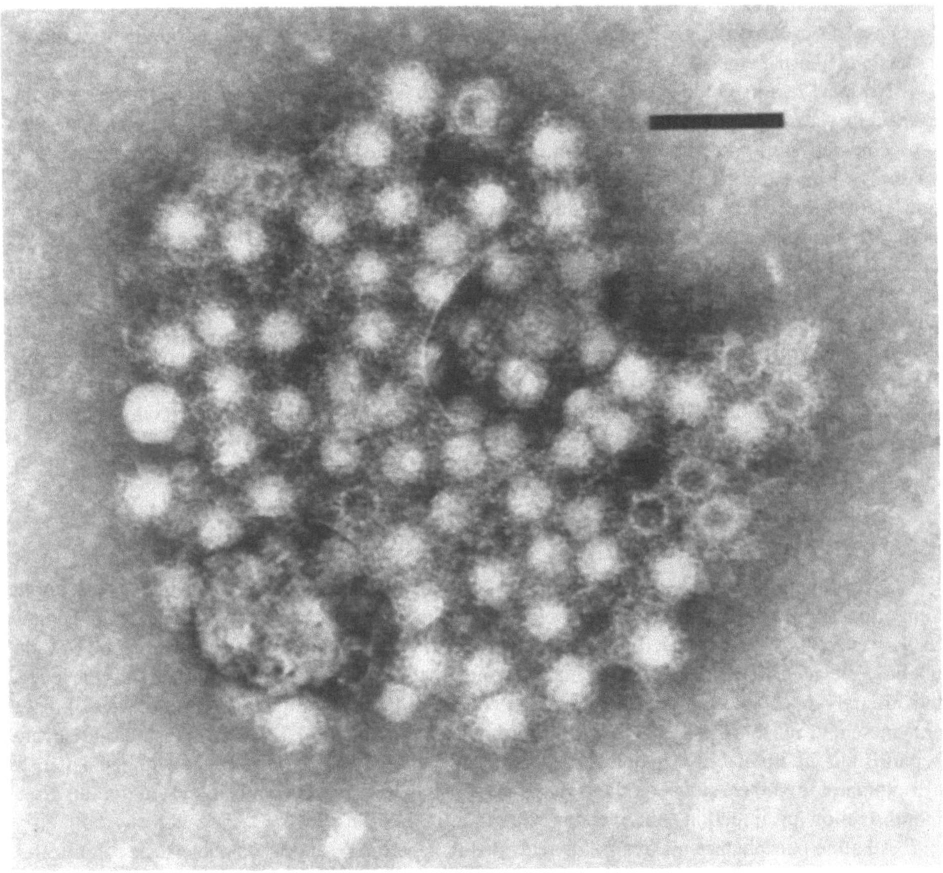

Figure 2. Electron micrograph of HAV particles aggregated by antibody. Bar = 100 nm.

antibody and the resulting complexes examined by electron microscopy. Particles reacting with the antibody are aggregated and surrounded by antibody. These features can be used to quantitate roughly the amount of antibody in different preparations and to distinguish HAV from other particulate material. Using IEM and other less cumbersome serologic techniques, the virologic and immunologic events of HAV infection were described (Fig. 3). Following infection, HAV is excreted in the stool early in the disease, usually peaking at about the time of the appearance of jaundice. Serum antibody to HAV also appears concurrent with the onset of clinical disease, and viral shedding rapidly declines at that time. While both IgG and IgM antibody seem to be produced early in the disease, most of this early antibody is IgM. If a patient first seeks medical attention because of the appearance of dark urine and jaundice, viral shedding may no longer be detectable, but IgM antibody to HAV should be present. Thus, the detection of IgM anti-HAV forms the basis for the serodiagnosis of acute hepatitis A.

Specific diagnostic tests for HAV can be divided into three categories: tests for the virus, tests for total antibody, and tests for IgM antibody. Testing for the virus has limited value for diagnostic purposes, because about one half the patients no longer have detectable virus in their stools when they first seek medical attention. Most tests for HAV are immunologic, beginning with IEM.[36] IEM can be a very sensitive test if the microscopist is skilled and is willing to spend considerable time

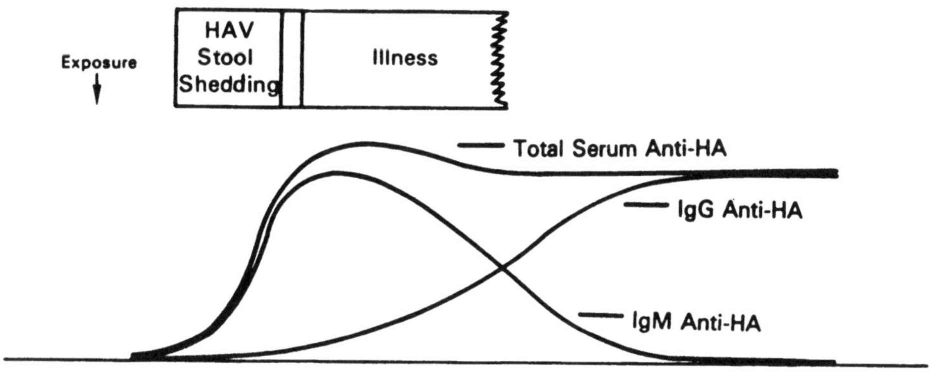

Figure 3. Diagrammatic representation of the clinical, virologic, and serologic events that occur in HAV infections.

examining one specimen, but it is usually stated that IEM requires approximately 10^6 viral particles per ml to be positive. RIA[38,39] and enzyme immunoassays (EIA)[40] for HAV antigen have been developed and may be able to detect as little as 10^5 particles per ml. Cell culture is the most sensitive method for detecting many viruses; however, wild-type strains of HAV often replicate poorly on the initial passages in cell culture; therefore, cell culture cannot be relied on to detect HAV in clinical specimens. Inoculation of susceptible animals may be as sensitive as cell culture but, because the major models for HAV infection are chimpanzees and marmoset monkeys, this is not a practical approach.

The recent cloning of the HAV RNA genome as cDNA now permits the production of specific molecular hybridization probes for HAV.[41] Using this system, Ticehurst et al.[42] have been able to detect as little as 10^4 or even 10^3 HAV particles. Tassopoulos and colleagues[43] used this system to look for HAV in the stools of patients in Greece. They were able to detect the virus shedding for longer periods than with the conventional solid-phase RIA.[43]

There has been some specificity problem using molecular probes on stool samples, but Jansen et al.[44] have combined immunoaffinity and molecular hybridization to overcome this specificity problem.

Even though these new technologic approaches to diagnostics offer heretofore unachievable sensitivity, in the case of hepatitis A there remain too many false-negative results for these tests to be useful except for research purposes.

While many tests for antibody to HAV have been developed, beginning again with IEM, most of the tests in use today are RIA or EIA.[38–40] The typical RIA or EIA anti-HAV test is based on blocking the attachment of a labeled specific antibody to HAV by the test serum. All classes of antibody may block the labeled anti-HAV; therefore, blocking tests measure total serum antibody. These tests are generally sensitive enough to detect antibody in virtually 100% of patients infected by HAV, even if the infection occurred many years before. Therefore, a positive result in the total antibody test in a patient with a viral hepatitis syndrome is of no value, because it cannot be determined whether the antibody was from a much earlier, perhaps inapparent, infection. Testing paired serum specimens on a patient may not demonstrate rising levels of total antibody, because as the IgG levels begin to rise, IgM levels may begin to fall. In addition, clinical decisions, such as whether to give immune serum globulin to contacts, cannot be put off until the late serum can be collected and tested. Therefore, the primary purpose of the total antibody test is for the determination of immunity and epidemiologic investigations.

The problem of rapid diagnosis of HAV infections using a single serum collected during the acute phase of the illness is solved by the use of tests for IgM-class specific anti-HAV. Locarnini et al.[37] in Melbourne first detected IgM anti-HAV by IEM, whereby this class of antibody can be recognized morphologically. When early acute-phase serum was used in their IEM experiments, these workers noted that HAV particles were coated and aggregated by large-antibody molecules, some of which formed staplelike bridges. It was demonstrated specifically that there was both IgM and IgG antibody in patients' serum by immunoferritin staining and by separating the serum into the 19S IgM-containing component from the slower sedimenting 7S IgG-containing component. Several types of RIA and EIA tests have subsequently been developed for IgM class-specific anti-HAV.[46–48] Most commercial tests are of the capture type, in which highly specific antiserum to human IgM is bound to the solid phase[46,48,49] (Fig. 4). The test serum is reacted with this anti-IgM/solid phase, which binds the IgM in the serum. HAV is then added, followed by a labeled anti-HAV IgG detector. The quantity of labeled IgG that is bound is an indirect measure of the amount of specific anti-HAV IgM present in the test serum. These tests have proved highly sensitive and are positive in nearly 100% patients with acute HAV infections at their first clinical presentation. In fact, the commercial tests are actually run at a reduced sensitivity so that IgM anti-HAV will no longer be detectable 6 months after the onset of disease. On occasion, a patient such as a family contact of a clinical case tested early in the course of illness, will have no detectable IgM anti-HAV test. If hepatitis A is strongly suspected, a later serum should be tested for both IgM and total antibody to HAV. Thus, the serodiagnosis of HAV is now rapid and highly sensitive and can be performed on a single acute phase serum sample.

8. VIROLOGY AND PATHOGENESIS OF HEPATITIS A

Hepatitis A virus is a member of the picornavirus family, which includes rhinoviruses and enteroviruses of humans and animals, the cardioviruses of mice, and the aphthoviruses (foot-and-mouth-disease virus) of cattle. While HAV shares many characteristics with enteroviruses, it has several unique features that appear to place it into a category by itself. Relative to enteroviruses, HAV is highly resistant to heat and can survive 60°C for 1 hr.[50,51] In cell culture, HAV grows slowly, is generally not cytolytic, and does not seem to reduce the rate of host protein or RNA synthesis. Poliovirus, as an example of an enterovirus, replicates in hours, quickly and efficiently shuts down host macromolecular synthesis, and lyses the cell in which it is growing.[52–54] It seems likely that these in vitro growth characteristics of HAV are important in the pathogenesis of hepatitis A.

Hepatitis A virus is generally infectious by the fecal–oral route. Because the virus is resistant to acid, it may pass the stomach and replicate somewhere in the lower intestine; but despite limited evidence of replication of HAV in the small intestine, we still do not have a clear picture of the primary site of replication of HAV. It may be anywhere in the alimentary tract, or HAV may

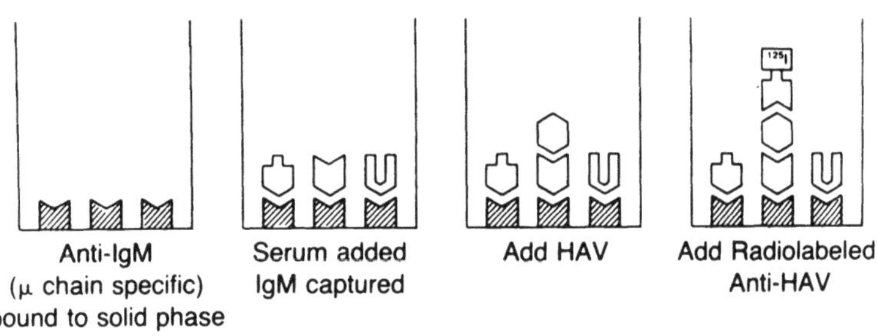

Figure 4. Diagrammatic representation of the solid phase capture test for specific IgM antibody to HAV.

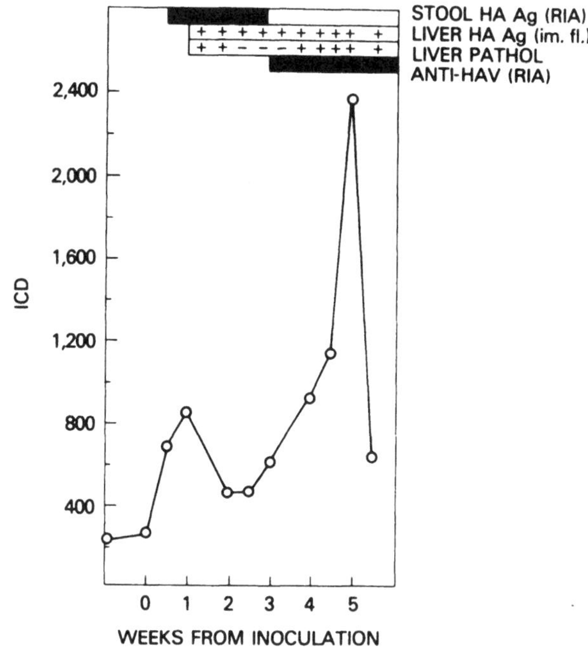

Figure 5. Biphasic enzyme elevations in a marmoset inoculated with 10^8 infectious units of HAV. The second enzyme elevation occurs at about the time of the appearance of serum antibody.

somehow be transported to the liver without prior replication in the host. HAV, like many other picornaviruses, is very organ specific, which may be based on highly specific receptors on the hepatocytes. Although HAV antigen has been detected by immunofluorescence in cells other than hepatocytes, particularly cells of the reticuloendothelial system (RES), it is not known whether the virus grows in these cells.[14] No extrahepatic pathology is recognized in HAV infections. When marmosets (*Saguinas labiatus* or *S. mystax*) are inoculated, we can observe HAV antigen in almost every hepatocyte; however, as in cell culture, we do not observe generalized necrosis of the infected hepatocytes. How, then, does HAV cause disease?

When we inoculated marmosets with 10^8 infectious dose of HAV, we observed abnormal liver-function tests and HAV antigen in the liver within 1 week (Fig. 5). The enzymes stabilized or even declined a little until the third week when, coincident with the appearance of serum antibody, we observed a second, higher, peak of liver enzyme elevation. The obvious explanation is that the early mild hepatitis was a viropathic effect, but the second, more severe, disease was an immunopathic effect. Krawczynski et al.[55] were unable to detect deposits of Ig or complement components in liver biopsies of marmosets infected with HAV; however, Kurane et al.[56] showed that mononuclear cells with characteristics of natural killer (NK) cells from nonimmune donors will lyse HAV-infected tissue culture cells, and Vallbracht et al.[57] showed that lymphocytes from convalescent patients produced cytotoxic changes in their own epidermal cell lines infected with HAV.

Therefore, it seems possible that HAV infections produce only a mild cytopathic effect in hepatocytes but that the major injury is a result of the cell-mediated immune response. Circulating antibody may be important in limiting the spread of virus to uninfected or recovered cells, and other factors such as interferon (INF) may also be important for recovery.

Although hepatitis A is caused by a member of a well-recognized viral family—picornaviruses—and the disease is self-limited without chronic sequelae, there remains much to learn about both the virus and the disease. Finally, vaccines for the prevention of this disease are now being developed, and control of hepatitis A may soon be practical.

REFERENCES

1. Dienstag JL, Gust ID, Lucas CR, et al: Mussel-associated viral hepatitis, type A: Serological confirmation. *Lancet* **1**:561–563, 1976.
2. Purcell RH, Feinstone SM, Ticehurst JR, et al: Hepatitis A virus, in Vijars GN, Dienstag JL, Hoofnagle JH (eds): *Viral Hepatitis in Liver Diseases*. Grune & Stratton, Orlando, 1984, pp. 9–22.
3. Skinhoj P, Gluud C, Ramsoe K: Traveller's hepatitis. Origin and characteristics in cases in Copenhagen 1976–1978. *Scand J Infect Dis* **13**:1–9, 1981.
4. Hadler S, Erben J: in Szmuness W, Alter HJ, Maynard JE (eds): *Viral Hepatitis*. Franklin Institute Press, Philadelphia, 1982, pp. 740–741.
5. Morse LJ, Bryan JA, Hurley JP, et al: The Holy Cross College football team hepatitis outbreak. *JAMA* **219**:706–708, 1972.
6. Friedman LS, O'Brien TF, Morse LJ, et al: Revisiting the Holy Cross football team hepatitis outbreak (1969) by serological analysis. *JAMA* **254**:774–776, 1985.
7. McNeill M, Hoy JF, Richards MJ, et al: Etiology of fatal hepatitis in the Melbourne. *Med J Aust* **2**:637–640, 1984.
8. Provost PJ, Bishop RP, Gerety RJ, et al: New finding in live, attenuated hepatitis A vaccine development. *J Med Virol* **20**:165–175, 1986.
9. Karron RA, Daemer PJ, Ticehurst J, et al: Studies in prototype live HAV vaccine in primate models. *J Infect Dis* **157**:338–345, 1988.
10. Havens WP Jr, Kushlan SD, Green MR: Experimentally induced infectious hepatitis: Roentgenographic and gastroscopic observations. *Arch Intern Med* **79**:457–464, 1947.
11. Knight WA, Cogswell RC: Preliminary observations of the gastric mucosa in patients with infectious hepatitis. *JAMA* **128**:803–804, 1945.
12. Gordon SC, Reddy KR, Schiff L, et al: Prolonged intrahepatic cholestatis secondary to acute hepatitis A. *Ann Intern Med* **101**:635–637, 1984.
13. Routenberg JA, Dienstag JL, Harrison WO, et al: Food borne epidemic of hepatitis A: Clinical and laboratory features of acute and protracted illness. *Am J Med Sci* **278**:123–137, 1979.
14. Mathieson L, Feinstone SM, Purcell RH, et al: Detection of hepatitis A antigen by immunofluorescence. *Infect Immunol* **18**:524–530, 1977.
15. Schiff L: The use of steroids in liver disease. *Medicine (Baltimore)* **45**:565–573, 1966.
16. Bamber M, Thomas HC, Bannister B, et al: Acute type A, B, and non-A, non-B hepatitis in a hospital population in London. Clinical and epidemiological features. *Gut* **24**:561–564, 1983.
17. Gruer LD, McKendrick MW, Beeching NJ, et al: Relapsing hepatitis associated with hepatitis A virus. *Lancet* **2**:163, 1982.
18. Chiriaco P, Guadalupi C, Armigliato M, et al: Polyphasic course of hepatitis type A in children. *J Infect Dis* **153**:378–379, 1986.
19. Sjögren MH, Tanno H, Fay O: Hepatitis A virus in stool during clinical relapse. *Ann Intern Med* **106**:221–226, 1987.
20. Giles JP, Leibhaber H, Krugman S, et al: Early viremia and viruria in infectious hepatitis. *Virology* **24**:107–108, 1964.
21. Krugman S, Ward R, Giles JP: The natural history of infectious hepatitis. *Am J Med* **32**:717–728, 1962.
22. Barker LF, Dienstag JL, Lorenz DF, et al: Serologic and animal inoculation studies of a communal outbreak of viral hepatitis, type A. *Am J Med Sci* **274**:247–253, 1977.
23. Francis T Jr, Frisch AW, Quilligan JJ Jr: Demonstration of infectious hepatitis virus in presymptomatic period after transfer by transfusion. *Proc Soc Exp Biol Med* **61**:276–280, 1946.
24. Harden AG, Barondess JA, Parker B: Transmission of infectious hepatitis by transfusion of whole blood. *N Engl J Med* **253**:923–925, 1955.
25. Meyers JD, Huff JC, Holmes KK, et al: Parenterally transmitted hepatitis A associated with platelet transfusions: Epidemiologic study of an outbreak in a marrow transplantation center. *Ann Intern Med* **81**:145–151, 1974.
26. Meyers JD, Dienstag JL, Purcell RH, et al: Parenterally transmitted non-A, non-B hepatitis: An epidemic reassessed. *Ann Intern Med.* **87**:57–59, 1977.
27. Seeberg S, Brandberg A, Hermodsson, S, et al: Hospital outbreak of hepatitis A secondary to blood exchange in a baby. *Lancet* **1**:1155–1156, 1981.

28. Barbara J, Howell D, Briggs M, et al: Post-transfusion hepatitis A. *Lancet* **1**:738, 1982.
29. Skidmore S, Boxhall E, Ala F: A case report of post-transfusion hepatitis A. *J Med Virol* **10**:223, 1982.
30. Hollinger FB, Khan NC, Oefinger PE, et al: Post-transfusion hepatitis type A. *JAMA* **250**:2313–2317, 1983.
31. Sheretz RJ, Russell BA, Reuman PD: Transmission of hepatitis A by transfusion of blood products. *Arch Intern Med* **144**:1579–1580, 1984.
32. Giles JP, Krugman S: Viral hepatitis. Immunoglobulin response during the course of the disease. *JAMA* **208**:497–503, 1968.
33. Iwarson S, Holmgren J: Patterns of immunoglobulins in acute viral hepatitis: Relation to hepatitis-associated antigen. *J Infect Dis* **125**:178–182, 1972.
34. Peters CJ, Johnson KM: Serum immunoglobulins in acute viral hepatitis: Relation to hepatitis-associated antigen. *Clin Exp Immunol* **11**:381–391, 1972.
35. Zhuang H, Kaldor J, Locarnini SA, et al: Serum immunoglobulin levels in acute A, B and non-A, non-B hepatitis. *Gastroenterology* **82**:549–553, 1982.
36. Feinstone SM, Kapikian, AZ, Purcell RH: Hepatitis A: detection by immune electron microscopy of a virus-like antigen associated with acute illness. *Science* **182**:1026–1028, 1973.
37. Locarnini SA, Ferris AA, Stott AC, et al: The relationship between a 27 nm virus-like particle and hepatitis A as demonstrated by immune electron microscopy. *Intervirology* **4**:110–118, 1974.
38. Hollinger FB, Bradley DW, Maynard JE, et al: Detection of hepatitis A viral antigen by radioimmunoassay. *J Immunol* **115**:1464–1466, 1975.
39. Purcell RH, Wong DC, Moritsugu Y, et al: A microtiter solid-phase radioimmunoassay for hepatitis A antigen and antibody. *J Immunol* **116**:349–356, 1976.
40. Mathieson LR, Feinstone SM, Wong DC: Enzyme-linked immunosorbent assay for detection of hepatitis A antigen in stool and antibody to hepatitis A antigen in sera: Comparison with solid-phase radioimmunoassay, immune electron microscopy and immune adherence hemagglutination assay. *J Clin Microbiol* **7**:184–193, 1978.
41. Ticehurst JR, Racaniello VR, Baroudy BM, et al: Molecular cloning and characterization of hepatitis A virus cDNA. *Proc Natl Acad Sci USA* **80**:5885–5889, 1983.
42. Ticehurst J, Feinstone SM, Chestnut T, et al: Detection of hepatitis A virus RNA by molecular hybridization. *J Clin Microbiol* **25**:1822–1829, 1987.
43. Tassopoulos NC, Papaevangelou GJ, Ticehurst JR, et al: Fecal excretion of Greek strains of hepatitis A virus in patients with hepatitis A and in experimentally infected chimpanzees. *J Infect Dis* **154**:231–257, 1986.
44. Jansen RW, Newbold JE, Lemon SM: Combined immunoaffinity cDNA–RNA hybridization assay for detection of hepatitis A virus in clinical specimens. *J Clin Microbiol* **22**:984–989, 1985.
45. Locarnini SA, Ferris AA, Lehmann NF, et al: The antibody response following hepatitis A infection. *Intervirology* **8**:309–318, 1977.
46. Locarnini SA, Coulepis AG, Stratton AM, et al: Solid-phase enzyme immunoassay for detection of hepatitis A specific immunoglobulin M. *J Clin Microbiol.* **9**:459–465, 1979.
47. Anderson DA, Coulepis AG, Chenoweth MP et al: Indirect immunofluorescence assay for the detection of hepatitis A virus-specific serum immunoglobulins. *J Clin Microbiol* **24**:163–185, 1986.
48. Duermeyer W, Wielaard F, van der Veen J: A new principle for the detection of specific IgM antibodies applied in an ELISA for hepatitis A. *J Med Virol* **4**:25–32, 1979.
49. Roggendorf M, Frösner GG, Deinhardt F: Comparison of solid phase test systems for demonstrating antibodies against hepatitis A virus (anti-HAV) of the IgM-class. *J Med Virol* **5**:47–62, 1980.
50. Parry JV, Mortimer PP: The heat sensitivity of hepatitis A virus determined by a single tissue culture method. *J Med Virol* **14**:277–283, 1984.
51. Siegl G, Weitz M, Kronauer G: Stability of hepatitis A virus. *Intervirology* **22**:218–226, 1984.
52. Provost PJ, Hilleman MR: Propagation of human hepatitis A virus in cell culture in vitro. *Proc Soc Exp Biol Med* **160**:213–221, 1979.
53. Locarnini SA, Coulepis AG, Westaway AG, et al: Restricted replication of human hepatitis A virus in cell culture: Intracellular biochemical studies. *J Virol* **37**:216–225, 1981.
54. Wheeler C, Fields HA, Schable CA, et al: Absorption and growth characteristics of hepatitis A virus strain HA5-15 propagated in fetal rhesus monkey kidney cells (FRhK-4). *J Clin Microbiol* **23**:434–440, 1986.

55. Krawczynski KS, Bradley DW, Murphy BL, et al: Pathogenic aspects of hepatitis A virus infection in enterally inoculated marmosets. *Am J Clin Pathol* **76**:698–706, 1981.
56. Kurane I, Binn LN, Bancroft WH, et al: Human lymphocyte responses to hepatitis A virus-infected cells: Interferon production and lysis of infected cells. *J Immunol* **135**:2140–2144, 1985.
57. Vallbracht A, Gabriel P, Maier K, et al: Cell-mediated cytotoxicity in hepatitis A virus infection. *Hepatology* **6**:1308–1314, 1986.

2

Hepatitis A Infection: Pathology

Kamal G. Ishak

The hepatitis A virus was first detected by immune electron microscopy by Feinstone et al.[1] Hepatitis A is an acute self-limited illness, but a protracted course and severe cholestatic features may occur.[1–4] Relapses (biphasic course) are rare.[5–8] It does not lead to chronic liver disease or a carrier state. Infection results in lifelong immunity. Hepatitis B carriers can be superinfected by hepatitis A without any effect on their clinical course,[9,10] and acute hepatitis B and A can occur simultaneously.[10]

The diagnosis of hepatitis A is made by testing for immunoglobulin M (IgM) anti-HAV, an antibody that appears at the onset of the clinical illness and persists for only 6–12 months.[2–4] With time, IgG antibody rises and persists for life.

A number of investigators have described the morphologic changes in hepatitis A[11–18] (Figs. 1–8). The changes in mild cases may be nonspecific.[17–18] Kryger and Christoffersen[14] found no qualitative differences between the histophathologic changes in acute hepatitis A, B, and non-A, non-B (NANB). However, the degree of focal necrosis and portal inflammation was less pronounced in the NANB cases, as compared with the A or B cases. Also, 25% of NANB cases showed steatosis, as compared with 10% and 6% of the hepatitis A and B cases, respectively. Bridging necrosis only occurred in liver biopsies from patients with acute hepatitis B and NANB. Degenerative bile duct lesions were found only in acute NANB hepatitis (6.6%). A later study by Okuno et al.[15] also found no differences in the pathologic features of acute hepatitis A and B within 30 days of the onset of the illness. Sciot et al.[16] emphasized the cholestatic features in their cases, which included bile casts, cholestatic liver rosettes (pseudoglands), and ductular transformation of hepatocytes (as shown by keratin and S-100 immunostaining). By contrast, most studies of the pathology of hepatitis A have emphasized the periportal predominance of the injury.[11–13,16–18] The periportal necrosis may play a role in the cholestatic features of some cases of hepatitis A by disruption of canalicular connections to the canals of Hering. Teixeira et al.[13] drew attention to the resemblance of the portal/periportal changes to those of chronic active hepatitis (CAH), but in my experience the two diseases can be readily distinguished (Table I). The histopathology of the various

---

Kamal G. Ishak • Department of Hepatic Pathology, Armed Forces Institute of Pathology, Washington, D.C. 20306-6000. The opinions or assertions contained herein are the private views of the author and are not to be construed as official or as reflecting the views of the Department of the Army or the Department of Defense.

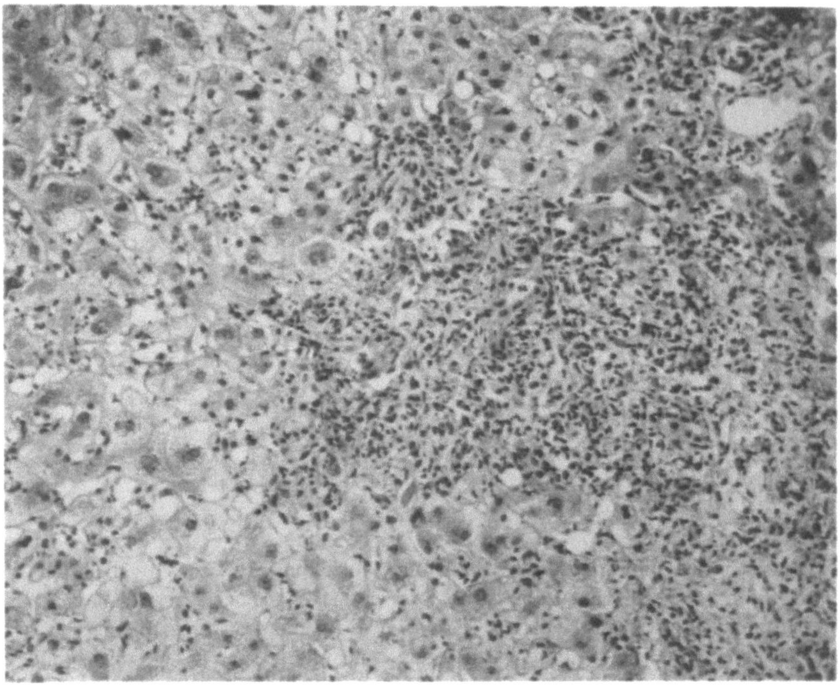

Figure 1. Marked portal and periportal inflammation with acute periportal necrosis. (H&E, ×160)

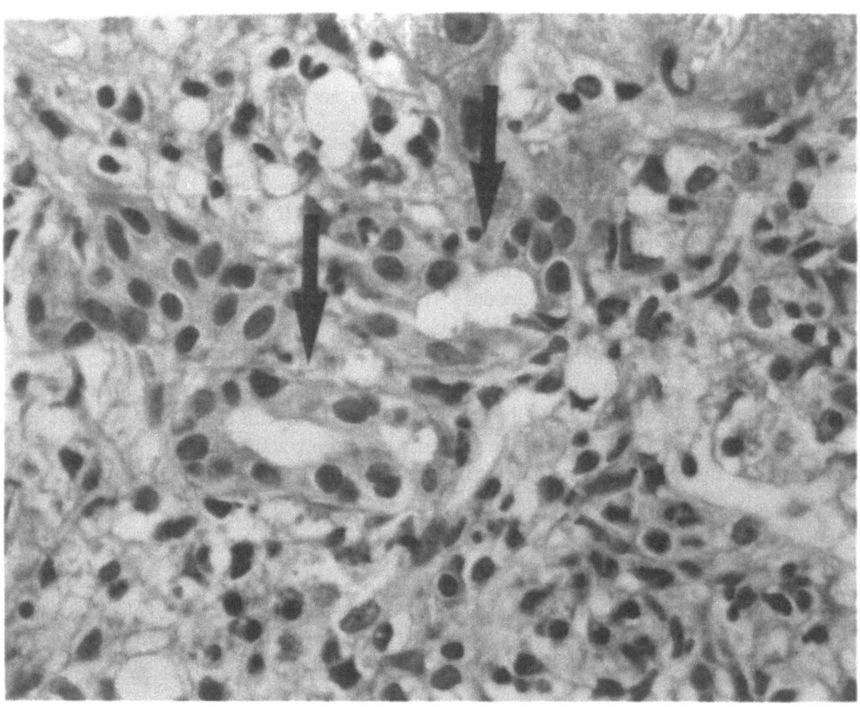

Figure 2. Periportal 'cholangiolar' proliferation (arrows). (H&E, ×630)

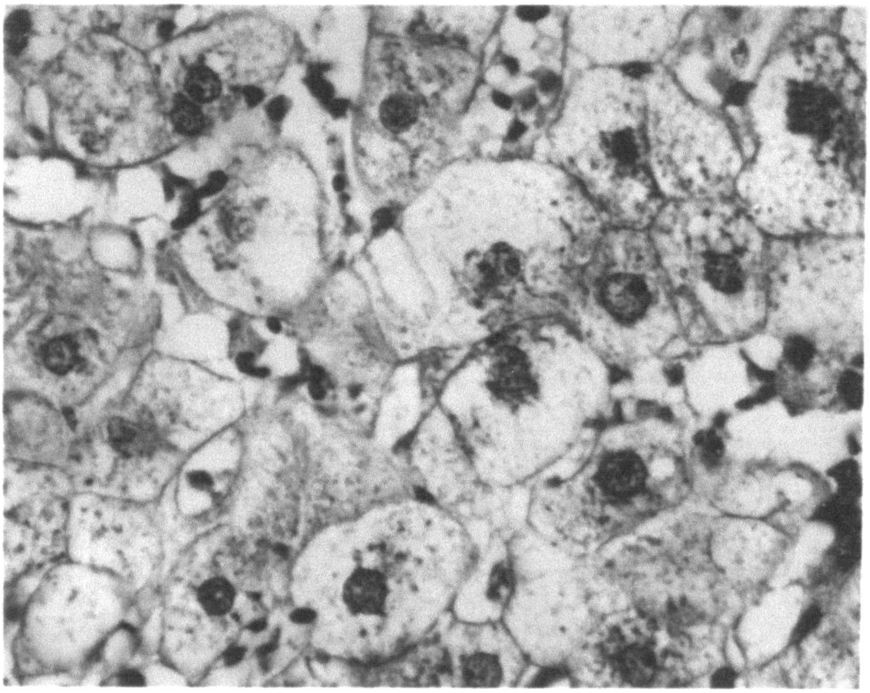

Figure 3. Same case illustrated in Fig. 1. Liver cells adjacent to zone of necrosis show prominent ballooning degeneration. (H&E, ×630)

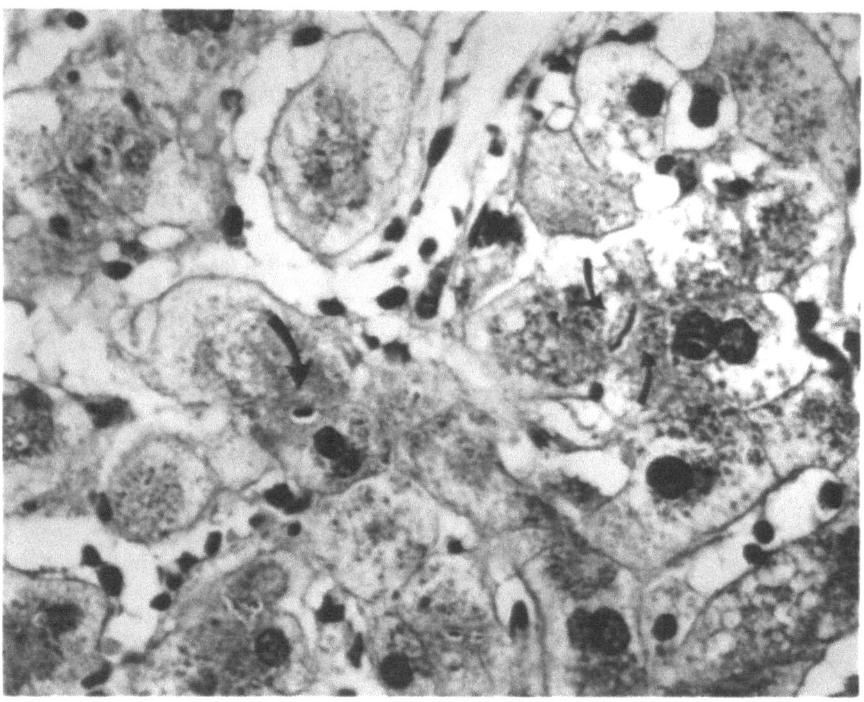

Figure 4. Same case illustrated in Figs. 1 and 2. Marked cholestasis both cytoplasmic and canalicular (arrows) is present. (H&E, ×630)

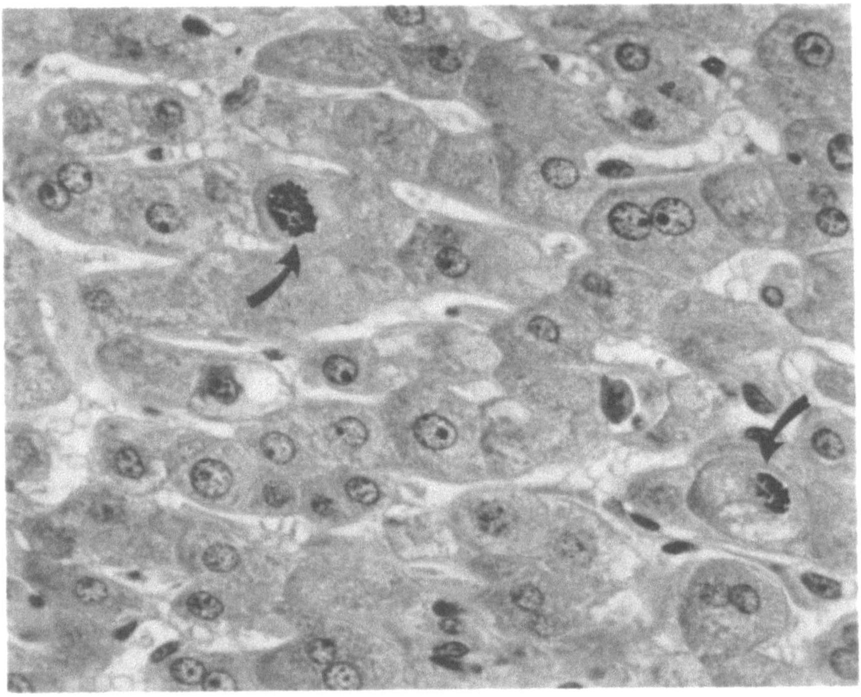

Figure 5. Liver cells show mitoses (arrows). A sinusoidal acidophilic body is present (H&E, ×630)

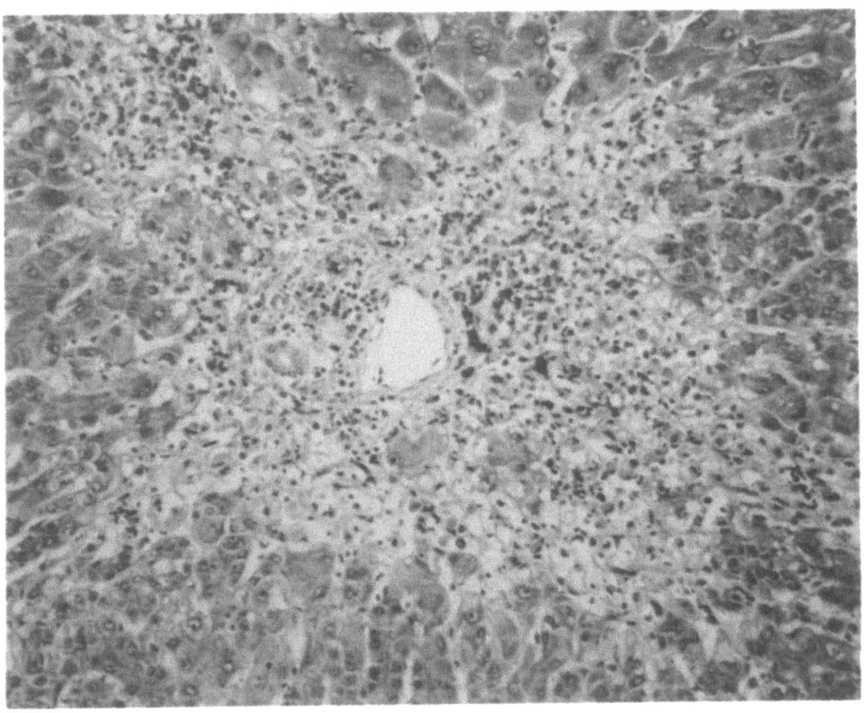

Figure 6. Fatal case of hepatitis A with acute necrosis of zone 1. A portal vein branch is present in the center of the field. (H&E, ×160)

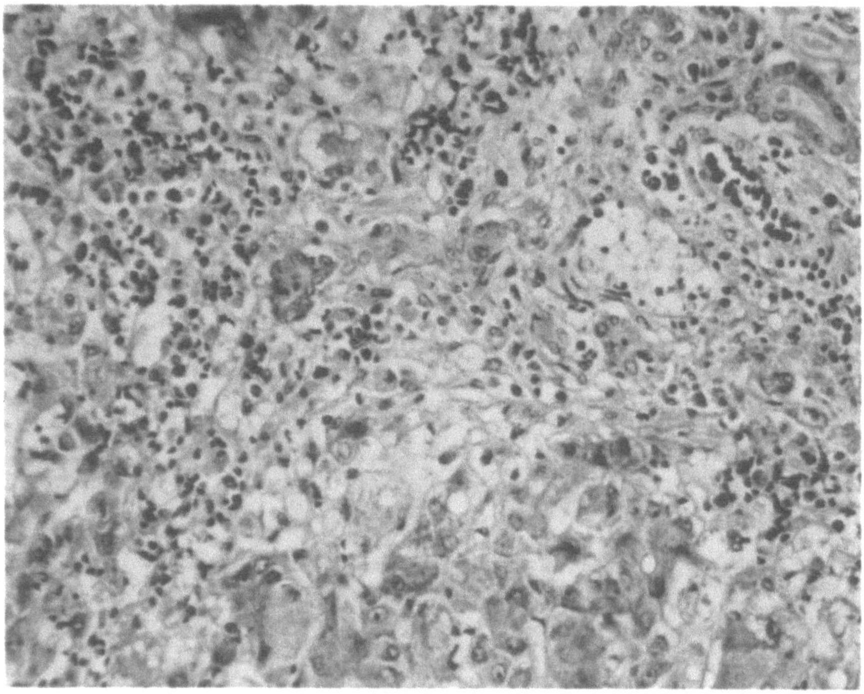

Figure 7. Same case illustrated in Fig. 4. There is drop out of liver cells in zone 1 and marked inflammation. A portal area occupies the upper right corner of the photomicrograph. (H&E, ×250)

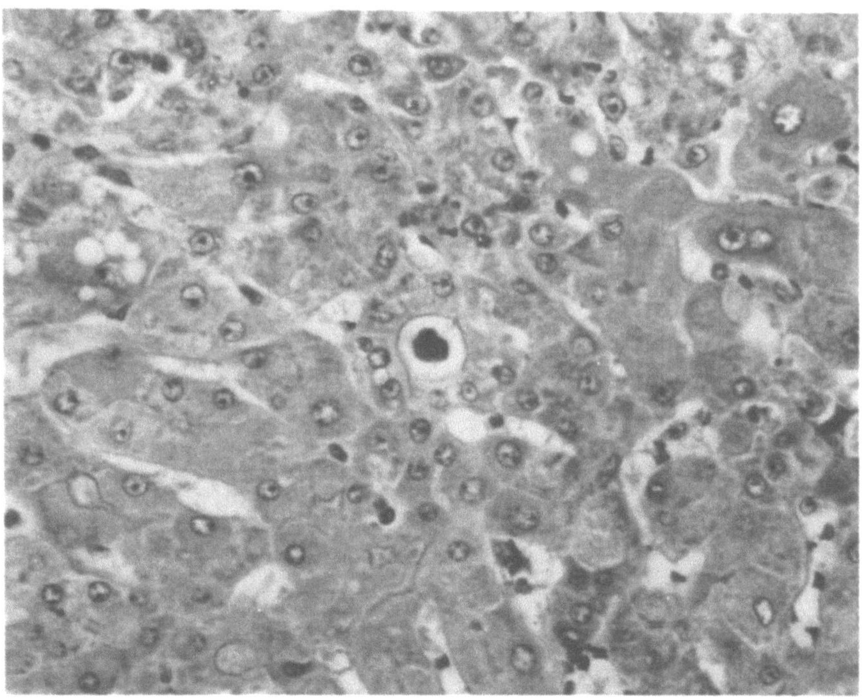

Figure 8. Same case illustrated in Figs. 4 and 5. The spared parenchyma (zones 2 and 3 in this case) showed marked cholestasis, as exemplified by a large bile plug in a pseudogland. (H&E, ×400)

Table I. Comparison of Histopathology of Acute Hepatitis A and Chronic Active Hepatitis

Histopathologic change	Acute hepatitis A	Chronic active hepatitis
Spotty necrosis, panacinar[a]	+	+
Ballooning, zone 1 (with or without dropout)	+	−
Collapse of reticulin fibers, zone 1	+	−
Hypertrophy of Kupffer cells with pigment (lipofuscin and/or iron)	+	−
Apoptosis, zone 1	±	+
Multiacinar necrosis	−	+
Cholestasis with or without pseudoglands	+	− (usually)
Fibrosis (stellate), zone 1	−	+
Fibrous entrapment of isolated hepatocytes	−	+
Basement membrane in Disse spaces, zone 1	−	+
Rosette formation, zone 1	−	+
Thick plates, zone 1	−	+
Nodular regeneration	−	+
Portal/periportal inflammation[b]	P,E,L,N	P,L
Peripolesis/emperipolesis (P,L)	−	+
Bile duct degeneration	−	± (NANB)
Ground-glass cells, Shikata stain+	−	+ (hepatitis B)

[a]Includes apoptosis, unicellular acidophilic degeneration and ballooning, and focal necrosis.
[b]N, neutrophils; E, eosinophils; L, lymphocytes; P, plasma cells.

Table II. Comparison of Histopathology of Different Types of Acute Viral Hepatitis

			Hepatitis NANB	
Histopathologic change	Hepatitis A	Hepatitis B	Parenteral	Enteral (epidemic or sporadic)
Spotty necrosis[a]	+	+	+	±
Zone 3 ballooning and necrosis	−	±	±	−
Zone 1 ballooning and necrosis	+	−	−	+ (1 report)
Marked cholestasis with or without pseudoglands	+	−	−	+
Kupffer cell hypertrophy with iron and/or lipofuscin	+	+	+	−
Kupffer cell hypertrophy with bile accumulation	±	−	−	+
Portal inflammation	+	+	+	+
Types of inflammatory cells[b]	P,L,E,N	L,P.	L,P	N,L
Cholangiolar proliferation	±	−	−	±
Bile duct degeneration	−	−	±	−

[a]Includes apoptosis, unicellular acidophilic and ballooning degeneration, and focal necrosis.
[b]L, lymphocytes; P, plasma cells; N, neutrophils; E, eosinophils.

types of acute viral hepatitis is compared and contrasted in Table II. With the exception of a single report of hepatitis A-like lesions in sporadic NANB hepatitis,[19] the periportal predilection of injury appears to be characteristic. Rarely, drug-induced liver injury can lead to changes resembling those of acute viral hepatitis A. For example, Benjamin et al.[20] found that pattern of injury in eight of 77 cases of halothane-associated hepatotoxicity. The clinical setting and serologic testing should readily distinguish such cases from hepatitis A.

Lymphocyte subsets in acute hepatitis A have been studied and compared with those of chronic hepatitis B.[21] Helper/inducer T cells (admixed with B cells and plasma cells) in acute hepatitis A were considered to represent the morphologic expression of a humoral immune response. By contrast, the presence of numerous suppressor/cytotoxic T cells in the piecemeal necrosis of chronic hepatitis B represents the morphologic expression of a cellular immune response.

Hepatitis A virus was detected by immunofluorescence in liver biopsies from 11 of 17 patients with type A hepatitis by Mathiesen et al.[22] The viral particles were seen in the cytoplasm of hepatocytes and probably of Kupffer cells. Positive cells were found in clusters, and the proportion of cells involved varied from very few cells to nearly all the cells in a given biopsy specimen.

Experimental studies with HAV have revealed the presence of viral particles (24–28 nm in diameter) with both solid and empty forms in the endoplasmic reticulum of liver cells as well as in lysosomes in Kuppfer cells and in bile canaliculi,[23–27] and recently, in epithelial cells of intrahepatic bile ducts.[28] In one study, the predominant localization of viral particles or antigen to liver cells undergoing cytolysis suggested a direct cytopathic effect.[25] Most experimental studies, however, favor immunopathologic processes in the liver injury associated with HAV infection.[26–29] Vallbracht et al.[29] provided strong evidence that cytolytic T cells play an important role in the pathogenesis of HAV infection.

REFERENCES

1. Feinstone SM, Kapikian AZ, Purcell RH: Hepatitis A: Detection by immune electron microscopy of a viruslike antigen associated with acute illness. *Science* **182:**1026–1028, 1973.
2. Mathiesen LR: The hepatitis A virus infection. *Liver* **1:**81–109, 1981.
3. Lemon SM: Type A viral hepatitis. New developments in an old disease. *N Engl J Med* **313:**1059–1067, 1985.
4. Feinstoen SM: Hepatitis A. *Prog Liver Dis* **8:**299–310, 1986.
5. Jacobson IM, North BJ, Dienstag JL: Relapsing viral hepatitis A. *J Med Virol* **16:**163–169, 1985.
6. Cobden I, James OFW: A biphasic illness associated with acute hepatitis A virus infection. *J. Hepatol* **2:**19–23, 1986.
7. Sjogren MH, Tanno H, Fay O, et al: Hepatitis A in stool during clinical relapse. *Ann Intern Med.* **106:**221–226, 1987.
8. Tanno H, Fay O, Rojman, JA, et al: Biphasic form of hepatitis A infection: A frequent variant in Argentina. *Liver* **8:**53–57, 1988.
9. Conteas C, Kao H, Rakela J, et al: Acute type A hepatitis in three patients with chronic HBV infection. *Dig Dis Sci* **28:**684–686, 1983.
10. Zachoval R, Roggendorf M, Deinhardt F: Hepatitis A infection in chronic carriers of hepatitis B virus. *Hepatology* **3:**528–531, 1983.
11. Abe H, Ikejiri N, Sata M, et al: Histological findings of the liver in viral hepatitis type A. A comparison with viral hepatitis type B. *Acta Hepatol Jpn* **22:**22–31, 1981.
12. Abe H, Beninger PR, Ikejiri N, et al: Light microscopic findings of liver biopsy specimens from patients with hepatitis type A and comparison with type B. *Gastroenterology* **82:**938–947, 1982.
13. Teixeira MR Jr, Weller IVD, Murray A, et al: The pathology of hepatitis A in man. *Liver* **2:**53–60, 1982.
14. Kryger P, Christoffersen P: Liver histopathology of the hepatitis A virus infection: A comparison with hepatitis type B and non-A, non-B. *J. Clin Pathol* **36:**650–654, 1983.
15. Okuno T, Sano A, Deguchi T, et al: Pathology of acute hepatitis A in humans. Comparison with acute hepatitis B. *Am J Clin Pathol* **81:**162–169, 1984.

16. Sciot R, Van Damme B, Desmet VJ: Cholestatic features in hepatitis A. *J. Hepatol* **3:**172–181, 1986.
17. Korb G: Morphologische Befunde bei der menschlichen Virus-A-hepatitis. *Verh Dtsch Ges Pathol* **68:**540, 1984.
18. Korb G: Dic Virus-A-hepatitis. *Dtsch Med Wochenschr* **109:**110–112, 1984.
19. Dienes HP, Hutteroth T, Bianchi L, et al: Hepatitis A-like non-A, non-B hepatitis: Light and electron microscopic observations of three cases. *Virchows Arch Pathol Anat* **409:**657–667, 1986.
20. Benjamin SB, Goodman ZD, Ishak KG, et al: The morphologic spectrum of halothane-induced hepatic injury: Analysis of 77 cases. *Hepatology* **5:**1163–1171, 1985.
21. Sciot R, Van Den Oord JJ, De Wolf-Peeters C, et al: *In situ* characterization of the (peri)portal inflammatory infiltrate in acute hepatitis A. *Liver* **6:**331–336, 1986.
22. Mathiesen LR, Fauerholdt, L, Moller AM, et al: Immunofluorescence studies for hepatitis A virus and hepatitis B surface and core antigen in liver biopsies from patients with acute viral hepatitis. *Gastroenterology* **77:**623–628, 1979.
23. Huang S-N, Lorenz D: Electron and immunoelectron microscopic study on liver tissues of marmosets infected with hepatitis A virus. *Lab Invest* **41:**63–71, 1979.
24. Moriyama M: Detection of HAV in the epithelial cells of interlobular bile ducts of marmosets with acute hepatitis A. *Acta Hepatol Jpn* **26:**867–876, 1985.
25. Krawczinski KK, Bradley DW, Murphy BL, et al: Pathogenetic aspects of hepatitis A virus infection in enterally inoculated marmosets. *Am J Clin Pathol* **76:**698–706, 1981.
26. Inoue O: Morphological studies on the mechanism of hepatocellular injury during acute phase of infection in marmosets inoculated with hepatitis A virus. *Acta Pathol Jpn* **35:**1319–1331, 1985.
27. Karayiannis P, Jowett, T, Enticolt M et al: Hepatitis A virus replication on Tamarins and host immune response in relation to pathogenesis of liver cell damage. *J Med Virol* **18:**261–276, 1986.
28. Hirose S: Experimental infection of hepatitis A virus in marmoset monkeys: growth kinetics of the virus and the mechanism of liver cell destruction in vivo. *Acta Hepatol Jpn* **29:**16–23, 1988.
29. Vallbracht A, Gabriel P, Maier K et al: Cell mediated cytotoxicity in hepatitis A virus infection. *Hepatology* **6:**1308–1314, 1986.

3

Acute and Chronic Hepatitis B

Raymond S. Koff

1. INTRODUCTION

Acute hepatitis B is a systemic infection in which the liver is the predominant, if not necessarily the sole, target organ of the infectious agent, the hepatitis B virus (HBV). Regardless of whether extrahepatic tissues participate in the replication of this DNA virus, the liver is the principal organ site of the host response to HBV infection. Infection by HBV, one of at least six agents responsible for the disorder known as viral hepatitis, produces a broad spectrum of acute and chronic illness with a wide array of outcomes. In acute hepatitis B infection, this ranges between asymptomatic anicteric self-limited infections at one end and fulminant fatal hepatitis at the opposite end. When HBV infection is persistent, the spectrum of disease also varies strikingly between an asymptomatic HBV carrier state at one extreme and progressive chronic hepatitis B with or without the development of cirrhosis or primary hepatocellular carcinoma at the other.

2. VIROLOGY

2.1. Hepadnaviruses

Long thought to be unique among animal viruses, HBV is now understood to belong to a family of unusual viruses, termed the hepadnaviruses (hepatotrophic DNA viruses).[1] In addition to HBV, currently classified as hepadnavirus type I, similar viruses have been identified in other species (Table I). It seems likely that other family members may be identified as investigations of the animal world for markers of hepadnaviruses are further explored. While HBV is the sole member of this family known to infect human beings and nonhuman primates (chimpanzees), HBV-related variants have been postulated to be responsible for some human hepatitis B-like infections in which conventional markers of HBV infection have not been found.[2,3] The characterization of the latter variants remains incomplete, and their existence has yet to be fully confirmed, despite reports of successful experimental transmission studies in chimpanzees.[3]

The five established agents—HBV, woodchuck hepatitis virus (WHV), ground squirrel hepatitis virus (GSHV), tree squirrel hepatitis virus (TSHV), and duck hepatitis B virus (DHBV)—appear

Raymond S. Koff • Department of Medicine, Framingham Union Hospital, Framingham, Massachusetts 01701; Hepatology Section, Boston University School of Medicine, Boston, Massachusetts 02118.

Table I. The Hepadnaviruses

Agent	Number of nucleotides in genome
Hepatitis B virus (HBV)	3188
Woodchuck hepatitis virus (WHV)	3320
Ground squirrel hepatitis virus (GSHV)	3311
Tree squirrel hepatitis virus (TSHV)	?
Duck hepatitis B virus (DHBV)	3021

to have morphologic and antigenic similarities; to contain partially double-stranded partially single-stranded circular DNA molecules with similar nucleotide length (see Table I); and to replicate in the liver, and possibly in other tissues, by mechanisms used by retroviruses. Some homology has been demonstrated between the DNA of HBV and the DNA of the other hepadnaviruses[4] and between the DNA of HBV and that of the recently postulated HBV-related variants.[3]

2.2. Structure of HBV

Hepatitis B virus is a 42-nm double-shelled spherical particle comprising a 27-nm icosahedral nucleocapsid inner core and a surrounding 7-nm detergent-sensitive envelope.[5] The envelope consists of a lipid component, derived from host lipids, and at least three polypeptides: the large protein, the middle protein, and the major protein. The major protein is the dominant structural component of the envelope and is termed hepatitis B surface antigen (HBsAg). HBsAg and the middle protein are also found in the sera of HBV-infected patients in the form of nucleic acid free particles that are smaller, 22-nm spherical, tubular, and incomplete. The large protein appears to be present in relatively increased amounts in the envelope of the HBV particle and in the tubular forms, as compared with its distribution in the small, 22-nm spherical particle. These noninfectious but immunogenic HBsAg spheres and tubular particles are produced in extraordinary amounts, well in excess of intact HBV particles.

The major HBsAg protein, comprising 226 amino acids, exists in both glycosylated and nonglycosylated forms, as do the large and middle proteins. The HBsAg polypeptide and smaller linear or circularized peptides derived from the major protein or synthesized chemically are immunogenic; they induce formation of the protective antibody to the HBsAg, i.e., anti-HBs. The other envelope polypeptides also are immunogenic, and one of these may enhance the immunogenicity of HBsAg.

The nucleocapsid of HBV contains the circular, partially double-stranded, partially single-stranded DNA and displays endogenous DNA polymerase and protein kinase activity. The full-length minus DNA strand is ~3200 (3180–3220) nucleotides long, while the short plus DNA strand is ~1700–2800 nucleotides. The DNA polymerase appears to repair the single-stranded region and to render it double-stranded by adding nucleotides to one end; whether it also serves as a reverse transcriptase remains uncertain. The protein kinase is believed to phosphorylate the proteins of the nucleocapsid core.[6] The major antigenic protein expressed on the surface of the core is hepatitis B core antigen (HBcAg). A third antigenic component of the nucleocapsid core of HBV is hepatitis B "e" antigen (HBeAg). This soluble nonparticulate protein appears to be an internal component or cryptic degradation product of HBcAg. HBeAg is seldom found in HBsAg-negative sera; its presence indicates ongoing viral replication (HBV DNA and intact HBV in sera), and it serves as an indirect marker of infectivity.

The HBV genome has been cloned in a variety of vectors, including bacterial, yeast, and mammalian cells; several nucleotide segments comprising open reading frames (or genes) on the long minus DNA strand have been identified (Table II). One open reading frame, termed the S gene, codes for the 226 amino acid major protein of HBsAg. Upstream or preceding the S gene are two gene regions labeled pre-S1 and pre-S2, which encode for the large and middle proteins, each containing HBsAg and additional peptides. These larger proteins may be more immunogenic than HBsAg per se; a role in viral attachment, viral assembly, secretion of HBsAg, infectivity, and recovery from infection has been postulated, but available data are too limited to characterize their full importance.[7–9]

The second open reading frame, termed the C gene, specifies the HBcAg polypeptide and includes the coding region for HBeAg. Pre-C regions have been described, but their function remains uncertain. They may serve to target HBcAg to cytoplasmic membranes and to promote the secretion of HBeAg.[10] Partial deletion of some pre-C sequences appears to inhibit secretion but not synthesis of HBeAg.[11] The third and longest open reading frame is the P gene, which overlaps with the others and is thought to specify the HBV DNA polymerase protein. The fourth open reading frame, the X gene, encodes for a protein of uncertain function. A relationship to primary hepatocellular carcinoma has been hypothesized.[12]

2.3. Concepts of HBV Replication

The minus strands of HBV DNA are believed to be generated by reverse transcription of HBV RNA intermediates. The plus strands are thought to be generated from templates of minus DNA strands. In infected hepatocytes, in addition to HBV DNA and HBV-specific RNA, superhelical closed circular duplex DNA and incomplete HBV DNA forms comprising protein-linked minus DNA strands, with or without plus strands, may be detected. These incomplete forms and similarly identified HBV RNA–DNA hybrids appear to be intermediates in the synthesis of the HBV genome.[13] Hybridization analysis of HBV RNA transcripts in the liver of persistently infected patients showed the presence of either 29S RNA (messenger RNA of HBcAg) and 21S RNA (messenger RNA of HBsAg) or only 21S RNA. Expression of these transcript patterns could be correlated with the presence of free viral DNA or integrated viral DNA, respectively.[14]

Although conventional thought has suggested that replication of HBV is limited to the hepatocyte, extrahepatic synthesis of HBV has been postulated in light of recent evidence supporting the replication of hepadnaviruses in other tissues and the demonstration of HBV DNA in extrahepatic sites. Active replication of DHBV in duckling liver is followed by replication in

Table II. Hepatitis B Virus Genes, Specified Gene Products, and Their Amino Acid Residues[a]

Gene	Specified gene products	Amino acid residues
Pre-S1	Large protein	400
Pre-S2	Middle protein	281
S	HBsAg	226
C	HBcAg/HBeAg	183–214
P	DNA polymerase	832–845
X	HBxAg	145–154

[a]HBsAg, hepatitis B surface antigen; HBcAg, hepatitis B core antigen; ABeAg, hepatitis B "e" antigen; HBxAg, hepatitis B "x" antigen.

pancreas, kidney, and spleen.[15] If the sites of replication are similar for human HBV and the other members of this family of viruses, these agents should not be considered strictly hepatotrophic. Evidence supporting the presence of human HBV DNA or HBV antigens in human bone marrow cells, peripheral leukocytes, spleen, kidney, pancreas, bile duct epithelium, and vascular elements has been reported in recent years.[16–21] Despite these observations, suggesting that HBV may replicate at least to some extent in extrahepatic tissues, it is likely that the term hepadnavirus, although imperfect, will persist in the literature.

2.4. Growth of HBV In Vivo

Early attempts to grow HBV in cell culture failed or resulted in equivocal production of the virus. Attempts at transfection of cell lines with cloned circular HBV DNA capable of transmitting infection to nonhuman primates[22] also proved frustrating. Following the demonstration that DHBV could grow in primary cultures of duck hepatocytes,[23] continuous propagation of HBV in vitro has been achieved through the introduction of cloned circular HBV DNA into a human hepatocellular cell line that closely resembles differentiated human hepatocytes.[24]

3. SEROLOGY

3.1. Acute HBV Infection

The first identifiable serologic marker of HBV infection is the appearance of HBsAg, days to weeks after exposure to HBV, but prior to the onset of serum aminotransferase elevations, symptoms, or jaundice (Fig. 1). Circulating HBsAg persists for a variable period of a few weeks to several months after the symptomatic or icteric phase and then becomes undetectable. In 92–98% of adults, HBsAg has been cleared within 6 months. The persistence of HBsAg beyond 6–12 months indicates that HBV infection has become chronic.

The second serologic marker to appear, concurrent with or a few days after HBsAg, is HBeAg. The presence of HBeAg signals the replicative phase of HBV infection in which HBV DNA can be detected in a nonintegrated form within the hepatocyte; HBV DNA, HBV DNA polymerase, and intact HBV particles are present in the serum. Although available data are limited, pre-S proteins and antibodies to pre-S proteins also may appear in the circulation during this replicative phase. In

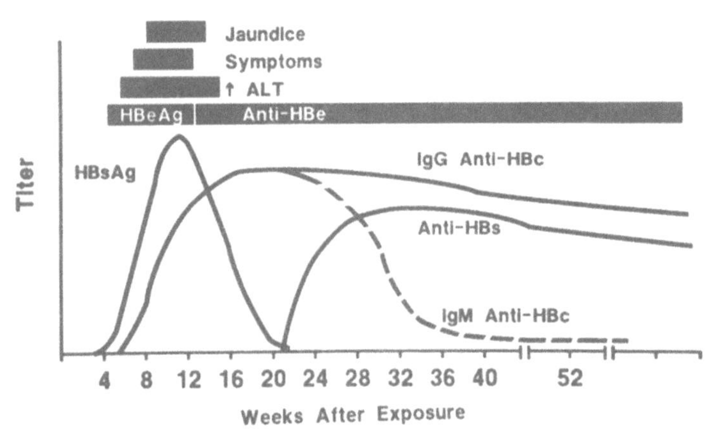

Figure 1. Sequence of serologic events and clinical and laboratory features seen in typical acute hepatitis B.

acute HBV infection, HBeAg disappears before the disappearance of HBsAg and is followed by the appearance of its corresponding antibody, anti-HBe.

The first antibody to appear in acute HBV infection is anti-HBc, which is usually detected within 1 or 2 weeks of the appearance of HBsAg, well before recognition of anti-HBe. Initially, the anti-HBc belongs to both immunoglobulin M (IgM) and IgG classes, with a predominance of the IgM anti-HBc. By 4–6 months later, the titer of this IgM antibody has fallen dramatically, and IgG anti-HBc is predominant. Total anti-HBc persists for prolonged periods in gradually declining titers. After HBsAg disappears, anti-HBs becomes detectable, usually during the recovery phase, and this neutralizing protective antibody persists indefinitely. In a small proportion of patients who have recovered fully and who are immune to reinfection, anti-HBs cannot be detected in convalescent sera.

3.2. Persistent HBV Infection

Persistent HBV infection is recognized by the continuing detection of circulating HBsAg for more than 6–12 months (Fig. 2). Affected persons are labeled HBsAg carriers. Although anti-HBs was rarely detected in HBsAg carriers in the early years after the development of serologic assays for this antibody, increased sensitivity of the present assays appears to be responsible for the finding that 10–40% of HBsAg carriers have positive tests for anti-HBs.[25] The anti-HBs found in such patients is present in low titer and represents heterotypic antibody, directed against HBsAg subdeterminants not present on the HBsAg in the serum of the carrier. The heterotypic anti-HBs may disappear on follow-up in some but not all affected carriers. The presence or disappearance of this anti-HBs in HBsAg carriers has no clinical significance; the patient must be considered a true HBsAg carrier.

All HBsAg carriers have positive tests for anti-HBc and IgG anti-HBc is the predominant Ig class found in their sera. Distinction between acute and persistent HBV infection based on IgM anti-HBV may require quantitation, since low levels of IgM anti-HBc may persist in some persons with chronic HBV infections.[26] In the so-called replicative phase of persistent HBV infection, in which HBV replication is highly active, HBeAg may remain detectable for a prolonged period, and the carrier may remain highly infectious during this phase. In a variable proportion of carriers, evidence of active hepatic inflammation and necrosis, i.e., chronic hepatitis, may be striking and appears to be closely correlated with ongoing viral replication. When HBV replication diminishes, presumably

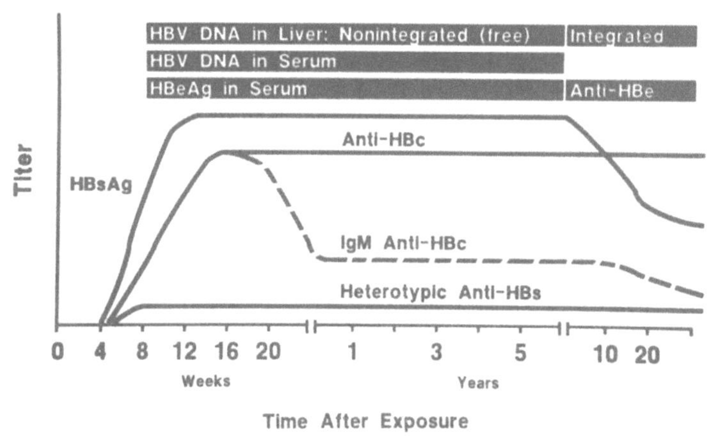

Figure 2. Sequence of serologic events and status of hepatitis B virus (HBV) DNA in liver and serum seen in persistent HBV infection.

concurrent with the integration of HBV DNA into the genome of the hepatocyte, HBeAg is usually lost, and anti-HBe can be detected in the circulation. HBeAg seroconversion to anti-HBe occurs at an annual rate reported to vary between 3 and 25% in different studies.[27] The so-called non-replicative phase of persistent HBV infection, in which HBV DNA becomes integrated into the genome of the host hepatocyte, closely follows HBeAg seroconversion and may persist for several decades. Even in this nonreplicative low-level HBV infection, replication may persist, and some intact HBV particles may be released into the circulation. In most cases, hepatic inflammation and necrosis become quiescent during this phase, but cirrhosis, if present, remains unchanged. A small proportion of HBsAg carriers, in the range of 1–2% per year, may lose detectable circulating HBsAg and develop anti-HBs.

4. EPIDEMIOLOGY

Hepatitis B virus infection may be transmitted to susceptible contacts by either acutely or persistently infected persons. The latter, recognized by the persistence of HBsAg in sera (HBsAg carriers), are believed to constitute the major reservoir and source of HBV infection throughout the world. The HBV carrier rate varies considerably from area to area; e.g., in the United States less than 0.5% of the general population are carriers, while in sub-Saharan Africa and parts of the Far East, carrier rates in excess of 20% have been described. Carrier rates also vary among specific population groups within a single country. For example, in the United States, HBsAg carrier rates in excess of 5% (10 times that of the general population) have been found in Asian Americans, in homosexual men, in parenteral drug addicts, and in persons with Down syndrome residing in large institutions, to name but a few of the high-prevalence groups.

In addition to the classic percutaneous routes of HBV transmission, typified in the past by transfusion-associated HBV and currently by HBV infection in needle-using drug addicts, two nonpercutaneous modes of spread have been recognized to have a profound impact on the epidemiology of HBV infection: sexual contact and maternal–neonatal transmission. Considerable evidence indicates that in addition to blood, the semen and saliva of infected persons may contain intact HBV and that close intimate contact can lead to transfer of HBV across mucosal surfaces and efficient transmission of HBV infection. Sexual contacts of acutely infected and persistently infected patients are at high risk of HBV infection, as are sexually promiscuous persons, such as promiscuous homosexual men. Maternal–neonatal transmission is a critical factor in perpetuating the high prevalence of the carrier state in the Far East and in some developing nations. About 90% of newborn infants of HBsAg-carrier mothers who also are HBeAg positive will become infected, and about 90% of these acute infections, although largely asymptomatic, will become persistent. Available information suggests that most episodes of maternal–neonatal transmission occur at the time of delivery or shortly thereafter. Breast feeding does not play a role and only about 5–10% of perinatal infections are acquired in utero.

Despite increased understanding of the epidemiology of HBV infection, it is nonetheless true that an exposure episode preceding infection is identified in only 50–60% of patients with acute HBV infection. Unrecognized or inapparent percutaneous and nonpercutaneous routes of transmission must be responsible for these sporadic cases of acute HBV infection.

5. ACUTE HEPATITIS B

5.1. Clinical and Laboratory Features

The average incubation period of hepatitis B is 60–90 days, with a range of 30–180 days. About 1–5% of patients with HBV infection may have a preicteric prodromal serum sickness-like syndrome characterized by symptoms and signs of arthritis, rash, angioedema, and, less frequently, hematuria and proteinuria. Affected patients are invariably HBsAg positive and may have elevated serum aminotransferase levels. This immune-complex-mediated disorder is followed by the development of constitutional and gastrointestinal (GI) symptoms and in about 20–25% of patients by the appearance of dark urine, light stools, and scleral icterus. The serum aminotransferases rise during the late prodromal phase, reaching peak levels (10–100 times the upper limits of normal) shortly after jaundice is recognized. During the recovery phase, serum aminotransferases and bilirubin decline progressively, reaching normal levels within 3–4 months in most patients. In less than 1% of patients, symptoms of hepatic encephalopathy and marked prolongation of the prothrombin time signal the development of fulminant HBV infection due to massive hepatic necrosis. Among those patients who develop fulminant HBV infection, as many as 75% with severe encephalopathy will succumb, despite aggressive intensive management.

5.2. Management

No specific antiviral chemotherapy is available. Most patients recover, regardless of whether they receive medical care, and very few require hospitalization. Restrictions of physical activity are set by the patient, who also selects the diet most desired. Treatment of fulminant hepatitis is mainly supportive; liver transplantation has been attempted in a number of instances, but its role remains ambiguous.

6. CHRONIC HEPATITIS B

6.1. Frequency and Classification

The frequency of chronic hepatitis B is largely dependent on the frequency with which acute HBV infection becomes persistent. A large number of studies suggest that the major determinant of the HBsAg carrier state is the age at which acute HBV infection occurs. Among infected neonates and infants, nearly 90% become carriers, while among children about 20% will develop the carrier state. In sharp contrast, only 2–8% of acutely infected adults develop persistent HBV infection. Recent studies suggest that even these low percentages may be too high and that the risk in the adult population has been overestimated.[28]

Point prevalence surveys of adult HBsAg carriers suggest that about one half are asymptomatic with neither serum aminotransferase elevations nor histologic evidence of chronic hepatitis B on liver biopsy. In most of these asymptomatic HBsAg carriers, markers of viral replication are absent or diminishing, and short-term follow-up suggests a stable uneventful course in the absence of spontaneous or induced reactivation of HBV infection or superinfection by the hepatitis D (delta) virus or other hepatitis viruses.[27] A variable but important proportion of asymptomatic carriers, some of whom have cirrhosis despite the absence of clinical and laboratory evidence of chronic liver disease, will eventually develop primary hepatocellular carcinoma (see Chapter 32). It is assumed that earlier in the course of their HBV infections, many of these persons may have had clinically mild chronic hepatic inflammation and necrosis, associated with markers of ongoing HBV replication. Longitudinal follow-up studies of large numbers of such patients are not yet available, and current concepts of the natural history of chronic hepatitis B may require revision as more data accumulate.

Three major histopathologic entities have been associated with chronic hepatitis B, as defined by positive tests for HBsAg and elevated serum aminotransferases for 6–12 months or longer. These include chronic active hepatitis, chronic persistent hepatitis, and chronic lobular hepatitis.

6.2. Clinical and Laboratory Features

Persistent serum aminotransferase elevations accompanied by histologic features of acute hepatitis B characterize the infrequently recognized patient with chronic lobular hepatitis.[29] Patients with chronic persistent hepatitis and chronic lobular hepatitis in remission (relapses and remissions may occur over a period of years) may appear entirely normal; they have few complaints and only minimal aminotransferase elevations to confirm the existence of chronic liver disease.

The clinical and laboratory features of chronic active hepatitis B vary widely. Most patients appear to be asymptomatic and are identified through multiphasic health screening, in which elevated serum aminotransferase levels suggest the presence of liver disease. In a few patients, chronic fatigue, mild jaundice, or signs of liver disease such as edema and ascites are the presenting features. Laboratory abnormalities may include, in addition to elevation of both alanine and aspartate aminotransferases (2–20 times the upper limits of normal), prolongation of the prothrombin time, reduction of serum albumin, and increased levels of serum bilirubin. The latter three abnormalities suggest that the disease process is severe and possibly progressive. The presence of cirrhosis should be considered if edema, ascites, splenomegaly, or other symptoms and signs of portal hypertension are evident.

6.3. Sequelae

Limited studies suggest that patients with chronic persistent and chronic lobular hepatitis due to persistent HBV infection generally run a nonprogressive course that rarely evolves into cirrhosis or leads to hepatic failure. Nonetheless, such patients may remain at risk of primary hepatocellular carcinoma. Patients with HBV-associated CAH are also at risk of developing hepatocellular carcinoma and may suffer considerable morbidity and mortality as a consequence of continuing disease activity, leading to hepatic failure and cirrhosis with clinical manifestations of portal hypertension. In a large proportion of patients who develop cirrhosis, cirrhosis is present within a year of the initial clinical presentation. In some patients in whom the development of cirrhosis appears to be delayed, the late progression to cirrhosis appears to be a consequence of superinfection by the hepatitis D or non-A, non-B (NANB) hepatitis viruses. Other factors may also influence the natural history of CAH B but remain poorly understood.

6.4. Management

Effective therapy for CAH B is not yet available.[30] Experimental regimens, involving combinations of antiviral drugs given sequentially or together, appear to reduce markers of HBV replication, and perhaps in a few instances may lead to the transient or prolonged clearance of HBsAg from the circulation. Whether such regimens influence disease activity and the long-term sequelae of HBV infection remains uncertain because many of the studies have involved asymptomatic subjects and follow-up periods have been relatively short. Sadly enough, uncontrolled trials of antiviral chemotherapy in virus-induced chronic hepatitis continue to appear in the medical literature, even in prestigious journals.[31] Administration of hepatitis B vaccine has no therapeutic efficacy in HBsAg-positive patients. While the role of liver transplantation in the treatment of patients with CAH B remains controversial, in some centers such patients are considered appropriate candidates. Only limited short-term and long-term survival data are currently available.

7. PREVENTION OF HBV INFECTION

The keystone to the prevention of HBV infection is the appropriate use of active and passive immunoprophylaxis. Pre-exposure active immunization with hepatitis B vaccines, composed of

HBsAg particles derived from plasma or produced in yeast by recombinant DNA technology, has been shown to be highly effective, safe, and capable of providing protection for several years. The plasma-derived and recombinant vaccines appear to be comparable in many respects, including market price.[32] Vaccine characteristics are compared in Table III.

The plasma-derived vaccine available in the United States is given to adults in a 20-μg dose, while the recombinant yeast-derived vaccine is given in a 10-μg dose. Both vaccines are given by intramuscular injection into the deltoid in adults or the anterolateral thigh muscle in infants, rather than in the buttock, in a three-dose schedule, at 0, 1, and 6 months. In healthy young adults about 90–95% will respond to the three-dose schedule by developing protective levels of anti-HBs. Older and immunodeficient persons have an impaired anti-HBs response. In infants and children, the response rate to either vaccine approaches 100%, even if one half the adult dose is given (10 μg plasma-derived of 5 μg recombinant vaccine).

The peak anti-HBs titer observed after vaccination occurs 1 or 2 months after the third vaccine dose and is highly predictive of the duration of anti-HBs persistence and protection against clinical infection.[33] Booster injections may be required between the fourth and fifth year after the primary vaccination series, since a small proportion of vaccinees will have lost protective anti-HBs levels. The duration of protection afforded by booster doses remains to be determined.

Pre-exposure active immunization with the plasma-derived or recombinant vaccine is recommended for health-care workers exposed to blood or other body fluids likely to be contaminated by HBV, for hemodialysis patients, and for recipients of high-risk blood products, e.g., clotting factor concentrates, illicit parenteral drug users, homosexual men, clients and staff of institutions for the mentally retarded, and heterosexual or household contacts of HBsAg carriers. In addition to these categories, vaccination should be considered in other settings in which the risk of HBV infection exists, e.g., in certain prison populations, in first responders, and in travelers to high-risk areas who are likely to have intimate contact with native carriers.

Postexposure prophylaxis involving administration of hepatitis B Ig and hepatitis B vaccine has been recommended for the newborn of HBsAg-positive women. In this setting, a protective efficacy rate for combined prophylaxis of 85–95% has been achieved.[34] While screening for HBsAg of high-risk pregnant women has been suggested by some authorities,[35] such screening will probably detect only about one half of the HBsAg-positive population. A case for screening of all pregnant women can be made.

Table III. Comparison of the Hepatitis B Vaccines

Characteristics	Plasma-derived	Recombinant yeast-derived
Isolation and purification	Ammonium sulfate precipitation	Yeast cell-disruption
		Chromatography
Procedures	Isopyknic banding in sodium bromide	Hydrophobic adsorption
		Nonimmune affinity
	Rate-zonal sedimentation in sucrose	Size exclusion
Chemical conversion		Disulfide bonding
Inactivation	Pepsin, urea, and formaldehyde	Formaldehyde
HBsAg	Glycosylated	No glycosylation
Subtype of HBsAg	ad[a]	ad[a]
Size of particle	22 nm	17–25 nm
Adjuvant	Alum	Alum
Preservative	Thimerosol	Thimerosol
Cost	Equal	Equal

[a]ad, the group specific "a" determinant and "d" subdeterminant of HBsAg.

Other settings in which postexposure prophylaxis has been recommended include accidental exposure to HBsAg-positive blood or short-term intimate contact with an HBsAg-positive person. Convincing evidence of protective efficacy for combined passive-active immunization with hepatitis B Ig and hepatitis B vaccine in each of these situations is not yet available. It is possible that efficacy for combined immunization will be no greater than that achieved with hepatitis B Ig alone. If repeated HBV exposures are likely to occur, combined immunoprophylaxis may be a reasonable approach.

REFERENCES

1. Gust ID, Burrell CJ, Coulepis AG, et al: Taxonomic classification of human hepatitis B virus. *Intervirology* **25:**14–29, 1986.
2. Fujita YK, Kamata K, Kameda H, et al: Detection of hepatitis B virus infection in hepatitis B surface antigen-negative hemodialysis patients by monoclonal radioimmunoassays. *Gastroenterology* **91:**1357–1363, 1986.
3. Wands JR, Fujita YK, Isselbacher KJ, et al: Identification and transmission of hepatitis B virus-related variants. *Proc Natl Acad Sci USA* **83:**6608–6612, 1986.
4. Mandart E, Kay A, Galibert F: Nucleotide sequence of a cloned duck hepatitis B virus genome: Comparison with woodchuck and human hepatitis B virus sequences. *J Virol* **49:**782–792, 1984.
5. Tiollais P, Pourcel C, Dejean A: The hepatitis B virus. *Nature (Lond)* **317:**489–495, 1985.
6. Feitelson MA, Marion PL, Robinson WS: Core particles of hepatitis B virus and ground squirrel hepatitis virus. II. Characterization of the protein kinase reaction associated with ground squirrel hepatitis virus and hepatitis B virus. *J Virol* **43:**741–748, 1982.
7. Persing DH, Varmus HE, Ganem D: Inhibition of secretion of hepatitis B surface antigen by a related presurface polypeptide. *Science* **234:**1388–1391, 1986.
8. Theilmann L, Klinkert M-Q, Gmelin K, et al: Detection of pre-S1 proteins in serum and liver of HBsAg-positive patients: A new marker for hepatitis B virus infection. *Hepatology* **6:**186–190, 1986.
9. Budkowska A, Dubreuil P, Capel F, et al: Hepatitis B virus pre-S gene-encoded antigenic specificity and anti-pre-S antibody: Relationship between anti-pre-S response and recovery. *Hepatology* **6:**360–368, 1986.
10. Ou J-H, Laub O, Rutter WJ: Hepatitis B virus gene function: The precore region targets the core antigen to cellular membranes and causes the secretion of the e antigen. *Proc Natl Acad Sci USA* **83:**1578–1582, 1986.
11. Roossinck MJ, Jameel S, Loukin SH, et al: Expression of hepatitis B viral core region in mammalian cells. *Mol Cell Biol* **6:**1393–1400, 1986.
12. Moriarty AM, Alexander H, Lerner RA, et al: Antibodies to peptides detect new hepatitis B antigen: Serological correlation with hepatocellular carcinoma. *Science* **227:**429–432, 1985.
13. Seeger C, Ganem D, Varmus HE: Biochemical and genetic evidence for the hepatitis B virus replication strategy. *Science* **232:**477–484, 1986.
14. Yokosuka O, Omata M, Imazeki F, et al: Hepatitis B virus transcripts and DNA in chronic liver disease. *N Engl J Med* **315:**1187–1192, 1986.
15. Tagawa M, Omata M, Yokosuka O, et al: Early events in duck hepatitis B virus infection. Sequential appearance of viral deoxyribonucleic acid in the liver, pancreas, kidney, and spleen. *Gastroenterology* **89:**1224–1229, 1985.
16. Romet-Lemonne JL, McLane MF, Elfassi E, et al: Hepatitis B virus infection in cultured human lymphoblastoid cells. *Science* **221:**667–669, 1983.
17. Zeldis, JB, Mugishima H, Steinberg HN, et al: In vitro hepatitis B virus infection of human bone marrow cells. *J Clin Invest* **78:**411–417, 1986.
18. Shen H-D, Choo K-B, Lee S-D, et al: Hepatitis B virus DNA in leukocytes of patients with hepatitis B virus-associated liver diseases. *J Med Virol* **18:**201–211, 1986.
19. Shimoda T, Shikata T, Karasawa T, ct al: Light microscopic localization of hepatitis B virus antigens in the human pancreas. Possibility of multiplication of hepatitis B virus in the human pancreas. *Gastroenterology* **81:**998–1005, 1981.
20. Blum HE, Stowring L, Figus A, et al: Detection of hepatitis B virus DNA in hepatocytes, bile duct epithelium, and vascular elements by in situ hybridization. *Proc Natl Acad Sci USA* **80:**6685–6688, 1983.

21. Dejean A, Lugassy C, Zafrani S, et al: Detection of hepatitis B virus DNA in pancreas, kidney and skin of two human carriers of the virus. *J Gen Virol* **65:**651–655, 1984.
22. Will H, Cattaneo R, Koch HG, et al: Cloned HBV DNA causes hepatitis in chimpanzees. *Nature (Lond)* **299:**740–742, 1982.
23. Tuttleman JS, Pugh JC, Summers JW: In vitro experimental infection of primary duck hepatocyte cultures with duck hepatitis B virus. *J Virol* **58:**17–25, 1986.
24. Sureau C, Romet-Lemonne J-L, Mullins JI, et al: Production of hepatitis B virus by differentiated human hepatoma cell line after transfection with cloned circular HBV DNA. *Cell* **47:**37–47, 1986.
25. Tsang, T-K, Blei AT, O'Reilly DJ, et al: Clinical significance of concurrent hepatitis B surface antigen and antibody positivity. *Dig Dis Sci* **31:**620–624, 1986.
26. Gerlich WH, Uy A, Lambrecht F, Thomssen R: Cutoff levels of immunoglobulin M antibody against viral core antigen for differentiation of acute, chronic, and past hepatitis B virus infections. *J Clin Microbiol* **24:**288–293, 1986.
27. Seeff LB, Koff RS: Evolving concepts of the clinical and serologic consequences of hepatitis B virus infection. *Semin Liver Dis* **6:**11–22, 1986.
28. Koff RS: Natural history of acute hepatitis B in adults re-examined. *Gastroenterology* **92:**2035–2037, 1987.
29. Liaw Y-F, Chu C-M, Chen T-J, et al: Chronic lobular hepatitis: Clinical pathological and prognostic study. *Hepatology* **2:**258–262, 1982.
30. Seeff LB, Koff RS: Therapy for chronic active hepatitis. *Adv Intern Med* **29:**109–145, 1984.
31. Hoofnagle JH, Mullen KD, Jones DB, et al: Treatment of chronic non-A, non-B hepatitis with recombinant human alpha interferon. A preliminary report. *N Engl J Med* **315:**1575–1578, 1986.
32. Zajac BA, West DJ, McAleer WJ, et al: Overview of clinical studies with hepatitis B vaccine made by recombinant DNA. *J Infect* **13**(suppl A):39–45, 1986.
33. Hadler SC, Francis DP, Maynard JE, et al: Long-term immunogenicity and efficacy of hepatitis B vaccine in homosexual men. *N Engl J Med* **315:**209–214, 1986.
34. Stevens CE, Taylor PE: Hepatitis B vaccine: Issues, recommendations, and new developments. *Semin Liver Dis* **6:**23–27, 1986.
35. Centers for Disease Control: Recommendations for protection against viral hepatitis. *MMWR* **34:**313–335, 1985.

4

Pathology and Immunopathology of Acute and Chronic Hepatitis B

Michael A. Gerber

1. INTRODUCTION

This chapter describes the pathologic characteristics of acute and chronic hepatitis B, as derived from our current knowledge of the biology of hepatitis B virus (HBV)[1] and of the immunopathology of the disease.[2] Since the precise mechanism of hepatocyte necrosis by HBV is still unknown, some of the information presented here is speculative.

Several lines of evidence indicate that HBV is not directly cytopathic for hepatocytes. First, there is no correlation between the amount of HBV antigens in the serum or liver of patients with hepatitis B and the severity of liver damage.[3–6] In fact, the relationship is often inverse.[7–10] Second, infected hepatocytes containing HBV or its antigens show only minor, if any, degenerative changes at light and electron microscopic levels.[11] Many HBV carriers have normal liver morphology and function, although their hepatocytes frequently express abundant amounts of HBV or its antigens.[12–14] Third, there is no cytopathic effect in cultured human hepatoma cells that actively replicate HBV and produce mature infectious Dane particles, as recently reported by several groups of investigators.[15–17]

2. ACUTE HEPATITIS

In the absence of a direct viropathic effect, it is likely that the immune response of the patient mediates hepatocyte injury in acute and chronic HBV infection. This is supported by the predominance of lymphocytes and macrophages rather than polymorphonuclear leukocytes in the infected liver. In acute hepatitis B, conspicuous numbers of lymphocytes and other mononuclear cells infiltrate portal tracts and sinusoids throughout the hepatic lobules and are often in apposition to hepatocytes. The latter show evidence of cell injury that may present in two forms, i.e., ballooning degeneration and cytolysis or coagulative necrosis and formation of acidophilic or apoptotic bodies. Lymphocytes are sometimes seen within the cytoplasm of hepatocytes (emperipolesis).[18] Close contact between lymphocytes and damaged hepatocytes (peripolesis) or acidophilic bodies (Fig. 1)

Michael A. Gerber • Department of Pathology, Tulane University School of Medicine, New Orleans, Louisiana 70112.

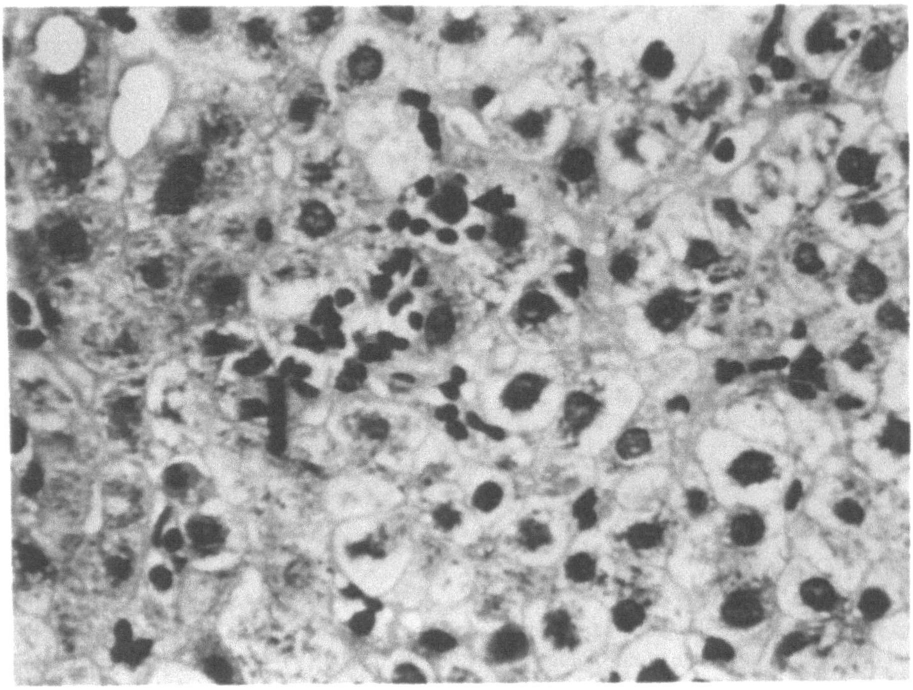

Figure 1. Acute viral hepatitis B showing pleomorphism of hepatocytes due to ballooning degeneration and coagulation necrosis as well as infiltration by mononuclear inflammatory cells. An acidophilic body (arrow) is surrounded by several lymphocytes (peripoesis). (H&E, ×250)

has been described as a characteristic finding in hepatitis B in contrast to one form of non-A, non-B hepatitis, which may be mediated by a direct viropathic mechanism. Regeneration in acute viral hepatitis is reflected in mitoses and bi- or multinucleation of hepatocytes. The combination of these features, i.e., hepatocyte degeneration and regeneration, sinusoidal cell activation, and diffuse inflammation result in the characteristic overall picture of lobular disarray, hepatocyte pleomorphism, and hypercellularity.[19–28]

What is the phenotype, target, and effect of the lymphocytes in the liver of patients with hepatitis B? The life cycle of HBV may shed some light on these questions. Studies of the natural history of hepatitis B suggest that HBV infection proceeds through two stages: an early replicative (permissive) stage and a later nonreplicative (nonpermissive) stage.[29–31] During acute infection and the initial period of chronic infection, the viral DNA is present in episomal (free or extrachromosomal) form, and the virus replicates in the hepatocyte with complete transcription of the genome resulting in production of mature infectious virions, HBV DNA, DNA polymerase, HB surface antigen (HBsAg), HB core antigen (HBcAg), and HB e antigen (HBeAg). HBV replication appears to occur primarily in the cytoplasm,[32] with concomitant expression of HBcAg or HBeAg on the cell surface.[33] This replicative phase of HBV infection is associated with progressive liver disease.[34–37]

Immunohistochemical studies of lymphocyte subsets in liver sections demonstrated that CD8 positive lymphocytes accumulated in areas of focal necrosis in acute hepatitis B and of piecemeal necrosis in chronic active hepatitis B.[38–46] These cells probably represent cytotoxic T lymphocytes, which recognize HBcAg or HBeAg on the surface of infected cells in the context of class I HLA antigens[2] (Fig. 2A,B). A series of cytotoxicity studies of peripheral blood lymphocytes against

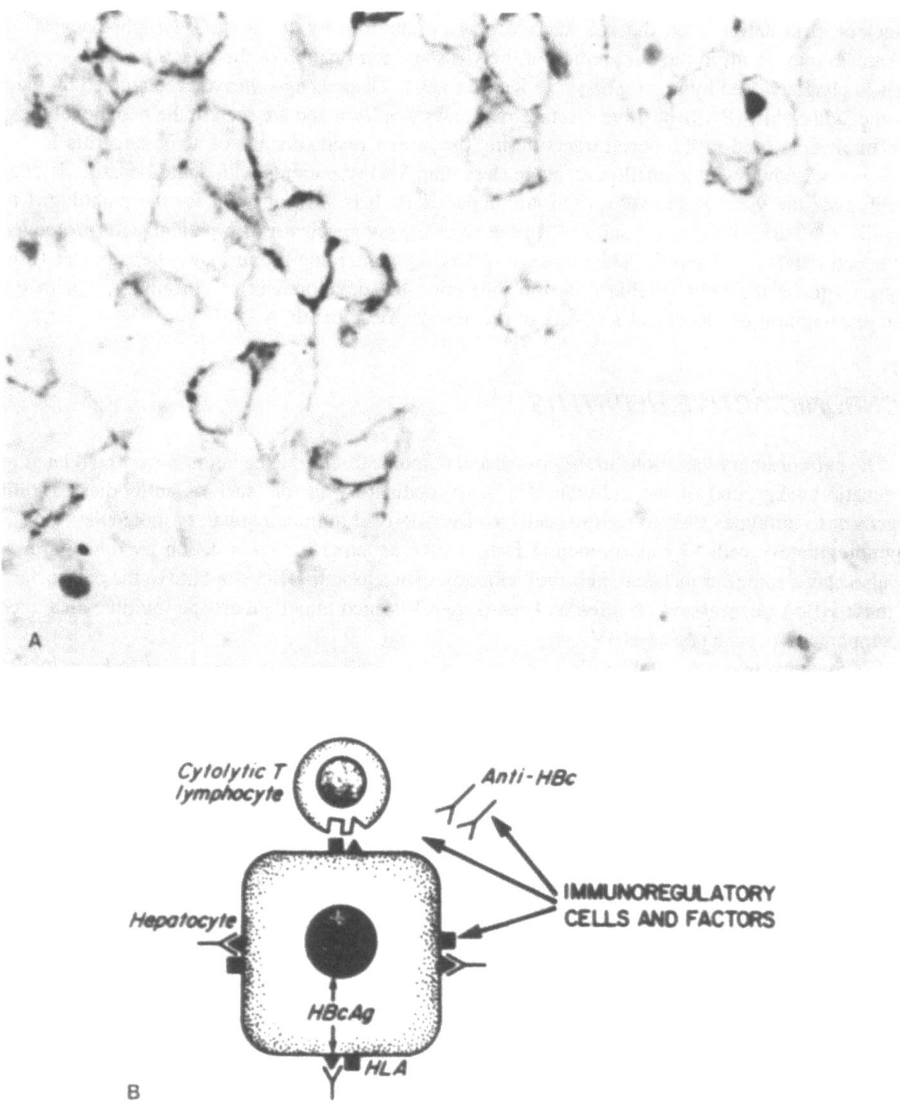

Figure 2. (A) Demonstration of β_2-microglobulin in the plasma membranes of hepatocytes in chronic hepatitis B. β_2-Microglobulin represents the light chain of class I HLA antigens. (Immunoperoxidase staining with antiserum to β_2-microglobulin, $\times 250$) (B) Model of hepatocyte lysis in viral hepatitis B. Hepatocyte with replicating HBV expresses HBcAg or HBeAg together with HLA class I molecules on the cell surface. This molecular complex represents the target antigen for cytolytic T lymphocytes. The reaction is modulated by immunoregulatory cells or factors such as antibodies.

autologous hepatocytes in patients with chronic HBV infection suggested that T lymphocytes were cytotoxic for hepatocytes with HBcAg or HBeAg, but not for hepatocytes with HBsAg, on the cell surface.[47–52] If confirmed, it follows that hepatocytes with active HBV replication and expression of nucleocapsid antigens on the cell surface may be attacked by cytotoxic T lymphocytes. This mechanism may result in the elimination of the virus and termination of the infection. The necrotic debris is phagocytosed by macrophages or Kupffer cells. These phagocytes are recognized by their periodic acid-Schiff (PAS)-positive diastase-resistant cytoplasm and are seen in the hepatic lobules, often in clusters, and in the portal tracts during the late or residual stage of acute hepatitis B.

It is not known why a small percentage (less than 5%) of patients with acute hepatitis B does not eliminate the virus and develops chronic hepatitis B. It is very difficult for the pathologist to recognize the "transition to chronicity" in the liver biopsy specimen of a patient with prolonged viral hepatitis B[53–56] (Table I). The presence of HBsAg-containing ground-glass hepatocytes (Fig. 3) appears to be the only reliable criterion indicating the development of chronicity,[53] with the possible exception of piecemeal necrosis in the absence of hepatitis A.[55]

3. CHRONIC ACTIVE HEPATITIS

The extraordinary variations in the course and outcome of chronic hepatitis B may be related to the genetic background of the individual[57–59]; to modulatory factors such as antibodies to viral antigens or to idiotypes,[60,61] to serum-, cell-, or liver-derived immunoregulatory molecules[62]; or to immunoregulatory cells.[63] Environmental factors such as super- or co-infection by other viruses may also play a role. For instance, antiviral antibodies such as anti-HBc, can bind to the cell surface and mask HBcAg expression on infected hepatocytes,[33] which may then escape immune clearance and support the persistence of HBV.

Continued active viral replication will result in the development of chronic active hepatitis B. HBV replication is probably a major cause of active and progressive liver disease.[35–37,64] Depending on factors that are still unknown, HBV DNA will become integrated into the chromosomes of increasing numbers of hepatocytes with conversion to the nonreplicative phase of HBV infection.[30,31] This period of HBeAg/anti-HBe conversion is often preceded by increased necroinflammatory activity in chronic active hepatitis B.[65–68] The morphologic hallmark of this disease represents piecemeal necrosis,[69,70] i.e., extension of the inflammatory infiltrate from the portal tracts (as the sites of entry) into the surrounding limiting plate with destruction of single or grouped hepatocytes (Fig. 4). Hepatocytes at the edge of portal tracts and septa often show peripolesis and emperipolesis by lymphocytes. $CD8^+$ cytotoxic T lymphocytes predominate among the inflammatory cells, but macrophages, plasma cells, and scattered polymorphonuclear leukocytes are also present. The portal tracts are expanded by the periportal zone of piecemeal necrosis, inflammatory infiltration, and fibrosis, with the formation of septa. Increased synthesis of collagen and prolifera-

Table I. Histologic Findings Suggested to Predict Transition to Chronicity in Prolonged Viral Hepatitis

HBsAg-containing ground-glass hepatocytes
Piecemeal necrosis
Bridging necrosis
Bile duct damage
Plasma cells in portal tracts
Lymphoid follicles in portal tracts

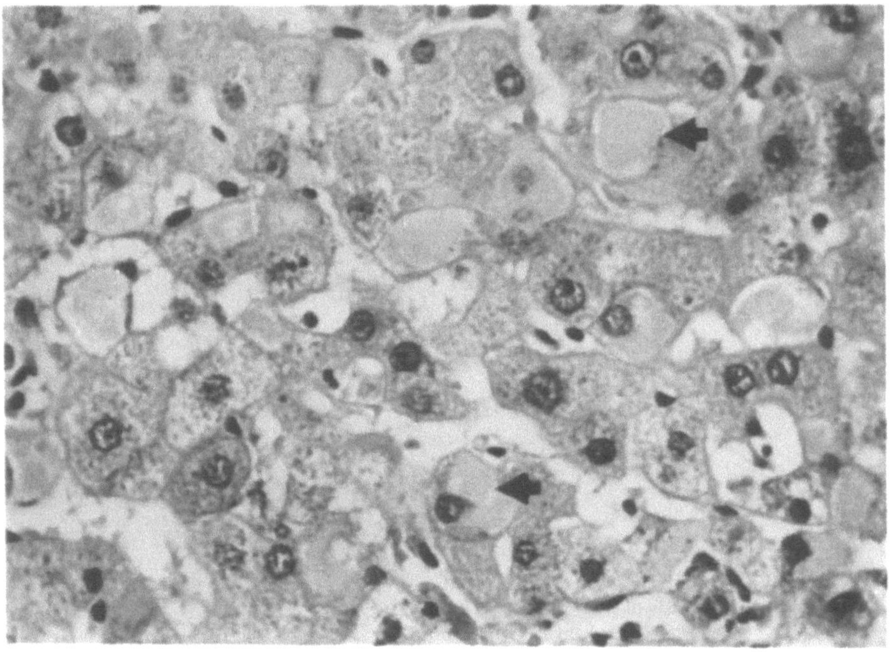

Figure 3. Ground-glass hepatocytes (arrows) in the liver of a patient with chronic hepatitis B. The ground-glass appearance of the cytoplasm of hepatocytes is due to the accumulation of HBsAg. (H&E, ×250).

tion of bile ductules are probably secondary phenomena mediated by lymphokines or monokines. The progressive fibrosis extends from the portal tracts to and around the periportal hepatocytes with the formation of pseudorosettes and septa, which eventually connect portal tracts with terminal hepatic venules leading to loss of the normal lobular architecture and to the development of cirrhosis.[19–25,73–78] Increased activity may also be reflected in irregular necroinflammatory foci in the hepatic lobules[69] and around the terminal hepatic venules, in the formation of bridging necrosis between portal tracts and terminal hepatic venules[79–82] (Fig. 5) or in multilobular necrosis and collapse (Fig. 6) of liver parenchyma.[83] These processes, particularly the circumscribed lobular alterations,[31] which may mimic acute hepatitis and may be followed by seroconversion to anti-HBe,[65–68] probably hasten the development of cirrhosis and may be precipitated by reactivation of latent HBV infection (or "reversion")[5,89,90,64] or superinfection by other viruses[84–88] (Table II).

Immunohistochemical studies demonstrated that scattered hepatocytes express HBsAg in the cytoplasm and/or along the plasma membrane and HBcAg in the nuclei and/or cytoplasm or plasma membranes.[91] The cytoplasmic localization of HBcAg appears to correlate best with increased necroinflammatory activity in chronic active hepatitis B.[92]

In the nonreplicative phase of HBV infection, the integrated viral genome often shows deletions or rearrangements resulting in incomplete viral gene expression and transcription, mainly of the S gene and little or no production of HBcAg, HBeAg, free HBV DNA, DNA polymerase, and complete virus.[93] This phase is usually associated with anti-HBe in the serum and remission of disease activity in the liver, which may show chronic persistent hepatitis or inactive cirrhosis.[31,35,94–96] If it is true that HBcAg or HBeAg represent the major target antigens for cytotoxic T lymphocytes, the lack of production of these antigens during the nonreplicative phase would explain the decreased activity.

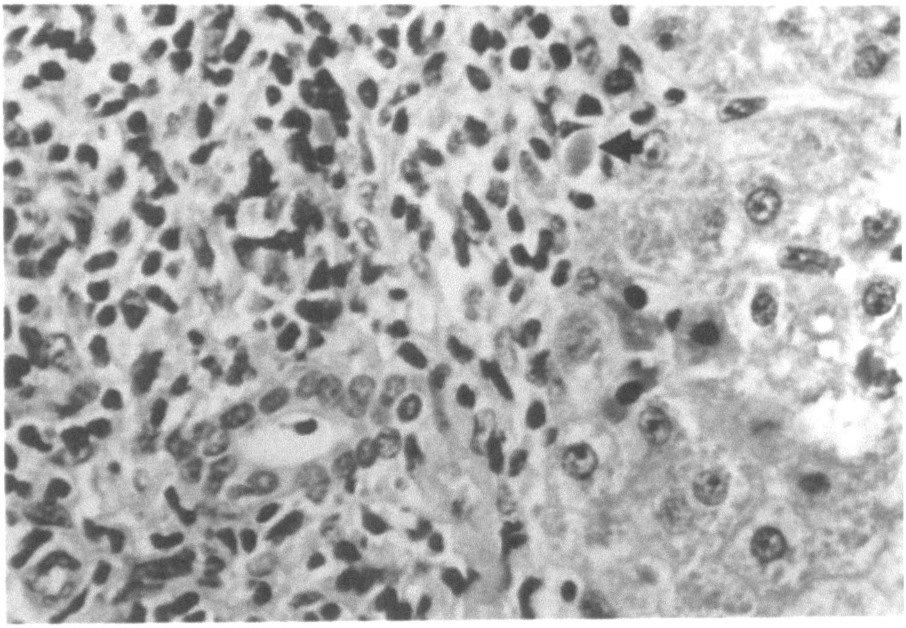

Figure 4. Piecemeal necrosis in the liver of a patient with chronic active hepatitis B. The border between the portal tract (left) and the hepatic parenchyma (right) is irregular due to infiltration of mononuclear inflammatory cells into the limiting plate with necrosis of individual hepatocytes (arrow). (H&E, ×250)

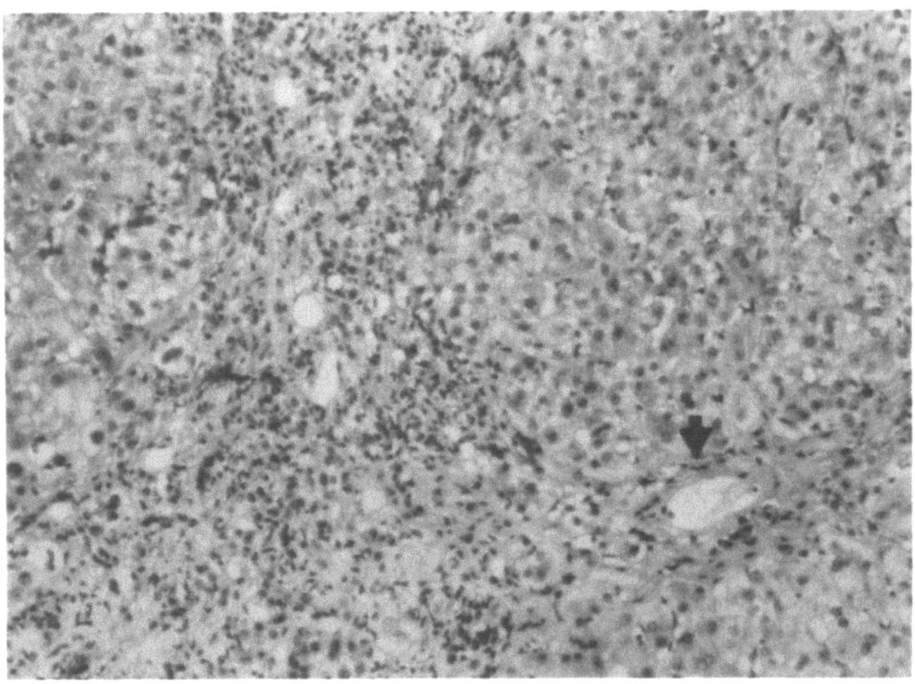

Figure 5. Bridging necrosis in the liver of a patient with chronic active hepatitis B. The expanded portal tract (left) and the central vein (arrow) are connected by a band of necrotic and collapsed hepatic parenchyma. (H&E, ×100)

Table II. Events That May Be Related to Intralobular Necroinflammation in Chronic Active Hepatitis B

Increased immune elimination of HBV infected hepatocytes (HBeAg → anti-HBe)
Reactivation of HBV replication ("reversion") (anti-HBe → HBeAg)
Superinfection by other viruses (HAV, HDV, non-A, non-B, ? HIV)

4. CHRONIC PERSISTENT HEPATITIS

Chronic persistent hepatitis B is characterized by little necroinflammatory activity in the hepatic parenchyma and at the limiting plate, which remains intact[73,74,97] (Fig. 7). The mononuclear cell infiltrate is confined to the portal tracts which are expanded, but usually do not show significant fibrosis or proliferation of bile ductules. The lobular architecture is preserved, and the sinusoidal lining cells are activated to varying degrees. By contrast, chronic septal hepatitis[98] and inactive cirrhosis are characterized by fibrosis, while inflammation and necrosis are minimal. Histochemical (orcein or Victoria blue) or immunohistochemical stains often show large numbers of HBsAg-positive ground-glass hepatocytes in chronic persistent hepatitis and inactive cirrhosis, while little or no HBcAg is demonstrable.[91] It should be noted that the separation between chronic

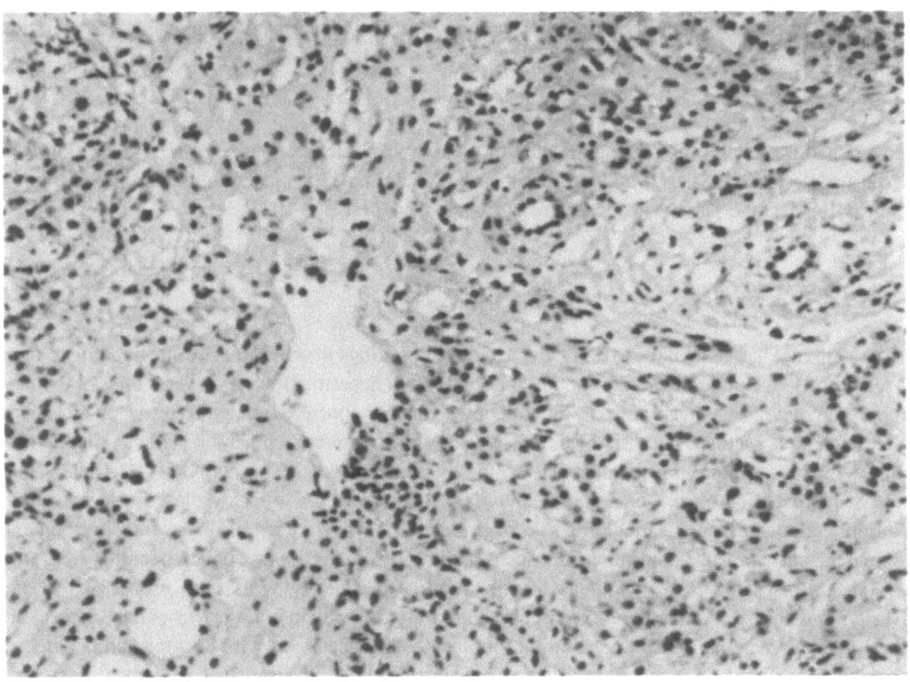

Figure 6. Multilobular collapse in the liver of a patient with chronic active hepatitis B. All hepatocytes of an entire lobule have been replaced by a mononuclear inflammatory cells with collapse of the preexisting framework of the liver. (H&E, ×100)

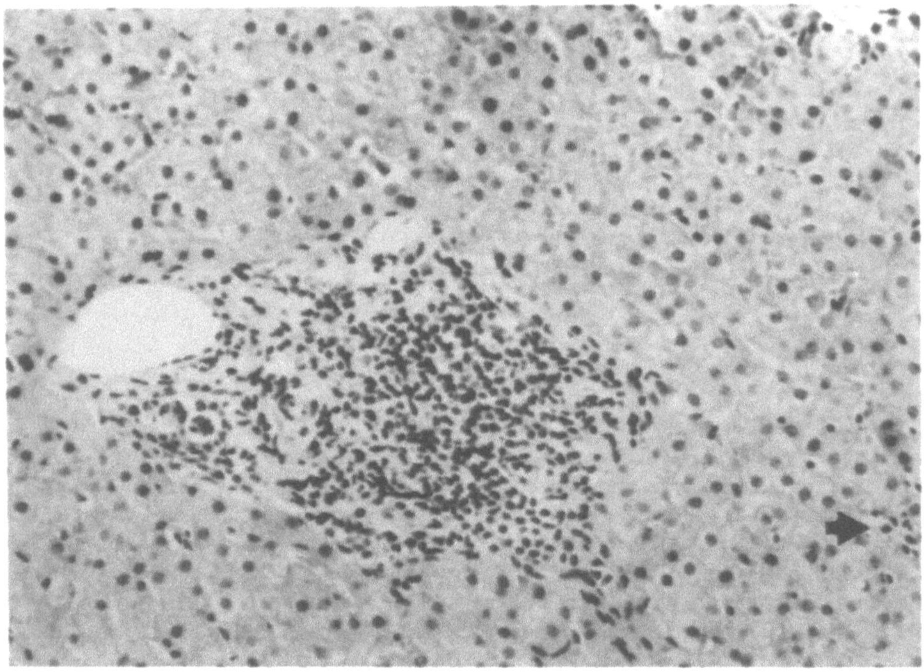

Figure 7. Chronic persistent hepatitis B characterized by expansion of the portal tract by mononuclear inflammatory cells without significant fibrosis or piecemeal necrosis. The hepatic parenchyma shows a focal necrosis (arrow). (H&E, ×100)

active hepatitis and chronic persistent hepatitis and between the two phases of HBV infection is not sharp; i.e., serum HBV DNA and/or intrahepatic HBcAg have been found in a significant number of anti-HBe-positive patients with severe chronic active hepatitis B.[29,94,99–101]

5. CONCLUSIONS

An attempt has been made to relate the pathologic findings in acute and chronic hepatitis B to our current knowledge of the life cycle and immunobiology of hepatitis B virus. Several lines of evidence support the hypothesis that cytotoxic T lymphocytes that recognize HBcAg or HBeAg on the surface of infected cells mediate necrosis of hepatocytes with active viral replication. Other immune reactions, such as humoral mechanisms,[102] antibody-dependent cellular cytoxicity (ADCC), macrophage-mediated cytolysis, or natural killer (NK) cell activity,[63,103] may play a role as well. In addition, genetic influences, including sex-linked factors,[104] hormones, life-style and environmental parameters, such as drugs, and superimposed infections by other viruses, such as hepatitis A, D, non-A, non-B viruses[84–88,105] as well as human immune deficiency virus may influence the type, severity, and course of hepatitis B. Lymphocytotoxicity rather than a direct viropathic effect would explain the characteristic histologic finding of close contact between lymphocytes and hepatocytes throughout the lobular parenchyma in acute hepatitis B and in the areas of piecemeal necrosis in chronic active hepatitis B. Histologically, deposition of collagen distinguishes acute from chronic hepatitis B. Chronic persistent hepatitis does not show significant necroinflammatory activity and may occur de novo or during the nonreplicative phase of HBV infection.

During this decade, much progress has been made in our knowledge of HBV, including recent success in the propagation of the virus in vitro. The mechanism of hepatocyte injury and the pathogenesis of acute and chronic hepatitis B, however, remain major unsolved problems in this worldwide disease.

ACKNOWLEDGMENTS. I am grateful to Ms. Nancy Ruiz for secretarial assistance and to Steve Mortillo for technical assistance.

REFERENCES

1. Gerber MA, Thung SN: Molecular and cellular pathology of hepatitis B. *Lab Invest* **52**:572–590, 1985.
2. Gerber MA: Immunopathology of chronic hepatitis, in Phillips MJ, and Farber E (eds): *Pathogenesis of Liver Diseases*. IAP Monograph No. 28. Williams & Wilkins, Baltimore, 1986, pp. 54–64.
3. Alberti A, Tremolada F, Fattovich G, et al: Virus replication and liver disease in chronic hepatitis B virus infection. *Dig Dis Sci* **28**:961–996, 1983.
4. Bonino F, Hoyer B, Nelson J, et al: Hepatitis B virus DNA in the sera of HBsAg carriers: A marker of active hepatitis B virus replication in the liver. *Hepatology* **1**:386–391, 1981.
5. Davis GL, Hoofnagle JH, Waggoner JG: Spontaneous reactivation of chronic hepatitis B virus infection. *Gastroenterology* **86**:230–235, 1984.
6. Sjögren M, Hoofnagle JH, Gerin JL: IgM antibody to hepatitis B core antigen in patients with chronic type B hepatitis. *Gastroenterology* **89**:252–258, 1985.
7. Alberti A, Realdi G, Tremolada F, et al: Liver cell surface localization of hepatitis B antigen and of immunoglobulins in acute and chronic hepatitis and in liver cirrhosis. *Clin Exp Immunol* **25**:396–402, 1976.
8. Lamothe F, Laurencin-Piché J, Cote J, et al: Detection of surface and core antigens of hepatitis B virus in the liver of 164 human subjects. *Gastroenterology* **71**:102–108, 1976.
9. Portmann B, Galbraith RM, Eddleston ALWF, et al: Detection of HBsAg in fixed liver tissue: use of a modified immunofluorescence technique: Comparison with histochemical methods. *Gut* **17**:1–9, 1976.
10. Ray MB: Hepatitis B virus Antigens in Tissues. MTP Press, Lancaster, England, 1979.
11. Gerber MA, Thung SN: Pathobiology of hepatitis B virus. *Pathobiol Annu* **11**:197–228, 1981.
12. Hadziyannis S, Gerber MA, Vissoulis C, et al: Cytoplasmic hepatitis B antigen in "ground-glass," hepatocytes of carriers. *Arch Pathol Lab Med* **96**:327–330, 1973.
13. Gerber MA, Hadziyannis S, Vissoulis C, et al: Electron-microscopy and immunoelectron microscopy of cytoplasmic hepatitis B antigen in hepatocytes. *Am J Pathol* **75**:489–502, 1974.
14. Gerber MA, Hadziyannis S, Vernace S, et al: Incidence and nature of cytoplasmic hepatitis B antigen in hepatocytes. *Lab Invest* **32**:251–256, 1975.
15. Sureau C, Romet-Lemonne JL, Mullins JI, et al: Production of hepatitis B virus by a differentiated human hepatoma cell line after transfection with cloned circular HBV DNA. *Cell* **47**:37–47, 1986.
16. Tsurimot T, Fujiyama A, Matsubara K: Stable expression and replication of hepatitis B virus genome in an integrated state in a human hepatoma cell line transfected with the cloned viral DNA. *Proc Natl Acad Sci USA* **84**:444–448, 1987.
17. Sells MA, Chen M-L, Acs G: Production of hepatitis B virus particles in Hep G2 cells transfected with cloned hepatitis B virus DNA. *Proc Natl Acad Sci USA* **84**:1005–1009, 1987.
18. Bechtelsheimer H, Gedigk P, Muller R, et al: Aggressive Emperipolese bei chronischen Hepatitiden. *Klin Wochenschr* **54**:137–140, 1976.
19. Gerber MA, Thung SN: Viral hepatitis: Pathology, in Berk JE, Haubrich WS, Kalser MH, Roth JLA, Schaffner F (eds): *Bockus Gastroenterology*, Vol. V: *The Liver*, 4th ed. WB Saunders, Philadelphia, 1985, pp. 2225–2235.
20. Ishak KG: Light microscopic morphology of viral hepatitis. *Am J Clin Pathol* **65**:787–827, 1976.
21. Bianchi L, Simmerli-Ning M, Gudat F: Viral hepatitis, in MacSween RNM, Anthony PP, Scheuer PJ (eds): *Pathology of Liver*. Churchill Livingstone, Edinburgh, 1979, pp. 164–191.
22. MacSween RNM: Pathology of viral hepatitis and its sequelae. *Clin Gastroenterol* **9**:23–45, 1980.
23. Scheuer PJ: *Liver Biopsy Interpretation*, 3rd ed. Balliere Tindall, London, 1980.
24. Review by an International Group: Morphological criteria in viral hepatitis. *Lancet* **1**:333–337, 1971.

25. Review by an International Group: Acute and chronic hepatitis revisited. *Lancet* **2**:914–919, 1977.
26. Popper H, Dienstag JL, Feinstone SM, et al: Pathology of viral hepatitis in chimpanzees. *Virchows Arch A Pathol Anat Histol* **387**:91–106, 1980.
27. Peters RL: Viral hepatitis: A pathological spectrum. *Am J Med Sci* **270**:17–31, 1975.
28. Phillips MJ, Poucell S: Modern aspects of the morphology of viral hepatitis. *Hum Pathol* **12**:1060–1084, 1981.
29. Hadziyannis SJ, Lieberman HM, Karvountzis GG, et al: Analysis of liver disease, nuclear HBcAg viral replication, and hepatitis B virus DNA in liver and serum of HBeAg, vs. anti-HBe positive carriers of hepatitis B virus. *Hepatology* **3**:656–662, 1983.
30. Hoofnagle JH: Chronic type B hepatitis. *Gastroenterology* **84**:422–424, 1983.
31. Shafritz DA, Rogler CE: Molecular characterization of viral forms observed in persistent hepatitis infections, chronic liver disease and hepatocellular carcinoma in woodchucks and humans, in Vyas GN, Dienstag JL, Hoofnagle JH (eds): *Viral Hepatitis and Liver Disease*. Grune & Stratton, Orlando, Florida, 1984, pp. 225–243.
32. Burrell CJ, Gowans EJ, Jilbert AR, et al: Hepatitis B virus DNA detection by in situ cytohybridization: Implications for viral replication strategy and pathogenesis of chronic hepatitis. *Hepatology* **2**(suppl):85S–91S, 1982.
33. Trevisan A, Realdi G, Alberti A, et al: Core antigen-specific immunoglobulin G bound to the liver cell membrane in chronic hepatitis B. *Gastroenterology* **82**:218–222, 1982.
34. Alter HJ, Seef LB, Kaplan PM, et al: Type B hepatitis: the infectivity of blood positive for e antigen and DNA polymerase after accidental needlestick exposure. *N Engl J Med* **295**:909–913, 1976.
35. Hoofnagle JH, Alter HJ: Chronic viral hepatitis, in Vyas GN, Dienstag JL, Hooffnagle JH (eds): *Viral hepatitis and Liver Disease*. Grune & Stratton, Orlando, Florida, 1984, pp. 97–113.
36. Smith JI, Murphy BI, Auslander MO, et al: Studies of the "e" antigen in acute and chronic hepatitis. *Gastroenterology* **71**:208–219, 1976.
37. Yokosuka O, Omata M, Imazeki F, et al: Hepatitis B virus RNA transcripts and DNA in chronic liver disease. *N Engl J Med* **315**:1187–1192, 1986.
38. Colucci G, Colombo M, Del Ninno E, et al: In situ characterization by monoclonal antibodies of the mononuclear cell infiltrate in chronic active hepatitis. *Gastroenterology* **85**:1138–1145, 1983.
39. Eggink HF, Houthoff HJ, Huitema S, et al: Cellular and humoral immune reactions in chronic active liver disease. I. Lymphocyte subsets in liver biopsies of patients with untreated idiopathic autoimmune hepatitis, chronic active hepatitis B and primary biliary cirrhosis. *Clin Exp Immunol* **50**:17–24, 1982.
40. Govindarajan S, Uchida T, Peters RL: Identification of T lymphocytes and subsets in liver biopsy cores of acute viral hepatitis. *Liver* **3**:13–18, 1983.
41. Husby G, Blomhoff JP, Elgio K, et al: Immunohistochemical characterization of hepatic tissue lymphocyte subpopulations in liver disease. *Scand J Gastroenterol* **17**:855–860, 1982.
42. Montano L, Aranguibel F, Boffill M, et al: An analysis of the composition of the inflammatory infiltrate in autoimmune and hepatitis B virus-induced chronic liver disease. *Hepatology* **3**:292–296, 1983.
43. Nishihara T: Intrahepatic distribution of T cell subsets in cases with type B chronic liver disease by peroxidase-labeled antibody method using monoclonal antibodies. *Gastroenterol Jpn* **18**:320–329, 1983.
44. Pape GR, Rieber EP, Eisenburg J, et al: Involvement of the cytotoxic suppressor T-cell subset in liver tissue injury of patients with acute and chronic liver diseases. *Gastroenterology* **85**:657–662, 1983.
45. Si L, Whiteside TL, Van Thiel DH, et al: Lymphocyte subpopulations at the site of "piecemeal" necrosis in end stage chronic liver diseases and rejecting liver allografts in cyclosporine-treated patients. *Lab Invest* **50**:341–347, 1984.
46. Thomas HC, Montano L, Goodall A, et al: Immunological mechanisms in chronic hepatitis B virus infection. *Hepatology* **2**(suppl):116S–121S, 1982.
47. Eddleston ALWF, Mondelli M, Mieli-Vergani G, et al: Lymphocyte cytotoxicity to autologous hepatocytes in chronic hepatitis B virus infection. *Hepatology* **2**(suppl):122S–127S, 1982.
48. Mieli-Vergani G, Vergani D, Portmann B, et al: Lymphocyte cytotoxicity to autologous hepatocytes in HBsAg positive chronic liver disease. *Gut* **23**:1029–1036, 1982.
49. Mondelli M, Eddleston AL: Mechanisms of liver cell injury in acute and chronic hepatitis B. *Semin Liver Dis* **4**:47–58, 1984.
50. Mondelli M, Mieli-Vergani G, Alberti A, et al: Specificity of T lymphocyte cytotoxicity to autologous hepatocytes in chronic hepatitis B virus infection: evidence that T cells are directed against HBV core antigen expressed on hepatocytes. *J Immunol* **129**:2773–2778, 1982.

51. Naumov NV, Mondelli M, Alexander GJ, et al: Relationship between expression of hepatitis B virus antigens in isolated hepatocytes and autologous lymphocyte cytotoxicity in patients with chronic hepatitis B virus infection. *Hepatology* **4**:63–68, 1984.
52. Thomas HC, Lok AS: The immunopathology of autoimmune and hepatitis B virus-induced chronic hepatitis. *Semin Liver Dis* **4**:36–46, 1984.
53. Houthoff HJ, Niermeijer P, Gips CH, et al: Hepatic morphologic findings and viral antigens in acute hepatitis B. *Virchows Arch A Pathol Anat Histol* **389**:153–166, 1980.
54. Dietrichson O, Juhl T, Christoffersen P, et al: Acute viral hepatitis: Factors possibly predicting chronic liver disease. *Acta Pathol Microbiol Scand A* **83**:183–188, 1975.
55. Vanstapel MJ, van Steenbergen W, de Wolf-Peeters C, et al: Prognostic significance of piecemeal necrosis in acute viral hepatitis. *Liver* **3**:46–57, 1983.
56. Sherlock S. Predicting progression of acute type-B hepatitis to chronicity. *Lancet* **2**:354–356, 1976.
57. Milich DR, Chisari FV: Genetic regulation of the immune response to hepatitis B surface antigen (HBsAg). I. H-2 restriction of the murine humoral immune response to the a and d determinants of HBsAg. *J Immunol* **129**:320–325, 1982.
58. Milich DR, Leroux-Roels GG, Chisari FV, et al: Genetic regulation of the immune response to hepatitis B surface antigen (HBsAg). IV. Distinct H-2 linked Ir genes control antibody responses to different HBsAg determinants on the same molecule and map to the I-A and I-C subregions. *J Exp Med* **159**:41–56, 1984.
59. Milich DR, Peterson DL, Chisari FV: Comparison of T cell and B cell immune recognition of HBsAg, in Vyas GN, Dienstag JL, Hoofnagle JH (eds): *Viral Hepatitis and Liver Disease*. Grune & Stratton, Orlando, Florida, 1984, pp. 573–582.
60. Kennedy RC, Adler-Storthz K, Henkel RD, et al: Immune response to hepatitis B surface antigen: Enhancement by prior injection of antibodies to the idiotype. *Science* **221**:853–855, 1983.
61. Kennedy RC, Melnick JL, Dreesman GR: Antibody to hepatitis B virus induced by injecting antibodies to the idiotype. *Science* **223**:930–931, 1984.
62. Chisari FV: Regulation of lymphocyte function and viral transformation by hepatic bioregulatory molecules. *Hepatology* **2**(suppl):97S–106S, 1982.
63. Dienstag JL: Immunologic mechanisms in chronic viral hepatitis, in Vyas GN, Dienstag JL, Hoofnagle JH (eds): *Viral Hepatitis and Liver Disease*. Grune & Stratton, Orlando, Florida, 1984, pp. 135–166.
64. Davis GL, Hoofnagle JH: Reactivation of chronic hepatitis B virus infection. *Gastroenterology* **92**:2028–2031, 1987.
65. Liaw Y-F, Pao CC, Chu C-M, et al: Changes of serum hepatitis B virus DNA in two types of clinical events preceding spontaneous hepatitis B e antigen seroconversion in chronic type B hepatitis. *Hepatology* **7**:1–3, 1987.
66. Realdi G, Alberti A, Rugge M, et al: Seroconversion from hepatitis B e antigen to anti-HBe in chronic hepatitis B virus infection. *Gastroenterology* **79**:195–199, 1980.
67. Hoofnagle JH, Dusheiko GM, Seeff LB, et al: Seroconversion from hepatitis B e antigen to antibody in chronic type B hepatitis. *Ann Intern Med* **94**:744–748, 1981.
68. Liaw YF, Chu CM, Su IJ, et al: Clinical and histological events preceding hepatitis B e antigen seroconversion in chronic type B hepatitis. *Gastroenterology* **84**:216–219, 1983.
69. Popper H: Changing concepts of the evolution of chronic hepatitis and the role of piecemeal necrosis. *Hepatology* **3**:758–762, 1983.
70. Kerr JF, Cooksley WGE, Searle J, et al: The nature of piecemeal necrosis in chronic active hepatitis. *Lancet* **2**:827–828, 1979.
71. Baggenstoss AJ, Summerskill WHK, Ammon HV: The morphology of chronic hepatitis, in Schaffner F, Sherlock S, Leevy CM (eds): *The Liver and Its Diseases*. Intercontinental Medical Book, New York, 1974, pp. 199–206.
72. Popper H, Schaffner F: Chronic hepatitis: Taxonomic, etiology and therapeutic problems, in Popper H, Schaffner F (eds): *Progress in Liver Diseases*. Grune & Stratton, Orlando, Florida, 1977, pp. 531–558.
73. Popper H, Schaffner F: The vocabulary of chronic hepatitis. N Engl J Med **284**:1154–1156, 1971.
74. De Groote J, Desmet VJ, Gedigk P, et al: A classification of chronic hepatitis. *Lancet* **2**:626–628, 1968.
75. Ludwig J: A review of lobular, portal and periportal hepatitis. *Hum Pathol* **8**:269–276, 1977.
76. Scheuer PJ: Liver biopsy in chronic hepatitis: 1968–1978. *Gut* **19**:554–557, 1978.
77. Christofferson P, Dietrichson O: Histological changes in liver biopsies from patients with chronic hepatitis. *Acta Pathol Microbiol Scand A* **82**:539–546, 1974.
78. Scheuer PJ: Chronic hepatitis. A problem for the pathologist. *Histopathology* **1**:5–19, 1977.

79. Boyer JL, Klatskin G: Pattern of necrosis in acute viral hepatitis. Prognostic value of bridging (subacute hepatic) necrosis. *N Engl J Med* **283:**1063–1071, 1970.
80. Boyer JL: The diagnosis and pathogenesis of clinical variants in viral hepatitis. *Am J Clin Pathol* **65:**898–908, 1976.
81. Bianchi L: Acute viral hepatitis B with bridging necrosis: A follow-up study. *Liver* **1:**222–229, 1981.
82. Ware AJ, Eigenbrodt EH, Combes B: Prognostic significance of subacute hepatic necrosis in acute hepatitis. *Gastroenterology* **68:**519–524, 1975.
83. Baggenstoss AH, Soloway RD, Summerskill WHS, et al: Chronic active liver disease, the range of histologic lesions, their response to treatment and evolution. *Hum Pathol* **3:**183–198, 1972.
84. Dienes HP, Purcell RH, Popper H, et al: Simultaneous infection of chimpanzees with more than one hepatitis virus. *Hepatology* **1:**506, 1981. (abst).
85. Marmion BP, Burrell CJ, Tonkin RW, et al: Dialysis-associated hepatitis in Edinburgh, 1969–1978. *Rev Infect Dis* **4:**619–637, 1982.
86. Popper H, Thung SN, Gerber, MA, et al: Histologic studies of severe delta infection in Venezuelan Indians. *Hepatology* **3:**906–912, 1983.
87. Rizzetto M: The delta agent. *Hepatology* **3:**729–737, 1983.
88. Liaw YF, Tai DI, Chu C-M, et al: Acute exacerbation in chronic type B hepatitis: Comparison between HBeAg and antibody-positive patients. *Hepatology* **7:**20–23, 1987.
89. Perrillo RP, Campbell CR, Sanders GE, et al: Spontaneous clearance and reactivation of hepatitis B virus infection among male homosexuals with chronic type B hepatitis. *Ann Intern Med* **100:**43–46, 1984.
90. Lok AS, Lai C-L, Wu P-C, et al: Spontaneous hepatitis B e Antigen to antibody seroconversion and reversion in Chinese patients with chronic hepatitis B virus infection. *Gastroenterology* **92:**1839–1843, 1987.
91. Gerber MA, Thung SN: The diagnostic value of immunohistochemical demonstration of hepatitis viral antigens in liver. *Hum Pathol* **18:**771–774, 1987.
92. Chu CM, Liaw YF: Intrahepatic distribution of hepatitis B surface and core antigen s in chronic hepatitis B virus infection. *Gastroenterology* **92:**220–225, 1987.
93. Omata M, Yokosuka O, Imazeki F, et al: Correlation of hepatitis B virus DNA and antigens in the liver. A study in chronic liver disease. *Gastroenterology* **92:**192–196, 1987.
94. Brechot C, Scotto J, Charnay P, et al: Detection of hepatitis B virus DNA in liver and serum: a direct appraisal of the chronic carrier state. *Lancet* **2:**765–770, 1981.
95. Hoofnagle JH, Dusheiko GM, Seeff LB, et al: Seroconversion from hepatitis B e antigen to antibody in chronic type B hepatitis. *Ann Intern Med* **94:**744–748, 1981.
96. Realdi G, Alberti A, Ruzzi M, et al: Seroconversion from HBe antigen to anti-HBe in chronic HBV infection. *Gastroenterology* **79:**195–199, 1980.
97. Becker MD, Baptista A, Scheuer PJ, et al: Prognosis of chronic persistent hepatitis. *Lancet* **1:**53–57, 1970.
98. Gerber MA, Vernace S: Chronic septal hepatitis. *Virchows Arch A Pathol Anat Histol* **363:**303–309, 1973.
99. Kam W, Rall LB, Smuckler EA, et al: Hepatitis B viral DNA in liver and serum of asymptomatic carriers. *Proc Natl Acad Sci USA* **79:**7522–7526, 1982.
100. Lieberman HM, LaBrecque DR, Kew MC, et al: Detection of hepatitis B virus DNA directly in human serum by a simplified molecular hybridization test: Comparison to HBeAg anti-HBe status in HBsAg carriers. *Hepatology* **3:**285–291, 1983.
101. Scotto J, Hadchouel M, Hery C, et al: Detection of hepatitis B virus DNA in serum by a simple spot hybridization technique: Comparison with results for other viral markers. *Hepatology* **3:**279–284, 1983.
102. Nowoslawski A, Krawczynski K, Nazarewicz T, et al: Immunopathological aspects of hepatitis type B. *Am J Med Sci* **270:**229–239, 1975.
103. Chisari FV, Edginton TS, Routenberg JA, et al: Cellular immune reactivity in HBV-induced liver disease, in Vyas GN, Cohen SN, Schmid R (eds): *Viral Hepatitis*. The Franklin Institute Press, Philadelphia, 1978, pp. 245–266.
104. Craxi A, Montano L, Goodall A, et al: Genetic and sex-linked factors influencing HBs antigen clearance. I. Nonimmune clearance in inbred strains of mice. *J Med Virol* **9:**117–123, 1982.
105. Tassopoulos N, Papaevangelou GZ, Sjögren MH, et al: A: Natural History of acute hepatitis B surface antigen-positive hepatitis in Greek adults. *Gastroenterology* **92:**1844–1850, 1987.

5

Delta Hepatitis and the Hepatitis Delta Virus

Jay H. Hoofnagle

1. INTRODUCTION

Since its discovery in 1977 by Rizzetto and co-workers from Turin, Italy, the hepatitis delta virus (HDV) has become a focus of worldwide interest—interest almost equal to its worldwide importance.[1,2] The delta antigen, which first appeared to be a poorly explained finding of immunofluorescence staining in liver biopsies from Italian chronic hepatitis B surface antigen (HBsAg) carriers, has now been shown to be the nucleocapsid antigen of a startlingly unique and important viral agent. HDV is a "defective" RNA virus that can replicate only in the presence of HBsAg, the helper function provided by hepatitis B virus (HBV). For this reason, delta hepatitis occurs only in patients who have HBsAg in serum. Acute delta hepatitis occurs either as co-infection, simultaneous with acute hepatitis B, or as superinfection, in which acute delta hepatitis is superimposed on a chronic hepatitis B or an HBsAg carrier state. Delta superinfection commonly leads to chronic delta hepatitis, which ultimately leads to cirrhosis in more than 50% of cases.[3] Delta hepatitis also has a peculiar epidemiology, commonly occurring in prolonged severe outbreaks in isolated communities.[4] Delta hepatitis is most likely an old disease; indeed, the fulminant hepatitis syndromes known as Labrea fever and the hepatitis of Sierra Nevada de Santa Marta, described in South America for the past 50 years, probably present severe forms of acute delta hepatitis.[5] This chapter summarizes recent advances made in the understanding of delta hepatitis and HDV.

2. THE HEPATITIS D VIRUS

Hepatitis delta virus is a 35-nm double-shelled particle that looks very similar electron microscopically to the Dane particle of HBV[2] (Fig. 1). HDV has an external coat antigen of HBsAg provided by the genome of HBV and an internal antigen called delta antigen (HDV Ag), provided by the genome of HDV. Associated with HDV Ag is a small single-stranded molecule of RNA.[6] The HDV RNA isolated from virions in serum exists as a covalently closed circular molecule. Small amounts of a nicked linear form of this circle give a doublet of RNA on electrophoretic sizing gels;

Jay H. Hoofnagle • Liver Diseases Section, Digestive Diseases Branch, National Institute of Diabetes and Digestive and Kidney Diseases, National Institutes of Health, Bethesda, Maryland 20892.

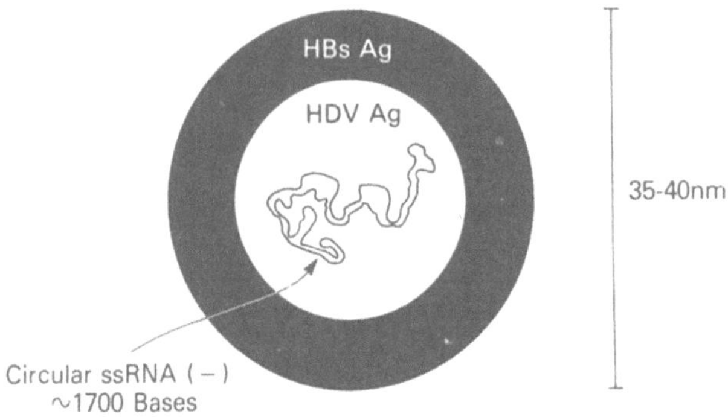

Figure 1. The hepatitis delta virus (HDV).

one molecular species of delta RNA is 1900 and one is 1750 nucleotides in length.[7–9] This virion form of HDV RNA is not polyadenylated and is not translatable using in vitro systems, for which reasons it is believed to be the negative (−) strand of the viral RNA. For the HDV RNA to be translated into a protein antigen, it must, therefore, be transcribed into a positive (+) strand RNA. Positive strands of HDV RNA are not detectable in serum.

HDV RNA isolated from infected liver exists in both genomic (−) and antigenomic (+) strands of HDV RNA.[6–9] Furthermore, some of the HDV RNA is present in longer-than-genomic length forms that are both linear and circular. Such findings suggest that HDV replicates its RNA by the double-rolling circle model[10] (Fig. 2). The (−) strand RNA enters the liver cell and a (+) strand is transcribed by an unknown RNA polymerase. One and perhaps two proteins are translated from the (+) RNA strand, which also serves as a further template for transcription of (−) RNA strands that are then associated with delta antigen and encapsidated by HBsAg to form virions. The need for HBsAg is obvious from this schema of replication; whether HDV also needs the polymerase of HBV is both unknown and unlikely.

Several groups of investigators have prepared complementary DNA (cDNA) clones from delta virion RNA.[7–9] Houghton and co-workers from Chiron Corporation isolated and sequenced multiple clones which demonstrated overlapping sequences, allowing for the sequencing of the whole genome.[7] They have suggested that HDV RNA is a single-stranded covalently closed molecule of RNA that is 1678 nucleotides in length. The RNA has a high CG content (60%) that has many areas of internal complementarity. The complementarity allows for the RNA molecule to self-anneal by internal base pairing (of the single strand to itself) and thereby yields a great stability and secondary structure to the RNA molecule.

It is uncertain what proteins are produced by the HDV RNA. Bergmann and Gerin[11] have done immunoblotting (Western blots) on purified preparations of HDV particles that reveal two polypeptide bands, one 24,000 (p24) and one 27,000 (p27) in molecular weight. Both polypeptides are found together, usually in similar amounts. Preliminary studies using monoclonal antibodies suggest that p24 and p27 are similar antigenically.[12] Bonino et al.[13] have also identified two HDV polypeptides by immunoblotting but characterized them as 27,000 and 29,000 daltons in size. These proteins probably represent the solubilized forms of delta antigen and are encoded for by a large open reading frame on the antigenomic strand of HDV RNA. The HDV RNA has multiple open reading frames and enough nucleotides to code for at least one more small protein, but it remains uncertain whether it does.

The structure and replicative cycle of HDV place it outside of any known family of animal viruses. Indeed, one must go to plant virology to find similar viral agents—those most closely resembling HDV being the plant satellite viruses.[14,15] Satellite viruses are small defective RNA viruses that typically have single-stranded RNAs with negative polarity and sizes ranging from 800 to 1700 nucleotides (Table I). Each satellite virus cannot replicate without the specific helper

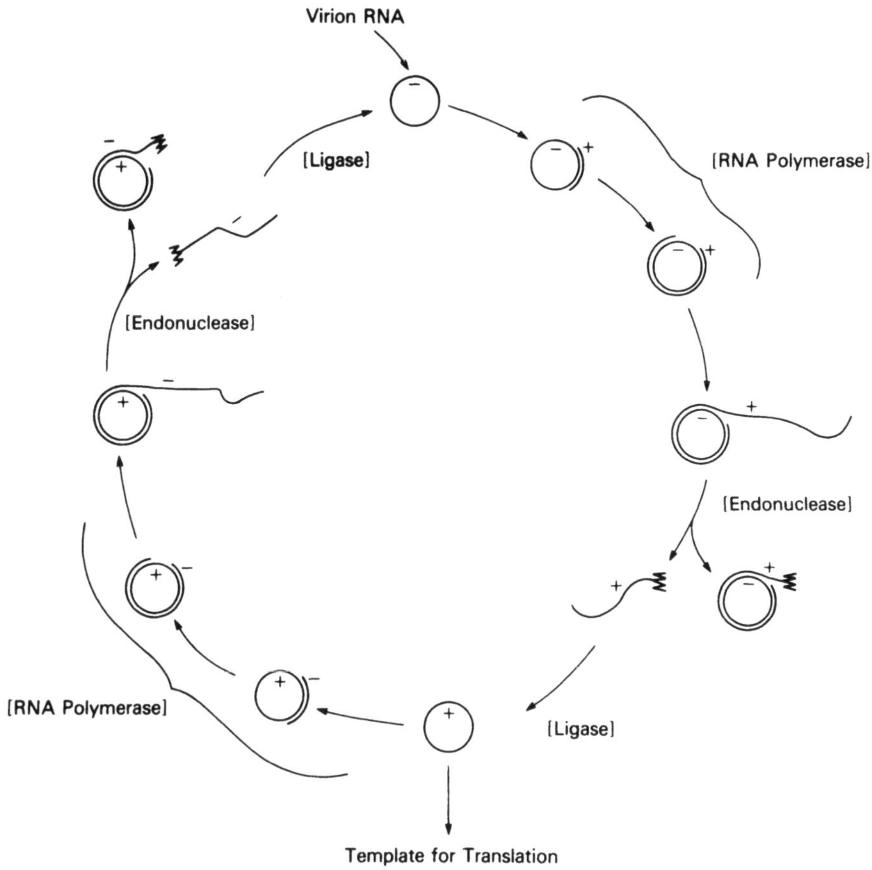

Figure 2. The proposed replicative cycle of the hepatitis delta virus: the double rolling circle.

Table I. Comparison of Hepatitis Delta Virus and Plant Satellite Viruses[a]

Feature	Delta hepatitis	Satellite viruses
Replication	Defective ?Rolling circle	Defective Rolling circle
Genome	RNA	RNA
Polarity	Negative	Negative
Size	1.7 kb	0.9–1.7 kb
Helper virus	HBV, WHBV, DHBV	Plant viruses
Effect on helper virus	Inhibits and changes virulence of HBV	Inhibits and changes virulence of helper virus

[a]From Rizzetto[2] and Bonino et al.[13]

Table II. Nomenclature

Hepatitis delta virus (HDV)
Hepatitis delta virus antigen (HDV Ag)
Antibody to HDV (anti-HDV)
Type D hepatitis: delta hepatitis

function of another virus. This helper function is often to provide an envelope protein. Furthermore, satellite viruses often inhibit the replication of the helper virus and change its pathogenicity. Thus, the satellite virus of the tomato black ring virus changes this benign infection of tomatoes into a virulent fatal illness. A similar effect on viral replication and pathogenicity is often seen when HDV infects a human HBsAg carrier.[1–3]

The HDV is suitably well characterized to warrant an official nomenclature. The terms used in this chapter for the antigens and antibodies and their abbreviations are given in Table II.

3. EXPERIMENTAL HEPATITIS DELTA VIRUS INFECTION

Acute and chronic delta hepatitis have been transmitted to several animal species. Chimpanzees, which are susceptible to human HBV infection, can also be infected with HDV.[16] Chimpanzees without immunity to hepatitis B have developed acute type B and delta hepatitis simultaneously (co-infection) upon inoculation with infectious serum. Chronic HBsAg carrier chimpanzees have invariably developed an acute, superimposed delta hepatitis (superinfection) following inoculation. Chimpanzees that are negative for HBsAg and that have antibody (anti-HBs) have resisted infection with delta hepatitis. Most chimpanzees, even the chronic HBsAg carriers, infected with HDV have had acute delta hepatitis and recovered without developing chronic infection. Most of these chimpanzees have been young and have had high levels of HBV replication with HBeAg in serum. Interestingly, the sole chimpanzee in which chronic delta hepatitis developed was an animal with low levels of HBV replication and antibody to HBeAg (anti-HBe) in serum.[17] These data suggest that risk factors for the development of chronic delta hepatitis are the chronic HBsAg carrier state with low levels of HBV replication (anti-HBe rather than HBeAg in serum). Preliminary findings in humans support these conclusions.

Delta hepatitis has now been transmitted to the Eastern American woodchuck (*Marmona Monax*) infected with the woodchuck hepatitis virus (WHV).[18] WHV is a hepadnavirus-like HBV that shares many similarities with the human virus. The animals could be infected with HDV using inocula from human and chimpanzee HDV carriers.[18] The woodchucks developed acute hepatitis along with HDV RNA and antigen in serum and liver. The HDV that appeared in serum was encapsidated with the surface antigen of the woodchuck virus (WHsAg) rather than the HBsAg from chimpanzees or humans. Thus, the HDV captured the surface antigen of the helper virus present in the liver, even though it infected that liver with the surface antigen of another helper virus. Woodchuck-associated HDV has recently been transmitted back to chimpanzees. As might be expected, the HDV then recaptured HBsAg from the helper virus of the infected chimpanzee. HDV has also recently been transmitted to another species that harbors an HBV-like hepadnavirus—the Pekin duck.[19]

Hepadnavirus-infected animals may provide an important role in defining the biology, immunology, pathogenesis, and course of HDV infection. Recent studies in chronic HBsAg carrier chimpanzees have suggested that immunity to HDV infection may not be absolute. Most HBsAg carrier chimpanzees that were inoculated developed acute superinfection without developing chronic delta hepatitis. Purcell et al.[20] recently rechallenged several of these chimpanzees, 4–5 years after the initial infection. Three of four animals inoculated redeveloped biochemical and histologic evidence of hepatitis. However, delta antigen was not detected in liver or serum, although acute-phase sera were infectious, transmitting delta hepatitis to susceptible animals. Whether human chronic HBsAg carriers also do not develop solid immunity to HDV infection remains to be shown.

4. ACUTE DELTA HEPATITIS

Acute delta hepatitis occurs in two forms: co-infection and superinfection (Table III). Co-infection signifies the simultaneous occurrence of acute hepatitis B and acute delta infection. Superinfection signifies the appearance of acute HDV infection in a chronic HBV carrier. Both forms of acute delta hepatitis tend to be severe; they cannot be distinguished from each other by clinical or serum biochemical findings alone. However, the outcomes of both and their serologic markers are quite different.

Acute delta co-infection is usually self-limited; it rarely leads to chronic hepatitis. Obviously, a patient with acute co-infection of HBV and HDV who recovers from the acute hepatitis B and clears HBsAg will also recover from the acute delta hepatitis and clear HDV from the liver. In prospectively following a large cohort of parenteral drug abusers from Milan, Italy, Caredda et al.[21] found that only 2.4% of 208 cases of acute delta co-infection developed chronic delta hepatitis; the remainder cleared both HBsAg and HDV.

By contrast, acute delta superinfection often leads to chronic hepatitis. In a patient who has a previous chronic HBsAg carrier state or chronic hepatitis B, delta superinfection will often result in persistence of HDV. In the prospective study conducted by Caredda et al., 33 patients who were chronic HBsAg carriers developed acute delta superinfection, and 30 of these (91%) developed chronic delta hepatitis. Thus, most cases of chronic delta hepatitis probably arise from acute delta superinfection.

The clinical course and severity of acute delta hepatitis has been documented in several studies of patients with acute HBsAg-positive hepatitis. In studies from Milan, cases of acute delta co-infection and superinfection were compared with cases of acute uncomplicated hepatitis B.[21] The two diseases did not differ in average height of serum aminotransferase activities, bilirubin, or prothrombin time, but delta infection was typically a more severe disease than acute type B hepatitis, as assessed by average time of stays in hospital, frequency of prolonged illness, and frequency of markedly elevated prothrombin time. The mortality rate of acute delta hepatitis was approximately 5% compared with that of acute type B hepatitis, which was approximately 1%. These findings agreed with data from De Cock et al.[22] from Los Angeles, who reported the

Table III. Two Forms of Acute Delta Hepatitis

Characteristic	Co-infection	Superinfection
HBV infection	Acute	Chronic
HDV infection	Acute	Acute to chronic
Mortality rate	1–2%	1–5%
Chronicity rate	1–3%	>75%
HBsAg in serum	+, transient	+, usually persists
IgM anti-HBc	+	–
Anti-HDV	±, transient low titer	+, usually persists, rising titers
IgM anti-HDV	+, transient	+, usually persists
HDV RNA in serum	+, transient	+, usually persists
HBV Ag in liver	+, transient	+, usually persists

mortality rate of their delta cases to be 4.7%. Thus, acute delta hepatitis is, on average, a more severe illness than acute hepatitis B.

Acute delta hepatitis often has a biphasic course. In the series from Milan, 32% of patients with acute delta co-infection had two distinct peaks in serum aminotransferase activity and bilirubin levels.[21] This biphasic course occurred in only 16% of cases of acute hepatitis B. The first peak in activity was usually due to hepatitis B, the second peak to delta. A similar frequency of biphasic illness (23%) has also been reported by De Cock et al. from Los Angeles.[22]

5. CHRONIC DELTA HEPATITIS

Approximately 2% of cases of acute delta co-infection and more than 90% of cases of acute delta superinfection result in chronic HDV infection and residual chronic liver disease.[21] Chronic delta hepatitis is an important form of chronic liver disease and accounts for a large proportion of cases of HBsAg-positive cirrhosis.[3] Like acute delta hepatitis, chronic delta hepatitis tends to be more severe than uncomplicated type B hepatitis. The early course and natural history of chronic delta hepatitis have been described.[2,3,23–28] The long-term consequences of this disease are now being defined in several ongoing studies of chronic delta hepatitis.

Bonino et al.[23] from Turin, Italy, analyzed the long-term natural history of chronic delta hepatitis among 176 cases followed in their institution since 1972. In this series, men outnumber women 2.6 : 1, and the average age at onset of disease was 39 years; patients were followed for 6–16 (mean: 12) years. The initial liver biopsies revealed cirrhosis in 42%, chronic active hepatitis in 30%, chronic persistent hepatitis in 14%, and other diagnoses in 14%. Patients with cirrhosis tended to be older and to have had the disease for longer than those with chronic active or persistent hepatitis. Nevertheless, chronic delta hepatitis was the most common cause for juvenile cirrhosis in their hospital and clinic population. The ultimate course of the patients disease was rated as either severe (15%), moderate (65%), or mild (15%). Patients with severe disease developed cirrhosis within 1–2 years of onset of disease, and the mortality rate was high. In patients with moderate disease, the course was more protracted; patients developed cirrhosis gradually, and deaths occurred after one to two decades of disease activity. A final group was rated as mild, and the chronic delta hepatitis either went into remission or remained subclinical and mild.

The poor prognosis of chronic delta hepatitis has been well substantiated.[24–28] It is estimated that 60–70% of patients with chronic delta hepatitis ultimately develop cirrhosis,[3] in contrast to only 15–25% of patients with chronic hepatitis B or non-A, non-B hepatitis. The mortality rate of chronic delta hepatitis is also high.[22] Causes of death in chronic delta hepatitis have been similar to those in chronic type B hepatitis: variceal bleeding (35%), liver failure (25%), and primary hepatocellular carcinoma (35%), in the series by Bonino et al.[23]

6. SEROLOGIC DIAGNOSIS OF DELTA HEPATITIS

Acute co-infection and superinfection also differ in the pattern of development of serologic markers and the ease with which they can be diagnosed. The pattern of development of serologic markers during acute HDV infection were carefully analyzed by Aragona and Farci from Cagliari, Turin, and Milan, Italy, using serial serum samples collected from prospectively followed patients with acute delta hepatitis.[29,30] The diagnosis of acute delta hepatitis usually rests on the finding of either HDV antigen or antibody (anti-HDV) in the serum of a patient with acute HBsAg-positive hepatitis, but none of several serologic tests was found to be entirely satisfactory in making the diagnosis.

Acute delta co-infection is particularly difficult to diagnose correctly (Fig. 3). Conventional radioimmunoassays and enzyme-linked immunsorbent assays (ELISA) are not particularly sensitive

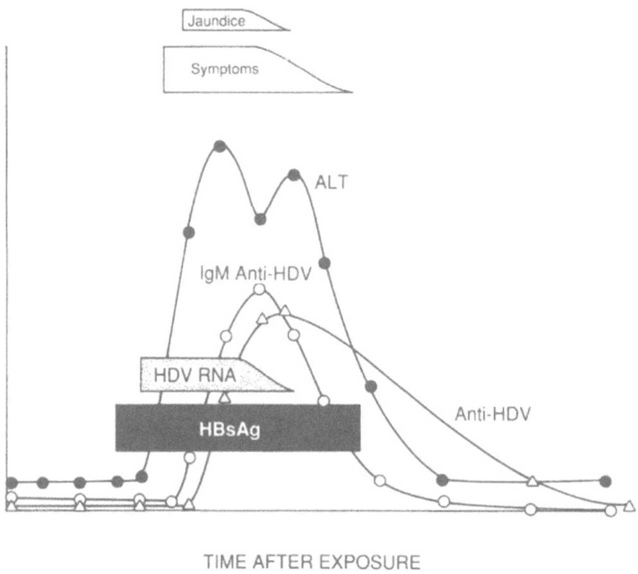

Figure 3. A typical serologic course of acute delta co-infection based on data presented in refs. 29–31.

in detecting HDV antigen during the course of acute or chronic delta infection, being found in only a small proportion of cases of acute infection. In the studies conducted in Italy, only one third of patients with acute delta co-infection had detectable HDV antigen in the serum at the onset of illness; when present, it was invariably short-lived (persisting for less than 1 week).[29,30] In addition, while most patients with acute co-infection developed anti-HDV, they usually did not have the antibody detectable at the onset of disease. Anti-HDV took up to 6–8 weeks to develop and persisted for only a few weeks.

Tests for IgM anti-HDV were better than tests for anti-HDV alone in detecting serologic evidence of HDV infection. However, the IgM antibody was also often late-appearing, short-lived, and transient. Farci et al.[30] have rightly stressed that adequate assessment for delta hepatitis requires testing of multiple samples, preferably for HDV antigen, anti-HDV, and IgM anti-HDV during the acute and convalescent phase of illness.[30] Unfortunately, the only commercially available assay in the United States is a blocking RIA (Delta Test: Abbott Laboratories, North Chicago, Illinois), whose sensitivity in detecting cases of acute delta coinfection is as yet unreported.

Acute delta superinfection is a simpler disease to diagnose correctly than delta coinfection (Fig. 4). In the series of cases studied from Italy, only a small proportion of patients had HDV antigen detectable in serum, but all developed both IgM anti-HDV and anti-HDV, and titers of these antibodies often rose rapidly to high levels.[29] However, not all patients had detectable levels of these antibodies at the onset of symptoms, stressing again the importance of testing acute and convalescent serum samples for anti-HDV for adequate assessment of delta infection. Co-infection can be separated from superinfection by testing for IgM anti-HBc, the serologic marker of acute type B hepatitis (Table IV). Patients with HBsAg, IgM anti-HBc and serologic evidence of HDV infection have acute delta co-infection, and those who lack IgM anti-HBc should be suspected of have acute delta superinfection and have serial samples tested for anti-HDV.

The diagnosis of chronic delta hepatitis usually rests on the finding of delta antigen in liver. Serum testing is preferable, but conventional serum tests are only partially accurate in diagnosis of chronic HDV infection. Patients with chronic delta hepatitis do not have HDV antigen detectable in serum by immunoassays but invariably have high titers of anti-HDV. The finding of anti-HDV at a

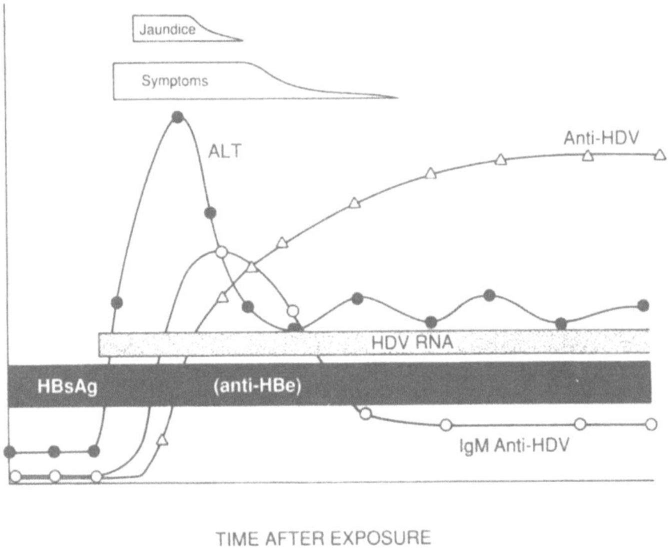

Figure 4. A typical serologic course of acute delta superinfection followed by chronic delta hepatitis based on data presented in refs. 29–31.

titer of greater than 1 : 100 by RIA in an HBsAg carrier is suggestive of chronic delta hepatitis. In establishing the diagnosis of chronic and ongoing HDV infection without resorting to liver biopsy, three new research serum assays are promising: immunoassay for IgM anti-HDV, Northern blotting for HDV RNA, and Western blotting for HDV antigen.

Immunoglobin M (IgM) anti-HDV almost invariably appears in serum within a few weeks of onset of acute delta (either co-infection or superinfection).[29,30,32] If HDV persists, IgM anti-HDV persists. Therefore, the finding of IgM anti-HDV in a chronic HBsAg carrier strongly supports the diagnosis of chronic delta hepatitis. The pattern of persistence of IgM anti-HDV resembles that of IgM anti-HBc in that IgM anti-HBc appears in high titer during acute hepatitis B and disappears soon after recovery but persists in patients who develop chronic hepatitis B.[33] These features can help in evaluating patients with chronic HBsAg-positive hepatitis who have anti-HDV in serum. Is

Table IV. Serologic Diagnosis of Hepatits Delta Virus Infections

Diagnosis	Suggested by	Confirmed by
Acute co-infection	HBsAg +, and IgM anti-HBc +, and anti-HDV +[a]	IgM anti-HDV +[a]
Acute superinfection	HBsAg +, and IgM anti-HBc −, and anti-HDV +[a]	IgM anti-HDV +[a]
Chronic	HBsAg + (6 months), and IgM anti-HBc −, and anti-HDV + (titer >1 : 100 or IgM anti-HDV >6 months)	HDV Ag in liver, or HDV Ag in serum, or HDV RNA in serum

[a]A minimum of one acute and convalescent sera should be assayed for anti-HDV, as this antibody can be transient, low titered, and late in arising during the acute illness.

the disease activity due to HBV, or to HDV replication? The presence of IgM anti-HBc would indicate that hepatitis B is the cause of the disease activity. The presence of IgM anti-HDV would indicate that delta hepatitis is the cause.

Smedile and co-workers recently summarized data on the testing of serum of patients with acute and chronic delta hepatitis for HDV RNA.[34,35] Delta RNA can be detected by molecular hybridization (northern blotting) using a complementary DNA (cDNA) probe in the serum of most patients with acute and chronic delta hepatitis. Indeed, the finding of HDV RNA in serum proves that HDV replication is occurring, making this assay a valuable noninvasive method of assessing viral replication in studies on the natural history and treatment of delta hepatitis. Although HDV RNA testing may be the most specific, it is not the most sensitive assay for HDV infection. Delta antigen can be detected in liver in some patients with HBsAg and anti-HDV in serum but with no detectable HDV RNA. This is particularly true in patients with cirrhosis or advanced forms of chronic delta hepatitis. The absence of detectable HDV RNA is probably due to lack of sensitivity of northern blotting techniques.

Smedile et al.[36] attempted to increase the sensitivity of HDV RNA assays by using different (larger) cDNA probes and by employing the riboprobe method, which uses RNA rather than cDNA as a probe in the hybridization reaction. Preliminary results indicate that the riboprobe technique increases the sensitivity of detecting HDV RNA in serum by 10- to 100-fold. Thus, assays for delta RNA that are of equivalent sensitivity to assays for HBV DNA may soon become available.

Another assay of great promise in assessing HDV infection is immunoblotting techniques for the detection of delta antigen in serum.[11] Subjecting serum and liver homogenates from patients with acute and chronic delta hepatitis to gel electrophoresis and staining of the gels using human anti-HDV has indicated two distinct polypeptides of delta antigen. Preliminary results indicate that this means of assaying delta antigen is far more sensitive than RIA for HDV antigen in detecting ongoing HDV infection. At least 50% of patients with chronic delta hepatitis and HDV antigen in liver have HDV antigen detectable in serum by these Western blot techniques. Improvements and applications of this technique may provide important help in diagnosis of delta hepatitis and in assessing the natural history of this infection.

Thus, the newly developed assays for detection of HDV RNA and antigen in serum may provide the needed specificity and sensitivity lacking in current serologic assays to make the diagnosis of delta hepatitis reliable and easy (Table IV).

7. IMMUNOLOGY OF HEPATITIS DELTA VIRUS INFECTION

Hepatitis B virus can exist and replicate in the liver with minimal or no injury to the liver cells. For this reason, HBV is believed to be a noncytopathic virus, and the injury in hepatitis B is thought to be immunologically mediated. In this regard, HDV may be quite different from HBV. Chronic delta hepatitis tends to progress regardless of immunologic status. The severity of delta hepatitis in children, in renal dialysis patients, and in patients on immunosuppressive agents suggests that the immune system is less important in delta than in hepatitis B in determining the course and outcome of disease.[2,3,37] Histologic studies have indicated a close association between active HDV replication and liver injury[5]; the nature of the liver cell injury with a marked eosinophilic necrosis and relatively mild lymphocytic inflammation further supports the cytopathic qualities of HDV infection.

However, the claim that delta is a cytopathic virus may be an oversimplification. Instances of mild changes in the liver with readily detectable delta antigen have been reported by Hadziyannis et al.[38] from Greece. Furthermore, electron and immune electron microscopic studies reported by Kojimo et al.[39] from Leuven, Belgium, indicate that cells containing HDV antigen are frequently otherwise normal histologically. The HDV antigen is usually detected in hepatocyte nuclei, in a spotty localization sparing nucleoli. HDV antigen can also be detected on ribosomes, either free or membrane bound.

The possible role of the immune system in delta hepatitis was most recently invoked by the finding of autoantibodies in patients with HDV infection. Several autoantibodies have been described in patients with chronic delta hepatitis, including liver–kidney microsomal antibody (anti-LKM)[40,41] and basal cell membrane antibody (anti-BCL).[42] In a series of patients with chronic delta hepatitis studied by Pisi et al.[43] from Rome, 13% had anti-LKM and 49% had anti-BCL, rates far higher than those found in patients with chronic hepatitis B (4% and 5%, respectively). The anti-BCL activity has been intensively analyzed by Magnius et al.[44] from Malmo, Sweden. These workers found that anti-BCL also reacts with thymic epithelial cells that express the BCL antigen in a stellate epithelial cell on dendritic processes. Testing of serial samples from patients who developed delta hepatitis indicated that anti-BCL appeared at the same time that anti-HDV arose. The significance of this autoantibody in defining the pathogenesis and course of delta hepatitis awaits further analyses.

8. EPIDEMIOLOGY OF HEPATITIS DELTA VIRUS INFECTIONS

The epidemiology of delta hepatitis is every bit as complex as its biology and natural history. Since HDV infection is linked to HBV infection, its epidemiology is also linked to the epidemiology of hepatitis B. Maps of the world showing the frequency of delta hepatitis are far more difficult to design than those for hepatitis B.[45] Delta hepatitis generally occurs in three epidemiologic patterns: as an endemic disease occurring in a large proportion of chronic HBsAg carriers, as an epidemic disease striking isolated communities of HBsAg carriers, and as a disease that occurs only in certain high-risk populations (Table V).

Delta hepatitis is endemic in certain populations of the world. Large-scale screening of populations and then testing of HBsAg carriers for anti-HDV has shown that this infection is common in the Mediterranean area and the Middle East,[45,46] the highest prevalence being reported from Kuwait and Saudi Arabia (where 20–40% of carriers have anti-HDV). Lower rates of prevalence are found in Southern Italy and Northern Africa. Delta is rare in Northern Europe and the United States and in most of South and Central America. Interestingly, delta infection is also uncommon in HBsAg carriers in Southeast Asia and China, where the prevalence of the HBsAg carrier rate is the highest.[47,48] This distribution of delta hepatitis infections remains unexplained.

Delta hepatitis also occurs as epidemics in certain populations, usually isolated populations in underdeveloped areas of the world. The most well-defined outbreaks have occurred in Northern South America and the Amazon Basin.[4,5,49,50] Recently similar outbreaks have been described in Central Asia and Africa.[51] How HDV becomes introduced into these populations is unknown. Indeed, delta hepatitis has probably been common in Northern South America for several decades,

Table V. Epidemiology of Hepatitis Delta Virus Infection

Pattern	Description	Geographic areas
Endemic	High rate of HDV among HBsAg carriers in general population	Middle East (Kuwait, Saudi Arabia, Egypt) Mediterranean countries (Italy, Greece)
Epidemic	Outbreaks of severe hepatitis in isolated populations	Venezuela, Columbia, Brazil, Peru, Central Africa
Sporadic	Most cases occur sporadically or as outbreaks in certain high-risk populations (drug addicts, hemophiliacs)	United States, Western Europe, Asia

in that the disease known in these areas as Labrea fever, or black fever, or hepatitis of the Sierra Madre de Santa Marta is probably acute delta superinfection.[5] This has been suggested by serologic and immunopathologic studies on cases from these areas that demonstrate delta antigen in most liver-biopsy samples and anti-HDV in a high percentage of serum samples from these outbreaks. The disease in these outbreaks tends to be severe with sudden onset of fulminant hepatitis and rapid course. In addition, the disease occurs most frequently in children, and the mortality rate (10–20%) is far higher than in typical outbreaks of acute hepatitis A or B. Popper and co-workers[5] recently stressed the characteristic histologic features of this form of fulminant delta hepatitis, which are almost diagnostic for this disease. There is a prominent microvesicular (small-droplet) fat and an intense eosinophilic degeneration that is distinctly unlike the findings in other forms of fulminant hepatitis, such as yellow fever or hepatitis B. The cause of this unusual presentation and course of delta hepatitis in these populations is unknown.

In Northern Europe and the United States, delta hepatitis is an uncommon disease, occurring largely in certain high-risk groups, such as intravenous (IV) drug addicts, patients receiving multiple transfusions, and patients with hemophilia. Indeed, this pattern is typical for most of the world, including Central and South America as well as Asia.[52,53] Thus, in most of the world, delta hepatitis is a rare disease among HBsAg carriers, with the exception of certain subgroups of patients, especially those with severe hepatitis, IV drug abusers, and hemophiliacs. Why this disease is common in these groups and is rare in other high-risk persons (medical care workers, male homosexuals) is not clear.

The epidemiology of delta hepatitis is closely linked to that of hepatitis B but has peculiarities that make it one of the most intriguing viral infections known. Indeed, recent reports suggest that delta hepatitis usually occurs in outbreaks, and instances in which it appears to be endemic often represent the manifestation of an indolent and prolonged outbreak. Thus, the high rate of delta hepatitis among drug addicts in Sweden was shown to be due to a prolonged outbreak of this disease among the HBsAg carrier addicts that began during the middle-1970s; before 1975, delta hepatitis was not present in the Swedish drug addict population.[54] Similar outbreaks among drug addicts and institutionalized persons have been reported from several other areas of the world.[2,45] Recently, an outbreak of severe hepatitis among drug addicts and their contacts was carefully studied and reported from Worcester, Massachusetts.[55] Popper referred to delta hepatitis as a migrating disease, a term that captures the peculiar spread of this disease as outbreaks in defined populations.

The means by which HDV is transmitted are only partially known. This virus is obviously spread by the parenteral route. In outbreaks, the role of contaminated needles, scarification, biting insects, and skin disorders is often discussed. Sexual spread of delta hepatitis must also occur. Cases have been transmitted by parenteral drug abusers to their sexual contacts.[55] Furthermore, intrafamilial spread from HDV-positive carriers to other family members who are carriers was conclusively shown in studies by Rocca et al.[56] from Italy in which an excess of cases of delta hepatitis occurred in sexual partners of HDV carriers. Other means of spread are less well defined. Vertical transmission is extremely rare.[57]

9. PREVENTION OF DELTA HEPATITIS

Delta hepatitis is inexorably linked to type B hepatitis; therefore, prevention of delta hepatitis should begin with attempts at preventing hepatitis B. Patients immune to hepatitis B, who have anti-HBs either as a result of previous infection or HBV vaccination, should be considered immune to delta hepatitis. Patients susceptible to hepatitis B who are seronegative for anti-HBs and anti-HBc should be considered susceptible to delta hepatitis as well. The severity of delta hepatitis provides a further impetus for immunization with HBV vaccine. Thus, in areas of the world in which delta hepatitis is common, such as northern South America, where severe epidemics of fulminant delta hepatitis occur, HBV vaccination should be recommended for all newborns or infants.[5] In areas of the world where delta hepatitis is not endemic but occurs only in high-risk groups (e.g., the United States and Western Europe), routine HBV vaccination should be recommended for patients in these high-risk groups, such as parenteral drug abusers and patients with hemophilia.

Actually, patients who are most in need of preventive measures against delta hepatitis are not persons who are susceptible to hepatitis B but rather those who are HBsAg carriers. Unfortunately, there are no known means of preventing HDV superinfection other than avoidance of contact. Patients who are chronic HBsAg carriers should be warned of the dangers of HDV superinfection and advised against further exposure, in the form of either continued drug abuse or even continued promiscuity.

Passive immunization has been shown to be effective in preventing both hepatitis A and B. There have been no studies of passive immunization against delta hepatitis. Commercial preparations of immune serum globulin (ISG) often have detectable levels of anti-HDV.[58] Yet it is unlikely that this anti-HDV will prevent delta hepatitis. Anti-HDV is directed against an internal antigen of the virus and therefore, like anti-HBc, is unlikely to neutralize infectious virus particles. Furthermore, titers of anti-HDV in ISG, similar to titers of anti-HBc, have been falling in recent years. The highest levels of anti-HDV are found in preparations of ISG made before 1972, when routine screening of plasma for HBsAg was introduced. Obviously, the highest titers of anti-HDV are found in chronic HBsAg-positive delta carriers. Thus, ISG made from donors who are screened for HBsAg should have only low levels or be devoid of anti-HDV. Furthermore, the presence of high titers of anti-HDV in plasma products such as ISG should be considered evidence of contamination of the donor plasma pools with units of plasma that are infectious for delta hepatitis.

10. TREATMENT OF DELTA HEPATITIS

There is no established therapy for acute or chronic delta hepatitis. Retrospective studies have suggested that corticosteroids are not effective in ameliorating the course and preventing the progression of this disease.[3,59] Recent studies have focused on the possible use of antiviral agents in chronic delta hepatitis.

Three groups of investigators have used α-interferon (IFNα) in chronic delta hepatitis. Preliminary results indicated that IFNα inhibited HDV replication and that a prolonged course of therapy could improve the associated liver injury. Hoofnagle et al.[60] treated six patients with chronic delta hepatitis and achieved remissions in disease in one half. In each instance, improvement in the liver disease was accompanied by a disappearance of HDV RNA and Ag from the serum and loss of HDV Ag from the liver. Unfortunately, 1–6 months after IFNα was discontinued, HDV RNA and Ag reappeared in the serum, and the liver disease relapsed with a return of serum aminotransferase elevations and worsening of liver biopsy histology (Fig. 5).

Similar pilot studies using lymphoblastoid IFNα have been reported from England.[61] Thomas et al. reported treating five patients with chronic delta hepatitis. Serum levels of HDV RNA fell in all patients and became undetectable in three. The serum aminotransferase levels and hepatic histology improved in some but not all treated patients. All patients remained positive for HBsAg and continued to have unchanging titers of IgM anti-HDV. These results supported the findings of other studies that IFNα inhibits but does not regularly eradicate HDV replication.

On the basis of these preliminary findings, Rosina et al.[62] from Turin, Italy, conducted a randomized controlled trial of IFNα in 24 patients with chronic delta hepatitis. Twelve patients received a 12-week course of recombinant human IFNα, and 12 patients served as untreated controls. Serum HDV RNA decreased in most treated patients and became undetectable in eight (67%); serum aminotransferase activities improved in seven patients (58%). Importantly, none of the 12 control patients had appreciable improvements in serum aminotransferase activities, and all remained positive for HDV RNA during the period of evaluation. Unfortunately, all except one of

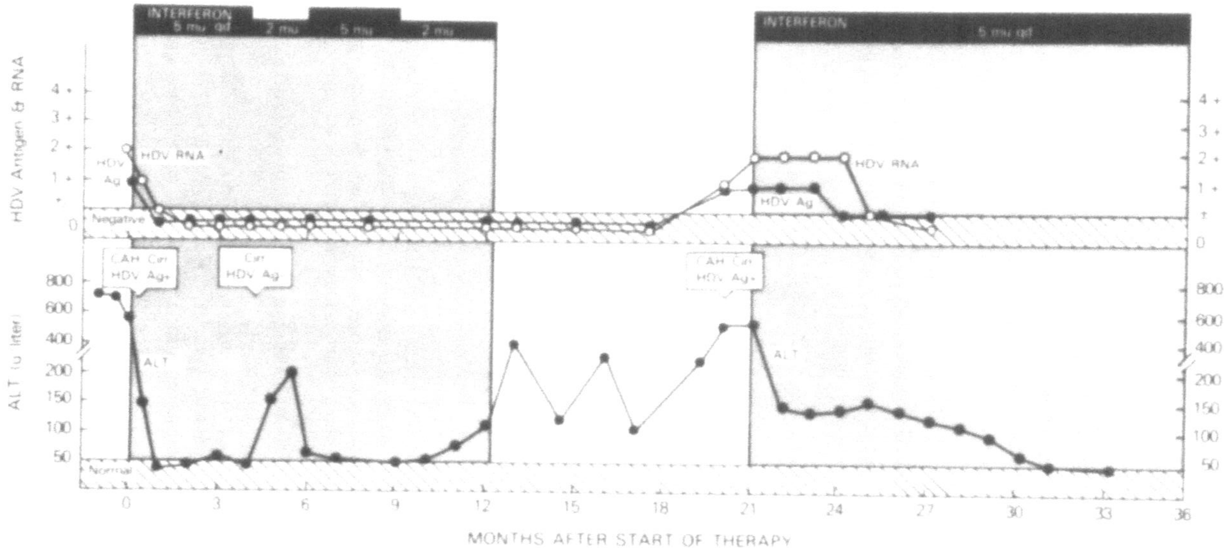

Figure 5. The clinical, serum biochemical, and serologic course of a patient with chronic delta hepatitis who was treated with recombinant human α-interferon (α-IFN). Liver biopsy taken before treatment showed an active cirrhosis with HDV Ag in hepatocytes. Liver biopsy taken after 4 months of therapy showed an inactive cirrhosis and no detectable HDV Ag, by immunofluorescence and immunoperoxidase staining. Serum ALT levels improved markedly and serum HDV Ag and RNA disappeared on α-IFN therapy, either 5 or 2 million units (mu) subcutaneously each day for 1 year. However, ALT levels increased when interferon was stopped and six months later HDV Ag and HDV RNA were again detected in serum. Repeat liver biopsy showed an active cirrhosis and HDV Ag in hepatocytes. Reinstitution of IFN therapy was followed by biochemical improvement in the liver disease and disappearance of HDV Ag and RNA from the serum.

the treated patients who demonstrated an improvement on interferon therapy had a relapse of disease when it was discontinued.

These results of small clinical trials have been encouraging. Approximately one half of treated patients have demonstrated unequivocal improvement in serum biochemical test results and liver histology with IFN therapy.' However, these improvements have not been sustained, even with therapy for 1 year. These findings suggest that therapy of chronic delta hepatitis will probably require long-term, and possibly permanent, therapy.

While antiviral therapy holds promise for many patients with chronic delta hepatitis, it has little hope of efficacy in patients with advanced disease and decompensated cirrhosis. Patients with cirrhosis do not tolerate IFNα well and are susceptible to the development of severe fatigue, diarrhea, and bacterial infectious complications when treated with IFN or immunosuppressive agents.[60] In patients with advanced and life-threatening disease, hepatic transplantation is the most worthwhile option. Results of liver transplantation for chronic delta hepatitis have been good.[63] Indeed, some long-term survivors have remained HBsAg and HDV negative after liver transplantation, suggesting that transplantation for chronic delta hepatitis may have a better prognosis than transplantation for chronic hepatitis B (after which most patients redevelop HBsAg and chronic HBV infection). Liver transplantation may also provide new clues to the interesting biology of HDV and the natural history of this chronic viral infection.

11. CONCLUSIONS

During the 10 years since the delta agent was discovered, major advances have been made into the understanding of its structure, genomic organization, replicative cycle, clinical course and epidemiology. The recent breakthroughs in cloning of the HDV genome and development of animal models for study of this agent promise to transform these advances in knowledge to advances in means of prevention and therapy of this severe form of acute and chronic liver disease.

REFERENCES

1. Rizzetto M, Canese MG, Arico S, et al: Immunofluorescence detection of new antigen-antibody system (δ/anti-δ) associated to hepatitis B virus in liver and serum of HBsAg carriers. *Gut* **18**:997–1003, 1977.
2. Rizzetto M: The delta agent. *Hepatology* **3**:729–737, 1984.
3. Rizzetto M, Verme G, Recchia S, et al: Chronic HBsAg hepatitis with intrahepatic expression of delta antigen. An active and progressive disease unresponsive to immunosuppressive treatment. *Ann Intern Med* **98**:437–441, 1983.
4. Hadler SC, de Monzon M, Ponzetto A, et al: An epidemic of severe hepatitis due to delta virus infection in Yucpa Indians of Venezuela. *Ann Intern Med* **100**:339–349, 1984.
5. Buitrago B, Popper H, Hadler SC, et al: Specific histologic features of Santa Marta hepatitis: A severe form of hepatitis delta-virus infection in northern South America. *Hepatology* **6**:1285–1291, 1986.
6. Rizzetto M, Hoyer B, Canese MG, et al: δ Agent: association of the δ antigen with hepatitis B surface antigen and RNA in serum of δ-infected chimpanzees. *Proc Natl Acad Sci USA* **77**:6124–6128, 1981.
7. Wang K-S, Choo Q-L, Weiner AJ, et al: Structure, sequence and expression of the hepatitis delta (δ) viral genome. *Nature (Lond)* **323**:508–514, 1986.
8. Chen PJ, Kalpana G, Goldberg J, et al.: Structure and replication of the genome of the hepatitis delta virus. *Proc Natl Acad Sci USA* **83**:8774–8778, 1986.
9. Makino S, Chang MF, Shieh CK, et al: Molecular cloning and sequencing of a human hepatitis delta virus RNA. *Nature (Lond)* **329**:343–346, 1987.
10. Branch AD, Robertson HD: A replication cycle for viroids and other small infectious RNAs. *Science* **223**:450–458, 1984.
11. Bergmann KF, Gerin JL: Antigens of hepatitis delta virus in the liver and serum of humans and animals. *J Infect Dis* **514**:702–705, 1986.
12. Pohl C, Baroudy BM, Bergmann KF, et al: A human monoclonal antibody that recognizes viral polypep-

tides and in vitro translation products of the genome of the hepatitis D virus. *J Infect Dis* **156**:622–629, 1987.
13. Bonino F, Heermann KH, Rizzetto M, Gerlich WH: Hepatitis delta virus: Protein composition of delta antigen and its hepatitis B virus-derived envelope. *J Virol* **58**:945–950, 1986.
14. Murant AF, Mayo MA: Satellites of plant viruses. *Annu Rev Phytopathol* **20**:49–70, 1982.
15. Diener TO: Autonomous and helper-dependent small pathogenic RNAs of plants: Viroids and satellites, in Rizzetto M, Gerin JL, Purcell RH (eds): *Hepatitis Delta Virus and Its Infection*. Liss, New York, 1987, pp. 3–18.
16. Rizzetto M, Canese MG, Gerin JL, et al: Transmission of the hepatitis B virus-associated delta antigen to chimpanzees. *J Infect Dis* **141**:590–602, 1980.
17. Fields HA, Govindarajan S, Margolis HS, et al: Experimental transmission of the delta virus to a hepatitis B chronic carrier chimpanzee with the development of persistent delta carriage. *Am J Pathol* **122**:308–314, 1986.
18. Ponzetto A, Cote PJ, Popper H, et al: Transmission of the hepatitis B virus-associated δ agent to the eastern woodchuck. *Proc Natl Acad Sci USA* **81**:2208–2212, 1984.
19. Ponzetto A, Rapicetta M, Forzani B, et al: Hepatitis delta virus infection in Pekin ducks chronically infected by the duck hepatitis B virus in Rizzetto M, Gerin JL, Purcell RH (eds): *Hepatitis Delta Virus and Its Infection*. Liss, New York, 1987, pp. 47–49.
20. Purcell RH, Satterfield WC, Bergmann KF, et al: Experimental hepatitis delta virus infection in the chimpanzee in Rizzetto M, Gerin JL, Purcell RH (eds): *Hepatitis Delta Virus and Its Infection*. Liss, New York, 1987, pp. 27–36.
21. Caredda F, Antinori S, Re T, et al: Course and prognosis of acute HDV hepatitis in Rizzetto M, Gerin JL, Purcell RH (eds): *Hepatitis Delta Virus and Its Infection*. Liss, New York, 1987, pp. 267–276.
22. De Cock KM, Govindarajan S, Chin KP, Redeker AG: Delta hepatitis in the Los Angeles area: A report of 126 cases. *Ann Intern Med* **105**:108–114, 1986.
23. Bonino F, Negro F, Baldi M, et al: The natural history of chronic delta hepatitis in Rizzetto M, Gerin JL, Purcell RH (eds): *Hepatitis Delta Virus and Its Infection*. Liss, New York, 1987, pp. 145–152.
24. Smedile A, Dentico P, Zanetti A, et al: Infection with the delta (δ) agent in chronic HBsAg carriers. *Gastroenterology* **81**:992–997, 1981.
25. Farci P, Smedile A, Lavarini C, et al: Delta hepatitis in inapparent carriers of hepatitis B surface antigen. *Gastroenterology* **85**:669–673, 1983.
26. Colombo M, Cambieri R, Rumi MG, et al: Long-term superinfection in HBsAg carriers and its relationship with the course of chronic hepatitis. *Gastroenterology* **85**:235–239, 1983.
27. Fattovich G, Boscaro S, Noventa F, et al: Influence of hepatitis delta virus infection on progression to cirrhosis in chronic hepatitis, type B. *J Infect Dis* **155**:931–935, 1987.
28. Verme G, Amoroso P, Lettier G, et al: Histological study of hepatitis delta virus liver disease. *Hepatology* **6**:1303–1307, 1986.
29. Aragona M, Macagno S, Caredda F, et al: IgM anti-HD in acute hepatitis D: Diagnostic and prognostic significance, in Rizzetto M, Gerin JL, Purcell RH (eds): *Hepatitis Delta Virus and Its Infection*. Liss, New York, 1987, pp. 243–248.
30. Farci P, Gerin JL, Aragona M, et al: Diagnostic and prognostic significance of the IgM antibody to the hepatitis delta virus. *JAMA* **255**:1443–1446, 1986.
31. Mushahwar IK, Gerin JL, Dienstag JL, et al: Interpretation of hepatitis B virus and hepatitis delta virus serologic profiles. *Pathologist* **38**:648–650, 1984.
32. Buti M, Esteban R, Jardi R, et al: Clinical and serological outcome of acute delta infection. *J Hepatol* **5**:59–64, 1987.
33. Sjogren M, Hoofnagle JH: Immunoglobulin M antibody to the hepatitis B core antigen in patients with chronic type B hepatitis. *Gastroenterology* **89**:252–258, 1985.
34. Denniston KJ, Hoyer BH, Smedile A, et al: Cloned fragment of the hepatitis delta virus RNA genome: Sequence and diagnostic application. *Science* **232**:873–875, 1986.
35. Smedile A, Rizzetto M, Denniston KJ, et al: Type D hepatitis: The clinical significance of hepatitis D virus RNA in serum as detected by a hybridization-based assay. *Hepatology* **6**:1297–1302, 1986.
36. Smedile A, Baroudy BM, Bergmann KF, Rizzetto M, et al: Clinical significance of HDV RNA in HDV disease, in Rizzetto M, Gerin JL, Purcell RH (eds): *Hepatitis Delta Virus and Its Infection*. Liss, New York, 1987, pp. 231–234.
37. Bortolotti F, Calzia R, Cadrobbi P, et al: Liver cirrhosis associated with chronic hepatitis B virus infection in childhood. *J Pediatr* **108**:224–227, 1986.
38. Hadziyannis SJ, Hatzakis A, Papaioannou C, et al: Endemic hepatitis delta virus infection in a Greek

community, in Rizzetto M, Gerin JL, Purcell RH (eds): *Hepatitis Delta Virus and Its Infection*. Liss, New York, 1987, pp. 181–202.
39. Kojimo T, Callea F, Desmyter J, Desmet VJ: Immune electron microscopy of hepatitis delta-antigen in hepatocytes. *Lab Invest* **55**:217–225, 1986.
40. Crivelli O, Lavarini C, Chiaberge E, et al: Microsomal autoantibodies in chronic infection with the HBsAg-associated delta agent. *Clin Exp Immunol* **54**:232–238, 1983.
41. Caredda F, de Bartolo G, Zampini L, et al: Detection and further characterization of a newly described microsomal autoantibody associated with chronic delta infection. *Digestion* **33**:181–188, 1986.
42. Zauli D, Fusconi M, Crespi C, et al: Close association between basal cell layer antibodies and hepatitis B virus-associated chronic delta infection. *Hepatology* **4**:1103–1106, 1984.
43. Pisi E, Zauli D, Crespi C: Autoantibodies in chronic hepatitis delta virus infection, in Rizzetto M, Gerin JL, Purcell RH (eds): *Hepatitis Delta Virus and Its Infection*. Liss, New York, 1987, pp. 249–256.
44. Magnius LO, Lenkei R, Norder H, et al: Autoantibodies to thymic epithelial cells in hepatitis B virus-associated delta infection. *J Infect Dis* **152**:232–236, 1985.
45. Ponzetto A, Forzani B, Parravicini PP, et al: Epidemiology of delta virus (HDV) infection. *Eur J Epidemiol* **1**:257–263, 1985.
46. Nordenfelt E, Hansson BG, Al Nakib B, et al: Frequency of delta agent infections in Kuwait. *J Infect Dis* **143**:768–769, 1984.
47. Chen DS, Lai MY, Sung JL: Delta agent infection in patients with chronic liver disease and hepatocellular carcinoma: An infrequent finding in Taiwan. *Hepatology* **4**:502–503, 1984.
48. Wang DQ, Cheng HH, Minuk GY, et al: Delta hepatitis virus infection in China. *Int J Epidemiol* **16**:79–83, 1987.
49. Buitrago B, Hadler SC, Popper H, et al: Epidemiologic aspects of Santa Marta hepatitis over a 40-year period. *Hepatology* **6**:1292–1296, 1986.
50. Bensabath G, Hadler SC, Soares MC, et al: Hepatitis delta virus infection and Labrea hepatitis: Prevalence and role in fulminant hepatitis in the Amazon Basin. *JAMA* **258**:479–483, 1987.
51. Lesbordes JL, Ravisse P, Georges AJ, et al: Studies on the role of HDV in an outbreak of fulminant hepatitis in Bangui (Central African Republic), in Rizzetto M, Gerin JL, Purcell RH (eds): *Hepatitis Delta Virus and Its Infection*. Liss, New York, 1987, pp. 451–459.
52. Lee SD, Wang JY, Wu JC, et al: Hepatitis B and D virus infection among drug abusers in Taiwan. *J Med Virol* **30**:247–252, 1986.
53. Liaw Y-F, Lin H-H, Chu C-M, et al: Hepatitis delta virus infection in Taiwan, in Rizzetto M, Gerin JL, Purcell RH (eds): *Hepatitis Delta Virus and Its Infection*. Liss, New York, 1987, pp. 479–483.
54. Hansson BG, Moestrup T, Widell A, Nordenfelt E: Infection with delta agent in Sweden: Introduction of a new hepatitis agent. *J Infect Dis* **146**:472–478, 1982.
55. Lattau LA, McCarthy JG, Smith MH, et al: Outbreak of severe hepatitis due to delta and hepatitis B viruses in parenteral drug abusers and their contacts. *N Engl J Med* **317**:1256–1262, 1987.
56. Rocca G, Poli G, Gerardo P, et al: Familial clustering of delta infection, in Verme G, Bonino F, Rizzetto M (eds): *Viral Hepatitis and Delta Infection*. Liss, New York, 1984, pp. 133–137.
57. Zanetti AR, Dentico P, Del Vecchio BC, et al: Multicenter tiral on the efficiacy of HBIG and vaccine in preventing perinatal hepatitis B. Final report. *J Med Virol* **18**:327–334, 1986.
58. Ponzetto A, Hoofnagle JH, Seeff LB: Antibody to the hepatitis B virus-associated delta agent in immune serum globulins. *Gastroenterology* **87**:1213–1216, 1984.
59. Sagnelli E, Manzillo G: Clinical aspects of delta agent infection in southern Italy, in Verme G, Rizzetto M, Bonino F (eds): *Viral Hepatitis and Delta Infection*. Liss, New York, 1984, pp. 195–202.
60. Hoofnagle JH, Mullen K, Peters M, et al: Treatment of chronic delta hepatitis with recombinant human alpha interferon, in Rizzetto M, Gerin JL, Purcell RH (eds): *Hepatitis Delta Virus and Its Infection*. Liss, New York, 1987, pp. 291–298.
61. Thomas HC, Lever AML, Scully LJ, Pignatelli M: Approaches to the treatment of hepatitis B virus and delta-related liver disease. *Semin Liver Disease* **6**:34–41, 1986.
62. Rosina F, Saracco G, Lattore V, et al: Alpha 2 recombinant interferon in the treatment of chronic hepatitis delta virus (HDV) hepatitis, in Rizzetto M, Gerin JL, Purcell RH (eds): *Hepatitis Delta Virus and Its Infection*. Liss, New York, 1987, pp. 299–303.
63. Rizzetto M, Chiaberge E, Negro F, et al: Liver transplantation in hepatitis delta virus disease. *Lancet* **2**:469–471, 1987.

6

Pathology of Acute and Chronic Hepatitis D

Michael A. Gerber

1. INTRODUCTION

Since the discovery of the delta antigen by Rizzetto et al.[1] 10 years ago, the pathology of delta hepatitis has been described in detail. In recent years, several studies recorded significant differences in the clinical course and pathologic findings of hepatitis delta virus (HDV) infection in South America as opposed to those in North America and Europe. This chapter summarizes these interesting observations.

2. FULMINANT DELTA HEPATITIS IN SOUTH AMERICA

An acute, often fatal, form of viral hepatitis is common in children, adolescents, and young adults of the indigent population of northern South America. This fulminant hepatitis, known as black fever or Labrea fever in Brazil and as Santa Marta hepatitis in Northern Columbia, was also observed among the Yucpa Indians in Western Venezuela. Recent epidemiologic and serologic studies indicate that these forms of hepatitis are often due to HDV infection.[2–4] We had the opportunity to study many liver specimens from these South American countries by histologic and immunohistochemical methods and observed characteristic, almost diagnostic pathologic features.[5,6]

During the early stage of the disease, almost all hepatocytes contained many fine fat droplets without displacing the nucleus resulting in the formation of so-called morula cells (Fig. 1). Some hepatocytes showed eosinophilic granulation of the cytoplasm, as well as karyorrhexis and formation of granular eosinophilic bodies. The sinusoidal lining cells were increased, particularly periodic acid-Schiff (PAS)-positive diastase-resistant macrophages. The portal tracts were expanded by a dense infiltrate of mononuclear cells, primarily lymphocytes and macrophages. Immunohistochemical staining demonstrated delta antigen in many hepatocyte nuclei in almost all cases.

Progression of the disease was characterized by more extensive eosinophilic necrosis of hepatocytes without zonal predominance (Fig. 2), limited collapse of the reticulin framework, and

---

Michael A. Gerber • Department of Pathology, Tulane University School of Medicine, New Orleans, Louisiana 70112.

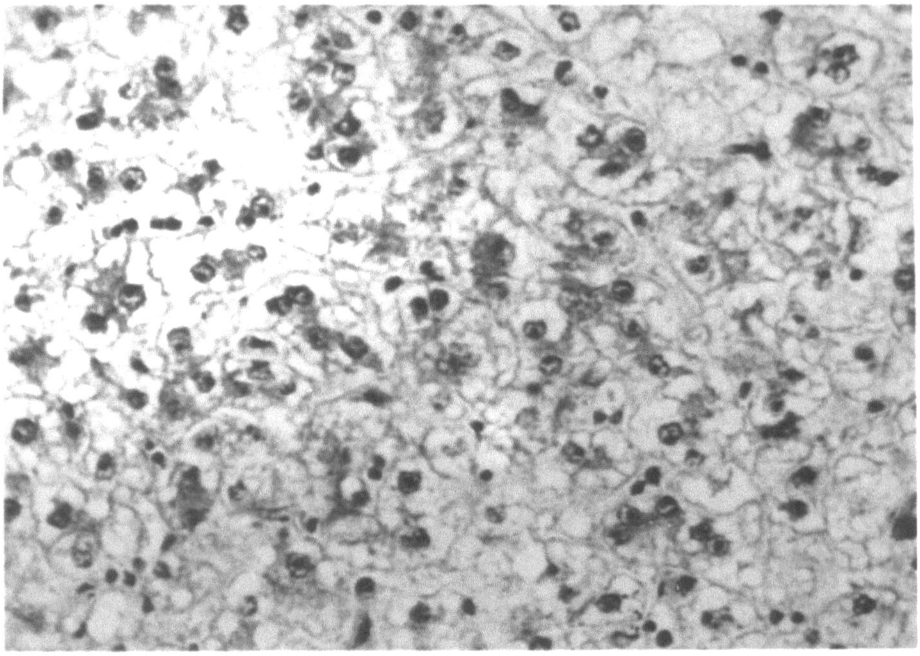

Figure 1. Early stage of fulminant delta hepatitis in a patient from Brazil. There is diffuse hepatocellular damage with numerous fine fat droplets in hepatocytes, but little necrosis and inflammation. (H&E, ×100)

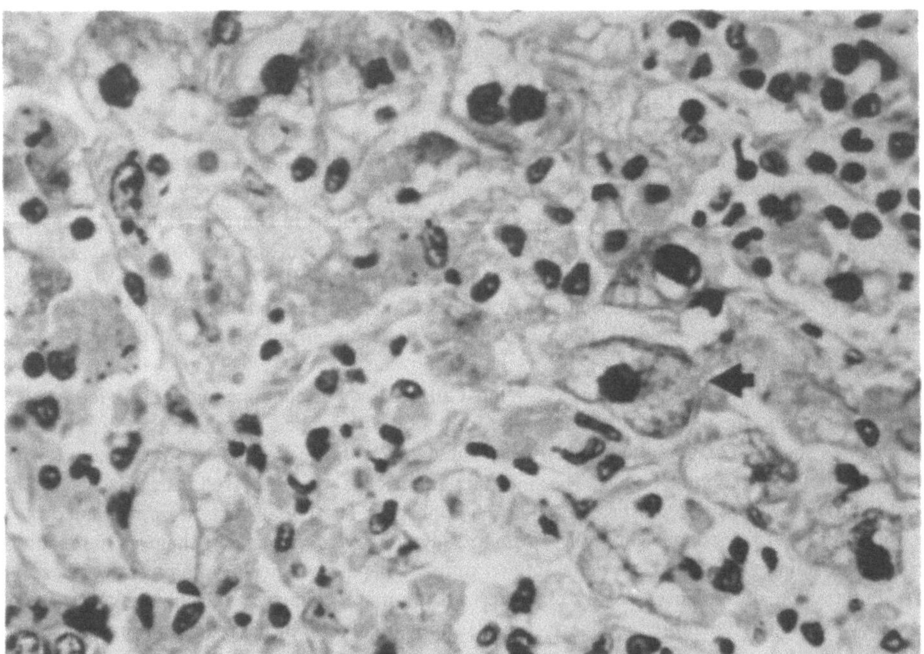

Figure 2. Advanced stage of fulminant delta hepatitis in a patient from Colombia. Many hepatocytes are necrotic and replaced by inflammatory cells, particularly macrophages. A hepatocyte containing many fine fat droplets without displacement of the nucleus, so-called morula cell (arrow), is also seen. (H&E, ×250)

increased infiltration of the lobules by lymphocytes and macrophages. This was accompanied by reduction of detectable delta antigen. In the late stage, regeneration was seen with formation of ductular hepatocytes and arrangement of hepatocytes in two-cell-thick plates. HB surface antigen (HBsAg) and HB core antigen (HBcAg) were detected in only 20% of these cases. Cholestasis was usually absent. Histologically, fulminant delta hepatitis resembled other diseases with microvesicular steatosis, such as acute fatty liver of pregnancy, some forms of drug-induced or toxic hepatitis, Reye syndrome, and yellow fever, but could be distinguished by the pattern and distribution of the granular eosinophilic necrosis.

In these cases, fulminant delta hepatitis was probably caused by HDV superinfection of hepatitis B virus (HBV) carriers rather than by co-infection by HDV and HBV. It is not known, however, why the clinical and histologic manifestations of the disease differ markedly from those usually observed in acute delta hepatitis in North America and Europe. It is also not known whether it can progress to chronic hepatitis and cirrhosis.

3. ACUTE AND CHRONIC DELTA HEPATITIS IN NORTH AMERICA AND EUROPE

3.1. Acute Co-Infection

Acute co-infection by HBV and HDV results in a self-limited acute hepatitis that frequently (about 25% of cases) has a fulminant and fatal course.[7–10] It has been reported that histologically acute delta hepatitis with or without submassive or massive hepatic necrosis cannot be distinguished from acute hepatitis A, hepatitis B, or non-A, non-B.[9] We have observed a case of acute delta hepatitis with unusual histologic features. The hepatocytes showed extensive hydropic swelling and vacuolization of the cytoplasm and granular acidophilic bodies. Only few intrasinusoidal lymphocytes but many PAS-positive diastase-resistant macrophages were identified (Fig. 3). These changes resembled to some degree the early stage of the South American type of delta hepatitis. However, extensive microvesicular steatosis and eosinophilic necrosis was absent from most cases of acute delta hepatitis in the United States and Europe. Delta antigen can often be demonstrated in hepatocyte nuclei but may be absent in fulminant delta hepatitis.[5,6,10]

3.2. Acute Superinfection

Acute HDV superinfection of chronic asymptomatic HBV carriers may present as acute delta hepatitis with focal bridging necrosis indistinguishable from acute hepatitis A, hepatitis B, or non-A, non-B.[9,11] However, the diagnosis could be established by immunohistochemical staining, because delta antigen was demonstrable in hepatocyte nuclei in 68–90% of cases.[11–13] In symptomatic HBV carriers with chronic persistent hepatitis or chronic active hepatitis, HDV superinfection clinically resembled an acute exacerbation[14] characterized by severe prolonged necroinflammatory changes or more extensive necrosis. The number of delta antigen-positive hepatocytes was inversely proportional to the extent of lobular inflammation in one study.[11] This form of delta hepatitis was characterized by rapid progression to severe chronic active hepatitis and cirrhosis in a short time.[12,13,15,16] In two studies, several patients with chronic delta hepatitis developed hepatocellular carcinoma,[10,17] but the frequency of HDV in HBsAg-positive tumors is low.

3.3. Chronic Delta Infection

Chronic hepatitis D may show histologic features of chronic active hepatitis with or without bridging necrosis, chronic lobular hepatitis, or cirrhosis.[10,11,18,19,20] Occasionally, chronic persistent hepatitis was observed.[10] No distinctive histologic features have been described for chronic

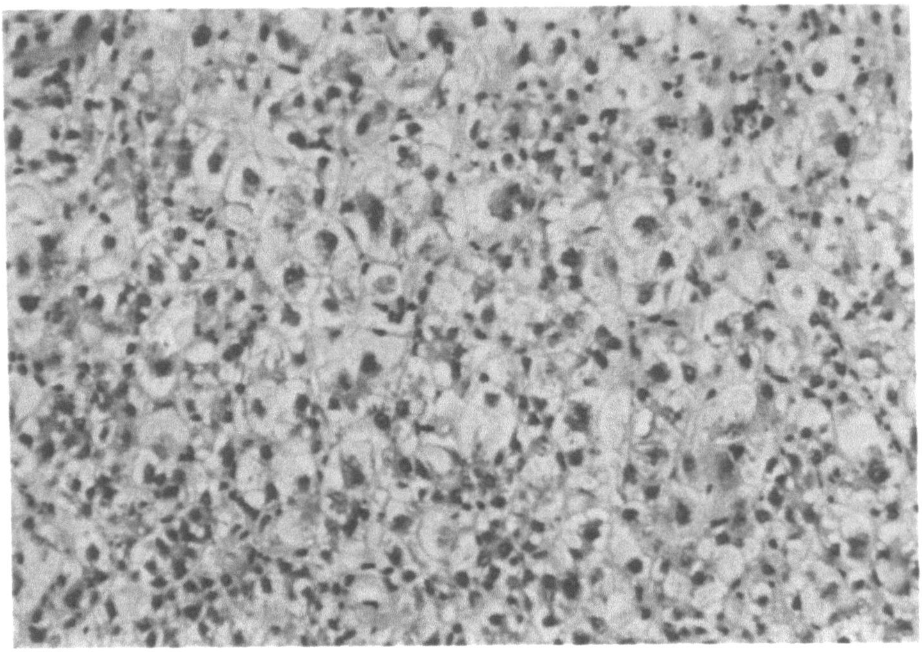

Figure 3. Acute delta hepatitis in a North American patient. The hepatocytes show extensive hydropic swelling and vacuolization of cytoplasm, but relatively few inflammatory cells in sinusoids. (H&E, ×100)

hepatitis D, but often eosinophilic granulation of hepatocyte cytoplasm, conspicuous acidophilic bodies, and a moderate to marked degree of diffuse lobular inflammation were seen[11] (Fig. 4). In most cases, delta antigen was found, usually in the nuclei, sometimes in the cytoplasm of apparently normal hepatocytes, and rarely in degenerated necrotic cells.[11,12,21–25] Several studies demonstrated suppression of HBV replication in hepatitis D with reduced amounts of HBV DNA, HBcAg, and HBsAg[22,23,26,27] in the liver, suggesting that the disease activity in delta antigen-positive HBV carriers was more related to persistent HDV infection than to continued HBV replication.[23]

4. ELECTRON MICROSCOPY

While HDV has been identified electron microscopically as 36-nm spherical particles in the serum of infected patients,[28] it has been difficult to demonstrate characteristic viral particles in infected hepatocytes. Delta antigen-positive nuclei contained 20- to 30-nm indistinct granular structures that bound specific antibody.[29–31] However, similar structures have been described in non-A, non-B hepatitis and were also present in delta antigen-negative nuclei.[31] In addition, cylindrical tubular structures and undulating membranes were found in the cytoplasm of HBV carrier chimpanzees infected with HDV[30,32,33] and showed striking resemblance to those in non-A, non-B hepatitis.

5. CONCLUSIONS

Acute delta hepatitis in the northern regions of South America and possibly in Central Africa is characterized by microvesicular steatosis and granular eosinophilic necrosis of hepatocytes. This

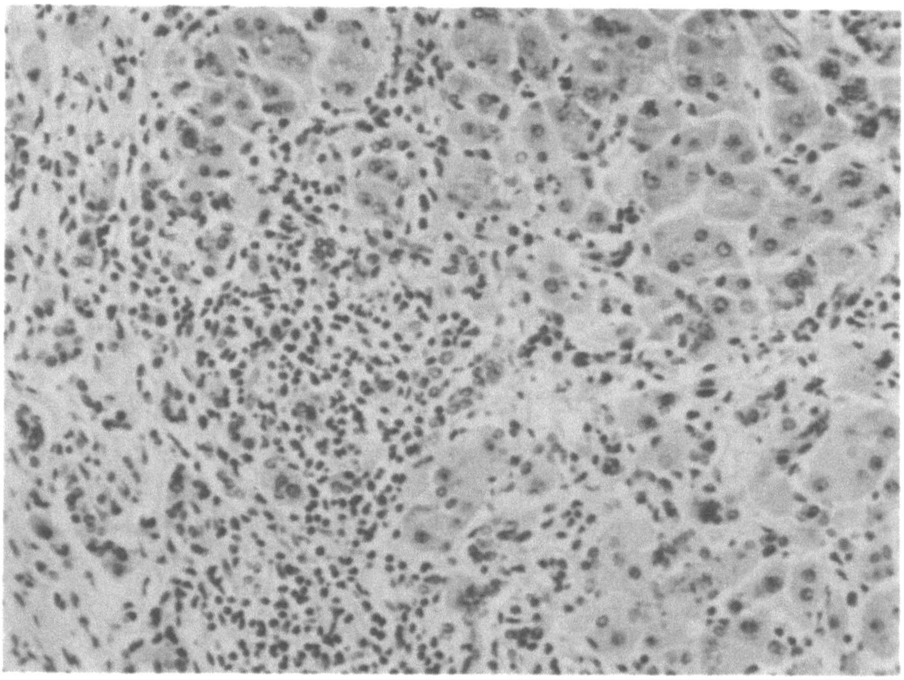

Figure 4. Chronic delta hepatitis in a hemophiliac patient from North America. The liver shows severe chronic active hepatitis with extensive piecemeal necrosis (left) as well as intralobular necrosis and inflammation. Hepatocytes and macrophages also contain iron as a result of many blood transfusions. (H&E, ×100)

histologic appearance is specific and diagnostic of this epidemic, often fatal form of delta hepatitis.[34] In the United States and Europe, acute or chronic delta hepatitis cannot be diagnosed histologically, although severe necroinflammatory changes are often seen. HDV superinfection of chronic HBV carriers usually produces more severe disease and more often chronicity than does coinfection by HDV and HBV.[34] Delta antigen in hepatocytes, as demonstrated by immunohistochemical methods, is a reliable and diagnostically useful marker of hepatitis D[35] because the serologic markers of HDV infection such as immunoglobin M (IgM) anti-HD or HDV RNA[25] are not always available.

In contrast to HBV, HDV is probably directly cytopathic[34] for hepatocytes for the following reasons: (1) the histologic features resemble those seen in cytotoxic liver injuries; (2) hepatocytes in acute delta hepatitis contain large amounts of delta antigen; and (3) conventional immunosuppressive treatment (prednisone or azathioprine) is without benefit,[18] but antiviral agents may be effective.

ACKNOWLEDGMENTS. I am grateful to Ms. Nancy Ruiz for secretarial assistance and to Steve Mortillo for technical assistance.

REFERENCES

1. Rizzetto M, Canese MG, Arico S, et al: Immunofluorescence detection of new antigen–antibody system (δ/anti-δ) associated to hepatitis B virus in liver and in serum of HBsAg carriers. *Gut* **18**:997–1003, 1977.
2. Hadler SC, Demonzon M, Ponzetto A, et al: Delta virus infection and severe hepatitis. An epidemic in the Yupca Indians of Venezuela. *Ann Intern Med.* **100**:339–344, 1984.

3. Ljunggren KE, Patarroyo ME, Engle R, et al: Viral hepatitis in Colombia: A study of the "Hepatitis of the Sierra Nevada de Santa Marta." *Hepatology* **5:**299–304, 1985.
4. Buitrago B, Hadler SC, Popper H, et al: Epidemiologic aspects of Santa Marta hepatitis over a 40-year period. *Hepatology* **6:**1292–1296, 1986.
5. Popper H, Thung SN, Gerber MA, et al: Histologic studies of severe delta agent infection in Venezuelan Indians. *Hepatology* **3:**906–912, 1983.
6. Buitrago B, Popper H, Hadler SC, et al: Specific histologic features of Santa Marta hepatitis: A severe form of hepatitis δ-virus infection in Northern South America. *Hepatology* **6:**1285–1291, 1986.
7. Smedile A, Verme G, Cargnel A, et al: Influence of delta infection on severity of hepatitis B. *Lancet* **2:**945–947, 1982.
8. Govindarajan S, Chin KP, Redeker AG, et al: Fulminant B viral hepatitis: Role of delta agent. *Gastroenterology* **86:**1417–1420, 1984.
9. Govindarajan S, De Cock KM, Peters RL: Morphologic and immunohistochemical features of fulminant delta hepatitis. *Hum Pathol* **16:**262–267, 1985.
10. De Cock KM, Govindarajan S, Chin KP, et al: Delta hepatitis in the Los Angeles area: A report of 126 cases. *Ann Intern Med* **105:**108–114, 1986.
11. Verme G, Amoroso P, Lettieri G, et al: A histological study of hepatitis delta virus liver disease. *Hepatology* **6:**1303–1307, 1986.
12. Govindarajan S, De Cock KM, Redeker AG: Natural Course of delta superinfection in chronic hepatitis B virus-infected patients: Histopathologic study with multiple liver biopsies. *Hepatology* **6:**640–644, 1986.
13. Kanel GC, Govindarajan S, Peters RL: Chronic delta infection and liver biopsy changes in chronic active hepatitis B. *Ann Intern Med.* **101:**51–54, 1984.
14. Chu C-M, Farci P, Liaw Y-F, et al: The role of delta superinfection in acute exacerbations of chronic type B hepatitis. *Liver* **6:**26–29, 1986.
15. Colombo M, Cambieri R, Rumi MG, et al: Long-term delta superinfection in hepatitis B surface antigen carriers and its relationship to the course of chronic hepatitis. *Gastroenterology* **85:**235–239, 1983.
16. Maggiore G, Hadchouel M, Sessa F, et al: A retrospective study of the role of delta agent infection in children with HBsAg-positive chronic hepatitis. *Hepatology* **5:**7–9, 1985.
17. Chen DS, Lai MY, Sung JL: δ Agent infection in patients with chronic liver diseases and hepatocellular carcinoma—An infrequent finding in Taiwan. *Hepatology* **4:**502–503, 1984.
18. Rizzetto M, Verme G, Recchia S, et al: Chronic hepatitis in carriers of hepatitis B surface antigen, with intrahepatic expression of the delta antigen. *Ann Intern Med* **98:**437–441, 1983.
19. Govindarajan S, Kanel G, Peters RL: Prevalence of delta-antibody among chronic hepatitis B virus infected patients in the Los Angeles area: Its correlation with liver biopsy diagnosis. *Gastroenterology* **85:**160–162, 1983.
20. Shiels MT, Czaja AJ, Taswell HF, et al: Frequency and significance of delta antibody in acute and chronic hepatitis B. A United States experience. *Gastroenterology* **89:**1230–1234, 1985.
21. Stocklin E, Gudat F, Krey G, et al: δ Antigen in hepatitis B: Immunohistology of frozen and paraffin-embedded liver biopsies and relation to HBV infection. *Hepatology* **1:**238–242, 1981.
22. Rizzetto M, Canese MG, Gerin JL, et al: Transmission of the hepatitis B virus-associated delta antigen to chimpanzees. *J Infect Dis* **141:**590–602, 1980.
23. Hadziyannis SJ, Sherman M, Lieberman HM, et al: Liver disease activity and hepatitis B virus replication in chronic delta antigen-positive hepatitis B virus carriers. *Hepatology* **5:**544–547, 1986.
24. Thung SN, Gerber MA: Immunohistochemical study of delta antigen in an American Metropolitan population. *Liver* **3:**392–397, 1983.
25. Smedile A, Rizzetto M, Denniston K, et al: Type D hepatitis: The clinical significance of hepatitis D virus RNA in serum as detected by a hybridization-based assay. *Hepatology* **6:**1297–1302, 1986.
26. Govindarajan S, Valinluck B: Serum hepatitis B virus-DNA in chronic hepatitis B and delta infection. *Arch Pathol Lab Med* **109:**398–399, 1985.
27. Krogsgaard K, Kryger P, Aldershvile J, et al: Delta infection and suppression of hepatitis B virus replication in chronic HBsAg carriers. *Hepatology* **7:**42–45, 1987.
28. Rizzetto M, Verme G, Gerin JL, et al: Hepatitis delta virus disease, in Popper H, Schaffner F (eds): *Progress in Liver Diseases,* Vol. 8. Grune & Stratton, Orlando, Florida, 1986, pp. 132–146.
29. Canese MG, Rizzetto M, Arico S, et al: An ultrastructural and immunohistochemical study on the δ antigen associated with the hepatitis B virus. *J Pathol* **128:**169–175, 1979.
30. Canese MG, Rizzetto M, Novara R, et al: Experimental infection of chimpanzees with the HBsAg-associated delta (δ) agent: An ultrastructural study. *J Med Virol* **13:**63–72, 1984.

31. Kojima T, Calles F, Desmyter J, et al: Immune electron microscopy of hepatitis δ-antigen in hepatocytes. *Lab Invest* **55**:217–225, 1986.
32. Kamimura T, Ponzetto A, Bonino F, et al: Cytoplasmic tubular structures in liver of HBsAg carrier chimpanzees infected with delta agent and comparison with cytoplasmic structures in non-A, non-B hepatitis. *Hepatology* **3**:631–637, 1983.
33. Shimizu YK, Purcell RH, Gerin JL, et al: Further studies by immunofluorescence of the monoclonal antibodies associated with experimental Non-A, Non-B hepatitis in chimpanzees and their relation to D hepatitis. *Hepatology* **6**:1329–1333, 1986.
34. Popper H, Buitrago B, Hadler SC, et al: Pathology of hepatitis delta infection in Amazon basin, in Rizzetto M, Gerin JL, Purcell RH (eds): *The Hepatitis Delta Virus and Its Infection.* Alan R. Liss, New York, 1987, pp. 121–128.
35. Gerber MA, Thung SN: The diagnostic value of immunohistochemical demonstration of hepatitis viral antigens in liver. *Hum Pathol* **18**:771–774, 1987.

7

Chronic Non-A, Non-B Hepatitis: The Pathologist's Perspective

Zachary D. Goodman

1. INTRODUCTION

A clinical diagnosis of chronic hepatitis is made when a patient has an elevation of serum aminotransferase activity that persists for 6 months or longer.[1] This may follow an otherwise typical acute viral hepatitis; it may be discovered incidentally in a patient being evaluated for some other reason; or the patient may present with symptoms of chronic liver disease. Frequently in this situation, the clinician is prompted to obtain a liver biopsy to confirm the diagnosis of chronic hepatitis and to gather information about the cause, the stage of the disease, and the prognosis. This raises the question of the value of the liver biopsy in providing that information.

To the pathologist, chronic hepatitis means chronic portal inflammation with variable amounts of parenchymal (i.e., intralobular) necrosis and inflammation and variable amounts of fibrosis. Pathologists, however, labor under the burden of an anachronistic terminology that developed before much was known about the causes and natural history of chronic hepatitis. The various morphologic lesions and patterns of injury were given names that implied pathogenesis and prognosis, often erroneously. For the past 10 years, the most frequently used classification of chronic hepatitis[2] has included two major morphologic entities: chronic persistent hepatitis (CPH) and chronic active hepatitis (CAH). It is important to realize, however, that chronic hepatitis has both a clinical and a morphologic spectrum.

It has been generally agreed that the pattern of injury known as CPH, characterized by chronic portal inflammation with minimal periportal injury, is a relatively benign lesion. By contrast, CAH, characterized by periportal injury as well as portal inflammation, has been regarded as a more serious lesion with the potential for progression to cirrhosis. This lesion is recognized by the presence of piecemeal necrosis, defined as "the destruction of liver cells at an interface between parenchyma and connective tissue, together with a predominantly lymphocytic or plasma cell infiltrate.[2] Piecemeal necrosis is recognized by the presence of individual cell necrosis at the edge of a portal area or along a fibrous septum (Fig. 1), by extension of the chronic portal inflammatory

Zachary D. Goodman • Department of Hepatic Pathology, Armed Forces Institute of Pathology, Washington, D.C. 20306. The opinions and assertions contained herein are the private views of the author and are not to be construed as official or as reflecting the views of the Department of the Army or the Department of Defense.

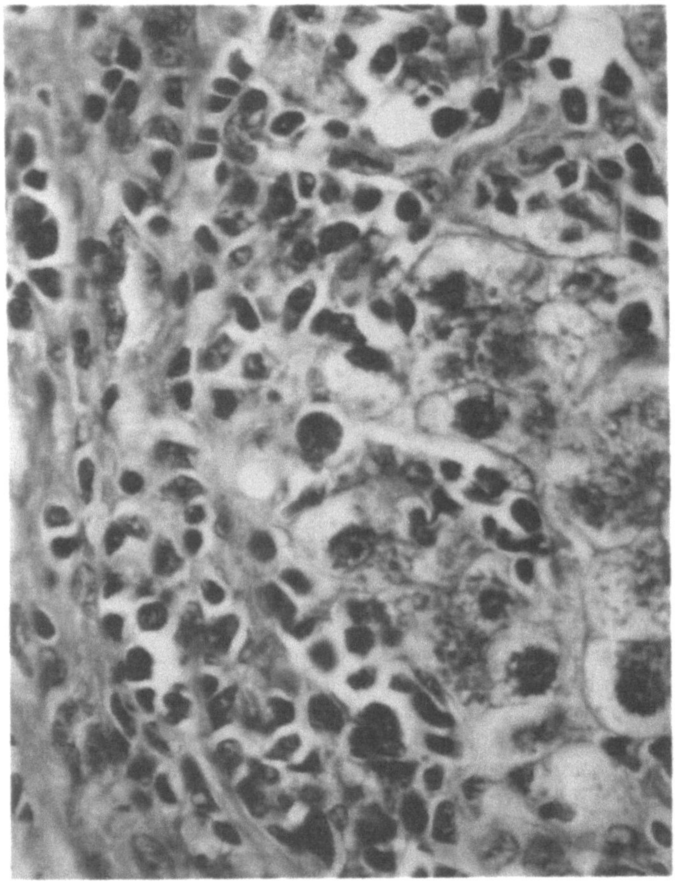

Figure 1. Periportal piecemeal necrosis in CAH. There is individual hepatocellular injury and necrosis at the edge of a portal area (left of photograph) with a lympho-plasmacytic inflammatory response. (H&E, ×630; AFIP neg. 87-5985)

infiltrate into the adjacent parenchyma (erosion of the limiting plate), or by trapping of small groups of hepatocytes within expanded portal areas. But within the spectrum of what has been called CAH, there is a wide range of severity, from borderline CPH/CAH to a markedly active cirrhosis. Furthermore, there are no firm guidelines as to where to draw the line between mild CAH and the severe form.

The following case illustrates the spectrum of what can be called CAH:

Case 1

This 34-year-old man had persistently elevated liver enzymes for at least 5 years. He had a history of yellow jaundice 5–6 years ago. He noted that this happened 5–6 weeks after using intravenous IV heroin with shared needles. During a recent visit to this physician, serum iron studies were ordered; all were normal except serum ferritin, which was moderately elevated. Liver biopsy was performed because of a suspicion of hemochromatosis. At the time of biopsy, LFTs included AST 62, ALT 102, bilirubin 0.5, Alk Phos 59, albumin 4.2, and normal PT and PTT. Serologic studies, including HB surface antigen (HBsAg), and anti-HBs, anti-HB core (HBc), HB e antigen (HBeAg), anti-HBe, and anti-HAV were all negative.

The biopsy shows no evidence of iron overload, despite the clinical suspicion (Fig. 2). There is, however, a mild degree of spotty hepatocellular dropout and focal inflammation. The portal areas are expanded with marked chronic inflammation, predominantly lymphocytes and plasma cells with a few eosinophils. Some portal areas contain lymphoid follicles with germinal centers. Bile ducts in some portal areas show epithelial injury, but all portal areas have a bile duct, and there are no features of chronic cholestasis. In some areas, the inflammation is confined to the portal tract, but many portal tracts have some areas in which the inflammation spills out into the surrounding parenchyma with occasional liver cell necrosis. The trichrome and reticulin stains show a moderate degree of portal–periportal fibrosis (Fig. 3). No bridging necrosis or fibrosis is present.

The histologic features in Case 1 are those of a relatively mild CAH biopsied during an inactive phase. The degree of irregularity of the limiting plate is too much for CPH, and the amount of fibrosis suggests that the disease has been more severe at some time in the past and is now in a relatively quiescent phase. Serologically, the patient has non-A, non-B (NANB) hepatitis.

The bile duct injury in this case (Fig. 2) raises the possibility of primary biliary cirrhosis, but the lack of cholestatis features and/or reduction in number of bile ducts rules this out. Bile duct injury in chronic active hepatitis, as described by Poulsen and Christoffersen,[3] is not specific for NANB, but it does seem to be much more frequent in that disease.[4] The cause and pathogenesis of this type of ductal injury have never been established. Despite the impressively destructive lesions that can be found (Figs. 4 and 5), there is no loss of ducts, in contrast to primary biliary cirrhosis.

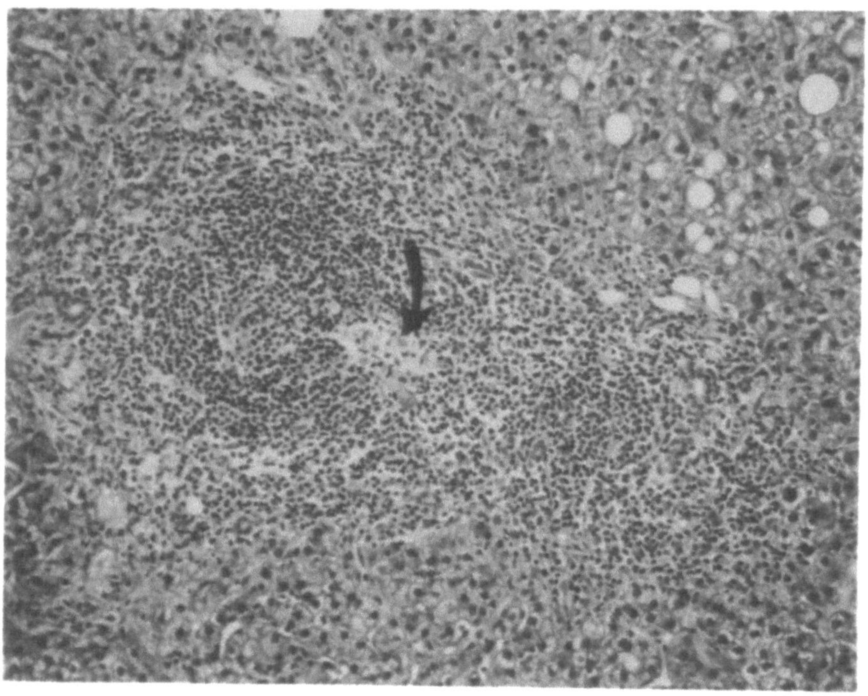

Figure 2. Mild NANB CAH (Case 1), showing intense chronic portal inflammation and foci of periportal piecemeal necrosis. An injured bile duct (arrow) is present within the portal inflammatory infiltrate. (H&E, ×160; AFIP neg. 87-5986)

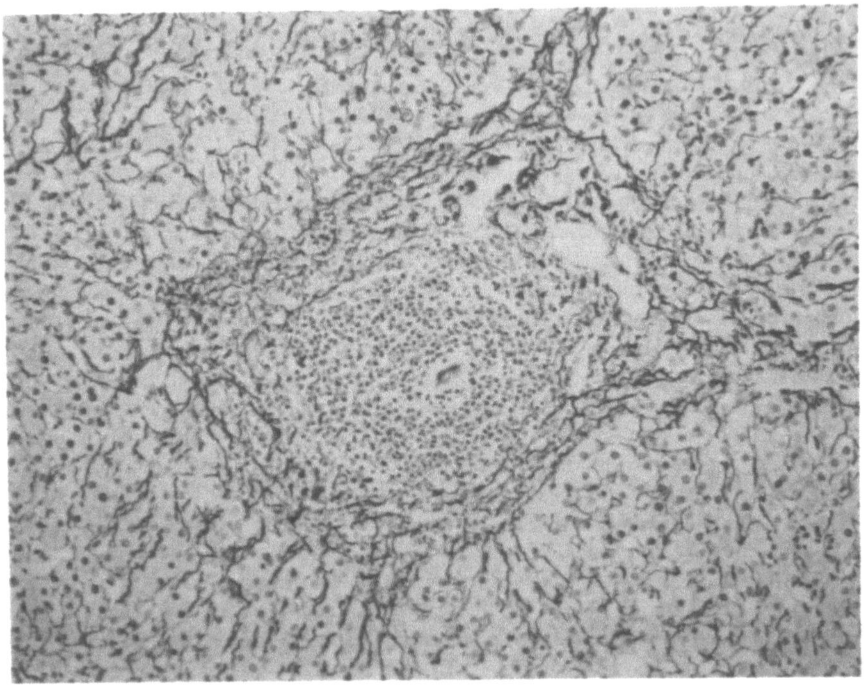

Figure 3. Mild NANB CAH (Case 1), showing a mild degree of periportal fibrosis. (Reticulin stain, ×160; AFIP neg. 87-5987)

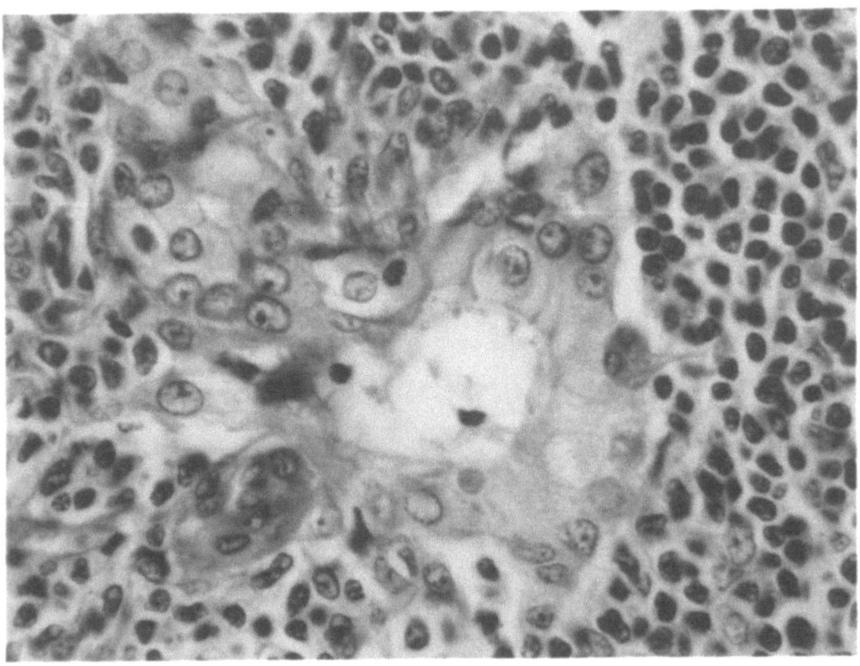

Figure 4. An injured bile duct (Poulsen lesion) in chronic NANB hepatitis. The duct shows disruption of the basement membrane, injury and necrosis of epithelial cells, and infiltration by chronic inflammatory cells. (H&E, ×630; AFIP neg. 87-5988)

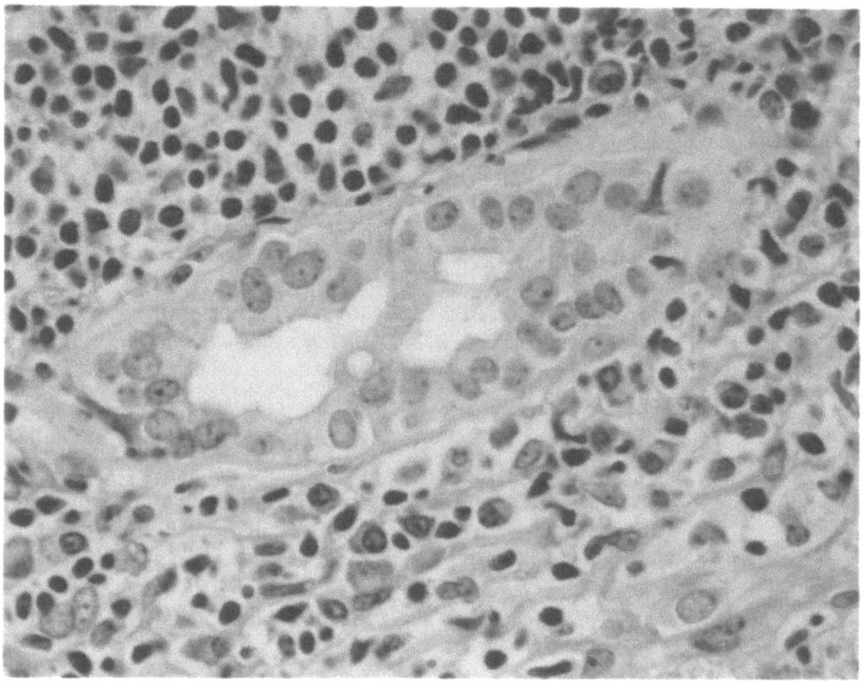

Figure 5. Another injured bile duct (Poulsen lesion) in chronic NANB. There is focal basement membrane disruption, pseudostratification of the bile duct epithelium, and a transluminal epithelial bridge. (H&E, ×630; AFIP neg. 87-5989)

2. PATHOLOGIC ASPECTS

Considering the relatively frequent occurrence of chronic NANB, there are surprisingly few detailed reports of its histopathologic features. In a recent review, Alter[5] compiled the histologic diagnoses in eight published series. Of the 102 cases described, 41% had CAH and 20% had cirrhosis. For most of these, no further histologic details are known. As far as is known, there are no definite features that permit an entirely specific histologic diagnosis of chronic NANB. The diagnosis remains one that can be made only after other causes of chronic hepatitis have been excluded, an exercise that is always intellectually unsatisfying. One study found no differences between chronic NANB and chronic HBV.[6] By contrast, bile duct injury has been found most often in NANB,[4] although it may also be seen occasionally in chronic HBV or in autoimmune (lupoid) hepatitis. Hepatocellular fat accumulation, sometimes quite impressive in amount, has also been frequently noted in chronic NANB. Peters[7] reported fat in 20% of NANB versus 10% of chronic HBV. But since these findings are not specific, the diagnosis of chronic NANB is most comfortably made when the onset of the disease follows transfusion or parenteral exposure.

There is no generally recognized point at which to separate mild CAH from severe CAH. This is in part because of the complexity of histologic features that make up the patterns of injury that fall within the spectrum of CAH. Every biopsy that can be called CAH has some degree of the following histologic features:

1. *Portal inflammation:* Consisting predominantly of lymphocytes and plasma cells, this can range from minimal inflammation, affecting relatively few portal areas, up to dense packing of all portal areas with chronic inflammatory cells.

2. *Periportal injury with or without bridging necrosis:* This can range from minimal piecemeal necrosis, with only occasional foci of periportal hepatocellular loss, to severe piecemeal necrosis, involving most of the circumference of all portal areas with expansion of the portal areas. In its most severe form, piecemeal necrosis can extend along a microcirculatory zone and produce a region of confluent hepatocellular necrosis that stretches from one portal area to the next or from a portal area to a terminal hepatic venule. Such zones of confluent necrosis are called bridging necrosis (Fig. 6).
3. *Intralobular injury.* This consists of acute hepatitis-like hepatocellular injury, ballooning degeneration, focal necrosis, acidophilic bodies, Kupffer cell hypertrophy, and sinusoidal lymphoplasmacytic inflammation.
4. *Fibrosis.* This represents the permanent largely irreversible component of the injury. Active fibrosis accompanies piecemeal necrosis and bridging necrosis, producing scarring that can link portal areas and lead to architectural distortion.

In published studies, it has been most unusual for all these features to be considered in distinguishing mild from severe CAH. A scoring system for assessing the histologic activity in CAH was devised by Knodell et al.[8] taking all the various features into account to arrive at a numerical Histology Activity Index. If widely used, this index might be very helpful in following individual patients and in comparing studies by different investigators. Unfortunately, this system has not become widely used. Most investigators have concentrated on one or another histologic feature, most often piecemeal necrosis and bridging necrosis in subdividing CAH. Whether this is appropriate is not known for certain. An argument can also be made for using the degree of fibrosis as a

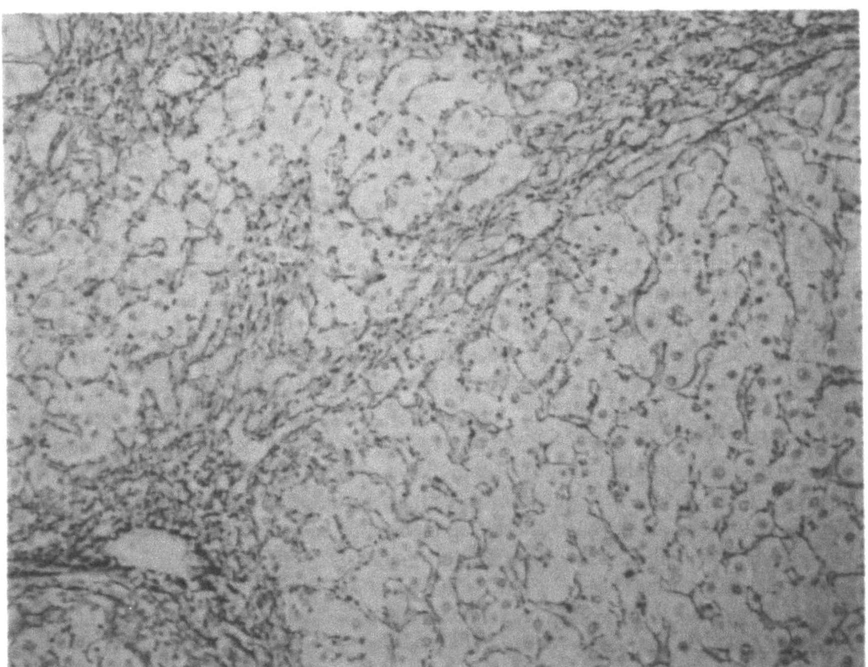

Figure 6. Bridging necrosis (and fibrosis) in a case of severe NANB CAH. An area of confluent hepatocellular necrosis, collapse, and early fibrosis stretches from the lower left to upper right. (Reticulin stain, ×160; AFIP neg. 87-5990)

marker of severity, since this indicates the amount of permanent damage and the degree of progression toward cirrhosis. The following case illustrates this problem:

Case 2

At the age of 76, this woman had required emergency surgery for a bleeding gastric ulcer. She underwent partial gastrectomy and required 2 units of whole blood intraoperatively. During the operation, the surgeon noticed a small lesion on the surface of the liver, which he biopsied. The lesion turned out to be a focal area of scarring and atrophy. The liver underlying the lesion was entirely normal. There was no evidence of any preexisting chronic liver disease.

The patient never developed symptomatic hepatitis. However, 5 months later, during follow-up evaluation, a routine chemistry panel showed a serum AST of 155 units (normal <40). No further evaluation was undertaken.

The patient was next evaluated 23 months later (2 years, 4 months after transfusion). She was still asymptomatic but this time had a serum AST activity of 219, with normal alkaline phosphatase, bilirubin, albumin, and total protein. HBsAg was negative, but anti-HBs and anti-HAV (IgG) were both positive, indicating previous infection with both hepatitis A and B. ANA, ASmA, and AMA were negative. A liver biopsy was performed.

The biopsy (Figs. 7 and 8) shows an established cirrhosis, with dense bands of scar tissue separating regenerative parenchymal nodules. Within the nodules, there is continuing active hepatocellular injury. Many hepatocytes are ballooned, and most contain cytoplasmic fat, which was not present in the previous biopsy. Acidophilic bodies are scattered throughout the nodules, and there is chronic inflammation with ongoing piecemeal necrosis along the fibrous septa. The histologic features are those of a cirrhosis that has evolved from an ongoing chronic active hepatitis.

3. PATHOLOGIC NATURAL HISTORY OF NANB

Clinically, there is little to distinguish the liver disease between the patients presented in Cases 1 and 2. Both were asymptomatic at biopsy. Pathologically, however, they represent the opposite extremes of what can be called CAH. They demonstrate the need for a liver biopsy to establish the stage of disease in an individual patient. Having established the stage, the question of prognosis arises.

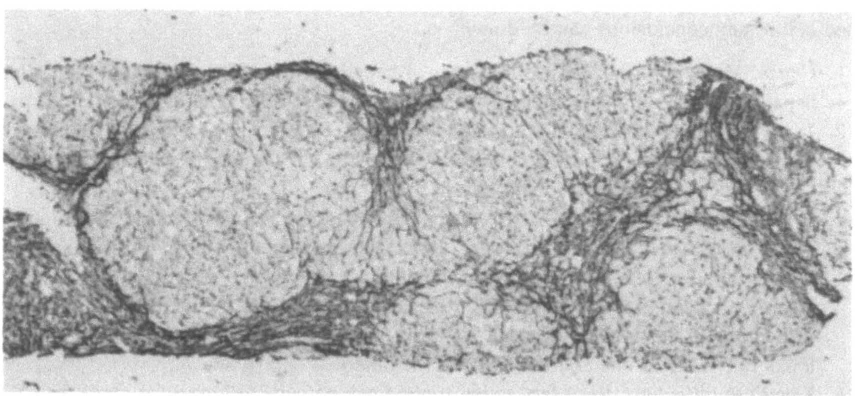

Figure 7. Cirrhosis in severe chronic NANB hepatitis (Case 2). There are small nodules of surviving parenchyma separated by fibrous scars. (Reticulin stain, ×40; AFIP neg. 87-5991)

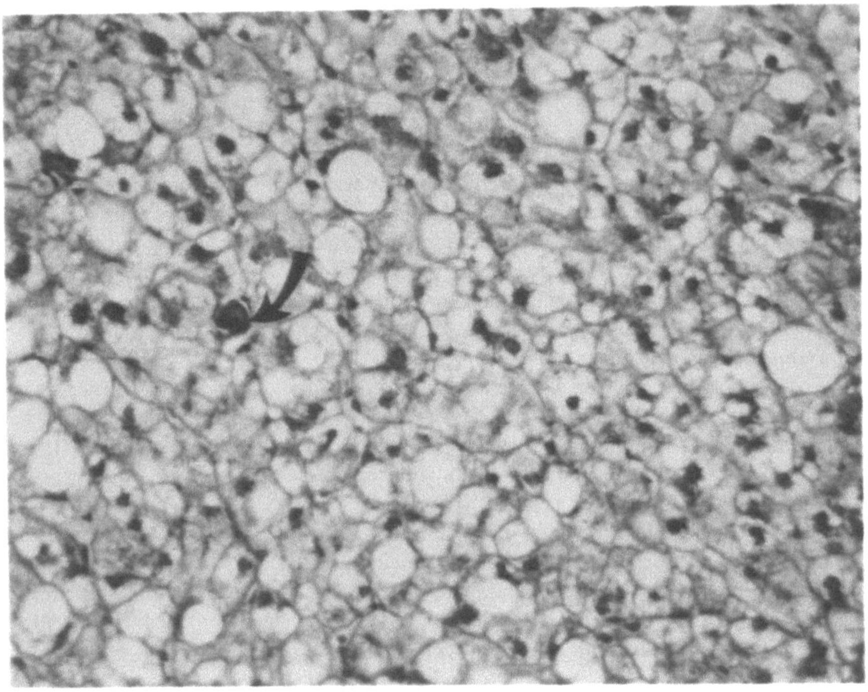

Figure 8. Severe chronic NANB with cirrhosis (Case 2). The surviving parenchyma shows scattered acidophilic bodies (arrow) and prominent fatty change. (H&E, ×250; AFIP neg. 87-5992)

Can a liver biopsy be used to gauge prognosis in CAH? This is a question that is not easily answered. Despite the number of published reports, none adequately addresses the issue of how the various morphologic lesions affect prognosis in the different diseases that can cause the patterns of injury recognized as CAH. A number of factors need to be taken into account in trying to understand the natural history of the various pathologic lesions. Unfortunately, most published studies do not give sufficient information to establish what the therapeutically unaltered course would be in patients in whom biopsies show the various lesions. Several confounding variables need to be defined before any conclusions can be drawn:

1. *Cause:* Many published series mix cases of hepatitis B, NANB, and autoimmune (lupoid) hepatitis, often indiscriminately.
2. *Treatment:* Most series contain no untreated control group. In particular, patients with the more severe histologic lesions and more severe clinical symptoms are more likely to have received corticosteroids or other therapy.
3. *Histologic criteria:* The criteria for diagnosis often differ between series, and sometimes it is not clear that the same criteria are applied to all patients within a given series. Some reports do not explain the criteria for diagnosis.
4. *Sampling:* Small biopsies may not be representative of the entire liver, but it is a rare paper that addresses this issue. Nevertheless, nearly every pathologist has seen a liver biopsy that looks like CAH at one end and CPH at the other.
5. *Length of follow-up:* Very few series contain any patients followed for more than 5 years and only rare patients followed for more than 10 years. However, since cirrhosis may develop very slowly in chronic NANB (20 years or longer), it may be premature to draw conclusions after a relatively brief follow-up.

Despite these problems, there are suggestions and some evidence in the literature indicating that patients whose biopsies show the most severe histologic lesions are the ones most likely to progress to cirrhosis, to have the highest mortality, and to run the most rapid clinical course. As part of the widely recognized Mayo Clinic controlled therapeutic trial, Baggenstoss et al.[9] reported on 41 precirrhotic patients, half of whom received corticosteroids. Six were HBsAg positive and 2 were later found to have primary biliary cirrhosis rather than CAH.[10] After 6 months to 4 years of follow-up evaluation, cirrhosis developed in 11 of 28 (39%) of those whose initial biopsy showed severe CAH (bridging or multilobular necrosis) but in only 1 of 10 (10%) of those with mild CAH (piecemeal necrosis only). Without steroid treatment, 7 of 11 (64%) of those with the severe lesions and 1 of 6 (17%) with mild CAH developed cirrhosis during the follow-up period. Schalm et al.[10] included these patients (except for those with PBC) in a larger series of 128 patients, most (approximately 66%) of whom probably had autoimmune (lupoid) hepatitis, rather than NANB. All the later patients received steroid treatment, but the conclusion was the same, i.e., that bridging and/or multilobular necrosis were the lesions most likely to progress to cirrhosis. However, 12% of patients with mild CAH progressed to cirrhosis while receiving steroids. Cooksley et al.[11] found that in a mixture of HBsAg-positive and -negative (presumably NANB) patients, many of them steroid-treated, 19% of those with bridging necrosis developed cirrhosis during a follow-up period of 3 months to 13 years, but no patients with mild CAH had this outcome. By contrast, De Groote et al.[13] followed a group of patients with moderate CAH without bridging for 2–15 years. One half were HBsAg positive, and all were steroid treated. Cirrhosis developed in 71% with hepatitis B and in 31% with non-B CAH. Furthermore, with longer follow-up of the Mayo Clinic patients, Davis et al.[13] found that in steroid-treated HBsAg-negative patients, 32% with mild CAH eventually developed cirrhosis compared with 43% with severe CAH. In a review of the subject, on the basis of these and several other studies, Combes[14] concluded that CAH, both with or without bridging, has the capacity to progress to cirrhosis, although bridging may indicate a more rapidly progressing disease or may be a stage in the evolution of the disease.

Since there is as yet no large group of untreated patients with well documented chronic NANB

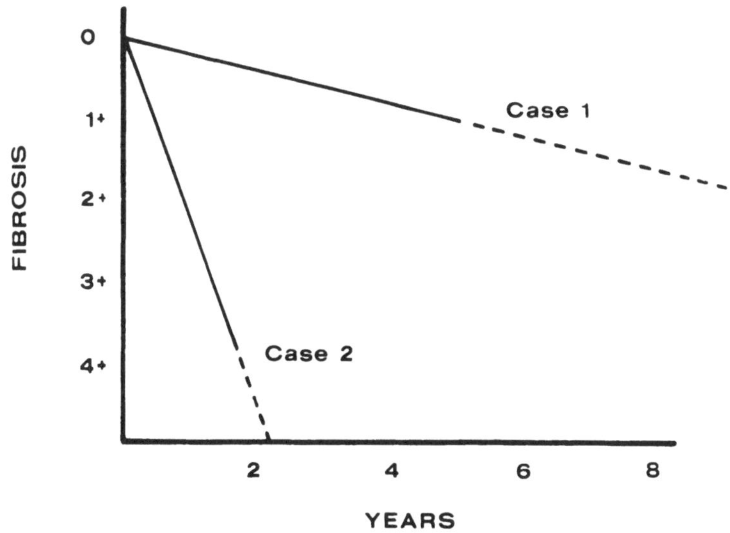

Figure 9. Graphic representation of presumed rate of progression of fibrosis in two cases of chronic NANB hepatitis. Case 1 went from a normal liver to mild fibrosis in 5 years. At that rate, it will be 20–30 years or more before he reaches end-stage liver disease. Case 2 progressed from a normal liver to cirrhosis in 2 years and will soon be in the end stages of the disease. (AFIP neg. 87-5993)

that has been followed with serial biopsies for as long as two to three decades, the true natural history of this disease remains to be determined. A practical although unproven approach to predicting prognosis from the liver biopsy is illustrated in Fig. 9. It seems reasonable to assume that for any given patient, the scarring due to chronic hepatitis progresses at a fairly constant rate over the years if nothing is done to alter the natural history of the disease. This is particularly true for chronic NANB, which does not seem to have the ability to undergo spontaneous resolution. There are marked differences between patients in the rate of progression, and within each patient there are periods of exacerbation alternating with periods of quiescence. However, the fibrosis, representing the permanent damage, tends to increase with time. Therefore, if we can estimate the amount of fibrosis at two points in time, we can try to predict how long it will take to reach end-stage liver disease. This is shown in Fig. 5 for the two cases presented here. Case 1 had progressed from a presumably normal liver to a stage of mild fibrosis after 6 years, and so we would predict that if his disease continues at this rate, cirrhosis will not develop for another 20 years or more. By contrast, Case 2 went from a normal liver to an advanced cirrhosis in only 2 years. We would predict the complications of end-stage liver disease to become evident very soon. This approach to predicting prognosis has not been subjected to a critical analysis or to experimental testing but, for the present, it is as good as anything we have to offer.

Of what use is a liver biopsy in chronic hepatitis? There are three questions that it can attempt to answer:

1. *Cause:* The cause of the chronic hepatitis can only be established with certainty if the agent is demonstrated in the liver. A positive immunostain for HBsAg or HBcAg or for delta antigen is evidence that the virus caused the chronic hepatitis. Fat and/or bile duct injury suggest NANB, but neither is entirely specific.
2. *Stage:* The liver biopsy is the best technique for establishing how much permanent damage has been done.
3. *Prognosis:* Although this has not been scientifically established, the liver biopsy seems to be as good a means as any in predicting the course of the disease.

REFERENCES

1. Boyer JL, Miller DJ: Chronic hepatitis, in Schiff L, Schiff ER (eds): *Diseases of the Liver.* JB Lippincott, Philadelphia, 1987, pp. 687–723.
2. Bianchi L, De Groote J, Desmet VJ, et al: Acute and chronic hepatitis revisited. *Lancet* **2**:914–919, 1977.
3. Poulsen H, Christoffersen P: Abnormal bile duct epithelium in chronic aggressive hepatitis and cirrhosis. A review of morphology and clinical, biochemical, and immunologic features. *Hum Pathol* **3**:217–225, 1972.
4. Bianchi L: Liver biopsy interpretation in hepatitis. Part II. Histopathology and classification of acute and chronic viral hepatitis/differential diagnosis. *Pathol Res Pract* **178**:180–213, 1983.
5. Alter HJ. Acute and chronic consequences of post-transfusion hepatitis, in Ostrow JD, Groszmann RJ, Hoofnagle JH (eds): *Hepatology Update—Portal Hypertension; Viral Hepatitis.* American Association for the Study of Liver Diseases, Chicago, 1986, pp. 219–228.
6. Thorne CHM, Higgins GR, Ulich TR, et al: A histologic comparison of hepatitis B with non-A, non-B chronic active hepatitis. *Arch Pathol Lab Med* **106**:433–436, 1982.
7. Peters RL. Viral inflammatory diseases, in Peters RL, Craig JR (eds): *Liver Pathology.* Churchill Livingstone, New York, 1986, pp. 73–123.
8. Knodell RG, Ishak KG, Black WC, et al: Formulation and application of a numerical scoring system for assessing histological activity in asymptomatic chronic active hepatitis. *Hepatology* **1**:431–435, 1981.
9. Baggenstoss AH, Soloway RD, Summerskill WHJ, et al: Chronic active liver disease. The range of histologic lesions, their response to treatment, and evolution. *Hum Pathol* **3**:183–198, 1972.
10. Schalm SW, Korman MG, Summerskill WHJ, et al: Severe chronic active liver disease. Prognostic significance of initial morphologic patterns. *Dig Dis* **22**:973–980, 1977.
11. Cooksley WGE, Bradbear RA, Robinson W, et al: The prognosis of chronic active hepatitis without cirrhosis in relation to bridging necrosis. *Hepatology* **6**:345–348, 1986.

12. De Groote J, Fevery J, Lepoutre L: Long-term follow-up of chronic active hepatitis of moderate severity. *Gut* **19**:510–513, 1978.
13. Davis GL, Czaja AJ, Ludwig J: Development and prognosis of histologic cirrhosis in corticosteroid-treated hepatitis B surface antigen-negative chronic active hepatitis. *Gastroenterology* **87**:1222–1227, 1984.
14. Combes B: The initial morphologic lesion in chronic active hepatitis, important or unimportant? *Hepatology* **6**:518–522, 1986.

8

Chronic Consequences of Non-A, Non-B Hepatitis

Harvey J. Alter

1. INTRODUCTION

There has existed a sequential skepticism regarding initially, the existence of, and subsequently, the clinical significance of non-A, non-B hepatitis (NANBH). Skepticism first centered on the question of whether NANBH is a viral disease or merely a transaminitis of nonviral etiology. This initial doubt was dispelled when it was demonstrated that NANBH could be transmitted to the chimpanzee, using acute- and chronic-phase human serum and then serially passaged in the chimpanzee model[1,2]; thus, the infectious nature of NANBH was unequivocally established. Accepting the transmissible nature of NANBH, the argument then turned to the clinical significance of the disease, as most cases were anicteric and asymptomatic in the acute phase. Did such mild acute disease merit serious consideration? When it later evolved that approximately 50% of NANBH cases progress to chronic hepatitis and that such progression was just as likely following asymptomatic as following overt icteric hepatitis, it became apparent that such mild cases could not be ignored.[3] Skepticism then shifted to another level; i.e., even if NANBH frequently results in chronic hepatitis, as judged by alanine aminotransferase (ALT), is this disease progression associated with any significant histologic outcome? There is a large body of evidence that indicates that approximately 20% of persons with chronic NANBH who are biopsied show histologic evidence of cirrhosis. Data supporting this are detailed in this chapter. Current skepticism revolves around the issue of the clinical importance of NANBH-related cirrhosis. Such cirrhosis appears to be clinically indolent compared with alcohol-induced cirrhosis, and the question has been raised as to whether NANB cirrhosis results in significant morbidity and mortality. This is a more difficult question to address, but certainly liver-related fatality has occurred in a variety of patient groups with chronic NANBH and cirrhosis.

This chapter addresses these issues and attempts to present evidence supporting the development and clinical significance of chronic NANB hepatitis.

Harvey J. Alter • Department of Transfusion Medicine, Warren G. Magnuson Clinical Center, National Institutes of Health, Bethesda, Maryland 20892.

2. EVIDENCE FOR CHRONIC NANBH FROM STUDIES OF TRANSFUSION-ASSOCIATED HEPATITIS

Most of what we know of NANBH and its causative agents derives from chimpanzee transmission studies and from prospective studies of transfusion-associated hepatitis (TAH). In the latter setting one can establish a normal pretransfusion ALT level, observe a discrete incubation period, establish a significant rise in ALT compared with baseline; obtain sequential ALT determinations to confirm the diagnosis, and follow the patient to establish the transaminase pattern and to determine the duration of ALT elevation. Chronic hepatitis is usually defined as an ALT elevation that persists greater than 1 year after disease onset. When a normal baseline has been established, when after an incubation period (generally 6–12 weeks) the ALT rises to at least 2½ times the upper limit of normal and persists at high level for at least 1 week, when other causes of ALT elevation such as alcohol and medications can be reasonably excluded and, when other viral disease of the liver can be serologically excluded, the diagnosis of NANBH assumes credibility, even in the absence of a serologic marker. If, in addition, there is the characteristic fluctuating ALT pattern and a prolonged duration of ALT elevation, the diagnosis assumes greater certainty and can usually be supported by liver biopsy; on rare occasions, it can be supported by transmission to the chimpanzee. By contrast, cases of sporadic hepatitis that lack a baseline of normality and an established incubation period and that have no known source of exposure leave a much greater degree of uncertainty as to the underlying cause of ALT elevation. This chapter focuses solely on transfusion-associated NANBH.

The pattern of ALT elevation has both diagnostic and prognostic value. Three primary patterns have been observed: monophasic, polyphasic (fluctuating), and plateau. In one study,[4] 42.5% of those with a monophasic peak in the acute phase developed chronic hepatitis, whereas 86.6% of those with a fluctuating pattern and 94.9% of those with a plateau pattern developed chronic NANBH. It has been observed that those with a plateau pattern tend to lack a distinct acute phase and seem to have the pattern of chronic hepatitis almost from the onset of their disease.

One of the earliest reports of chronic NANBH came from the follow-up evaluation of an outbreak of HB surface antigen (HBsAg)-negative hepatitis in a renal dialysis unit.[5] Of 29 patients who developed acute hepatitis, eight (28%) developed chronic ALT elevations dating from that time. Liver biopsy in seven of these patients indicated chronic aggressive (active) hepatitis (CAH) in three cases, two of which progressed to cirrhosis. While it is likely that NANBH was introduced into this dialysis unit as a result of blood transfusion, the circumscribed nature of the outbreak (1968–1970) suggests that spread could have occurred as the result of cross-contamination from hemodialysis machines, thus, this study differs from the prospective transfusion studies described below. Nonetheless, it does indicate that serially followed patients with acute HBsAg-negative hepatitis do progress to CAH and cirrhosis. One patient with cirrhosis manifested ascites and low serum albumin and died in hepatocellular failure.

In 1976, Koretz et al.[6] published their first analysis of a cohort of 47 patients who developed TAH during prospective follow-up. These patients received blood prescreened by first-generation tests for HBsAg but were only retrospectively tested by more sensitive assays; 85% of the blood transfused was from commercial sources, and every hepatitis case received at least 1 unit of commercial blood. The 47 patients who could be followed long term were derived from a total of 54 hepatitis cases that occurred. The overall incidence of TAH was 43% and ranged from 37% in recipients of HBsAg-negative blood to 66% in those found retrospectively to have received HBsAg-positive blood. In this study, chronic hepatitis was defined as the persistence of transaminase elevation greater than two times the upper limit of normal for at least 20 weeks. Using this criterion, 29 (62%) developed chronic hepatitis. When those with chronic hepatitis were compared with those who resolved their disease in less than 20 weeks, there was no significant difference in age, sex, number of units transfused, incubation period, presence or absence of symptoms, jaundice, the maximum transaminase, the development of HBsAg or HBs antibody or the underlying illness. Although there was no difference in the age of those who did or did not develop chronic hepatitis, both populations were generally middle-aged or elderly, with a mean age of 50 and 48 years, respectively.

Of the 29 patients in the Koretz study who developed chronic hepatitis, 15 had a liver biopsy obtained 26–59 weeks (average 31 weeks) after the onset of acute hepatitis. Nine of the 15 biopsied patients (60%) had a histologic diagnosis of CAH, two (13%) had chronic persistent hepatitis (CPH), and four (27%) had unresolved hepatitis. Koretz and colleagues stress the disparity between the histologic outcome and the clinical outcome. Five of nine patients with CAH had no significant symptoms of liver disease; the other four were managed with steroids and azothioprine, perhaps masking clinical systems, but only one of these four patients had symptoms related to their liver disease. None of the patients had bridging necrosis, but one had cirrhosis in the setting of CAH. At the time of this analysis, there were no hepatic deaths or cases of hepatitis induced liver failure. An extension and follow-up of this study are presented later in this discussion.

A placebo-controlled study of the efficacy of gamma globulin in the prevention of TAH was conducted by the U.S. Army.[7] This study generated 47 cases of TAH, 44 (94%) of which were classified as NANBH, serving as the basis for a subsequent analysis of the chronic sequelae of acute transfusion-associated NANBH. In this analysis, chronic hepatitis was defined as the persistence of elevated ALT for more than 12 months from the onset of disease. Ten of the 44 patients (23%) had evidence of chronic hepatitis by this criterion. Six additional patients had ALT elevations for greater than 6 months but had two consecutive normal values on follow-up and were considered to have a delayed resolution of their hepatitis. These patients were neither biopsied nor entered into long-term follow-up. The 10 patients with chronic ALT elevations were compared with the 34 patients with rapid or delayed resolution of serum transaminase abnormalities. There were no significant differences in age, sex, or pretransfusion prevalence of antibody to HAV, HBV, EBV, or CMV. Patients who developed chronic hepatitis, however, received significantly more blood transfusions ($p < 0.025$). Although patients who developed chronic hepatitis were more frequently symptomatic in the acute phase, there was no objective evidence for increased severity of the acute hepatitis as measured by the mean peak ALT or the maximum bilirubin elevation. A somewhat surprising outcome of this study was that immune serum globulin (ISG) and hepatitis B immunoglobulin (HBIG) appeared to influence the progression from acute to chronic liver disease. Of 22 patients who received the albumin placebo and developed TAH, nine (41%) developed chronic hepatitis, whereas chronicity developed in only one of 11 (9%) who received ISG and in none of 11 who received HBIG. The difference between globulin recipients and albumin recipients was significant ($p = 0.009$). To my knowledge, this potentially important link between preoperative gamma globulin administration and the subsequent development of chronic NANBH has not been examined in any subsequent study. Indeed, it is unlikely to be further examined in the future because of the lowered incidence of TAH from a variety of other interventive measures and because of the enormous cost and complexity of performing a randomized controlled trial that would require thousands of participants at current levels of hepatitis incidence.

Of the 10 chronic hepatitis cases in the Knodell study,[7] eight had CAH, one had CPH, and one had a mixed macronodular and micronodular cirrhosis that was relatively inactive. Knodell et al. concluded that acute NANBH often progresses to CAH and that preoperative gamma globulin significantly reduces that progression.

In 1979 Rakela and Redeker[8] studied 62 patients hospitalized with HBsAg-negative acute hepatitis of presumed viral origin and assessed both the epidemiologic setting in which the hepatitis had occurred and the long-term outcome. On the basis of antibody seroconversion to HBsAg or HAV, few cases were determined to be type B hepatitis and 13 type A hepatitis. The remaining 45 cases were classified as NANBH. None of these patients had evidence of prior liver disease, alcoholism, or exposure to hepatotoxic drugs; in each case, the minimal ALT elevation was 500 IU/liter. Among the 45 NANBH cases, 13 (29%) gave a history of blood transfusion during the preceding 6 months, 12 (27%) admitted to illicit drug use, and 20 (44%) had no obvious source of hepatitis exposure. In composite, 40% of the patients developed chronic transaminase elevation, which was highly dependent on the epidemiologic source of infection. Among transfusion recipients and addicts, the incidence of chronic hepatitis was 54% and 58%, respectively, whereas it was only 20% among those without known parenteral exposure (sporadic hepatitis). Interestingly, chronicity occurred more frequently in anicteric cases (5 of 6, 83%) than in icteric cases (13 of 39, 33%). Fourteen of the 18 patients with chronic hepatitis underwent liver biopsy, four (22%) had CAH, and the remainder had CPH. All four CAH cases occurred in the transfused population; the incidence of CAH in this group was 4 of 6 (66%). Of most significance, one patient with CAH progressed to cirrhosis and died in hepatic failure 42 months after the onset of acute hepatitis. This patient had been enrolled in a prospective study; it was therefore clearly documented by serial samples that no evidence of liver disease had existed prior to the acute hepatitis. Furthermore, two liver biopsies showed progressively severe CAH, and the autopsy demonstrated CAH with advanced cirrhosis. This documented progression of acute NANBH to fatal cirrhosis is integral to the theme of this manuscript and is further documented in several studies described below.

In 1979, Berman et al.[9] published the initial results of an ongoing National Institutes of Health (NIH) prospective study of the chronic sequelae of acute transfusion-associated NANBH. In this analysis, 46% of NANBH cases developed biochemical evidence of chronic liver disease; six of eight biopsied patients had CAH and one had early cirrhosis. This study has now been expanded to include 75 patients, 32 of whom have undergone liver biopsy for chronic transfusion-associated NANBH.[10] At initial biopsy, 19 (61%) had CAH and three (9%) had cirrhosis. Thirteen of the patients with CAH had a repeat biopsy 1–4 years later. While the majority demonstrated a stable or improving histologic pattern, 39% demonstrated progressive disease, with four additional patients developing cirrhosis while under observation. Overall, 7 of 32 biopsied patients (22%) had cirrhosis on initial or repeat biopsy; in three patients, progressive liver failure was the primary or complicating cause of death. The demonstration of cirrhosis in 10–20% of those who develop chronic post-transfusion hepatitis is a highly consistent finding, documented particularly in studies involving patients with hemophilia.

The progression of acute NANBH to cirrhosis was further demonstrated in case reports by Iwarson et al.[11] Two patients with histologically verified acute hepatitis were documented to have developed CAH within 2 years of the acute episode. One of these patients was still alive 8 years after the onset of disease but was too debilitated to work and had persisting biopsy evidence of CAH despite steroid therapy. The second patient showed elements of cirrhosis together with CAH on a biopsy obtained only 1 year after his acute hepatitis; he died of liver failure within 3 years of the acute NANBH. The importance of these cases is the histologic documentation of the acute hepatitis and the demonstration of the rapid progression to cirrhosis and death. In actuality, the two cases reported by Iwarson's group derived from nine cases of CAH in which the progression from acute hepatitis to chronic hepatitis had been histologically documented. Three of the nine CAH patients had hepatitis B markers in the serum and were classified as type B hepatitis; four additional patients had antibody to HAV, and these were classified as type A hepatitis. However, since type A hepatitis does not progress to chronic liver disease, it is more likely that these were NANBH cases with coincidental antibody to HAV. If the latter is true, then the Iwarson study involved 6 rather than 2 patients who progressed from acute NANBH to CAH.

A larger study of similar nature and outcome to the Iwarson study was conducted by Realdi et al.,[12] who obtained acute-phase liver biopsies in 15 patients with clinical evidence of acute post-transfusion hepatitis. Biopsies confirmed the acute nature of the illness. Eight of the 15 patients (53%) manifested persistent transaminase abnormalities and subsequently fulfilled biochemical criteria for the diagnosis of chronic hepatitis. Repeat liver biopsies in seven of these eight patients demonstrated chronic lobular hepatitis in two, CAH in three, and frank cirrhosis in two. One patient with cirrhosis died of gastrointestinal (GI) bleeding 18 months after the diagnosis of cirrhosis and 55 months after the onset of acute hepatitis.

Omata and co-workers[13] obtained acute-phase (within 3 months of onset) liver biopsies in 24 patients with NANBH. Thirteen (54%) developed biochemical evidence of chronic liver disease.

Histologic analysis of the acute-phase biopsies demonstrated that erosion of the limiting plate, hepatocellular degeneration, and poor regenerative activity were indicative of subsequent transition to chronicity. Five of the patients with chronic ALT elevations underwent a subsequent liver biopsy after a mean of 24 months; two demonstrated CPH, two demonstrated CAH, and one developed cirrhosis.

The rare provision of acute-phase biopsy data in the Iwarson et al.,[11] Realdi et al.,[12] and Omata et al.[13] studies establishes that the subsequent chronic liver disease was unrelated to a preexisting condition and documents the progression from acute to chronic liver disease over a relatively brief interval. The sometimes fatal outcome of chronic NANBH is also documented.

In a separate review of the long-term outcome of transfusion-associated NANBH, Realdi and co-workers[14] expanded their initial study[12] and analyzed 40 prospectively followed cardiac surgery patients who demonstrated ALT elevations for more than 1 year after their acute episode of TAH; in addition, 21 nonconsecutive open heart surgery patients developing hepatitis between 1975 and 1979 were entered into long-term follow-up. Forty-one of these 61 patients had a liver biopsy between 1 and 6 years after acute onset, and 12 of these patients had two or more biopsies. Of the 41 biopsied patients, five (12%) had chronic lobular hepatitis, eight (20%) had CPH, 14 (34%) had CAH, and 14 (34%) had cirrhosis. Thus, approximately two thirds of biopsied patients had significant histologic abnormalities and one third had cirrhosis. Five patients with CAH on initial biopsy progressed to cirrhosis during follow-up. Cirrhosis tended to appear between the third and sixth years of follow-up, but two patients manifested cirrhosis within 1 year of their acute hepatitis. The histologic progression to cirrhosis was noted in some patients despite an improving transaminase pattern and the suggestion of a slow biochemical resolution of their chronic hepatitis. One patient (also described by Realdi et al.[12]) died of GI bleeding 18 months after the diagnosis of CAH with cirrhosis had been made. No cases were described with ascites or hepatic encephalopathy. It is of interest that 92% of sporadic cases had spontaneous resolution of ALT compared with only 43% of transfusion-related cases.

Kiyosawa and co-workers[15] performed both a prospective and retrospective study of tranfusion-associated NANBH. In the prospective aspect of the study, 70 patients developed NANBH after transfusion for a variety of medical and surgical conditions; in contrast to all prior studies cited herein, none of these patients underwent open heart surgery. Of the 70 patients, 66% had elevated ALT for greater than 6 months and 46% for greater than 1 year. Liver biopsy was performed in 14 of 32 patients with ALT elevations of more than 1 year's duration; five were diagnosed as CAH, three as CPH, and six as unresolved hepatitis. The interval between the onset of acute disease and the time of biopsy was not stated except to indicate that it was greater than 1 year. If not greater than two years, as suggested by the high proportion of unresolved hepatitis cases, this might account for the absence of cirrhosis as compared with other published series. By contrast, their retrospective study suggests a distinct relationship between nonalcoholic, non-B cirrhosis (presumably NANBH) and a history of prior transfusion. In the retrospective study, patients hospitalized with a histologic diagnosis of chronic hepatitis, cirrhosis, or hepatocellular carcinoma (HCC) were analyzed first for the probable cause of their chronic liver disease and second for the relationship of their chronic liver disease to a history of prior transfusion. After exclusion of alcoholism and other nonviral causes of chronic liver disease, there were 399 patients with chronic viral hepatitis; of 116 with type B chronic hepatitis, 3.4% had a history of prior transfusion, whereas 43% of 283 patients with NANB-related chronic hepatitis had been previously transfused. The occurrence of prior transfusion in hepatitis B virus (HBV)-related cirrhosis was only 7.1% compared with 37% in NANBV-related cirrhosis. These significant differences ($p<0.01$) suggest that, at least in Japan, there are many cases of both chronic hepatitis and cirrhosis that appear to be NANBV related and in which transfusion appears to be an important etiologic determinant. By contrast, HBV-related chronic liver disease appears to be relatively independent of transfusion, consistent with its predominant transmission by maternofetal and sexual routes. There was no statistical link between NANBV-related HCC and prior transfusion.

Another interesting aspect of this Japanese study was the long interval between the time of transfusion and the ultimate diagnosis of chronic liver disease. Of 406 cases in which the time of transfusion was known, the mean interval to hospitalization for chronic hepatitis was 13.6 years, that to cirrhosis 17.0 years, and that to HCC 23.4 years. There are several implications of these prolonged intervals to disease diagnosis. First, the mean intervals may be spuriously prolonged because cases of early cirrhosis and death would not have been included in this retrospective analysis. From studies already cited herein, it is clear that while most cases of cirrhosis may take a long time to develop, some are apparent within 1–2 years of transfusion, and many within 3–6 years. The retrospective study conducted by Kiyosawa et al.[15] does not deal with when cirrhosis first appeared but with when it first resulted in hospital admission. What is significant is the relatively large number (4C6 cases in 8 years) of NANBH-related chronic liver disease cases requiring hospitalization in a single region of Japan. The second implication of the long interval between disease onset and clinical diagnosis is that many transfused patients may die of intercurrent illness before cirrhosis and its consequences become apparent. This is substantiated by two facts. First, transfused patients tend to be over 50 years of age, at which time a variety of serious illnesses become more prevalent. Second, acquired immune deficiency syndrome (AIDS) lookback studies, which have tried to trace prior recipients of blood from donors who subsequently developed AIDS or had anti-HIV antibody, indicate that 50% of multiply transfused patients die within 1 year of their transfusion need, not from AIDS, but from the underlying disease which necessitated the transfusion or from a complication of the surgery or hospitalization. If these high early mortality rates can be generally applied, the observed incidence of NANBH-related cirrhosis will be less than that projected from prospective studies. Hence, from one perspective, the number of transfusion-related cirrhosis cases in a population may seem smaller than expected because (1) many recipients have died of intercurrent disease, (2) the cirrhosis is often indolent until late in its course, and (3) cases have not been actively sought and for the most part go unreported. From another perspective, it is clear from the studies cited herein that patients unequivocally progress from acute TAH to cirrhosis and that some of these patients die of liver failure. The fact that a patient may die of other causes before this sequence is fulfilled is clearly of no solace to the patient and is to some degree irrelevant to decisions regarding transfusion practice. That practice should be dedicated to the principle that the patient will survive the disease for which the transfusion was mandated and to the principle that blood transfusion should not serve as a vehicle for infectious disease transmission.

In a crucial study, Koretz et al.[16] reviewed the first decade of follow-up in their prospective study of TAH. Sixty-nine patients who developed transfusion-associated NANBH were studied and analyzed for the persistence of ALT abnormalities and for the clinical and histologic outcome of this acutely benign disease. Chronic hepatitis, as biochemically defined, occurred in 46 (67%) of the patients. Using six consecutive normal ALT values as the criterion for biochemical resolution of disease, only 5 of 46% (11%) resolved their chronic hepatitis. An actuarial analysis for the entire 69 patients who developed NANBH revealed an approximate 50% chance of achieving biochemical resolutions over a 6- to 10-year interval. However, it was noted that even among patients with apparent resolution there were often continued sporadic ALT elevations. These findings are highly consistent with the NIH[10] and other series that document an approximate 50% chronicity rate based on persistent ALT and also demonstrate the difficulty of defining and establishing resolution because of the low grade and fluctuating nature of the enzyme abnormalities.

In contrast to the biochemical abnormalities, Koretz et al.[16] stress that virtually all the patients with chronic hepatitis were asymptomatic. It is thus essential to obtain liver biopsies and long-term clinical follow-up to establish the significance of the persistent biochemical indices of chronic inflammation. In this study,[16] one or more liver biopsies were obtained in 21 of the 46 patients with chronic hepatitis; four of 21 (19%) demonstrated cirrhosis in the setting of CAH. An analysis of these four patients is instructive. The first died of metastatic carcinoma shortly after her first biopsy and although liver failure was not present at that time, a sufficient interval had not elapsed (<1 year) for this to have evolved. The second patient had four biopsies and showed CAH with progressive fibrosis and eventual cirrhosis 5 years after the onset of disease. This patient did not have evidence of end-stage liver disease at this 5-year interval but had been on long-term low-dose corticosteroids for his chronic hepatitis and the possible ameliorating effect of this therapy cannot be assessed. The third patient had chronic leukemia and worsening neutropenia and thrombocytopenia which necessitated splenectomy 6 years after the onset of NANBH. At surgery, cirrhosis was macroscopically obvious and microscopically confirmed, and it seemed possible, if not probable, that portal hypertension and hypersplenism were primarily responsible for the patient's hematologic deterioration. The fourth patient developed an abnormal coagulation profile 1 year after NANBH and over the next 6 years demonstrated a progressive coagulopathy and hypersplenism. He died during surgical treatment of a bleeding duodenal ulcer, at which time postnecrotic cirrhosis was confirmed. Hence, in this study, cirrhosis occurred in 6% of the patients who developed acute NANBH, in 9% of those who developed chronic NANHB and in 19% of those who were biopsied. The cirrhosis appeared to be associated with portal hypertension and hypersplenism in two of the patients and was at least indirectly responsible for the death of one patient. These findings are highly consistent with other studies cited herein wherein approximately 20% of NANBH patients have cirrhosis on biopsy and wherein 20–25% of those with cirrhosis sustain a liver-related fatality (Table I). It is fair to state, however, that the majority of patients with chronic NANBH and even those with histologically documented cirrhosis tolerate their disease very well. Whether this reflects a truly benign chronic illness or whether a longer interval is required for the other patients with cirrhosis to manifest end-stage liver disease cannot be determined at this time.

3. CHRONIC HEPATITIS IN PATIENTS WITH CLOTTING FACTOR DISORDERS

A large body of data on chronic hepatitis has now accrued from studies of multiply transfused patients with congenital bleeding disorders. Ironically, the clotting factor concentrates that have been instrumental in transmitting hepatitis to these patients have now provided adequate coagulation support to safely allow for liver biopsy documentation of the chronic hepatitis they induced. The proportion of hemophiliac patients infected by blood products is astounding. In most studies,[17] 75–95% have serologic markers indicating current or past infection with HBV and 45–80% have chronic ALT elevations, suggesting a high prevalence of NANBH. This chapter concentrates only on those studies in which liver histology is available and in which the occurrence of NANBH can be inferred by serologic, morphologic, or histochemical exclusion of HBV.

The first report of liver biopsies in patients with hemophilia comes from Lesesne and coworkers,[18] who selected six patients for biopsy from their hemophilia cohort, in which 50% have chronic ALT elevations. These six patients were selected on the basis of a twofold elevation in ALT over a 6-month period combined with clinical symptoms compatible with chronic hepatitis; two of the six patients were HBsAg positive. On liver biopsy, three of six had CAH, and the remaining three had CPH; two of the three CAH cases were HBsAg positive. One of the three CAH cases had early postnecrotic cirrhosis, and a second patient subsequently developed clinical signs of progression to cirrhosis, including esophageal varices and ascites. The one patient with biopsy documented cirrhosis was HBsAg negative and presumably had chronic NANBH.

A series of reports on liver biopsies in hemophilia patients appeared in 1978 and can be summarized as follows: First, Spero et al.[19] examined 14 liver biopsies from 13 asymptomatic patients with chronic transaminase elevation; eight patients showed CPH, three had CAH, one nonalcoholic patient had fatty infiltration with advance portal fibrosis, and one had CAH with postnecrotic cirrhosis. None of these patients was HBsAg positive, and all had anti-HBs, suggesting recovery from past HBV infection. This serologic pattern would usually suggest that the chronic hepatitis was unrelated to HBV. However, using indirect immunofluorescence, Spero found nuclear and cytoplasmic fluorescence in eight of 12 liver biopsies reacted with antisera containing anti-HBs

Table I. Development of Chronic Hepatitis, Cirrhosis, and Liver-Related Fatality in Non-A, Non-B Hepatitis[a]

Setting	Investigators	Total NANBH cases	Number (%) with chronic hepatitis[e]	Histologic outcome: Number biopsied	Histologic outcome: Number CAH	Histologic outcome: Number (%) cirrhosis[f]	Liver-related fatality: Number	Liver-related fatality: Percent biopsied	Liver-related fatality: Percent of cirrhosis cases
Transfusion-associated	Knodell et al.[7]	44	10 (23)[g]	10	8	1 (10)	0	—	—
	Rakela and Redeker[8]	45[h]	18 (40)	14	3	1 (7)	1	7	100
	Alter and co-workers[9,10]	75	51 (68)	32	15	7 (22)[b]	2[i]	6	29
	Iwarson et al.[11]	NS	6[j]	6[c]	4	1 (17)[b]	1	17	100
	Realdi et al.[12,14]	NS	61	41[d]	14	14 (34)[b]	1	2	7
	Omata et al.[13]	24	13 (54)	5[c]	2	1 (20)	0	—	—
	Kiyosawa et al.[15]	70	32 (46)	14	5	0	0	—	—
	Koretz et al.[6,16]	69	46 (67)	21	NS	4 (19)[b]	1	5	25
	Totals in biopsied population			143	—	29 (20%)	6	4	21
Clotting factor-associated	Aledort et al.[24]	NS	155	155[k]	11 (7%)[l]	23 (15)	NS	—	—
	Hay et al.[25]	79	56 (71)	34	9	8 (24)[b,m]	2[n]	6	25
	Totals in biopsied population			189	20	31 (16%)	—	—	—

[a]CAH, chronic active hepatitis; Cirrh, cirrhosis; NS, not stated (usually because chronic NANBH cases selected from a population whose total number is not specified).
[b]Studies in which at least two chronic-phase liver biopsies were obtained.
[c]Studies in which acute- and chronic-phase biopsies were obtained.
[d]Acute-phase biopsy in 15 of 41.
[e]Chronic hepatitis generally defined as ALT elevations for greater than 1 year.
[f]Classified as cirrhosis if cirrhosis was present in conjunction with CAH or if cirrhosis subsequently developed in a patient originally categorized as having CAH.
[g]Some patients received immune serum globulin or hepatitis B immune globulin, which was stated to decrease the incidence of chronic hepatitis.
[h]Studies of patients hospitalized with NANBH; 54% of NANBH cases classified as transfusion related.
[i]Two cases in which death was directly attributable to liver failure and a third case in which liver failure was the indirect cause.
[j]Four cases had anti-HAV but are classified here as NANBH because the occurrence of chronic hepatitis A has not been documented.
[k]International collaborative study of Ad Hoc Hemophilia Study Group. Includes submitted biopsies from multiple centers, some of which reported in earlier publications.[18–23]
[l]These were severe CAH cases with considerable likelihood of progressing to cirrhosis.
[m]Includes seven cases of biopsy-documented cirrhosis and one case in which cirrhosis presumed on the basis of spider nevi, splenomegaly, and esophageal varices.
[n]In addition, three other cirrhotic patients had radiographic evidence of esophageal varices.

and/or anti-HBc. It is unclear whether this hepatic fluorescence indicates that the chronic hepatitis was HBV related or whether these fluorescence reactions were independent of the chronic disease, which was NANBV related.

Second, Mannucci et al.[20] performed liver biopsy in 11 patients with severe hemophilia that had three consecutive abnormal ALT values obtained over a 3-year interval; four patients had CPH, and one had a history and histologic pattern suggesting alcoholic liver disease. In the remaining six patients, five had CAH and one had postnecrotic cirrhosis. Furthermore, three of the five patients with CAH had severe histologic disease, with two showing central to portal bridging necrosis and one fibrous septa diagnosed as CAH in transition to cirrhosis.

Third, Preston et al.[21] performed a similar study in England in which liver biopsy was performed on eight symptom-free hemophiliac patients with persistent ALT abnormality; 50% of these patients had CAH (two cases) or micronodular cirrhosis (two cases). All but one patient was HBsAg negative, and HBsAg was not detected in the biopsy tissue.

These 1978 studies in composite demonstrate a recurrent pattern in the hemophilia population, which includes (1) elevated ALT in most patients, (2) minimal clinical symptoms to suggest underlying liver disease, (3) a histologic pattern that is considerably more severe than suggested by either clinical status or the degree of transaminase elevation, and (4) cirrhosis in 12.5%, with additional patients showing CAH in transition to cirrhosis.

By contrast, other studies in hemophiliac patients suggest the almost uniformly benign nature of the chronic hepatitis. In 1982, White et al.[22] reported liver biopsy results on 15 patients selected because of intermittent rather than continuous ALT elevations. None of the patients biopsied displayed evidence of liver disease by history or physical examination. On biopsy, 11 of 15 had CPH, three had mild portal inflammation, and one had CAH with mild fibrosis. White et al. stress the mild histologic picture as compared with the studies cited above, but it is to be noted that the investigators intent was to examine the histologic outcome in those with milder biochemical evidence of hepatitis, and they therefore excluded from biopsy those with persistent ALT elevations. Furthermore, the mean ALT in those biopsied was only 60 ± 52, compared with 136 ± 99 in the group that was not biopsied. No follow-up biopsies were reported.

In 1982, Mannucci et al.[23] emphasized the nonprogressive nature of chronic NANBH in hemophiliacs. This report consisted of follow-up biopsies in 11 hemophiliac patients whose initial biopsy was reported in 1978.[20] These 11 patients had had 3 years of persistent ALT elevations prior to their initial biopsy; the subsequent biopsy was obtained 3 years later. The second series of biopsies, compared with the initial series, showed continuation of chronic persistent hepatitis in four of 11 patients and a minor change from CPH to chronic lobular hepatitis in two patients. Hence, these six patients were essentially unchanged over the 3-year interval. Furthermore, four patients initially diagnosed as having CAH or as being in transition between CPH and CAH were found to have a lessened degree of inflammation on repeat biopsy. One patient, who initially had active cirrhosis, died of liver failure, but this patient was HBsAg positive and also had Delta antigen on liver biopsy. Manucci et al. conclude that progressive liver disease is not the usual outcome in hemophiliacs who have chronic NANBH.

The most comprehensive analysis of chronic liver disease among hemophiliacs was a collaborative study initiated by the Ad Hoc Hemophilia Study Group.[24] This group contacted the major hemophilia treatment centers throughout the world and collected biopsy specimens from 155 hemophiliac patients; 115 were percutaneous liver biopsies, and the other 40 were obtained at autopsy. These biopsies were submitted under code to a panel of four of the world's leading hepatopathologists. Most biopsies (64%) were classified as trivial, mild, or moderate and included cases of CPH and some mild forms of CAH. Of greatest significance in this analysis was the fact that 15% of patients had cirrhosis, and an additional 7% had severe CAH, which would presumably progress to cirrhosis. This finding of approximately 15–20% of patients with chronic hepatitis demonstrating cirrhosis or severe CAH is consistent with findings in posttransfusion hepatitis studies of nonhemophiliac patients. As in other studies, the results of hepatitic biochemical tests did not predict the degree of hepatic histologic change. Although in this analysis of 155 liver biopsies some patients were HBsAg positive, none of the biopsies showed the characteristic "ground-glass" cells of hepatitis B involvement, and the liver histology was most consistent with that of chronic NANBH. It was thus believed that all or at least most of these severe chronic cases were attributable to NANB viral infection. It cannot be determined from this composite study[24] how many of these 155 biopsies were from patients previously cited in other studies included in this review.[18–23] It seems clear however, that the majority of hemophiliac patients with chronic transaminase elevations have a mild form of chronic liver disease, but that approximately 20% have evidence of severe liver disease including cirrhosis and severe CAH. In contrast to the study of Mannucci et al.,[23] Hay et al.[25] present evidence for severe progressive liver disease in patients with hemophilia. This study from England documents the potentially devastating effects of chronic hepatitis in the hemophilia population. In this 8-year study of 79 unselected patients with hemophilia who had received clotting factor concentrates, 56 (71%) had persistently abnormal ALT levels. An initial biopsy was performed in 34 patients, showing CPH in 20, chronic lobular hepatitis in one, CAH in nine, and established cirrhosis in four; one of these four cirrhotic cases was believed to be related to alcoholic liver damage. Of greatest significance in this study were repeat liver biopsies in nine patients who had persistently abnormal ALT for at least 2 years after the initial biopsy. In this group, six of the nine patients showed progressive liver disease on their subsequent biopsy, and only one patient showed a lessening histologic lesion. Of greatest interest was the fact that four patients initially diagnosed as having CPH nonetheless went on to progressive disease, with two developing CAH and two developing cirrhosis. Two other cases of cirrhosis were noted in patients initially diagnosed as having CAH. Thus, in addition to the three cases of cirrhosis noted at initial biopsy, four additional cases occurred while under observation and overall, seven of 34 biopsied patients (21%) appeared to develop cirrhosis as a result of their chronic transfusion-induced hepatitis. In addition to these seven documented cases of NANBH-induced cirrhosis, an eighth patient developed spider nevi, splenomegaly, and esophageal varices and had probable cirrhosis, although not documented by biopsy. The clinical features in these patients were more devastating than in any other published report; two patients with cirrhosis died from intracerebral hemmorhage, one of whom had hepatic encephalopathy and esophageal varices at death. A total of five cirrhotic patients had radiologic evidence of esophageal varices. Overall, in the Hay study of 79 hemophiliac patients selected solely on the basis of previous exposure to blood products, 17 had evidence of progressive liver disease, with eight developing nonalcoholic cirrhosis and nine CAH. Serial liver biopsies showed progression of CPH and CAH to cirrhosis within a period of 2–6 years. The eight cases of virus-induced cirrhosis represented 10% of the 79 patients enrolled in the study, 14% of the 56 patients with persistently abnormal ALT and 24% of the 34 patients who underwent liver biopsy. None of the patients with severe disease in this study had histologic or serologic evidence to indicate that they were chronic HBV carriers. Most had histologic evidence of NANBH, including seven of the nine who underwent a second liver biopsy. As in all such studies, most hemophiliac patients had persistent or intermittently abnormal ALT elevations, and neither the degree of biochemical abnormality nor the physical signs predicted the nature or severity of the underlying liver disease.

Although the above-cited studies indicate that some hemophiliac patients with chronic NANBV-induced cirrhosis succumb to end-stage liver disease, it is difficult to obtain an accurate estimate of liver-related fatalities in this disease population. The current estimate is that 5–10% of hemophiliac patients die of chronic liver disease and that this proportion might increase as additional time elapses for the further development of transfusion-associated cirrhosis. In an analysis of data supplied by the National Center for Health Statistics, Aronson[26] assessed 949 death records from patients with hemophilia A. These data are based on death certificates filed by individual states for 1968–1979. It is unknown what proportion of diagnoses in hemophiliacs are confirmed by postmortem examination and hence included in this death certificate information, but in the general population, it is estimated that 16% of death diagnoses are based on postmortem examination. Within the limitations of this sampling error, Aronson found hepatitis to be the leading infectious cause of death in patients with hemophilia. These infectious deaths include acute infectious complications, primarily fulminant hepatitis, and do not include late sequelae, such as posthepatitic cirrhosis. Most cases of fulminant hepatitis occurred during 1968–1974 prior to the introduction of more sensitive screening test for HBsAg and probably represent acute fulminant type B hepatitis. Of the total 949 deaths, cirrhosis was stated to be the major cause of death in 36 cases (4%). The primary pathogenesis of these cirrhotic cases was thought to be virus-induced hepatitis. Cirrhosis was listed as an additional cause of death in another 40 patients, such that 8% of deaths in hemophiliacs were associated directly or indirectly with cirrhosis. While the number of deaths due to NANBH-associated cirrhosis will continue to accrue in the hemophilia population, since a large cohort already has chronic NANBH, the number of new NANBV infections should be greatly diminished by the advent of heat-treated clotting factor concentrates and by the probability that even more potent and effective inactivation procedures will soon be implemented. In the hemophilia population, there are some parallels between transfusion-associated AIDS and transfusion-associated chronic hepatitis. The former is obviously more devastating and of deeper concern, but the parallel is that both infections: (1) occurred primarily before the advent of specific assays, hence at a time when we were powerless to prevent them; (2) infected a large proportion of the hemophilia population; (3) have a long latent period to significant disease development, and (4) may be ultimately fatal, albeit to a much lesser extent in NANBH than in HIV infection. Extremely important is the fact that both HIV and NANBV are susceptible to inactivation procedures that are already in place and that will undoubtedly become even more effective in the near future. Therefore, new infections with these viruses will occur at diminishing and perhaps negligible rates and the long-term prognosis for hemophilia patients not yet infected with these agents is extremely encouraging. The combination of potent clotting factor concentrates, sensitive viral screening procedures, and effective inactivation procedures portends great optimism for the hemophilia population and suggests a continuing trend toward a normal life-style and a normal life span.

4. THE ASSOCIATION BETWEEN NON-A, NON-B HEPATITIS AND HEPATOCELLULAR CARCINOMA

There is now an unequivocal link between chronic HBV infection and the development of hepatocellular carcinoma (HCC). The epidemiologic studies that documented this association were highly dependent on the development of sensitive serologic markers to trace exposure to and persistence of HBV. In a remarkable study among Taiwanese government workers, Beasley et al.[27] demonstrated that HBsAg-positive persons were at a greater than 200-fold increased risk of developing HCC than were HBsAg-negative persons. In addition, there is a dramatic overlap in the areas of high prevalence of HBsAg and the areas of high prevalence of HCC. In the absence of a serologic marker for NANBV, such definitive epidemiologic studies cannot be performed. We are thus dependent on the observation of HCC developing in patients presumed to have chronic NANBH and in the analysis of HCC cases in which other known factors, such as alcoholism and HBV infection, can be reasonably excluded. Such indirect evidence of a relationship between NANBV and HCC is beginning to accumulate.

In a study by Tabor et al.[28] investigating hepatocellular carcinoma cases in the United States, approximately one fourth of nonalcoholic patients with HCC had no evidence of HBV markers, suggesting a possible role of other viruses in the pathogenesis of their HCC. In 1983, Resnick et al.[29] reported a single case of a 42-year-old woman who developed acute NANBH five weeks after the administration of 6 units of whole blood. During the following 15 years, anicteric chronic liver disease was repeatedly documented by serum transaminase but not by liver biopsy. In 1981, 16 years after the onset of her TAH, progressive jaundice, constitutional symptoms and a hard, nodular, enlarged liver resulted in hospital admission wherein a markedly elevated α-fetoprotein (AFP) was noted and liver scan and liver biopsy demonstrated a massive hepatocellular carcinoma.

The patient was consistently negative for hepatitis B viral markers and other potential causes of PHC, including alcoholism, anabolic steroids, hemochromatosis, and α_1-antitrypsin deficiency were excluded. In 1984, Gilliam et al.[30] reported a similar case, in which acute transfusion-associated NANBH was followed by the development of biopsy-proven CAH. Nine years after the onset of acute hepatitis, the patient became progressively ill and was found to have an enlarged liver with a firm irregular border and elevated AFP. Liver biopsy revealed cirrhosis with both macronodular and micronodular elements and hepatocelluar carcinoma. All hepatitis B markers were once again negative, including HBV DNA polymerase and HBV DNA. This case and that described by Resnick et al.[29] suggest that HCC may develop during the course of chronic NANB post-transfusion hepatitis. Sequential progression from acute TAH to HCC was most dramatically documented in a case reported by Kiyosawa et al.[31] in Japan. In this patient, biopsy-documented acute NANBH was followed by sequential histologic progression to CPH, CAH, CAH with bridging necrosis, cirrhosis, and finally to HCC. The interval from the development of acute hepatitis to HCC was 19 years. Although this represents only a single case report, the absence of hepatitis B markers, the absence of other known etiologic factors associated with HCC and the extremely well-documented histologic progression from acute hepatitis through cirrhosis to hepatocellular carcinoma makes an extremely strong case for an association between the NANB agent and this form of hepatic cancer.

A serologic analysis of 113 nonalcoholic patients with biopsy-proven HCC in Japan further supports the association between NANBH and HCC.[32] Of the 113 HCC patients, 35 were HBsAg positive, 23 were negative for all hepatitis B markers, and 55 were negative for HBsAg but positive for antibody to the surface and/or code proteins of HBV. Having excluded alcohol, immune liver disease, hereditary factors, and the HBV, it was suspected that the 23 seronegative cases of HCC were NANBV related. In addition, and for similar reasons, it is possible, if not probable, that the 55 HBsAg-negative cases with anti-HBs and/or anti-HBc were also NANBV related. In the Beasley study in Taiwan,[26] the incidence of hepatocellular carcinoma in patients with anti-HBs or anti-HBc in the absence of HBsAg was similar to the incidence in those who had no HBV markers. Thus, while anti-HBc and/or anti-HBs indicate past exposure to HBV in this population with HCC, these hepatitis B markers do not imply a causal relationship. It would have been of interest to have data on the presence of HBV DNA in its episomal or integrated form in the liver tissue of these HCC patients, but such data are not available. The strong potential association between NANBV and HCC in Japan is not inconsistent with other data from the United States indicating the inordinantly high frequency of NANBV-related chronic liver disease.

5. SUMMARY

It is apparent that acute NANBH is a frequent consequence of transfusion therapy, particularly among recipients of commercial clotting factor concentrates. It is also apparent that most individuals with NANBH develop a biochemical pattern indicative of chronic inflammatory disease of the liver. Liver biopsy in those with chronic transaminse elevations indicates that the predominant lesion is histologically benign but that 15–20% of biopsied patients have developed cirrhosis and that some of these patients with cirrhosis succumb to end-stage liver disease (see Table I). The primary unresolved issue is whether the histologic appearance of cirrhosis connotes a clinically severe outcome or whether such cirrhosis is compatible with a normal life span. It seems apparent from most studies that the cirrhosis that accompanies chronic NANBH is clinically indolent compared with classic alcoholic cirrhosis or that associated with autoimmune forms of chronic liver disease. Such comparisons, however, may reflect the total duration of disease and the likelihood of recurrent injury rather than the severity of the cirrhosis per se. In other words, the severe outcome recognized in alcoholic cirrhosis may reflect not only the major and recurrent injury induced by repeated alcohol abuse, but also an almost lifelong process that manifests itself only when the end stages become apparent. By contrast, except in the hemophiliac situation, post-transfusion hepatitis tends to be a disease occurring late in life, when the frequency of transfusion increases dramatically and is most commonly a single event related to a particular transfusion episode. The terminal cirrhotic events may therefore require a longer interval than has been attained in most prospective studies conducted thus far or will not be attained because death from intercurrent causes will intervene in this predominantly elderly population. Of interest in this regard is the Japanese study,[15] in which chronic hepatitis, cirrhosis, and HCC were retrospectively related to a history of prior blood transfusion; the interval to the need for hospitalization for cirrhosis was exceedingly long and in the range of 17 years. By contrast, the histologic transition from acute NANBH to chronic hepatitis and then to cirrhosis has often been documented to occur in less than a 4-year interval. The progression from acute to chronic hepatitis to cirrhosis has been histologically documented on sufficient occasions to establish this pathway unequivocally as a potential deleterious outcome of transfusion therapy. The residual argument relates to how often this progression occurs and to whether the interval to the clinical presentation of cirrhosis is so long that for most tranfusion recipients this potential consequence is clinically irrelevant. From the standpoint of national statistics and health planning, these are pertinent questions and important issues to resolve. However, from the standpoint of the individual blood recipient, particularly the young recipient, it is important to recognize that acute and chronic hepatitis are not uncommon consequences of transfusion therapy and that the chronic hepatitis may eventuate in cirrhosis, which in turn may be fatal or be associated with significant morbidity.

The long disease-free interval and the potential that some post-transfusion cirrhosis may not have a relentlessly progressive course makes this problem less than might be projected from prospective studies. Nonetheless, severe cirrhosis is a documented sequela of transfusion therapy, and all reasonable measures to prevent its occurrence should be instituted. Transfusion services have made major advances to confront this problem, including the adoption of an all volunteer donor system, testing for HBsAg, the more recent institution of testing donors for ALT and anticore antibody, and the now universal application of heat treatment for all products transfused to hemophiliac patients. In addition, screening measures instituted to prevent transmission of AIDS will also indirectly decrease the donor population at risk of transmitting viral hepatitis. While a specific NANB test does not appear to be imminent, a major effort is being advanced in the area of viral inactivation. This approach has already achieved considerable success for plasma and plasma derivatives, and methods must now be evolved which can inactivate viruses in cellular blood products. Some methods of nucleic acid inactivation have already been successful in preventing hepatitis transmission in the chimpanzee and could theoretically be applied to the cellular components of blood transfusion.

Despite the emphasis of this chapter on the serious chronic consequences of blood transfusion therapy, it is clear that such therapy is remarkably safer than it was a decade ago, or even 5 years ago, and that there is a realistic hope that in the near future blood transfusions will no longer be a significant mechanism for the transmission of infectious disease.

REFERENCES

1. Alter HJ, Purcell RH, Holland PV, et al: Transmissible agent in non-A, non-B hepatitis. *Lancet* **1**:459–463, 1978.
2. Bradley BW, Cook EH, Maynard JE, et al: Experimental infection of chimpanzees with anti-hemophiliac (Factor VIII) materials: Recovery of virus-like particles associated with non-A, non-B hepatitis. *J Med Virol* **3**:253–259, 1979.
3. Alter HJ, Hoofnagle JH: Non-A, non-B: Observations on the first decade, in Vyas GN, Dienstag JL, Hoofnagle JH (eds): *Viral Hepatitis and Liver Disease*. Grune & Stratton, Orlando, Florida, 1984, pp. 345–354.

4. Barcena R, Suarez-Garcia E, Gil LA: Posttransfusion non-A, non-B hepatitis: A prospective study. *Liver* **5**:71–76, 1985.
5. Galbraith, RM, Portmann B, Eddleston ALWF, et al: Chronic liver disease developing after outbreak of HBsAg negative hepatitis in hemodialysis unit. *Lancet* **2**:886–889, 1975.
6. Koretz RL, Suffin SC, Gitnick GL: Post-transfusion chronic liver disease. *Gastroenterology* **71**:797–803, 1976.
7. Knodell RG, Conrad NE, Ishak KG: Development of chronic liver disease after acute non-A, non-B post-transfusion hepatitis: Role of gamma globulin prophylaxis in its prevention. *Gastroenterology* **72**:902–909, 1977.
8. Rakela J, Redeker AG: Chronic liver disease after acute non-A, non-B viral hepatitis. *Gastroenterology* **77**:1200–1202, 1979.
9. Berman M, Alter HJ, Ishak KG, et al: The chronic sequelae of non-A, non-B hepatitis. *Ann Intern Med* **91**:1–6, 1979.
10. Alter HJ: Transfusion associated non-A, non-B hepatitis: The first decade, in Zuckerman AJ (ed): *Viral Hepatitis and Liver Disease*. Liss, New York, 1988, pp. 537–542.
11. Iwarson S, Lindberg J, Lundin P: Progression of hepatitis non-A, non-B to chronic active hepatitis: A histologic follow-up of two cases. *J Clin Pathol* **32**:351–355, 1979.
12. Realdi G, Alberti A, Rugge M, et al: Long-term follow-up of acute and chronic non-A, non-B post-transfusion hepatitis: Evidence of progression to liver cirrhosis. *Gut* **23**:270–275, 1982.
13. Omata M, Iwama S, Sumida M et al: Clinico-pathological study of acute non-A, non-B post-transfusion hepatitis: Histological features of liver biopsies in acute phase. *Liver* **1**:201–208, 1981.
14. Realdi G, Tremolada F, Bortolotti F, et al: The natural history of post-transfusion and sporadic non-A, non-B Hepatitis in Italy in Verme G, Bonino F, Rizzetto M (eds): *Viral Hepatitis and Delta Infection*. Liss, New York, 1983, pp. 55–66.
15. Kiyosawa K, Akahane Y, Nagata A, et al: Significance of blood transfusion in non-A, non-B chronic liver disease in Japan. *Vox Sang* **43**:45–52, 1982.
16. Koretz RL, Stone O, Mousa M, et al: Non-A, non-B posttransfusion hepatitis—A decade later. *Gastroenterology* **88**:1251–1254, 1985.
17. Seeff LB: Hepatitis in hemophilia: A brief review, in Burk PB, Chalmers TC (eds): *Frontiers in Liver Disease*. Thieme-Stratton, New York, 1981, pp. 231–241.
18. Lesesne HR, Morgan JE, Blatt PM, et al: Liver biopsy in hemophilia A. *Ann Intern Med* **86**:703–707, 1977.
19. Spero JA, Lewis JH, Van Thiel DH, et al: Asymptomatic structural liver disease in hemophilia. *N Engl J Med* **298**:1373–1378, 1978.
20. Mannucci PM, Ronchi G, Rota L, et al: A clinicopathological study of liver disease in hemophiliacs. *J Clin Pathol* **31**:779–783, 1978.
21. Preston FE, Triger DR, Underwood JCE, et al: Percutaneous liver biopsy in chronic liver disease in haemophiliacs. *Lancet* **2**:592–594, 1978.
22. White GC II, Zeitler KD, Lesesne HR, et al: Chronic hepatitis patients with hemophilia A: Histologic studies in patients with intermittently abnormal liver function tests. *Blood* **60**:1259–1262, 1982.
23. Mannucci PM, Colombo M, Rizzetto M: Nonprogressive course of non-A, non-B chronic hepatitis in multitransfused hemophiliacs. *Blood* **60**:655–658, 1982.
24. Aledort LM, Levine PH, Hilgartner M, et al: A study of liver biopsies and liver disease among hemophiliacs. *Blood* **66**:367–372, 1985.
25. Hay CRM, Preston FE, Triger DR, et al: Progressive liver disease in haemophilia: An understated problem? *Lancet* **1**:1495–1497, 1985.
26. Aronson DL: Cause of death in hemophilia A patients in the United States from 1968–1979. *Am J Hematol* **27**:7–12, 1988.
27. Beasley RP, Hwang LY, Lin CC et al: Hepatocellular carcinoma and hepatitis B virus: A prospective study of 22,707 men in Taiwan. *Lancet* 2:1129–1133, 1981.
28. Tabor E, Gerety RJ, Vogel CL, et al: Hepatitis B virus infection and primary hepatocellular carcinoma. *J Natl Cancer Inst* **58**:1197–1200, 1977.
29. Resnick RH, Stone K, Antonioli D: Primary hepatocellular carcinoma following non-A, non-B posttransfusion hepatitis. *Dig Dis Sci* **28**:908–911, 1983.
30. Gilliam JH, Geissinger KR, Richter JE: Primary hepatocellular carcinoma after chronic non-A, non-B posttransfusion hepatitis: *Ann Intern Med* **101**:794–795, 1984.

31. Kiyosawa K, Akahane Y, Nagata A, et al: Hepatocellular carcinoma after non-A, non-B posttransfusion hepatitis. *Am J Gastroenterol* **79**:777–781, 1984.
32. Okuda H, Obata H, Motoike Y, et al: Clinicopathological features of hepatocellular carcinoma—Comparison of hepatitis B seropositive and seronegative patients. *Hepatogastroenterology* **31**:64–68, 1984.

9

Acute Non-A, Non-B Hepatitis: The Pathologist's Perspective

Zachary D. Goodman

1. INTRODUCTION

The pathologist takes a somewhat different view of viral hepatitis than does the clinician. The pathologic view is colored by the circumstances in which tissue is obtained for examination. This in turn is often dictated by the clinical indications for biopsy with a relative increase in either atypical or chronic cases, or both, and it is also skewed toward the more severe cases seen at autopsy. The spectrum of such cases is illustrated by the consultations seen at the Armed Forces Institute of Pathology (AFIP). The Hepatic Department of the AFIP reviewed 119 cases, both biopsy and autopsy, during 1986 in which the likelihood of non-A, non-B (NANB) hepatitis was raised by the clinical circumstances (Table I). These were nearly all diagnoses of exclusion in which the morphologic patterns were consistent with viral hepatitis, the serologic studies excluded hepatitis A and B, and no drug likely to cause a hepatitis-like injury could be implicated. Of these cases, 23% showed an acute injury, with 15 cases (13%) of acute hepatitis and 12 cases (10%) of massive or submassive necrosis.

2. DIFFICULTIES IN INTERPRETATION

There is currently no indication for biopsy in a typical case of acute post-transfusion NANB viral hepatitis, and so cases that come to biopsy usually have some confusing clinical features that the biopsy is expected to resolve. The following case illustrates the problem as encountered in practice.

Case 1

A 38-year-old woman had noted increasing pain in her left hip for several years. This gradually became constant and severe, limiting her activities, and was not relieved by analgesics or glucocor-

Zachary D. Goodman • Department of Hepatic Pathology, Armed Forces Institute of Pathology, Washington, D.C. 20306. The opinions and assertions contained herein are the private views of the author and are not to be construed as official or as reflecting the views of the Department of the Army or the Department of Defense.

Table I. Morphologic Patterns in Presumed Non-A, Non-B Viral Hepatitis among Cases Seen in Consultation at the AFIP during 1986

Condition	*N*
Acute hepatitis	27
Submassive necrosis	12
Chronic persistent hepatitis	12
Chronic active hepatitis	54
Cirrhosis	26
Total cases	119

ticoid injections. She underwent surgical exploration, and a gray, friable tumor that proved to be a synovial sarcoma was found involving the hip joint and sciatic nerve. Approximately 400 g of tumor was removed. The patient lost a great deal of blood intraoperatively and through postoperative drains, and so she was transfused 2 units of whole blood.

After recovery from surgery, the patient was scheduled for radiotherapy and chemotherapy. There was no evidence of tumor metastasis. Radiation to the left hip began 5 weeks after surgery, with 6000 rad given over 6 weeks. Chemotherapy was begun 11 days after the start of radiation (46 days after surgery). The patient received cyclophosphamide 425 mg IV (one dose) on the first day, dacarbazine (DTIC) 200 mg IV daily for 5 days (days 1–5), and vincristine 1.5 mg IV (two doses) on the first and sixth days. The patient tolerated the chemotherapy well. However, elevated liver enzymes were noted on the last day of chemotherapy, and aspartate aminotransferase (AST) and alanine aminotransferase (ALT) ranged from two to three times normal over the next 3 weeks. Alkaline phosphatase and bilirubin were normal, and the patient had no symptoms of liver disease. Serum HBsAg, anti-HB core (anti-HBc), and anti-hepatitis A (anti-HAV) were all negative. Computed tomography (CT) of the liver showed no mass lesion. A laparoscopically directed liver biopsy was done with clinical suspicion of metastasis versus drug-induced liver injury.

The biopsy (Figs. 1–3) shows mild acinar zone 3 (centrilobular) ballooning degeneration, scattered focal necrosis, free acidophilic bodies, Kupffer cell hypertrophy, and mild to moderate patchy portal inflammation with a predominance of lymphocytes. The features are those of an acute hepatocellular injury. In addition, a mild degree of hepatocellular fat accumulation is scattered throughout the biopsy. There is no evidence of vascular damage and no tumor.

The differential diagnosis in this case included viral hepatitis, drug-induced hepatic injury, or metastatic tumor. The biopsy shows features of an acute hepatocellular injury with ballooning, acidophilic bodies, focal necrosis, spotty hepatocellular dropout, and resulting inflammatory response. These features are consistent with either a mild acute viral hepatitis or a mild drug-induced hepatitis-like injury. On the basis of literature precedents, none of the drugs received by the patient is likely to have caused this type of hepatocellular injury. Cyclophosphamide has very rarely been associated with hepatic injury in a handful of cases, apparently as an idiosyncratic hypersensitivity reaction.[1,2] Dacarbazine has caused veno-occlusive disease,[3] but the biopsy shows nothing to suggest that type of injury. The history of blood transfusion 7 weeks before the onset of the injury makes an acute post-transfusion NANB viral hepatitis much more likely. The presence of fat in the biopsy caused some concern when the case was originally reviewed and led some observers to favor a toxic, i.e., drug-induced, injury, despite its unlikelihood. However, fat may be seen in viral hepatitis[4,5] and should not dissuade one from the diagnosis.

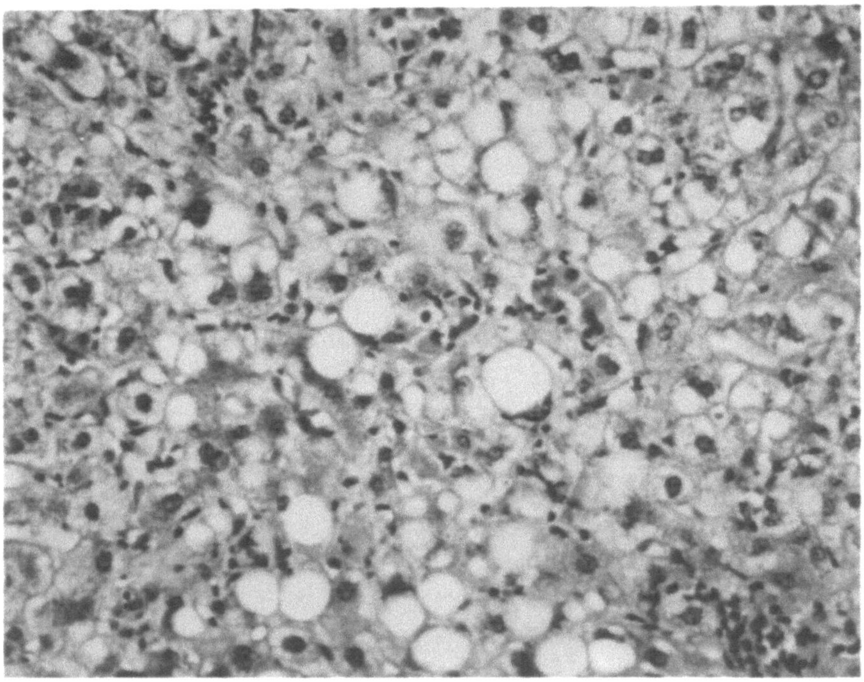

Figure 1. Liver biopsy in Case 1, showing fatty change in addition to diffuse hepatocellular injury and sinusoidal mononuclear inflammatory infiltrate. (H&E, ×250; AFIP neg. 87-5978)

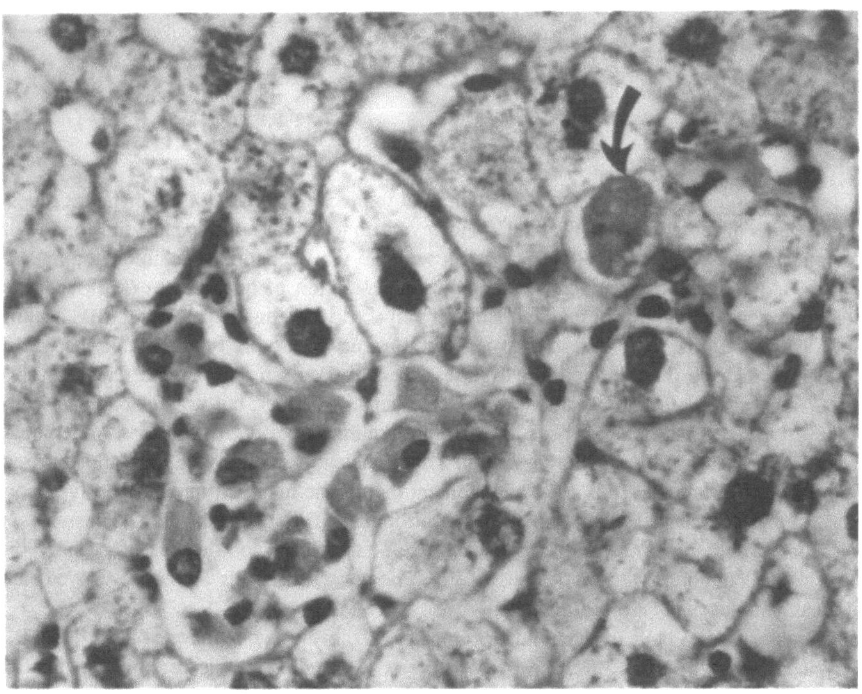

Figure 2. Acute NANB (Case 1) with hepatocellular ballooning degeneration, an acidophilic body (arrow), and a cluster of hypertrophied Kupffer cells and lymphocytes. (H&E, ×630; AFIP neg. 87-5979)

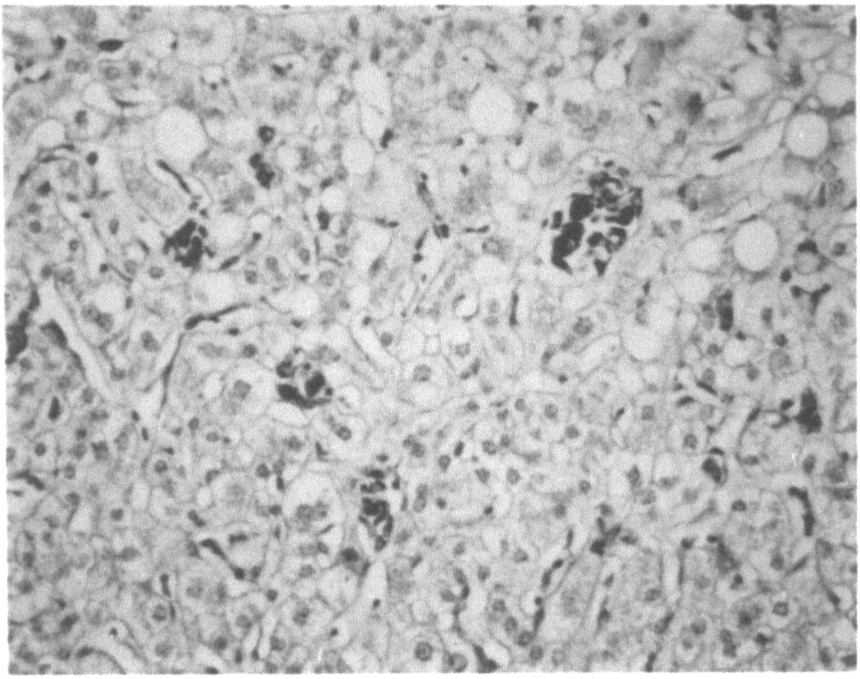

Figure 3. Spotty parenchymal necrosis in acute NANB hepatitis (Case 1). Clusters of hypertrophied lipofuscin-laden Kupffer cells (dark staining) mark foci of hepatocellular necrosis and dropout. (PAS stain after diastase digestion, ×250; AFIP neg. 87-5980)

3. COMPARATIVE HISTOLOGIC FINDINGS OF NANB INFECTION

Various histologic features have been suggested to be characteristic of the different types and causative agents of acute hepatitis (Table II). However, no feature is entirely specific, for any of the common viruses (A, B, D, and NANB) that cause acute viral hepatitis. Features cited as characteristic of NANB include prominent eosinophilic degeneration of hepatocytes (Fig. 4), a heavy sinusoidal mononuclear cell infiltrate and Kupffer cell activation, and hepatocellular fat accumulation (Fig. 1), but all may be found in biopsies from patients with other types of acute hepatitis.[4–6]

Injury of the bile duct epithelium, first described by Poulsen and Christoffersen in chronic hepatitis,[7] may also be found in patients with acute hepatitis. Most, but not all, patients with this lesion have NANB hepatitis, and these have a high likelihood of progression to chronic hepatitis. The lesion is characterized by swelling, vacuolization, nuclear irregularity, and pseudostratification of the biliary epithelial cells (Fig. 5). The basement membrane may be ruptured, and lymphocytes with occasional plasma cells and sometimes neutrophils infiltrate the duct. The lesion is very reminiscent of, and sometimes indistinguishable from, the florid duct lesions of primary biliary cirrhosis (PBC). In contrast to the lesions of PBC, however, the ducts are not destroyed, and so portal areas without ducts are seldom seen.

Two major studies have presented data comparing the histologic features of acute NANB with those of acute hepatitis A and B (Table III). Kryger et al.[5] studied the biopsies of 76 patients with acute NANB and compared them with 86 cases of hepatitis A and 78 cases of acute hepatitis B. Schmidt et al.[6] compared 24 cases of NANB with 15 each of hepatitis A and B. Neither study found

Table II. Morphologic Findings Frequently Noted in Different Types of Acute Viral Hepatitis or Hepatitis-like Drug Injury

Agent(s)	Morphologic features	References
Hepatitis A	Portal–periportal injury	5,6,10–12
	Plasma cells	
	Cholestasis	
Hepatitis B	Panlobular injury with or without central accentuation	5,6,11–13
	Lymphocytes	
Non-A, non-B	Acidophilic bodies	4–6,14
	Rhomboid cells	
	Sinusoidal inflammatory cells	
	Fat	
	Bile duct injury	
Hepatitis D (S. Am.)	Microvesicular fat	15–18
	Eosinophilic necrosis	
Drug	Zonal injury	1,19
	Eosinophils	
	Cholestasis	
	Granulomas	

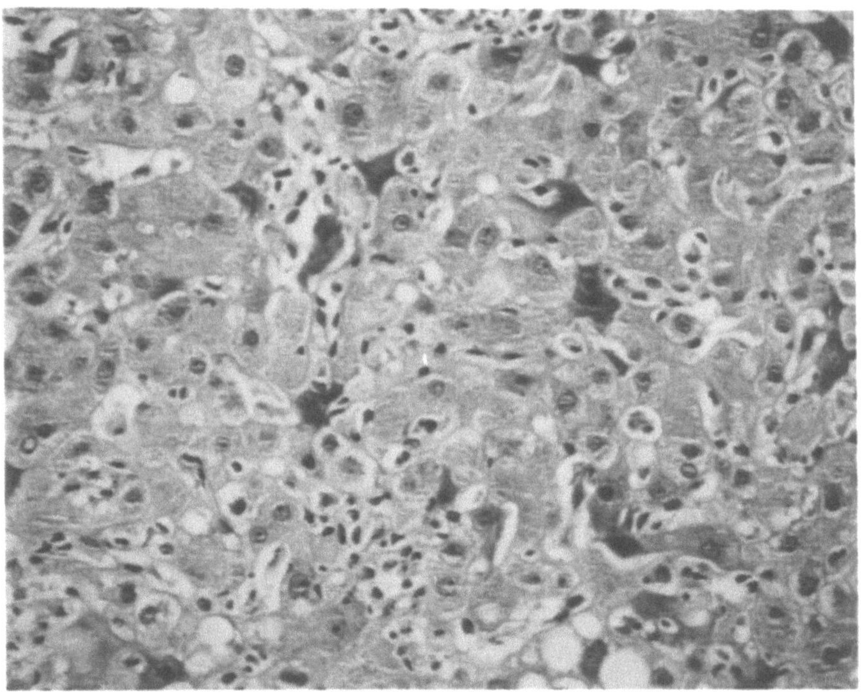

Figure 4. Acute hepatitis with prominent eosinophilic degeneration of hepatocytes and numerous sinusoidal inflammatory cells typical of some cases of NANB hepatitis. The degenerating hepatocytes frequently have an angulated or rhomboid outline. (H&E, ×300; AFIP neg. 87-5981)

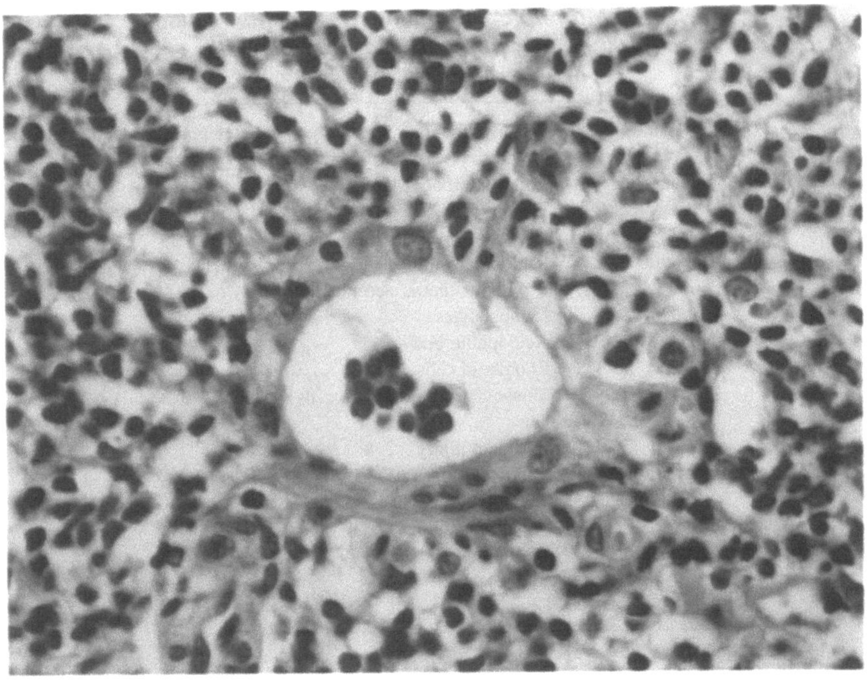

Figure 5. Bile duct lesion in NANB hepatitis. The interlobular bile duct shows marked injury of epithelium, disruption of basement membrane and lymphocytic inflammation. (H&E, ×630; AFIP neg. 87-5982)

any specific feature or pattern of injury to be specific for any type of hepatitis. Certain types of hepatocellular injury or inflammatory response tended to be more common or more severe in one type of hepatitis than another, but there was too much overlap for any of these to be of use in diagnosis of an individual case. For example, in the Danish study,[5] hepatocellular fat accumulation was seen in approximately 10% of biopsies in hepatitis A, 6% in hepatitis B, and 26% in NANB.

Table III. Incidence of Selected Histologic Features in Different Types of Acute Viral Hepatitis

	Virus		
Feature	A (%)	B (%)	NANB (%)
Fat			
Copenhagen	10	6	26
Zurich	—	—	—
Confluent or bridging necrosis			
Copenhagen	1	17	13
Zurich	27	40	58
Bile duct injury			
Copenhagen	1	1	4
Zurich	0	7	29

[a]Figures given are calculated from data published from 240 patients from Copenhagen[5] compared with 54 patients from Zurich.[6]

Thus, while fat is most frequent in NANB, its presence does not exclude A or B. Bile duct injury was only seen in five of the 240 cases in the Danish study, three with NANB and one each with A and B. On the other hand, Schmidt et al.[6] in Switzerland found bile duct injury in 29% of acute NANB and 7% of acute B but in no case of hepatitis A. Thus, while bile duct injury, like fat, suggests NANB, it is also not specific.

4. FULMINANT NANB

The other major setting in which material is available for pathologic examination in acute NANB is in patients with severe acute hepatitis and fulminant liver failure. In such patients, the liver is seldom biopsied but is often examined at autopsy or as a pretransplant hepatectomy specimen. The following case illustrates such a patient.

Case 2

A 15-year-old boy in previous excellent health presented with a 2-week history of malaise, fatigue, and the recent onset of jaundice. Laboratory studies showed AST 2000, bilirubin 8.0; negative HB surface antigen (HBsAg), anti-HB core (anti-HBc), anti-HBs, and anti-HAV; normal ceruloplasmin, serum, and urine copper. Over the next 4 weeks, the jaundice deepened, eventually reaching a level of 40 mg/dl, and the patient developed deep hepatic coma with a serum NH_3 of 710. Hepatic transplanation was performed, but the patient had a complicated postoperative course and died several weeks later.

The patient's liver removed prior to transplantation was shrunken, weighing 900 g, with a wrinkled capsule and a flabby consistency on sectioning. Microscopically, it showed large areas of confluent hepatocellular necrosis with stromal collapse and cholangiolar proliferation (Fig. 6). Some of the areas of collapse involved many adjacent acini (massive necrosis), while in others the acini had some surviving parenchyma in the periportal regions (submassive necrosis). The surviving hepatocytes showed continuing injury with frequent acidophilic bodies, Kupffer cell hypertrophy, lymphoplasmacytic infiltrate, cholestasis, and regenerative activity (Fig. 7).

The clinical features of this case are those of a fulminant hepatitis. Among the known causes of fulminant liver failure,[8] some, such as ischemia, certain viral infections (e.g., Herpes simplex, viral hemorrhagic fevers), and hepatic necrosis caused by toxins (e.g., CCl_4, Amanita mushrooms) have characteristic patterns different from that seen here. This appearance of confluent hepatocellular necrosis, dropout, and stromal collapse is typical of severe viral hepatitis due to the common hepatitis viruses (A, B, and NANB) and of the drug reactions that can mimic severe viral hepatitis (e.g., halothane, isoniazide). In the present case, no drugs could be implicated, and serologic markers for hepatitis A and B were negative. By exclusion, sporadic NANB viral hepatitis is most probable.

Fulminant hepatitis is an uncommon disease, but sporadic NANB, as in the present case, is one of the more common causes. At the Mayo Clinic between 1974 and 1982, NANB was responsible for 44% of cases of fulminant liver failure.[9] At the AFIP between 1980 and 1986, NANB was the presumed cause of 56% of American cases of fulminant hepatitis with this histologic pattern of submassive–massive necrosis (Table IV). Only four of the 63 patients had a history of blood transfusion or parenteral drug use. Fulminant NANB hepatitis is a disease of the young and the old. Approximately 46% of patients were under 40 years of age, while 43% were 60 or older (Table V). Two of the four patients in the 40 to 60-age range had a transfusion or parenteral exposure history. Many of the older patients with presumed NANB viral hepatitis had used medications, including therapeutic doses of acetaminophen, but none had a history to suggest fulminant drug-induced liver injury.

The two cases presented here illustrate the value and limitations of histopathology in establishing or suggesting a diagnosis of NANB hepatitis when the clinical circumstances are confusing.

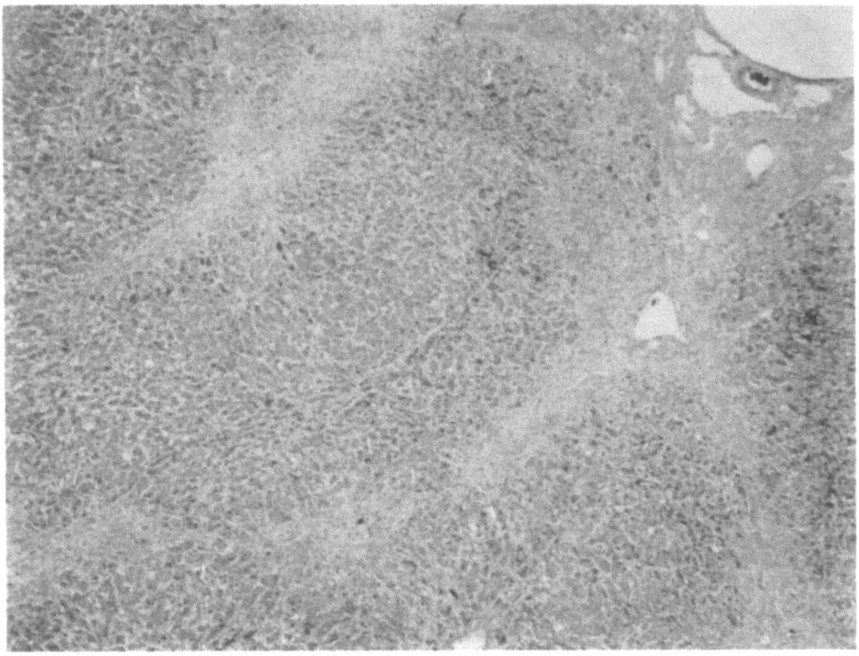

Figure 6. Submassive hepatic necrosis due to presumed sporadic NANB hepatitis (Case 2). Large areas of confluent hepatocellular necrosis and stromal collapse alternate with surviving and regenerating parenchyma. (H&E, ×25; AFIP neg. 87-5983)

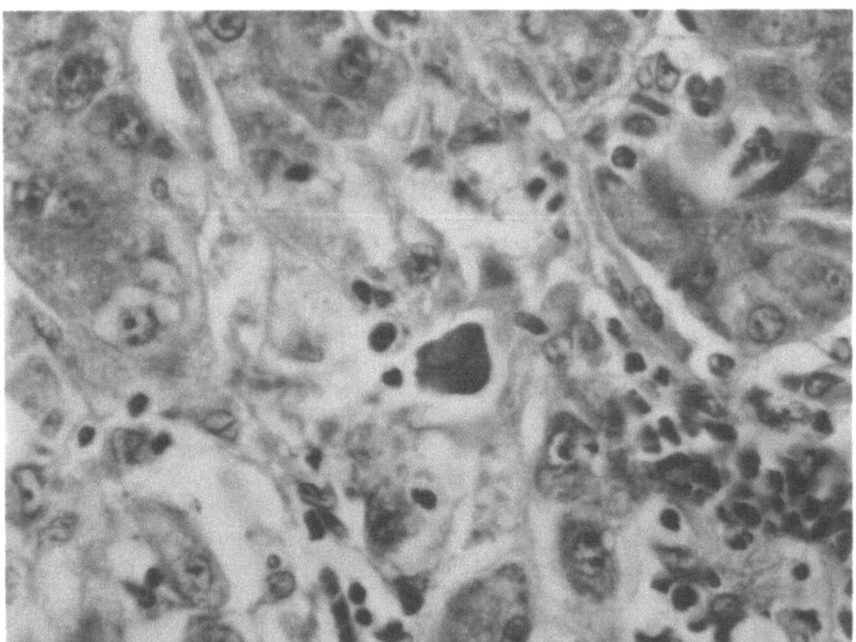

Figure 7. Fulminant NANB hepatitis (Case 2) with continuing acute hepatocellular injury, acidophilic bodies, lymphocytic inflammation, and regeneration in the areas of surviving parenchyma. (H&E, ×630; AFIP neg. 87-5984)

Table IV. Causes of Fatal Fulminant Hepatitis with Submassive Necrosis Reviewed at AFIP: 1980–1986[a]

Cause	Number of cases
Drug-induced	19
Hepatitis A	1
Hepatitis B (B + D)	8
Probable NANB	35

[a]American cases only.

Table V. Clinical Features in Fulminant NANB Hepatitis at AFIP: 1980–1986

Age	Number of cases	Sex M	Sex F	Transfusion or IV exposure	Nontoxic drug use[a]
20	6	3	3	—	—
20–39	10	4	6	—	2
40–59	4	1	3	2	2
60–84	15	4	11	2	9

[a]Heparin, metronidazole, papaverine, thyroxine, amphetamine, propranolol, hydrochlorthiazide, clonidine, oral contraceptives, prednisone, furosemide, theophylline, disopyramide, cimetidine, chlordiazepoxide, chlorpromazine, acetaminophen (therapeutic doses).

Whenever the biopsy shows an acute hepatocellular injury, as evidenced by ballooning and/or acidophilic degeneration with spotty necrosis, viral hepatitis must be considered in the differential diagnosis. Likewise, when a biopsy, autopsy, or hepatectomy shows severe massive or submassive hepatic necrosis with stromal collapse, viral hepatitis is the most likely cause. In their setting, serology should be obtained to evaluate the possibility of hepatitis A, B, and D; a drug history to evaluate the possibility of drug-induced injury; and a transfusion or parenteral exposure history to evaluate the likelihood of NANB viral hepatitis. Certain histologic features may suggest one or another agent, but the final diagnosis should be made in view of the serologic findings and history.

REFERENCES

1. Zimmerman HJ: Hepatotoxicity. The Adverse Effects of Drugs and Other Chemicals on the Liver. Appleton & Lange, E. Norwalk, Connecticut, 1978.
2. Stricker BHC, Spoelstra P. Drug-induced hepatic injury. Elsevier, Amsterdam, 1985.
3. Greenstone MA, Dowd PM, Mikhailidis DP, Scheuer PJ: Hepatic vascular lesions associated with dacarbazine treatment. *Br Med J* **282**:1744–1745, 1981.
4. Dienes HP, Popper H, Arnold W, Lobeck H: Histologic observations in human hepatitis non-A, non-B. *Hepatology* **2**:562–571, 1982.
5. Kryger P, and Christoffersen P. Light microscopic morphology of acute hepatitis non-A, non-B. A comparison with hepatitis type A and B. *Liver* **2**:200–206, 1982.
6. Schmidt M, Pirovino M, Altorfer J, et al: Acute hepatitis non-A, non-B: Are there any specific light microscopic features? *Liver* **2**:61–67, 1982.
7. Poulsen H, Christoffersen P: Abnormal bile duct epithelium in chronic aggressive hepatitis and cirrhosis. A review of morphology and clinical, biochemical, and immunologic features. *Hum Pathol* **3**:217–225, 1972.

8. Bernau J, Rueff B, Benhamou JP: Fulminant and subfulminant liver failure: Definitions and causes. *Semin Liv Dis* **6**:97–106, 1986.
9. Rakela J, Lange SM, Ludwig J, Baldus WP: Fulminant hepatitis: Mayo Clinic experience with 34 cases. *Mayo Clin Proc* **60**:289–292, 1985.
10. Teixeira MR, Weller IVD, Murray A, et al: The pathology of hepatitis A in man. *Liver* **2**:53–60, 1982.
11. Abe H, Beninger PR, Ikejiri N, et a: Light microscopic findings of liver biopsy specimens from patients with hepatitis type A and comparison with type B. *Gastroenterology* **82**:938–947, 1982.
12. Okuno T, Sano A, Deguchi T, et al: The pathology of acute hepatitis A in humans. Comparison with acute hepatitis B. *Am J Clin Pathol* **81**:162–169, 1984.
13. Houthoff HJ, Niermeijer P, Gips CH, et al: Hepatic morphologic findings and viral antigens in acute hepatitis B. A longitudinal study. *Virchows Arch A Pathol Anat Histol* **389**:153–166, 1980.
14. Omata M, Iwama S, Sumida M, et al: Clinico-pathological study of acute non-A, non-B post-transfusion hepatitis: Histological features of liver biopsies in acute phase. *Liver* **1**:201–208, 1981.
15. Popper H, Thung SN, Gerber MA, et al: Histologic studies of severe delta agent infection in Venezuelan Indians. *Hepatology* **3**:906–912, 1983.
16. Buitrago B, Popper H, Hadler SC, et al: Specific histologic features of Santa Marta hepatitis: A severe form of delta virus infection in northern South America. *Hepatology* **6**:1285–1291, 1986.
17. Govindarajan S, DeCock KM, Peters RL: Morphologic and immunohistochemical features of fulminant delta hepatitis. *Hum Pathol* **16**:262–267, 1985.
18. Lefkowitch JH, Goldstein H, Yatto R, Gerber MA: Cytopathic liver injury in acute delta virus hepatitis. *Gastroenterology* **92**:1262–1266, 1987.
19. Ishak KG: The liver, in Riddell RH (ed): *Pathology of Drug-Induced and Toxic Diseases*. Churchill Livingstone, New York, 1982, pp. 457–513.

II

Chronic Liver Disease, Including Cirrhosis

10

Portal Hypertension in Alcoholic Cirrhosis

Roberto J. Groszmann and Colin E. Atterbury

1. INTRODUCTION

Chronic progressive liver disease of various etiologies evolves into a final common pathway of circulatory and metabolic complications that eventually become the dominant aspects of the disease. Although the metabolic complications are themselves extensive, and in many cases life-threatening, the circulatory-related events are the most dramatic and the ones most likely to reflect the severity of the underlying liver disease. In fact, many of the metabolic abnormalities observed in chronic liver disease are initiated by a hemodynamic event: portal blood bypasses the liver through extrahepatic and intrahepatic shunts or through hepatic sinusoids that have decreased permeability both to essential nutrients and to toxins that require metabolism by the hepatocytes.[1,2]

In portal hypertension that occurs as a consequence of alcoholic liver disease, extrahepatic complications are initiated by intrahepatic morphologic changes. Early changes can be found in the sinusoids themselves. More than 20 years ago, Schaffner and Popper[3] coined the term *capillarization of the sinusoids* to convey the idea of the transformation of sinusoids from *leaky capillaries* into *tight capillaries*. It is essentially this transformation by means of collagenization of the sinusoids that initiates the intrahepatic circulatory abnormalities observed in alcoholic cirrhosis. These sinusoidal abnormalities impair not only the metabolic abilities of the liver but also induce an increased resistance to blood flow as well as decreased vascular compliance in response to changes in hepatic blood volume. These last two factors will eventually lead to the development of portal hypertension, the common denominator of all the major complications observed in chronic liver disease.

2. HEMODYNAMIC PRINCIPLES IN THE DEVELOPMENT OF PORTAL HYPERTENSION

Portal pressure is the result of the interelationship between portal blood flow and the resistance developed by the obstructed portal system (Fig. 1). In order to understand this relationship, it is necessary to apply the concepts of fluid dynamics that govern all systems, both living and nonliving,

---

Roberto J. Groszmann and Colin E. Atterbury • The Liver Center, Department of Internal Medicine, Yale University School of Medicine, New Haven, Connecticut 06510; Hepatic Hemodynamic Laboratory, Veterans Administration Medical Center, West Haven, Connecticut 06516.

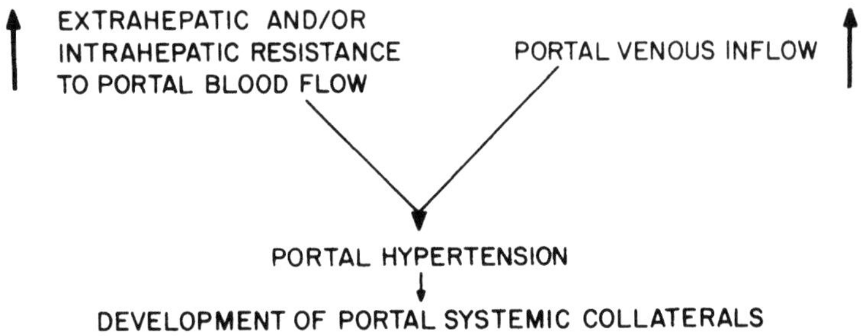

Figure 1. Factors that interrelate to produce portal hypertension.

Ohm's law as written for fluids defines the factors involved in the genesis of portal hypertension. The relationship between flow and resistance is expressed mathematically as

$$\Delta P = Q \times R$$

In this equation, ΔP is the perfusion pressure gradient along the vessel and is expressed as either millimeters of mercury (mm Hg or torr), newton per square meter (N/m^2 or pascal), or centimeters of water (cm H_2O); 1 mm Hg, or torr, equals 1.36 cm H_2O, or 133.3 N/m^2. Q is blood flow, expressed in units of volume per unit time (e.g., ml/min). R is the resistance opposing the flow of fluid and is expressed in dyne seconds per centimeters to the fifth power (dyne·sec/cm^5) or in millimeters of mercury minute per milliliter (mm Hg·min·ml^{-1}).

Whereas pressure and flow can be measured by a variety of techniques, resistance cannot be measured directly but may be calculated from the simultaneous measurements of flow and pressure gradient. The various factors affecting resistance in the vascular system are expressed by the familiar equation of Poiseuille's law:

$$R = \frac{8\eta l}{\pi r^4}$$

in which η is the coefficient of viscosity, r is the radius of the vessel, and l is its length.

When one substitutes these components for R in Ohm's formula, one obtains

$$P = Q\,\frac{8\eta l}{\pi r^4}$$

Since the length of blood vessels does not usually change and the viscosity of blood remains relatively constant with a stable hematocrit, the changes in vascular resistance are mainly represented by changes in the lumen of the vessels. Changes in pressure can then be accounted for by changes in the size of vessels and changes in flow. Minor changes in the former will have significant influence on the pressure gradient, since the pressure gradient is inversely related to the radius of the vessel raised to the fourth power. The contributions of changes in the size of vessels (i.e., resistance) or a change of flow are addressed separately.[4]

3. ROLE OF VASCULAR RESISTANCE

3.1. Site of Increased Vascular Resistance

It is clear from experimental data and clinical observations that an increased resistance to portal blood flow, whether intrahepatic or extrahepatic, will elevate portal venous pressure. Physiologic factors controlling resistance include (1) the opening of capillary beds, related to changes in metabolism, (2) passive dilation or contraction of vessels in response to changes in pressure, and (3) modifications in the contractile state of the smooth muscle in vascular walls mediated by vasomotor nerves, vascular receptors, and humoral substances.

Under physiologic conditions, the liver itself is the main site of resistance to portal flow. The vascular resistance within the liver is low and can accommodate large changes in portal blood flow with minimal changes in portal pressure. It must be emphasized, however, that the liver does not control the volume of portal flow; this is determined principally by the resistance vessels of the splanchnic organs that drain into the portal venous system.

The principal site of resistance within normal hepatic tissue is still debated. Proposed sites include the hepatic sinusoids, terminal hepatic venules, and small portal venules. More recently, at least in the cat, a hepatic vein sphincterlike structure within large hepatic veins has been described.[5] Hepatic venous manometric and radiologic studies in humans have not detected a high-pressure zone or sphinchterlike structure (S. Rolfe and R.J. Groszmann, unpublished data). Because accurate measurement within the hepatic parenchyma is fraught with technical difficulties, caution should be exercised when extrapolating animal data to humans.

Although the pathologic changes that may lead to the development of portal hypertension as a result of an increased resistance to portal blood flow could be located within the liver itself, they could also be at other levels of the portal system, such as within the portal vein itself or within hepatic drainage vessels. Increased resistance at the latter two sites could result from thrombosis of vessels; extravascular compression of the portal vein, hepatic vein, or venules by tumors; inflammation; or scarring. Different possibilities must be considered for the etiology of intrahepatic portal hypertension, which occurs in alcoholic cirrhosis.

3.2. Intrahepatic Resistance in the Cirrhotic Liver

In cirrhotic livers, the sites of increased resistance have not been conclusively determined. It has long been suggested that in alcoholic cirrhosis, postsinusoidal obstruction is present and is secondary to the compression of hepatic venules by regenerating nodules.[6] By contrast, a sinusoidal site for the increased resistance is supported by finding capillarized sinusoids in alcoholic cirrhosis characterized by deposition of collagen in the Disse space and formation of a basement membranelike structure. This view has been supported by recent micropuncture studies in the livers of rats with cirrhosis induced by a choline-deficient diet,[7] by morphometric studies in the baboon with alcohol-induced precirrhotic portal hypertension,[8] and more recently by scanning electron microscopy (SEM) studies in liver-biopsy specimens of chronic alcoholic patients wherein a decrease in the number of the sinusoidal fenestrations has been documented.[9] An alternative hypothesis suggests that hepatocyte enlargement is responsible for sinusoidal compression, hence, obstruction to blood flow.[10] However, the technique used to quantitate pressure in the latter study, the direct intrahepatic placement of a Chiba needle, has been questioned by others.[11]

3.3. Potentially Reversible Resistance

It has been assumed that the increase in vascular resistance induced by the above-mentioned mechanical factors is fixed and probably irreversible. There is increasing evidence, however, that even in cirrhotic livers there may be reversible components. For example, there may be an element of active constriction. In the normal animal, β_2-adrenoreceptors may modulate the luminal diameter of the sinusoids. Constriction of endothelial cells has been shown during administration of epinephrine and relaxation with the administration of isoproterenol, a β_2-adrenoreceptor agonist. These endothelial cells seem to be the main local modulators of sinusoidal perfusion under normal conditions.[12]

Another reversible mechanism for resistance has been suggested by the observation that the calcium channel blocker verapamil decreases portal resistance and increases the capability of albumin to diffuse into the extravascular space in the isolated perfused cirrhotic liver.[13] Verapamil may exert its effect by increasing the size or number of endothelial fenestrations, or both. Considering the nature of sinusoidal capillarization, it is unlikely that verapamil acts by dilating the fenestrae once they are occluded. An alternative explanation could be that verapamil could act by relaxing the fenestrae or endothelial cells or both that are in a state of increased constriction induced by endogenous constrictors. This effect may be due to increased circulating constrictors or to an enhanced response to normal levels of humoral constrictors, or a combination of both.

The role played by myofibroblasts in contributing to intrahepatic resistance may also be subject to reversal.[14] Myofibroblasts have been shown to exist in fibrous septa around sinusoids and in terminal hepatic venules in cirrhotic livers. These cells contain bundles of actin microfilaments within their cytoplasm and are believed to be responsible for the contraction of maturing scar tissue. Myofibroblasts within the cirrhotic liver are distributed around the sinusoids and thin walled venules within fibrous septa (Fig. 2). It has been suggested that by maintaining an increased contractile state, myofibroblasts may contribute to the increased resistance to portal flow in cirrhosis. Vasodilators acting on these myofibroblasts may decrease intrahepatic resistance to portal blood flow.[15] The area of reversible elements in intrahepatic resistance obviously requires further investigation because of the potential benefits that could be achieved if the intrahepatic resistance in cirrhosis is still amenable to pharmacologic manipulation.

4. ROLE OF BLOOD FLOW

4.1. Backward- versus Forward-Flow Hypotheses

As a direct consequence of the obstruction to blood flow, portal pressure increases and collateral vessels develop that result in portal-systemic shunting. These shunts, in some instances, may divert most of the portal flow out of the portal venous system into the systemic circulation. Despite this extensive collateral network, which tends to decompress the portal venous system, portal hypertension persists. Guido Banti, in 1883, described several patients with splenomegaly, anemia, and leukopenia. From this observation, Banti postulated that splenomegaly, portal hypertension, and cirrhosis could be accounted for primarily by increased splenic blood flow, i.e., the forward flow of blood is primarily responsible for portal hypertension. Since Banti's time, the pendulum of opinion about the role for an increased inflow into the portal system in the pathogenesis of portal hypertension and its complications has gone back and forth several times.[2]

The opposite view is that portal hypertension may be dependent solely on an increased intrahepatic or extrahepatic resistance to portal venous blood flow. This is the *backward-flow* hypothesis. In this construct, any reduction in resistance induced by portal-systemic shunting would be matched by a further increase in hepatic resistance. As a corollary, passive congestion of the portal venous system and its collateral vessels occurs. The result of the backward-flow theory would be a hypodynamic splanchnic and systemic circulation.

By contrast, the *forward-flow* theory would predict a hyperdynamic splanchnic and systemic circulation with a high portal vein inflow. Under the circumstances of the forward-flow theory, an elevated portal pressure may also be sustained through increased blood flow from the splanchnic bed into the portal system and collateral vasculature. It is widely accepted, however, that with few exceptions (e.g., splanchnic arteriovenous fistulas) portal hypertension is initiated by an obstruction at various levels of the portal system. Controversy remains about the roles of flow and resistance in maintaining portal hypertension during the development of portal-systemic collaterals. Recent evidence indicates that both factors—increased resistance to portal flow and increased portal blood flow—are involved in maintaining portal hypertension.

Decreased portal flow has been found during measurements performed with electromagnetic

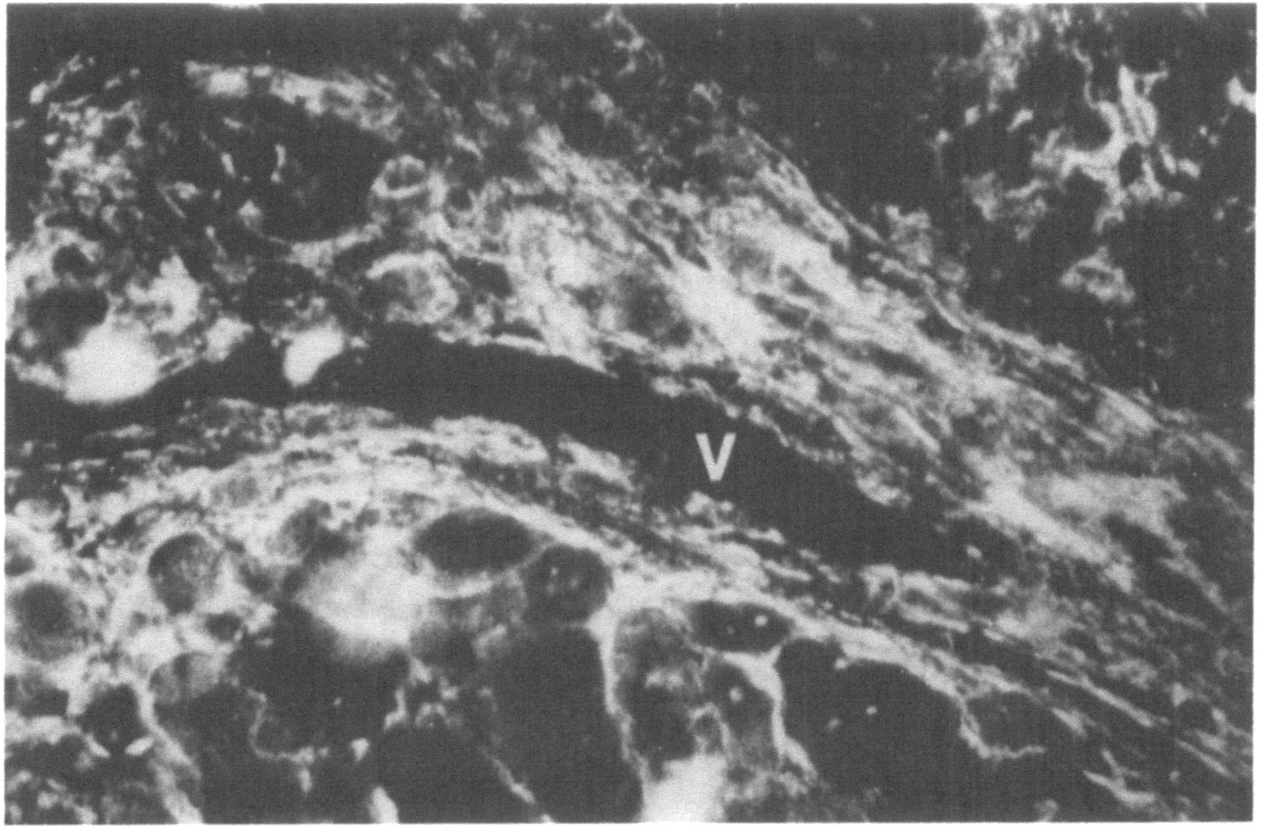

Figure 2. Cryostat section of cirrhotic rat liver (stained with antiactin serum) using the indirect immunofluorescent method. Numerous myofibroblasts are seen aligned in the axis of the fibrous septum and in a perivenular (v) distribution. Fluorescing cells are also seen in a perisinusoidal location. (From Bhathal and Grossman.[15]) (×500)

flowmeters in the portal vein of patients with cirrhosis of various etiologies.[16] Elevated portal pressure with decreased portal flow implies an increased resistance to splanchnic inflow. These flowmeter measurements support the backward-flow theory that there is increased resistance without any contribution of abnormally increased portal venous blood flow. Nevertheless, several pieces of information have been accumulated over the years in favor of the forward-flow theory of portal hypertension: (1) the finding of a hyperdynamic systemic circulation in patients with cirrhosis, (2) the shortening of the mean transit times of labeled albumin in the splanchnic circulation of cirrhotic patients, (3) the observation of an increase in splenic blood flow in cirrhosis, and (4) an increase in hepatic blood flow in patients with alcoholic hepatitis.[2]

Some of the conclusions supporting the backward-flow theory are misleading, owing to the misconception that in portal hypertension, portal flow, or even total hepatic blood flow, provides sufficient data for interpreting the changes that occur in the splanchnic circulation. In portal hypertension, the total amount of blood flow entering into the portal system is much greater than the amount of blood perfusing the liver.

In advanced liver disease, when portal blood flow perfusing the liver is measured, portal flow is generally decreased, even though splanchnic blood flow is probably increased. Since the collateral circulation in most patients with portal hypertension carries a large percentage of the total portal blood flow, erroneous conclusions can be reached unless all elements of this complex circulation are taken into account.

4.2. Hyperdynamic Circulation

Recently, several laboratories have accumulated evidence for the existence of a hyperdynamic splanchnic and systemic circulation, which would be predicted by the forward flow hypothesis in experimental models of chronic portal hypertension.[2] Elevated splanchnic blood flow and reduced splanchnic arteriolar resistance accompany chronic elevations in portal venous pressure. This hyperdynamic splanchnic circulation is accompanied by a hyperdynamic systemic circulation characterized by a high cardiac index and a low systemic arteriolar resistance.

The mechanism responsible for the hyperdynamic circulation is still undefined. Previous views suggested that the development of a collateral circulation, acting as an arteriovenous fistula, accounted for the appearance of a hyperdynamic state. However, a hyperdynamic circulation develops in the portal vein-constricted rat in spite of unchanged percentages of portal-systemic shunting. It has been recently postulated that the mediators of the hyperdynamic syndrome are circulating vasodilators, of which glucagon could account for 40% of the splanchnic hyperdynamic effect. No correlation between the glucagon blood levels and the portal venous inflow was observed in another study. Increased levels of serum bile acids, which are splanchnic arterial vasodilators, may also be implicated. It has also been reported that following chronic portal vein stenosis, the sympathetic vascular tone in the intestinal circulation may be impaired. This last finding could also explain, at least in part, the intestinal hyperemia associated with portal hypertension.

Several studies in experimental models and in patients with portal hypertension have suggested that the vascular resistance of the collateral circulation, although lower than the resistance of the obstructed portal system, is higher than that of normal liver.[2] Therefore, in portal hypertension we are confronted with the unusual combination of an increased resistance and an increased blood flow within the same vascular bed. The role that each of these factors plays in the maintenance of a portal hypertensive state may change at different stages of the disease process.[17] However, even at the peak of the hyperdynamic circulatory state, the importance of the increased blood flow may be limited. A reduction of the increased portal venous inflow to normal levels reduces portal pressure by no more than 15%, thus, even at the hyperdynamic stage, the increase in resistance to portal flow plays a dominant role in maintaining portal hypertension.[18]

The increase in portal pressure is the hallmark of the portal hypertensive syndrome; the hyperdynamic circulation plays a limited but definite role in the maintenance of the increased portal pressure. However, the increased blood flow through the portal-collateral system may induce changes in the collateral vessels that go beyond the pure effect of an increased pressure. Recent investigations suggest that a flow-oriented stress, i.e., a wall shear stress exerted by the adjacent flow velocity, may play a role not only in dilating the vessel but also in inducing endothelial lesions that may further weaken the wall of the vessel.[19] It is known that the collateral blood flow is increased in portal hypertensive patients. Whether the magnitude of the collateral blood flow, independent of the rise of portal pressure, plays any role in the dilatation of the collateral bed and the subsequent development of gastro-esophageal varices must be investigated.

In summary, portal pressure is determined by the interaction of an increased portal venous inflow and an increased resistance offered by the intrahepatic and portocollateral bed to that flow, but neither the forward-flow theory nor the backward-flow theory can be applied solely to explain the portal hypertensive syndrome. For the present, the evidence seems sufficiently compelling to postulate that chronic portal hypertension is the result not only of an increased resistance to portal flow but also of a hyperdynamic circulation, whereby an increase in blood flow beyond the normal range plays a limited but distinct role in the maintenance of the syndrome.

5. COMPLIANCE OF THE PORTAL VASCULAR SYSTEM

The classic factors governing portal pressure, flow, and resistance are strictly applicable only when a homogeneous fluid flows through a rigid tube of constant radius with a steady pressure applied to that fluid. The behavior of blood flow through the vascular system, although still qualitatively described by these relationships, nonetheless departs from these simple physical conditions. Blood flow in a vessel increases with an increase in pressure. Over wide ranges, however, the relationship between the two quantities is not as linear in a blood vessel as in a rigid tube. An elastic blood vessel, compared with a simple rigid tube, will distend, offering less opposition to flow as the pressure within the vessel increases. The relationship between the change in volume of a blood vessel for a given change in transmural pressure is known as compliance. Mathematically, compliance is expressed by

$$C = \frac{\Delta V}{\Delta TP}$$

where C is compliance, V is volume change (ml) and TP is transmural pressure change (mm Hg). From this equation, we derive

$$\Delta TP = \frac{\Delta V}{C}$$

Increases in volume and decreases in compliance can therefore be expected to result in increases in the transmural pressure gradient.

The normal liver is a highly compliant organ; the portal vascular resistance of a normal liver will decrease with increases in blood flow owing to further distention of the normal compliant vessels in response to the increased blood flow. This compensatory mechanism will maintain a normal portal pressure within a wide range of portal flow. This same phenomenon is not observed in portal hypertensive states. In portal hypertension, compliance of the vasculature is probably greatly reduced. At the same time, splanchnic blood volume in cirrhosis is often increased. Both the increase in volume and the decrease in compliance may play an additional role in perpetuating portal hypertension. However, these factors have not been sufficiently evaluated, owing to the limitations of current techniques for their study, which are both invasive and cumbersome.[2]

6. CONSEQUENCES OF COLLATERAL DEVELOPMENT: VARICEAL FORMATION AND HEMORRHAGE

6.1. Formation of Varices

Once portal hypertension becomes established, spontaneous portal-systemic collaterals develop in an attempt to decompress the portal system. In humans, these communications occur between the coronary and short gastric veins and among the intercostal, esophageal, and azygous veins; the superior hemorrhoidal vein and the middle and inferior hemorrhoidal veins; the paraumbilical plexus and veins of abdominal organs in contact with retroperitoneal or abdominal wall structures; and connections to the left renal vein from the splanchnic, adrenal, and spermatic veins. These communications probably result from dilation of preexistent embryonic channels, although angioneogenesis cannot be excluded. In humans, there is an area of the distal esophagus extending 2–5 cm from the gastroesophageal junction, where veins are primarily in the lamina propria rather than the submucosa. Dilation of these preexisting venous channels, owing to the increased portal flow and pressure, will eventually result in the development of esophageal varices, which are the most threatening complication of portal hypertension. Postmortem studies of the human esophageal microvasculature have demonstrated in patients with portal hypertension compared with controls an increase in vessel size in the lamina propria in this area. These studies further support the concept that varices are formed by dilation of preexistent channels and provide the anatomic explanation for the endoscopic observation of the predominantly distal location of esophageal varices.[20,21]

Initial dilation of the esophageal collaterals probably depends on a threshold portal pressure below which varices do not develop.[2] In addition, the volume of blood flow through the gastroesophageal collaterals and local anatomic factors may also play a role. Subsequently, progressive distension will depend on intrinsic properties of the varix wall and surrounding tissue support.

In patients with intrahepatic portal hypertension, primarily secondary to alcoholic cirrhosis, varices rarely, if ever, occur with portal pressure gradients (i.e., portal minus free hepatic vein pressure) of less than 11–12 mm Hg.[22] However, patients with portal pressure gradients above this level do not invariably develop varices.[22] Thus, this increased pressure gradient is necessary but insufficient for the development of esophageal varices.

6.2. Portal Pressure Elevation and Variceal Size as Predictors of Hemorrhage

A threshold pressure also appears to be necessary for variceal hemorrhage to occur. This threshold appears to be a hepatic venous pressure gradient above 12 mm Hg.[22] Since this is the same threshold as observed for the development of varices, it would seem that the portal pressure necessary for varices to form is sufficient to cause varices to bleed. Whereas one often sees higher, sometimes much higher, portal pressures in patients who bleed from varices, the large overlap in pressures between patients who bleed from varices and patients who have varices but do not bleed from them indicates that elevated portal pressure alone is a poor predictor of hemorrhage.

The inadequacy of the degree of elevation of portal pressure in predicting hemorrhage has challenged physicians to identify other factors that may be better predictors of variceal rupture and hemorrhage. One such factor has been variceal size. It has been observed and passed on from physician to physician that large varices are more likely to bleed than are small ones. There is investigative support for this observation. Figure 3 indicates that patients with large and small varices have similar portal pressures, but the incidence of variceal hemorrhage is significantly greater in patients with large varices. This observation lends support to the assumption that size is in fact an independent variable in the incidence of bleeding from varices. Nevertheless, size is not an absolute predictor because some patients with large varices do not bleed and some patients with

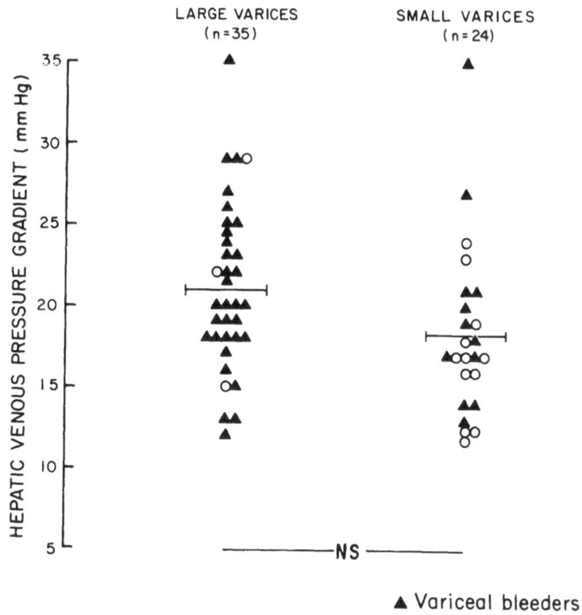

Figure 3. Patients with large and small varices have portal pressures that are not significantly different. However, the prevalence of variceal bleeding (triangles) is significantly greater in patients with large varices indicating that size may be an independent variable in the prevalence of bleeding varices.

small varices do bleed. Furthermore, local variceal signs seen at endoscopy (red wales, black dots, cherry red and hemocystic spots) also seem to be independent predictors of variceal bleeding.

The inability to identify a single factor predictive of variceal bleeding and the fact that pressure and size seem to be related to variceal bleeding suggest that the interaction of these factors may have a role in determining variceal rupture.[23]

6.3. Variceal Wall Tension as the Determinant of Varix Rupture

The decisive factor that may determine variceal rupture, and one that integrates observed phenomena, is the tension in the wall of the varix. The concept of tension is expressed as Frank's modification of LaPlace's law[20,23]:

$$T = TP \cdot \frac{r}{w}$$

where T is tension, TP is transmural pressure, r is radius, and w is wall thickness. Transmural pressure is the difference between intraluminal vessel pressure and esophageal luminal pressure. The transmural pressure is a component of LaPlace's law and therefore a determinant of variceal rupture.

The tension of a vessel wall, the left side of the equation, is an inwardly directed restraining force that opposes an outwardly directed expanding force ($TP \cdot r/w$), the right side of the equation (Fig. 4). The tension developed by the fibers of the wall of the vessel is an intrinsic property of the vessel wall. Increasing vessel distention results in increasing resistance to further distention. A balance is maintained as long as possible. Tension is in equilibrium with the expanding force (i.e., $TP \cdot r/w$). An increase in transmural pressure or in radius or a decrease in wall thickness will increase the expanding force of the vessel (Fig. 4). When this force exceeds wall tension, rupture will occur. At a certain point, small changes in volume or radius are associated with large changes in tension.

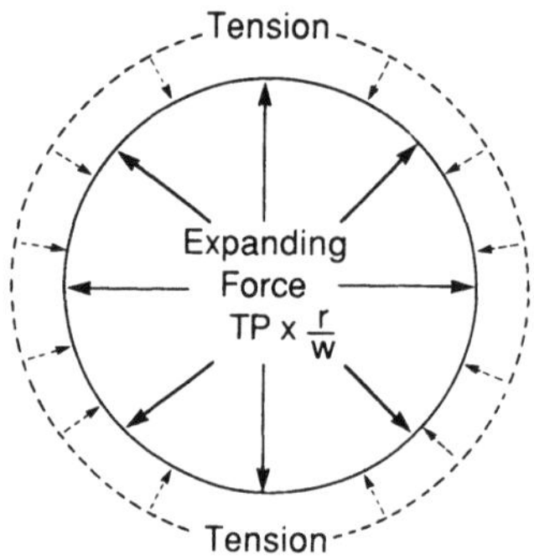

Figure 4. Tension, a property of the vessel wall, is an inwardly directed force. Tension opposes an outwardly directed force (*TP·r/w*). (From Groszmann and Polio.[24])

Beyond this point, where the elastic limit of the vessel wall is reached, further increases in radius do not generate a compensatory increase in tension.

It has been shown experimentally in blood vessels without tissue support that wall tension increases out of proportion to increases in transmural pressure because an increase in pressure causes an increase in the radius and a decrease in the wall thickness of the vessel. By contrast, at the same transmural pressure, a vessel embedded in tissue will have a smaller radius than one not embedded in tissue and will therefore have less wall tension. A vessel with no supporting tissue will be at a higher risk for rupture of its wall (Fig. 5).

Bursting at high pressures can only be avoided if a tissue support exists that can protect the wall from further distention. When there is no tissue support or when it is weak, as occurs with varices protruding into the esophageal lumen, the rupture point may occur at even relatively low pressures. During the course of events leading to rupture of varices, local factors and individual variations in vessel walls may change the tissue support, making wall thickness and radius more sensitive to changes in transmural pressure. The factors that determine wall tension may act either in opposition or in synergy, thereby preventing or hastening rupture (Fig. 6).

The interaction of these factors makes comparison of the risk of variceal bleeding among different patients difficult and may explain the contradictory results obtained in studies assessing the individual factors determining tension. It is conceivable that a patient with a lower portal pressure could have a higher risk of bleeding than a patient with a higher portal pressure, because of the severity of other factors. It is probable that a decrease in variceal pressure, by decreasing wall tension, would nonetheless reduce the risk of bleeding in all patients. All pharmacologic therapy for portal hypertension, in any event, is based on this hypothesis.

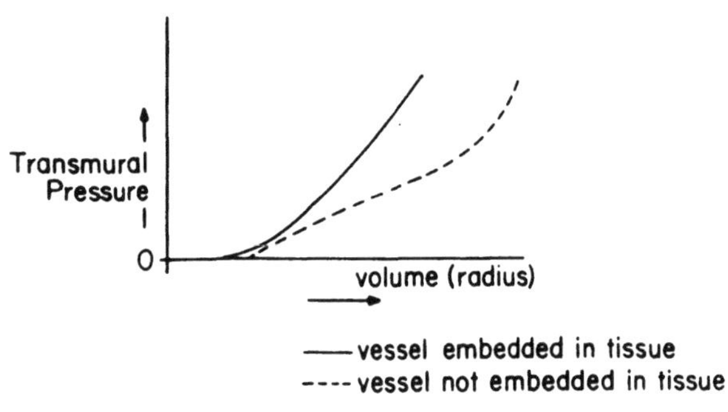

Figure 5. Vessel distention in response to changes in transmural pressure (*TP*). Comparison between a vessel embedded in tissue and a vessel without supporting tissue. At the same *TP*, the vessel not embedded in tissue has a greater radius and therefore greater wall tension. (From Polio and Groszmann.[20])

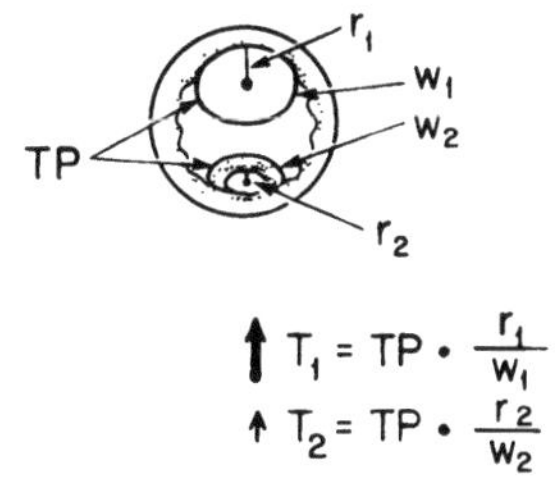

Figure 6. Variceal wall tension. In varices with the same transmural pressure (*TP*) but different radii ($r_1 > r_2$) and wall thickness ($w_1 < w_2$), wall tension (*T*) will be greatest in the varix with the largest radius (r_1) and thinner (w_1) wall. (From Polio and Groszmann.[20])

REFERENCES

1. Groszmann RJ: Portal hypertension: Circulatory and renal abnormalities. *Semin Liver Dis* **6**:275–276, 1986.
2. Groszmann RJ, Blei AT, Atterbury CE: Pathophysiology of portal hypertension, in Arias I, Popper H (eds): *The Liver: Biology and Pathobiology.* 2nd ed. Raven, New York, 1988, pp. 1147–1159.
3. Schaffner F, Popper H: Capillarization of hepatic sinusoids in man. *Gastroenterology* **44**:239–242, 1963.
4. Groszmann RJ, Atterbury CE: The pathophysiology of portal hypertension. A basis for classification. *Semin Liver Dis* **2**:177–186, 1982.
5. Lautt WW, Greenway CV, Legare DJ, et al: Localization of intrahepatic portal vascular resistance. *Am J Physiol* **151**:G375–G381, 1986.
6. Popper H, Zak FG: Pathological aspects of cirrhosis. *Am J Med* **24**:593–625, 1958.
7. Shibayama Y, Nakata K: Localization of increased hepatic vascular resistance in liver cirrhosis. *Hepatology* **5**:643–648, 1985.
8. Miyakawa H, Iida S, Leo MA, et al: Pathogenesis of precirrhotic portal hypertension in alcohol-fed baboons. *Gastroenterology* **88**:143–150, 1985.
9. Horn J, Christoffersen P, Henriksen J: Alcoholic liver injury: Defenestration in non-cirrhotic livers—A scanning electron microscopic study. *Hepatology* **7**:77–82, 1987.
10. Blendis LM, Orrego H, Crossley IR, et al: The role of hepatocyte enlargement on hepatic pressure in cirrhotic and noncirrhotic alcoholic liver disease. *Hepatology* **2**:539–546, 1982.
11. Fenyves D, Pomier-Layrargues G, Willems B, et al: Intrahepatic pressure: Not an accurate reflection of portal vein pressure. *Gastroenterology* **8**:211–216, 1988.
12. Reilly RD, Dimlich RVW, Cilento EV, et al: Hepatic microvascular regulatory mechanisms. III. Aminergic mechanisms as related to mast cells. *Int J Microcirc Clin Exp* **2**:61–73, 1983.
13. Reichen J, Le M: Verapamil favorably influences hepatic microvascular exchange and function in rats with cirrhosis of the liver. *J Clin Invest* **78**:448–455, 1986.
14. Bhathal PS, Grossman HJ: Reduction of the increased portal vascular resistance of the isolated perfused cirrhotic rat liver by vasodilators, *J. Hepatol.* **1**:325–337, 1985.
15. Bhathal PS, Grossmann HJ: Reduction of the increased portal vascular resistance of the isolated perfused cirrhotic rat liver by vasodilators. *J Hepatol* **1**:325–337, 1985.
16. Moreno AH, Burchell AR, Rousselot LM, et al: Portal blood flow in cirrhosis of the liver. *J Clin Invest* **46**:436–445, 1967.
17. Sikuler E, Kravetz D, Groszmann RJ: Evolution of portal hypertension and mechanisms involved in its maintenance in a rat model. 1. *Am J Physiol* **248**:G618–G625, 1985.
18. Kroeger RJ, Groszmann RJ: Increased portal venous resistance hinders portal pressure reduction during the administration of β-adrenergic blocking agents in a portal hypertensive model. *Hepatology* **5**:97–101, 1985.
19. Kamiya A, Togawa T: Adaptative regulation of wall shear stress to flow change in the canine carotid artery. *Am J Physiol Heart Circ Physiol* **239**:H14–H21, 1980.
20. Polio J, Groszmann RJ: Hemodynamic factors involved in the development and rupture of esophageal varices: A physiological approach to treatment. *Semin Liver Dis* **6**:318–331, 1986.
21. Spence RAJ: The venous anatomy of the lower esophagus in normal subjects and patients with varices: An image analysis study. *Br J Surg* **71**:739–744, 1984.

22. Garcia-Tsao G, Groszmann RJ: Fisher RL, et al: Portal pressure, presence of gastroesophageal varices and variceal bleeding. *Hepatology* **5**:419–424, 1985.
23. Groszmann RJ: Reassessing portal venous pressure measurements. *Gastroenterology* **80**:1611–1617, 1984.
24. Groszmann RJ, Polio J: Pathophysiologic mechanisms in esophageal variceal rupture, in Burroughs AK (ed): *Methodology and Review of Clinical Trials in Portal Hypertension*, Excerpta Medica, Amsterdam, 1987, pp. 263–272.

11

The Morphological Spectrum of Alcoholic Liver Disease

Lionel Rabin

1. INTRODUCTION

It is convenient to classify the manifestations of liver disease related to alcoholism into three types: (1) alcoholic fatty liver, (2) alcoholic hepatitis, and (3) cirrhosis. Light microscopic morphologic findings in these three categories, however, may coexist or overlap.[1–5] In addition, there is frequently a poor correlation between the clinical, biochemical, and morphological findings in patients with alcohol-related liver injury. Further difficulties in morphologic interpretation arise from the recognition of a variety of clinical settings or entities unrelated to alcohol ingestion that may mimic alcoholic liver disease, and from alterations superimposed on alcohol-related liver injury by causes, such as viral hepatitis, drug-induced hepatotoxicity, and biliary tract obstruction.

It is the purpose of this chapter to present a review of the light microscopic findings associated with alcoholic liver disease, emphasizing the so-called diagnostic criteria as well as features offering prognostic implications.

2. ALCOHOLIC FATTY LIVER

Alcoholic fatty liver or simple fatty liver is perhaps the most common alteration seen following moderate or significant alcohol ingestion.[6–8] Fat may accumulate within just a few days. Upon cessation of drinking, fat usually disappears within 3–4 weeks, even when the fatty change is diffuse and of a marked degree. Fatty change in alcoholic fatty liver is most often centrilobular to midzonal in distribution (zones 3 and 2, respectively, of the Rappaport acinus). It may also be diffuse or random. Sections of liver generally exhibit a predominantly large droplet type (macrovesicular) lipid accumulation in hepatocytes with displacement of the nucleus and cytoplasmic contents (Fig. 1A,B). The large droplet fat results from coalescence of small microvesicular droplets. Occasionally, large vacuoles may coalesce, forming fatty cysts.

An occasional (or sometimes more frequent) finding in alcoholic fatty liver is lipogranulomata.[9] It is claimed that lipogranulomata may be found in 30–50% of fatty livers. They generally consist of focal aggregates of macrophages, lymphocytes, fat vacuoles, and rarely, multinucleated

Lionel Rabin • Hepatic Pathology, Armed Forces Institute of Pathology, Washington, D.C. 20306-6000.

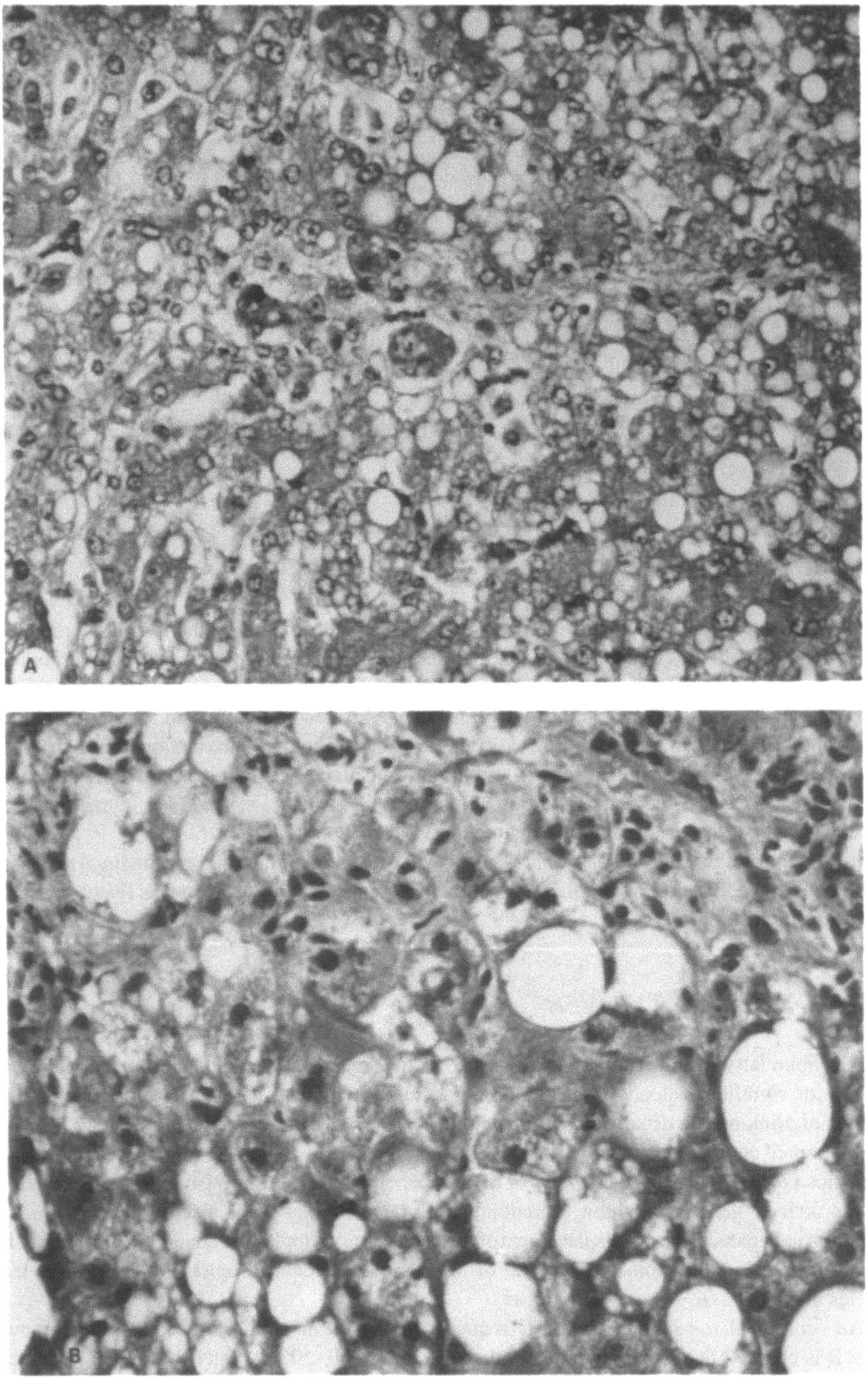

Figure 1. Alcoholic fatty liver. (A) Mixture of large, mid-, and small-sized fat vacuoles. Diffuse distribution. (H&E, ×300) (B) Alcoholic fatty liver. Predominantly large fat vacuoles in hepatocytes with a signet-ring appearance. (H&E, ×396)

giant cells. There may be associated fibrous connective tissue. The location of lipogranulomata is variable in the acinus; some may even involve terminal hepatic venules (central veins) and portal areas.

Alcoholic fatty liver is reversible. Simple alcholic steatosis is not accompanied by fibrosis or necrosis. Fatty liver in some instances may progress to cirrhosis in the absence of clinical documentation or histologic evidence of alcoholic hepatitis.[1,3,4] However, there are cases of sudden death associated with severe diffuse fatty change, usually resulting from continuous or "binge" alcohol imbibition.[10,11] In addition, there are some patients, usually middle-aged women with gross hepatomegaly and panlobular steatosis, who develop an acute cholestatic syndrome mimicking obstructive biliary tract disease, clinically and biochemically, that may lead to hepatic failure.[12]

In 1983, Uchida et al.[13] described a syndrome in chronic alcoholics characterized by microvesicular steatosis termed alcoholic foamy degeneration. This phenomenon may represent the initial episode of hepatic decompensation without evidence of portal hypertension or encephalopathy. Patients are usually jaundiced with persistently elevated serum alkaline phosphatase activity as well as transient but significantly elevated serum aminotransferase values. White blood cell (WBC) counts in peripheral blood are not elevated. Prognosis is good upon alcohol withdrawal, although occasional fatalities have been recorded.

On light microscopic examination, the liver with alcoholic foamy degeneration displays swelling of hepatocytes with microvesicular steatosis that is most intense in zone 3 (centrilobular areas), giving rise to a foamy appearance (Fig. 2). It is not uncommon to encounter spotty or occasional large vacuolar fat. Additional morphologic changes may include canalicular and hepatocellular cholestasis, occasional foci of necrosis, and giant or megamitochondria. Intralobular perisinusoidal

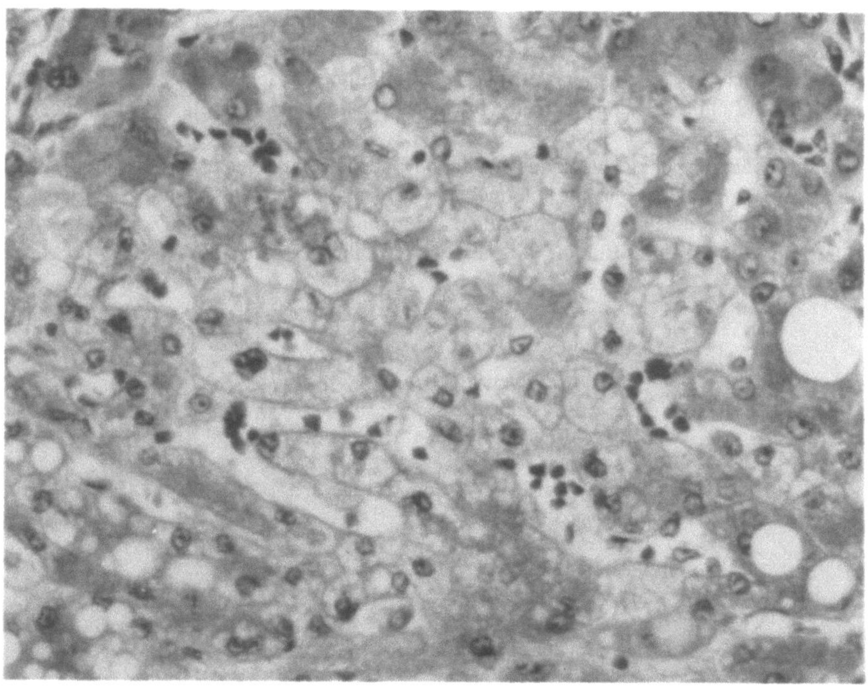

Figure 2. Alcoholic foamy degeneration. Note the predominance of the small vacuolar or microvescular cytoplasmic appearance of hepatocytes. Hepatocellular nuclei tend to be centrally located. (H&E, ×400)

fibrosis may be present as well as mild focal Kupffer cell hyperplasia. However, there is no acute inflammatory cell response.

Fatty change of the liver, whether macrovesicular or microvesicular, is not diagnostic of alcoholic liver disease. The causes of macrovesicular steatosis are many, including obesity, diabetes mellitus, nutritional disorders, and glucocorticoid and methotrexate therapy, to name a few. The microvesicular fatty change of alcoholic foamy degeneration may resemble acute fatty liver of pregnancy,[14,15] Reye syndrome,[16] Jamaican vomiting sickness, drug-induced injury (e.g., tetracycline,[17,18] valproate,[19] aspirin in children,[20] and several metabolic disorders (e.g., Wolman disease,[21,22] cholesteryl ester storage disease,[23] and disorders of ureogenesis[21] or fatty acid metabolism[24,25] (see Table I). The correct diagnostic interpretation is facilitated by the associated clinical and laboratory findings.

3. ALCOHOLIC HEPATITIS

Morphologically, alcoholic hepatitis is characterized by fatty change, acute inflammatory cell (polymorphonuclear) infiltration, liver cell necrosis, Mallory bodies (alcoholic hyalin), eventual collagen deposition, and fibrosis. No specific combination or single morphologic feature, however, is pathognomonic.[1–5]

Early changes in the liver in alcoholic hepatitis include ballooning of hepatocytes and occasional focal or individual cell necrosis. This histopathologic picture may even suggest hepatitis of viral etiology. Most commonly, patients exhibit fatty liver with focal polymorphonuclear cell infiltration and Mallory bodies (Fig. 3). The perivenular area (zone 3) of the hepatic acinus is predominantly affected in precirrhotic patients. Mallory bodies with chemotactic properties may attract polymorphonuclear leukocytes, giving rise to an appearance termed polymorphonuclear satellitosis. Mallory bodies, although a common and regular finding in alcoholic liver disease in general and alcoholic hepatitis in particular, are not required for the diagnosis of alcoholic hepatitis. Their presence, however, in combination with the acute inflammatory cell response and fatty change supported by the clinical history, greatly facilitates making the histopathologic diagnosis with confidence.

Mallory bodies are intracytoplasmic eosinophilic hepatocellular inclusions of variable size and shape resulting from damage to the intermediate filaments of the cytoskeleton.[26,27] Hepatocytes containing Mallory bodies are often swollen and, while their presence is neither specific for alcoholic injury nor required for the diagnosis, large numbers of Mallory bodies are generally

Table I. Differential Diagnosis of Microvesicular Steatosis

Alcoholic foamy degeneration
Reye syndrome
Acute fatty metamorphosis of pregnancy
Drug-induced
Parenteral tetracycline
Valproic acid
Acetylsalicylic acid overdose
Jamaican vomiting sickness
Inborn errors of metabolism
Defects in ureagenesis
Defects in fatty acid metabolism
Wolman disease and cholesteryl ester storage disease

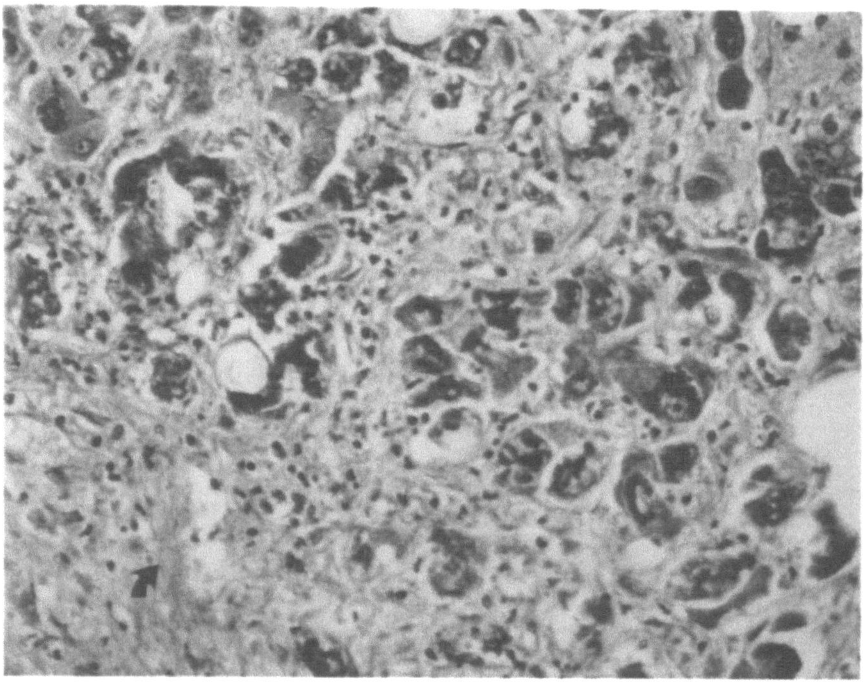

Figure 3. Alcoholic hepatitis. Many degenerating and swollen hepatocytes contain irregularly shaped Mallory bodies (alcoholic hyalin), which appear as black clumps. Note the presence of many polymorphonuclear leukocytes around many Mallory bodies. Arrow points to injured terminal hepatic vein (central vein). (H&E, ×300)

indicative of more severe injury and a worse prognosis.[1,4] Hepatocytes with Mallory bodies are considered viable, and the change is reversible.

The brunt of precirrhotic alcoholic hepatitis takes place in zone 3. Perivenular necrosis and the inflammatory cell response may be accompanied by damage to terminal hepatic venules (central veins), resulting in sclerotic change termed sclerosing hyalin necrosis or phlebosclerosis. In some cases, veno-occlusive alterations[28] may compromise hepatic venous outflow (Figs. 4A,B and 5). Perivenular collagen deposition may serve as a marker for an increased risk of progression to cirrhosis. Accompanying the perivenular fibrosis in many cases is intralobular pericellular collagenization and fibrosis, giving rise to a "chicken-wire," or latticelike, network (Fig. 6). With damage to the space of Disse, there is increased sinusoidal resistance, and functional interference between the hepatocellular membrane and blood in the sinusoids ensues. Deposition of immunoglobulin A (IgA) in hepatic sinusoids has been found, which according to Van de Wiel et al.,[29] provides an easy and reliable marker in diagnosis.

The hepatic alterations in alcoholic hepatitis described may be regarded major criteria for diagnosis. There are, however, additional nonspecific findings that, although less compelling or of minor diagnostic import, are nevertheless often associated with alcoholic liver disease, including alcoholic hepatitis. These changes include (1) giant or megamitochondria, (2) induced or ground-glass cytoplasmic change of hepatocytes, (3) oxyphil cells (oncocytes), (4) hemosiderosis, (5) portal–periportal cholangiolar proliferation with or without acute cholangiolitis, and (6) cholestasis.

In hematoxylin and eosin (H&E)-stained sections, giant or megamitochondria typically appear as round eosinophilic cytoplasmic inclusions in zone 3 hepatocytes. They are usually very small, in

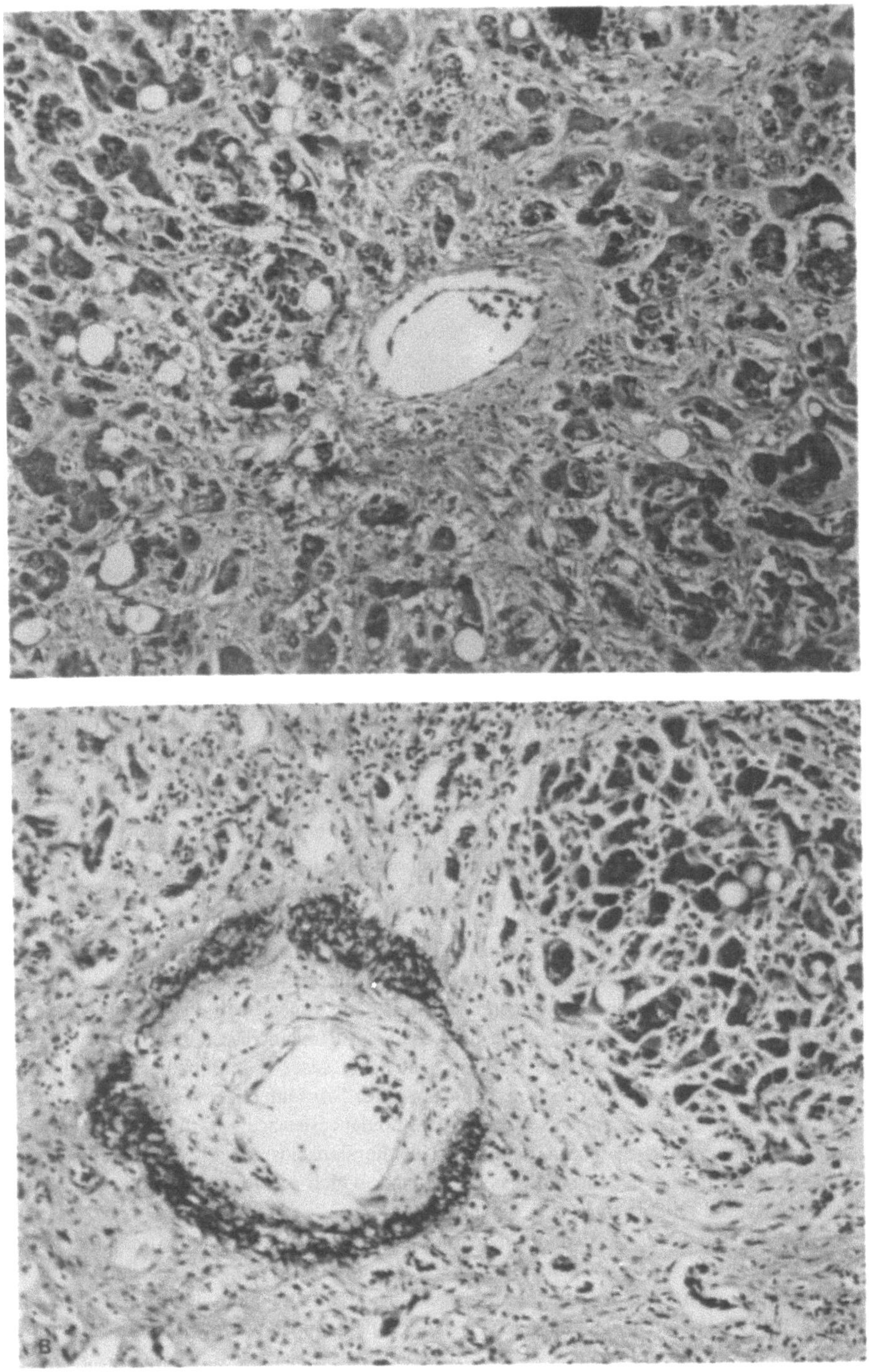

Figure 4. Alcoholic hepatitis. (A) Center of photograph exhibits early veno-occlusive changes of terminal hepatic vein. (H&E, ×150) (B) Alcoholic hepatitis with prominent veno-occlusive injury. (Movat, ×160)

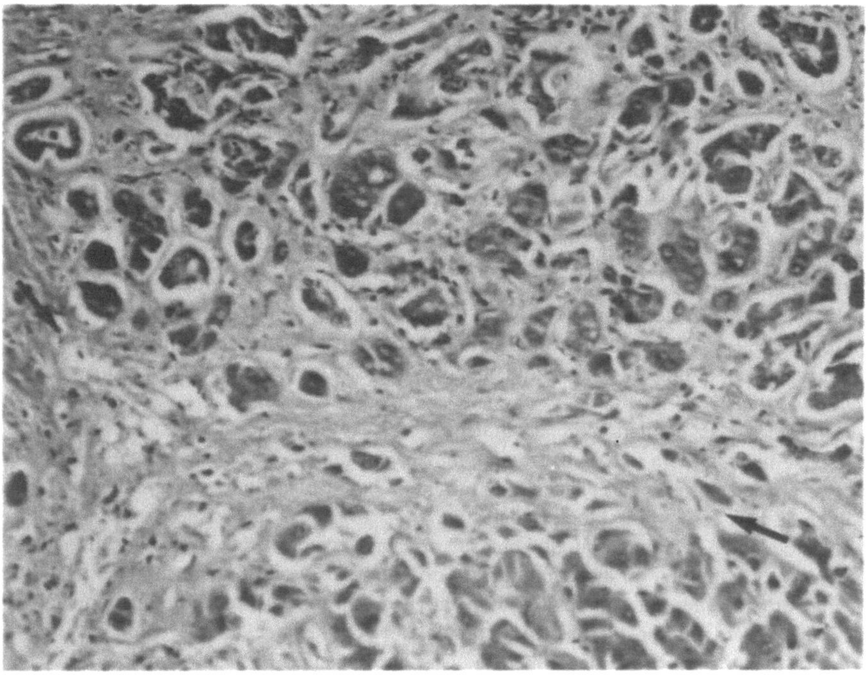

Figure 5. Alcoholic hepatitis. Sclerosed terminal hepatic vein between arrows (lower third of photomicrograph). Note presence of Mallory bodies and acute inflammatory cells upper half of field. (H&E, ×198)

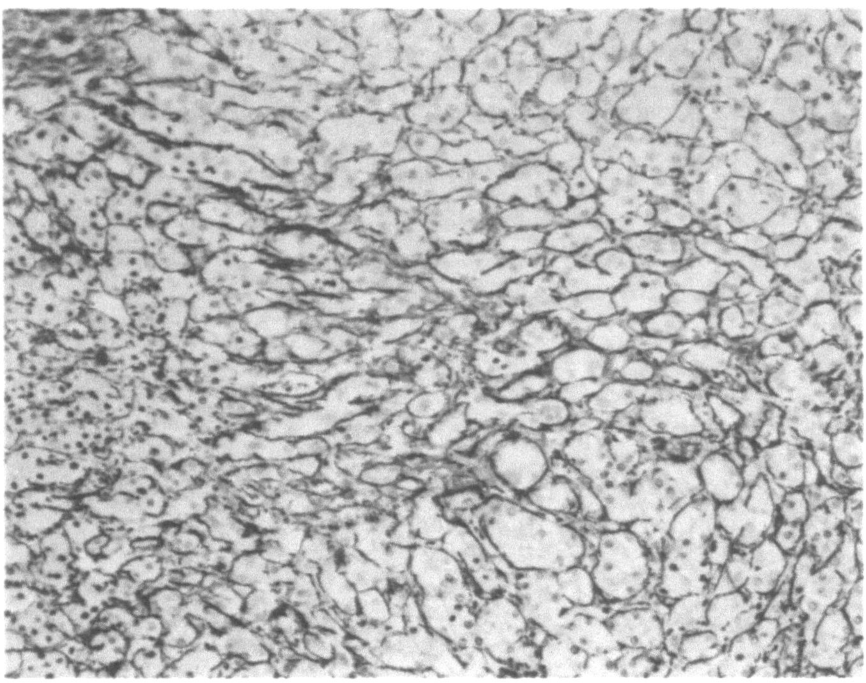

Figure 6. Alcoholic liver disease with diffuse pericellular fibrosis suggesting "chicken-wire" or latticelike pattern. (Reticulin, ×150)

the range of 1–2 μm in diameter but, on occasion, may be as large as a red blood cell (Fig. 7). In some cases, they assume a crystalline needlelike shape. Unlike α_1-antitrypsin globular inclusions, they are periodic acid-Schiff (PAS) negative. Giant mitochondria are found in approximately 25% of cases of alcoholic liver disease. Their presence is thought to be associated with a more favorable prognosis.[30,31]

Induced or ground-glass hepatocytes in alcoholism resemble the ground-glass change seen in chronic hepatitis B surface antigen (HBsAg) carriers. The ground-glass effect is due to adaptive smooth endoplasmic reticulum (SER) proliferation. Unlike the HBsAg carrier, the Shikata staining methods for HBsAg material are negative in alcohol-related ground-glass change.

Oxyphil cells or oncocytes appear as enlarged somewhat hypereosinophilic hepatocytes due to increased numbers of closely packed mitochondria in H&E-stained preparations. This change may be focal or extensive (Fig. 8).

Hemosiderin accumulation in alcoholic liver disease is variable. Both hepatocellular and reticuloendothelial system (RES) distribution may be encountered. The presence of hemosiderin in Kupffer cells and portal macrophages may provide a clue to hematologic complications, such as hemolytic anemia or possible blood transfusion.

Hepatocellular accumulation of hemosiderin may be correlated with constitutional hemochromatosis, or with the oral ingestion of iron, or with portosystemic shunt surgery, in addition to the iron overload syndrome mimicking idiopathic hemochromatosis related to alcoholism. In porphyria cutanea tarda, hemosiderin may accumulate in both hepatocytes and Kupffer cells.

Portal ductular proliferation, which may be accompanied by acute cholangiolitis, may be encountered in patients with recurrent episodes of alcoholic hepatitis. It results from the transformation of zone 1-limiting plate hepatocytes. With progressive injury, portal expansion with fibrosis

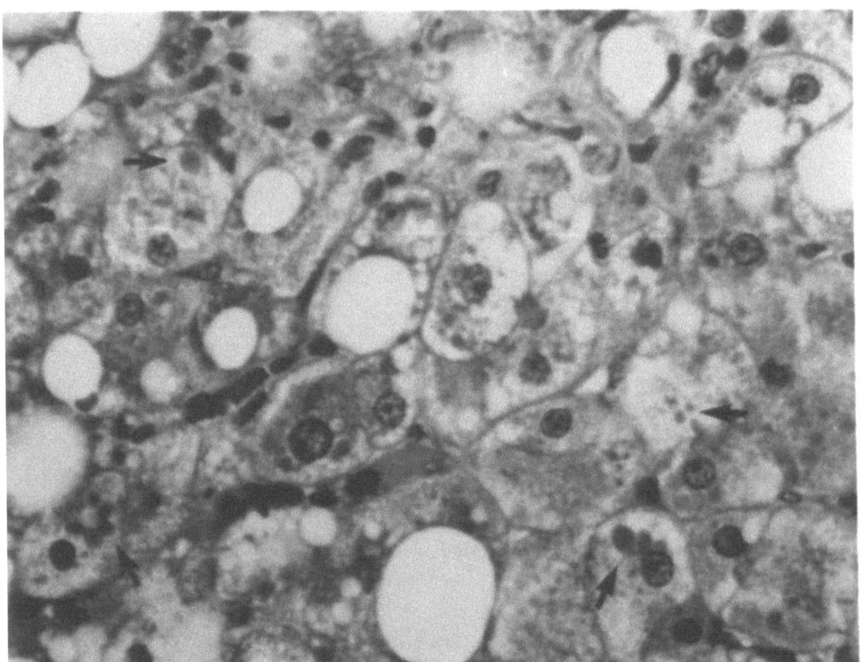

Figure 7. Alcoholic hepatitis with many swollen hepatocytes containing megamitochondria. Arrows point to several examples displaying variable size and distribution. (H&E, ×600)

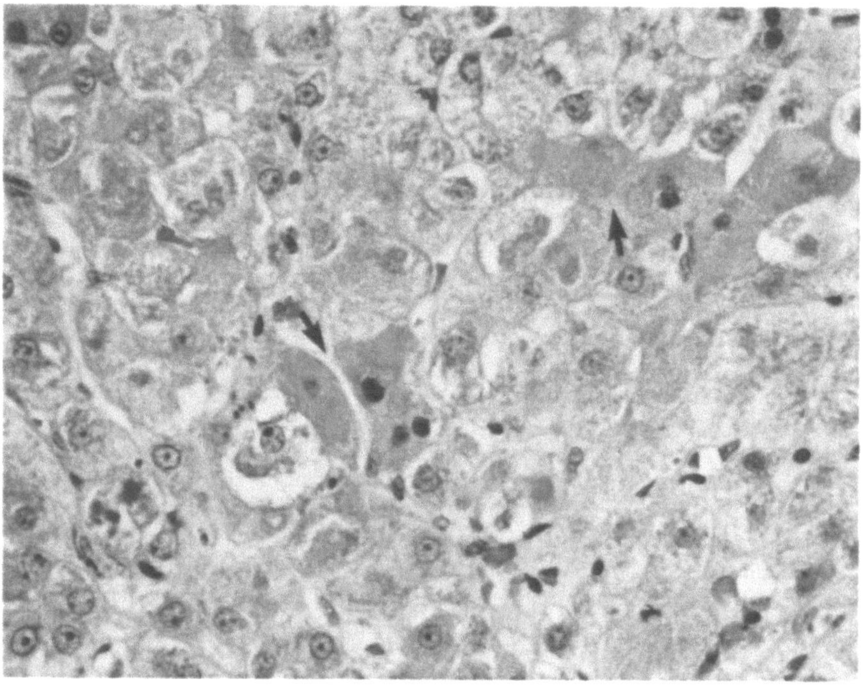

Figure 8. Alcoholic hepatitis. Arrows point to enlarged slightly darker staining hepatocytes (oncocytes) with a fine granular appearance. In occasional hepatocytes, irregular clumps and poorly formed aggregates of alcoholic hyalin are also present. (H&E, ×396)

occurs and, eventually, portal–portal bridging as well as portal–central bridging fibrosis develop.

Cholestasis, which may be present in any stage of alcoholic liver disease, is a frequent finding in alcoholic hepatitis. Most often, the bile pigment is seen in zone 3 bile canaliculi and to a much lesser extent in hepatocytes or Kupffer cells. Intrahepatic cholestasis in alcoholic hepatitis with acute cholangitis may suggest obstructive biliary tract disease due to concomitant alcohol-related acute pancreatitis.[32] The importance of recognizing cholestasis mimicking obstructive jaundice in alcoholic hepatitis cannot be overemphasized, in view of the increased surgical mortality risk in such patients.

4. PROGNOSTIC IMPLICATIONS

Continued alcohol ingestion most probably leads to cirrhosis and its complications.[33] In some cases, diffuse parenchymal injury may be severe enough to cause hepatic failure and death before cirrhosis is established. Diffuse or widespread Mallory body formation is indicative of more severe injury than occasional Mallory bodies.[1,4] Obliterative damage of hepatic venous outflow radicles may be severe enough to produce noncirrhotic portal hypertension.[28] Ultimately, it is the fibrosis that distorts the lobular architecture, leading to cirrhosis. Fibrous septa formation is more significant than pericellular "chicken-wire" fibrosis in the evolution to cirrhosis. Similarly, central–portal bridging fibrosis is more significant than central–central linkage in the progression to cirrhosis.

Although clinicopathologic correlation may be poor,[34] the morphologist evaluating liver biopsy material in alcoholic liver disease should record the severity of hepatic injury and activity to suggest prognostic implications as well as to serve as a basis for comparison with either previous or follow-up biopsy studies.

5. ALCOHOLIC CIRRHOSIS

In this discussion, cirrhosis is defined and classified according to the World Health Organization (WHO) report in 1977.[35] With progressive fibrosis, the normal lobular architecture undergoes pseudolobule formation and nodular regeneration, i.e., cirrhosis (Fig. 9). The nodular pattern of alcoholic cirrhosis is most often micronodular with nodules $\leq$3 mm in diameter surrounded by fibrous septa. In many instances, continuing regenerative activity gives rise to macronodules, with a resulting mixed micronodular–macronodular picture. A predominantly or purely macronodular cirrhosis in alcoholic liver disease is rather uncommon.

Morphologically, micronodular or mixed micromacronodular cirrhosis represents the end stage of liver disease, resulting from many causes. An alcoholic etiology is suggested by the presence of alcoholic fatty liver or the constellation of changes consistent with alcoholic hepatitis (Fig. 10). In patients who have stopped drinking alcohol, with eventual disappearance of fatty change, Mallory bodies, and inflammatory activity, establishing the cause of cirrhosis on purely morphologic grounds is virtually impossible. In occasional cases, focal accumulation of PAS-positive diastase-resistant α_1-antitrypsin globules or granules may be identified in the periseptal or periportal

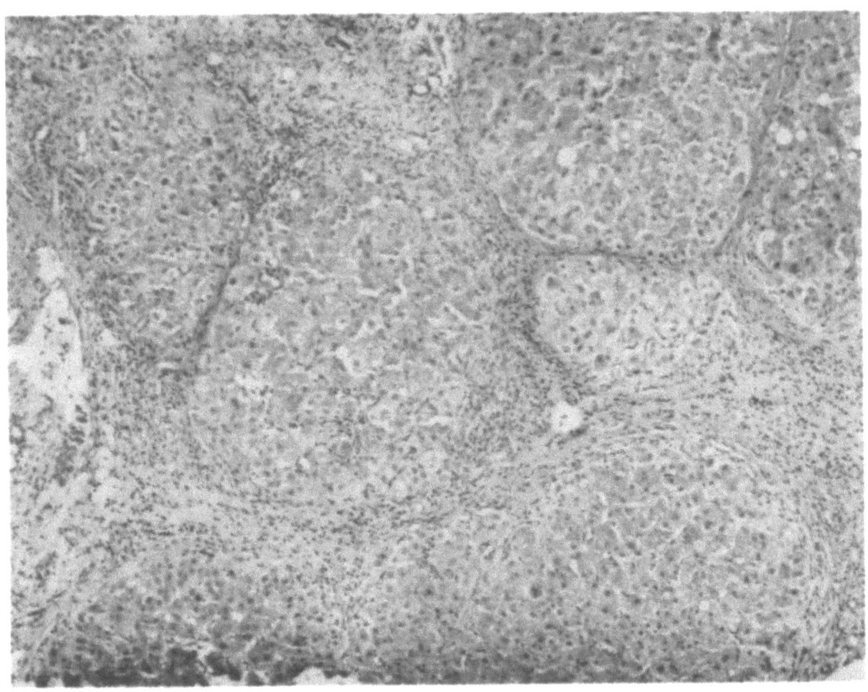

Figure 9. Alcoholic cirrosis. Note replacement of normal lobular architecture by regenerating micronodules. Minimal focal fatty metamorphosis present. Characteristic markers of alcoholic etiology not evident. (H&E, ×75)

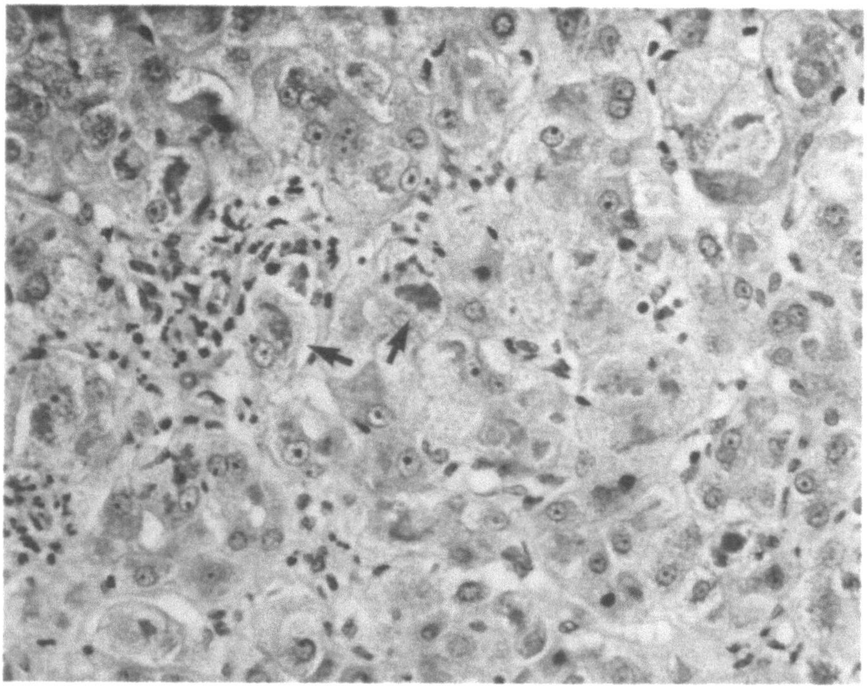

Figure 10. Portion of cirrhotic nodule with focal acute inflammatory cell infiltration several hepatocytes containing alcoholic hyalin (arrows). (H&E, ×300)

hepatocytes of patients who are phenotypically normal for α_1-antitrypsin[36] (Fig. 11). In known alcoholics, some cirrhotic livers without fatty change or alcoholic hyalin may contain portal and septal chronic inflammation, along with focal limiting plate irregularity that may be interpreted as having evolved from chronic active hepatitis (CAH) (Fig. 12). Indeed, alcoholism as a cause of CAH has been claimed in several published reports.[37–39] In more than one third of alcoholic cirrhotic livers, traces or even small amounts of copper or copper-associated protein may be detected with the aid of the rhodamine and the Shikata staining methods, respectively. In the inactive or end-stage alcoholic cirrhotic or precirrhotic liver, the presence of intralobular pericellular fibrosis, healed centrilobular sclerosing hyalin necrosis, or veno-occlusive changes, hemosiderosis and occasional portal, septal, or parenchymal lipogranulotoma may serve as clues to an alcoholic etiology.

6. DIFFERENTIAL DIAGNOSIS

It is relatively clear that, morphologically, there is no single pathognomonic light microscopic marker of alcoholic liver disease. As fatty liver is nonspecific, a presumptive diagnosis of alcoholism may be raised and seriously considered only if supported by reliable history and appropriate clinical signs, symptoms, or a blood alcohol determination.

The discovery in 1911 of alcoholic hyalin, synonymous with the Mallory body, provided a diagnostic marker for alcoholic liver injury. Over the next several decades, a number of nonalcoholic clinical settings and disease entities were recognized in which Mallory bodies could be

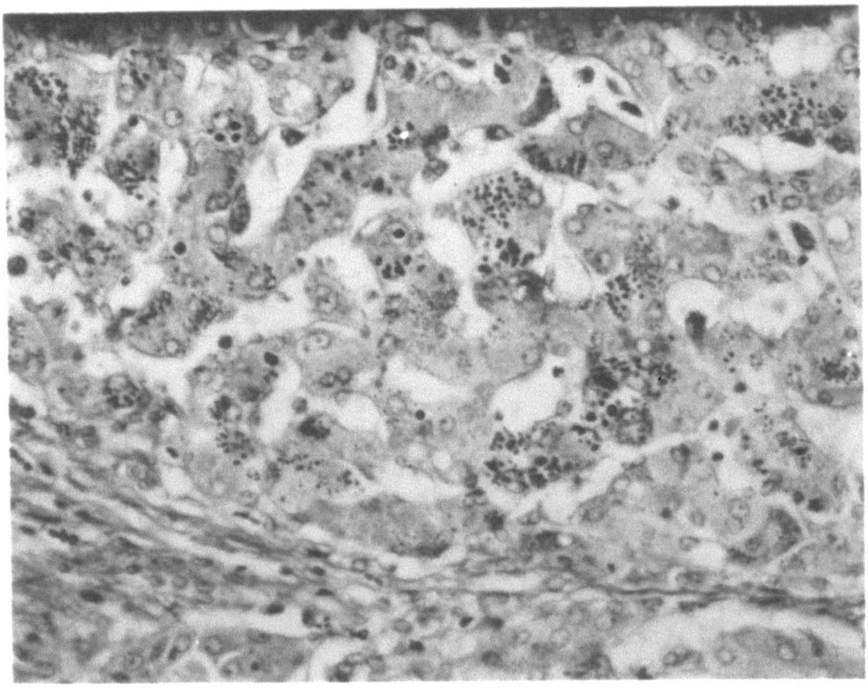

Figure 11. Alcoholic cirrhosis. Note presence of many diastase-resistant periodic acid-Schiff (PAS)-positive spherical cytoplasmic inclusions consistent with alpha-1-antitrypsin globules. Patient phenotypically normal. (PAS after diastase digestion, ×300)

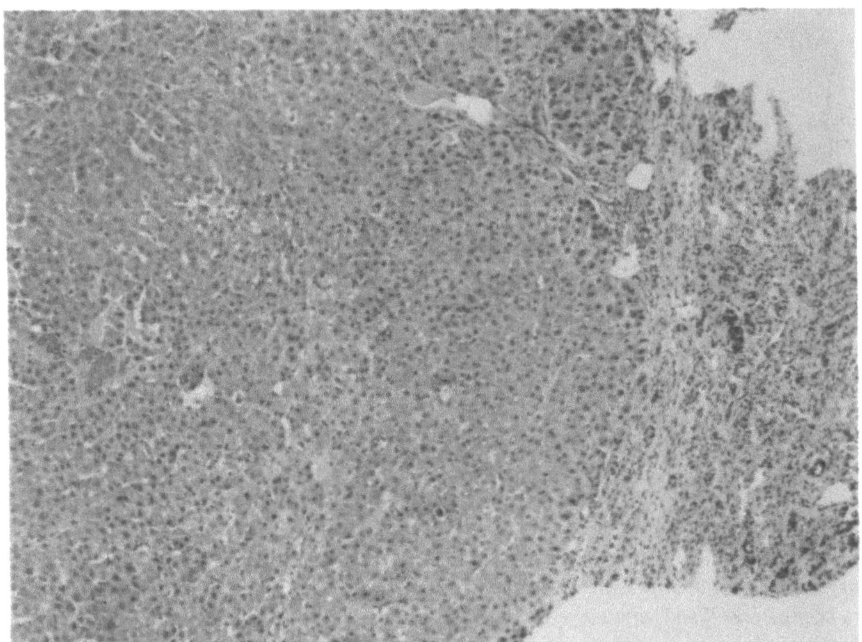

Figure 12. Alcoholic cirrhosis. The band of fibrosis containing portal area structures, ductular proliferation, chronic inflammation, slight limiting plate erosion, as well as a rare parenchymal free acidophilic body suggest chronic active hepatitis etiologically. (H&E, ×75)

found or in which changes mimicking the entire spectrum of alcohol liver injury were encountered, as summarized in Table II.

In recent years, changes resembling alcoholic fatty liver, alcoholic hepatitis, as well as cirrhosis have been observed in a number of susceptible obese and/or diabetic patients.[40–42] In some patients, well-formed Mallory bodies may be seen, but in most cases, the Mallory body material seems poorly formed or questionable at best. Whether Mallory bodies are present or not, the finding of fat, fibrosis, or cirrhosis may lead to an erroneous diagnosis in the absence of a relevant and reliable history. Similarly, a history of jejunoileal bypass surgery[43] or small bowel resection,[44] as well as an opportunity to compare pre- and postbypass liver sections should facilitate diagnostic interpretation.

Patients with porphyria cutanea tarda frequently have a history of heavy ethanol ingestion, that may contribute to the morphologic hepatic changes.[45] In addition to the possible accumulation of fat or the presence of Mallory bodies, the diagnosis may be made on the basis of iron overload and the presence of cytoplasmic acicular (needlelike) inclusions, along with the appropriate confirmatory ultraviolet (UV) tissue fluorescence and urinary uroporphyrin determination.[46] In his review on hepatic porphyrias, Bloomer[45] states that biopsy specimens in porphyria cutanea tarda lack the entire constellation of alcoholic hepatitis and that Mallory bodies are not seen.

The clinical setting and absence of fatty change in the liver should pose no difficulty in differentiating Indian childhood cirrhosis from alcoholic liver disease.[47] In cases of Wilson disease

Table II. Differential Diagnosis of Alcoholic Liver Disease[a]

Nonalcoholic steatohepatitis or steatonecrosis
Obesity[40–42]
Diabetes mellitus[40–42]
Postjejunoileal bypass surgery[43]
Short-gut syndrome[44]
Weber–Christian disease[65]
Abetalipoproteinemia[66]
Wilson's disease[48]
Porphyria cutanea tarde[45]
Drug-induced and chemical (therapeutic and experimental)
Amiodarone[52,53]
Perhexilene maleate[54,55]
Long-term glucocorticoid therapy[57]
Massive doses of synthetic estrogen[56]
Griseofulvin (experimental)[49]
Colchicine (experimental)[50]
Dieldrin (experimental)[51]
Chronic cholestatic syndromes
Primary biliary cirrhosis[58]
Primary sclerosing cholangitis[60]
Chronic progressive intrahepatic cholestasis of childhood[59]
Indian childhood cirrhosis[47]
Neoplasms and pseudotumors
Hepatocellular carcinoma[67]
Hepatocellular adenoma[62]
Focal nodular hyperplasia[68]
Nonhepatocelluar Mallory bodies
Biliary epithelium[62]
Pulmonary alveolar lining cells (asbestosis)[69]

[a]Selected references shown as superscript numbers.

that are not diagnosed until adolescence or during young adulthood, fatty change and portal fibrosis may raise the possibility of alcoholic liver injury.[48] If present, especially in early or established cirrhosis, the Mallory bodies in Wilson disease are periportal in distribution (zone 1). Staining for copper with supporting appropriate copper metabolism studies should resolve the diagnostic problem.

An important area in the differential diagnosis of alcoholic liver disease is the recognition of drug-induced pseudoalcoholic liver disease. Aside from experimental induction of Mallory bodies,[49–51] changes mimicking alcoholic liver disease have been documented with amiodarone,[52,53] perhexilene maleate therapy,[54,55] large doses of synthetic estrogens,[56] and long-term glucocorticoid therapy.[57] Amiodarone, an antiarrhythmic agent, has been shown to cause hepatic alterations similar to alcoholic liver disease including fatty change, Mallory bodies, fibrosis, and cirrhosis. In addition to alcohol-like liver injury, changes consistent with phospholipidosis may develop.[52,53] Although not available in the United States, perhexilene maleate, a cardiotherapeutic agent, also has the potential to induce pseudoalcoholic liver injury.[54,55]

While Mallory bodies may occur in chronic cholestatic syndromes, such as primary biliary cirrhosis (PBC)[58] and primary sclerosing cholangitis (PSC),[60] there should be little or no difficulty in differentiating these syndromes from alcoholic liver disease. In chronic cholestatic syndromes, Mallory body formation occurs relatively late in the clinical course when extensive fibrosis or biliary-type cirrhosis is present[59]; their distribution is in peripheral or periseptal hepatocytes (zone 1). The histopathologic diagnosis of PBC or PSC with intrahepatic involvement is based on recognizing or identifying chronic nonsuppurative destructive cholangitis and subsequent interlobular bile duct loss in the former and periductal fibrosis, eventually "strangling" interlobular bile ducts in the latter.

7. MALLORY BODIES

The nature and role of Mallory bodies in the diagnosis of alcoholic liver disease deserve special mention. The Mallory body, or alcoholic hyalin, is not pathognomonic of alcoholic liver disease. Despite the fact that Mallory bodies may be found or induced in a variety of conditions and circumstances, they are often considered a regular feature of alcoholic hepatitis. There is a sufficient body of evidence to conclude that they result from damage to the cytoskeleton and are composed of intermediate filaments.[27,60–62] Mallory body material contains several prekeratin-type polypeptides. Antibodies to epidermal cytokeratins have been shown to react with Mallory body prekeratins. Intact liver cells containing Mallory bodies appear to be viable. As a response to injury, the Mallory body change is reversible. Several studies suggest the following theories to explain Mallory body formation: (1) microtubular failure, (2) vitamin A deficiency, and (3) expression of preneoplasia.[60–62]

8. COMPLICATIONS

Alcoholic fatty liver, alcoholic hepatitis, and cirrhosis, alone or in combination, may result in hepatic failure and death, episodes of recurrent cholestasis, and iron overload. Portal hypertension is most commonly associated with cirrhosis but may be encountered in precirrhotic stages as a result of terminal hepatic venular and sublobular vein damage. Patients with alcoholic liver disease are at risk of superimposed drug injury such as acetaminophen[63] or toxic agents, such as carbon tetrachloride. Although deemed a controversial area, CAH and chronic persistent hepatitis have been attributed to alcoholism.[37–39] The significance of cytoplasmic accumulation of α_1-antitrypsin globules in hepatocytes in alcoholic patients with normal phenotypes for α_1-antitrypsin is not understood.

Last, but by no means least, the increased risk of primary hepatocellular carcinoma associated with alcoholic liver disease, even in the absence of cirrhosis, is well recognized. There is also well-documented evidence of cancer developing in other body sites in association with significant alcohol ingestion.[64]

REFERENCES

1. Baptista A, Bianchi L, DeGroote J, et al: Alcoholic liver disease: Morphologic manifestations. *Lancet* **1**:707–711, 1982.
2. French SW, Burbege EJ: Alcoholic hepatitis; clinical, morphologic, pathogenic and therapeutic aspects. *Prog Liver Dis* **6**:557–579, 1979.
3. Hall P: The pathological spectrum of alcoholic liver disease. *Pathology* **17**:209–218, 1985.
4. MacSween RNM, Burt AD: Histologic spectrum of alcoholic liver disease. *Semin Liver Dis* **6**:221–232, 1986.
5. Desmet VJ: Alcoholic liver disease. Histological features and evolution. *Acta Med Scand* **703**(suppl):111–126, 1985.
6. Lieber CS, Jones DP, DeCarli LM: Effects of prolonged ethanol intake: Production of fatty liver despite adequate diets. *J Clin Invest* **44**:1009–1021, 1965.
7. Rubin E, Lieber CS: Alcohol-induced hepatic injury in nonalcoholic volunteers. *N Engl J Med* **278**:869–876, 1968.
8. Lieber CS: Metabolism and metabolic effects of ethanol. *Med Clin North Am* **68**:3–31, 1984.
9. Christofferson P, Poulsen H: Alcoholic liver disease, in MacSween RNM, Anthony PP, Scheuer PF (eds): *Pathology of the Liver*. Churchill-Livingstone, Edinburgh, 1979, pp. 232–248.
10. Randall B: Sudden death and hepatic fatty metamorphosis. *JAMA* **243**:1723–1725, 1980.
11. Randall B: Fatty liver and sudden death. *Hum Pathol* **11**:147–153, 1980.
12. Popper H, Szanto RB: Fatty liver with hepatic failure in alcoholics. *J Mt Sinai Hosp* **24**:1121–1131, 1957.
13. Uchida T, Kao H, Quispe-Sjogren M, et al: Alcoholic foamy degeneration—A pattern of acute alcoholic injury of the liver. *Gastroenterology* **84**:683–692, 1983.
14. Kunelis CT, Peters RL, Edmondson HA: Fatty liver of pregnancy and its relationship to tetracycline. *Am. J Med* **38**:359–377, 1965.
15. Rolfes, DB, Ishak KG: Acute fatty liver of pregnancy. A clinicopathologic study of 35 cases. *Hepatology* **5**:1149–1158, 1985.
16. Bove KE, McAdams AJ, Partin JC, et al: The hepatic lesion in Reye's syndrome. *Gastroenterology* **69**:685–697, 1975.
17. Davis J: Liver damage due to tetracycline and its relationship to pregnancy, in Meyler L, Peck HM (eds): *Drug-Induced Diseases*. Excerpta Medica Foundation, Amsterdam, 1968, pp. 103–110.
18. Peters RL, Edmondson HA, Mikkelsen WP, et al: Tetracycline-induced fatty liver in non-pregnant patients. *Am J Surg* **113**:622–632, 1967.
19. Zimmerman HJ, Ishak KG: Valproate induced hepatic injury. Analysis of 23 fatal cases. *Hepatology* **2**:591–597, 1982.
20. Starko KM, Mullick FG: Hepatic and cerebral pathology findings in children with fatal salicylate intoxication. *Lancet* **1**:326–329, 1983.
21. Wolman M, Sterk VV, Gatt S, et al: Primary familial xanthomatosis with involvement and calcification of adrenals. *Pediatrics* **28**:742–745, 1961.
22. Miller R, Bialer MG, Rogers F, et al: Wolman's disease. Report of a case with multiple studies. *Arch Pathol Lab Med* **106**:41–45, 1982.
23. Schiff L, Schubert WK, McAdams A, et al: Hepatic cholesterol ester storage disease, a familial disorder. *Am J Med* **44**:538–546, 1968.
24. Walser M: Urea cycle disorders and other hyperammonemic syndromes, in Stanbury JB, Wyngaarden JB, Fredrickson DS, et al. (eds): *The Metabolic Basis of Inherited Disease*, 5th ed. McGraw-Hill, New York, 1983, pp. 402–438.
25. Glasgow AM, Eng G, Engel AG: Systemic carnitine deficiency simulating Reye's syndrome. *J Pediatr* **96**:889–891, 1980.
26. French SW: Present understanding of the development of Mallory bodies. *Arch Pathol Lab Med* **107**:445–450, 1982.
27. Denk H, Lockinger E, Vennigerholtz F: Pathology of the cytoskeleton of hepatocytes, in Popper H,

Schaffner F (eds): *Progress in Liver Diseases*, Vol. VIII. Grune & Stratton, Orlando, Florida, 1986, pp. 237–251.

28. Goodman ZD, Ishak KG: Occlusive venous lesions in alcoholic liver disease. A study of 200 cases. *Gastroenterology* **83**:786–796, 1982.
29. Van de Wiel A, Delacroix DL, Van Hattum J, et al: Characteristics of serum IgA and liver IgA deposits in alcoholic liver disease. *Hepatology* **7**:95–99, 1987.
30. Uchida T, Kronborg I, Peters RL: Giant mitochondria in alcoholic liver disease—Their identification, frequency and pathologic significance. *Liver* **4**:29–38, 1984.
31. Chedid A, Mendenhall T, Tosch T, et al: Significance of megamitochondria in alcoholic liver disease. *Gastroenterology* **90**:1858–1864, 1986.
32. Afroudakis A, Kaplowitz N: Liver histopathology in chronic common bile duct stenosis due to chronic alcoholic pancreatitis. *Hepatology* **1**:65–72, 1981.
33. Schenker S. Alcoholic liver disease: Evaluation of natural history and prognostic factors. *Hepatology* **4**:36S–43S, 1984.
34. Orrego H, Blake JE, Blendis LM, et al: Prognosis of alcoholic cirrhosis in the presence and absence of alcoholic hepatitis. *Gastroenterology* **92**:208–214, 1987.
35. Anthony PP, Ishak KG, Nayak NC, et al: The morphology of cirrhosis. *Bull WHO* **4**:521–540, 1977.
36. Pariente EA, Degott C, Martin JP, et al: Hepatocytic PAS-positive diastase resitant inclusions in the absence of alpha-1-antitrypsin deficiency—High prevalence in alcoholic cirrhosis. *Am J Clin Pathol* **76**:299–302, 1981.
37. Goldberg SJ, Mendenhall CL, Cannell AM, et al: "Nonalcoholic" chronic hepatitis in the alcoholic. *Gastroenterology* **72**:598–604, 1977.
38. Crapper RM, Bhatal PS, MacKay JR: Chronic active hepatitis in alcoholic patients. *Liver* **3**:327–337, 1983.
39. Nei J, Matsuda Y, Takada A: Chronic hepatitis induced by alcohol. *Dig Dis Sci* **28**:207–215, 1983.
40. Adler M, Schaffner F: Fatty liver hepatitis and cirrhosis in obese patients. *Am J Med* **67**:811–816, 1979.
41. Ludwig J, Viggiano TR, McGill DB, et al: Non-alcoholic steatohepatitis. *Mayo Clin Proc* **55**:434–438, 1980.
42. Schaffner F, Thaler H: Non-alcoholic fatty liver disease, in Popper H, Schaffner F (eds): *Progress in Liver Disease*, Vol. VIII. Grune & Stratton, Orlando, Florida, 1986, pp. 283–298.
43. Peters RL, Gary T, Reynolds TB: Post-jejunoileal bypass hepatic disease. Its similarity to alcoholic hepatic disease. *Am J Clin Pathol* **63**:318–331, 1975.
44. Craig RM, Newman T, Jeejeebhoy KN, et al: Severe hepatocellular reaction resembling alcoholic hepatitis with cirrhosis after massive small bowel resection and prolonged total parenteral nutrition. *Gastroenterology* **79**:131–137, 1980.
45. Bloomer JR: The hepatic porphyrias. *Gastroenterology* **71**:689–701, 1976.
46. Fakan F, Chlumska A: Demonstration of needle-shaped hepatic inclusions in porphyria cutanea tarda using the ferric ferricyanide reduction test. *Virchows Arch A* **411**:365–368, 1987.
47. Roy S, Ramalingaswami V, Nayak NC: An ultrastructural study of the liver in Indian childhood cirrhosis with particular reference to the structure of cytoplasmic hyaline. *Gut* **12**:693–701, 1971.
48. Sternlieb I: Evolution of the hepatic lesion in Wilson's disease (hepatolenticular degeneration), in Popper H, Schaffner F (eds): *Progress in Liver Diseases*, Vol. IV. Grune & Stratton, Orlando, Florida, 1979, pp. 511–525.
49. Denk H, Eckerstorfer R, Gschnait F, et al: Experimental induction of hepatocellular hyaline (Mallory bodies) in mice by griseofulvin treatment. I. Light microscopic observations. *Lab Invest* **35**:377–382, 1976.
50. Denk H, Eckerstorfer R: Colchicine-induced Mallory body formation in the mouse. *Lab Invest* **30**:563–565, 1977.
51. Meierhenry EF, Reubner BH, Gershwin ME, et al: Mallory body formation in hepatic nodules of mice ingesting dieldrin. *Lab Invest* **44**:392–396, 1981.
52. Lewis JH, Ranard RC, Caruso A, et al: Amiodarone hepatotoxicity: Incidence and clinical pathologic correlations among 104 patients. *Hepatology* in press, 1989.
53. Simon JB, Manley RN, Brien JF, et al: Amiodarone hepatotoxicity simulating alcoholic liver disease. *N Engl J Med* **311**:167–172, 1984.
54. Pessayre D, Bichara M, Feldmann G, et al: Perhexiline maleate-induced cirrhosis. *Gastroenterology* **76**:170–177, 1979.
55. Rosensztajn L, deSaint-Maus PP: Perhexiline maleate-associated hepatic injury. Prevalence and characteristics. *Digestion* **20**:145–150, 1980.

56. Seki K, Minami Y, Nishikawa M, et al: "Non-alcoholic steatohepatitis" induced by massive doses of synthetic estrogen. *Gastroenterol Jpn* **18:**197–203, 1983.
57. Itoh S, Igrashi M, Tsukada Y, et al: Non-alcoholic fatty liver with alcoholic hyaline after long term glucocorticoid therapy. *Acta Hepatogastroenterol* **24:**415–418, 1977.
58. Monroe S, French SW, Zamboni L: Mallory bodies in a case of biliary cirrhosis: An ultrastructural and morphogenetic study. *Am J Clin Pathol* **59:**254–262, 1973.
59. Jones EA, Rabin L, Buckley CH, et al: Progressive intrahepatic cholestasis of infancy and childhood. A clinicopathological study of a patient surviving to the age of 18 years. *Gastroenterology* **71:**675–682, 1976.
60. French SW: Present understanding of the development of Mallory bodies. *Arch Pathol Lab Med* **107:**445–450, 1983.
61. French SW: The Mallory body: Structure, composition and pathogenesis. *Hepatology* **1:**76–83, 1981.
62. Yokoo H, Minick OT, Batti F, et al: Morphologic variants of alcoholic hyalin. *Am J Pathol* **69:**25–40, 1972.
63. Seeff LB, Cuccherini BA, Zimmerman HJ, et al: Acetaminophen hepatotoxicity in alcoholics. A therapeutic misadventure. *Ann Intern Med* **104:**399–404, 1986.
64. Lieber C, Garro A, Leo MA, et al: Alcohol and cancer. *Hepatology* **6:**1005–1019, 1986.
65. Kimura H, Kako M, Yo K, et al: Alcoholic hyaline (Mallory bodies) in a case of Weber–Christian disease. *Gastroenterology* **78:**807–812, 1980.
66. Partin JS, Partin JC, Schubert WK, et al: Liver ultrastructure in abetalipoproteinemia: Evolution of micronodular cirrhosis. *Gastroenterology* **67:**107–118, 1974.
67. Keeley AF, Iseri OA, Gottlieb LS: Ultrastructure of hyaline cytoplasmic inclusions in human hepatoma: Relationship to Mallory's alcoholic hyaline. *Gastroenterology* **62:**280–293, 1972.
68. Wetzel WJ, Alexander RW: Focal nodular hyperplasia of the liver with alcoholic hyaline bodies and cytologic atypia. *Cancer* **44:**1322–1326, 1979.
69. Warnock ML, Press M, Churg A: Further observations on cytoplasmic hyaline in the lung. *Hum Pathol* **11:**59–65, 1980.

12

Autoimmune Chronic Active Hepatitis

Firas H. Al-Kawas

1. INTRODUCTION

Chronic active hepatitis is a clinicopathologic syndrome caused by a group of heterogeneous disorders that share in common a characteristic histologic picture (Table I). The clinical presentation, natural history, and response to treatment vary widely among the different etiologies. Clinically, the syndrome is defined by persistent necroinflammation in the liver for more than 6 months, as reflected by persistent elevation of serum aminotransferase levels. A group of patients with no viral markers, demonstrating hypergammaglobulinemia and a variety of non-organ-specific immunologic markers have been designated as having autoimmune or lupoid chronic active hepatitis and are responsible for approximately one third of all chronic hepatitis cases.[1]

The first description of this entity was by Waldenstrom[2] in Sweden, who reported a group of young women with cirrhosis, marked elevation of serum gammaglobulin, and plasma cell infiltration on liver biopsy. Later, other investigators described similar groups of patients,[3–5] many of whom had a positive lupus erythematosus (LE) cell test.[5,6] This led MacKay et al.[6] from Australia to suggest the name lupoid hepatitis. Many other names (Table II) have been used to describe this entity and were more a reflection of symptoms, pathology, or lack of understanding of the disease. More recently, some investigators have questioned the existence of the syndrome as a separate entity and suggested that these autoimmune markers may indicate a more active and severe liver disease.[7,8]

The following is an attempt to review the current literature in reference to this entity. The name autoimmune chronic active hepatitis will be used since it reflects both the serologic autoimmune markers and the histology encountered in this disease and does not in any way propose that this is a homogeneous entity. This discussion will be limited to the clinical and therapeutic aspects of the disease. Professor MacSween will discuss the pathologic aspects.

2. CLINICAL AND BIOCHEMICAL FEATURES

Since the initial description by Waldenstrom,[2] it was apparent that the majority of patients were women between the ages of 10 and 30 years. Nevertheless, the disease has been described

Firas H. Al-Kawas • Georgetown University School of Medicine, Division of Gastroenterology/Hepatology/Nutrition, Veterans Administration Medical Center, Washington, D.C. 20422.

Table I. Causes of Chronic Active Hepatitis

Autoimmune (lupoid)
Viral hepatitis (B, D, NANB)
Drugs
α_1-Antitrypsin deficiency
Hemochromatosis
Wilson's disease

in males,[9–11] and in postmenopausal women.[12] In early series, the onset in most patients was insidious,[3,9,11] but in approximately 25% the disease presented as an attack of acute hepatitis. In the early reports,[3,4,9] most patients were symptomatic, but the widespread use of automated autoanalyzers has led to the discovery of a growing number of asymptomatic or mildly symptomatic patients.[13–16] In the symptomatic group, easy fatiguability is a common finding. Jaundice is seen in 77% of patients, and a variety of endocrine manifestations, including amenorrhea and delayed menarche, are seen in young women. The most common presenting symptoms are listed in Table III.

The biochemical features reflect the necroinflammatory nature of the disease, with elevation of aminotransferase levels up to 500 IU/liter in most patients. Rarely, higher values similar to levels in acute hepatitis are seen, but most of these patients have clinical and biochemical findings suggestive of chronic liver disease.[17] Hyperbilirubinemia is present in most patients in the reported series. Alkaline phosphatase is usually less than twice the upper limit of normal except for the rare form of cholestatic chronic active hepatitis.[18] Hypergammaglobulinemia, sometimes to a striking level, is seen in approximately 80% of patients.[11]

The LE cell phenomenon is seen in up to 27% of patients[11] and a variety of non-organ-specific antibodies have been described.[19,20] These are listed in Table IV. Approximately 30% of patients will have more than one antibody.[11] Recently, a new classification based on the type of antibody detected has been proposed[20–22] and is listed in Table V. This subdivision identifies three different subgroups that may be immunologically different and that may serve in further identifying patients with autoimmune CAH. Patients with so-called classic autoimmune CAH have positive sera for antinuclear antibodies (ANA), while the presence of antiliver/kidney microsomal antibodies appear to identify younger patients with more active and advanced disease.[23] The titer of antibodies tends to decrease with treatment.[11] The value of this classification from a prognostic and therapeutic point of view is not clear. Also of interest is the high prevalence of seroimmunologic abnormalities in relatives of patients with autoimmune chronic active hepatitis.[24]

3. ASSOCIATED DISEASES

A large number of associated autoimmune disorders have been described in up to 63% of patients.[10,11,25] A partial list is presented in Table VI. Ulcerative colitis has been reported to have an adverse effect on the course of autoimmune hepatitis,[9] although many of the reported cases may have had sclerosing cholangitis. Overall, the associated autoimmune diseases do not seem to alter the course of hepatitis.

4. IMMUNOLOGY AND GENETICS

Patients with autoimmune CAH have many features that reflect a possible immune mechanism. These include infiltration of the portal area with plasma cells, elevation of the serum gammaglob-

Table II. Other Names for Autoimmune Chronic Active Hepatitis

Lupoid hepatitis
Chronic liver disease in young women
Active juvenile cirrhosis
Disproteinemic cirrhosis of unknown origin in women

Table III. Presenting Symptoms in Chronic Active Hepatitis

Easy fatiguability
Jaundice
Delayed menarche and amenorrhea
Pruritus
Myalgia
Anorexia

Table IV. Antibodies in Autoimmune Chronic Active Hepatitis

Antinuclear
Antismooth muscle (antiactin)
Anti liver/kidney microsomes (anti-LKMI)
Antimitochondrial
Antisoluble liver antigen (anti-SLA)

Table V. Classification of Autoimmune Chronic Active Hepatitis

Antiactin positive[a]
Anti-LKMI positive
Anti-SLA positive

[a]Anti-smooth muscle.

Table VI. Diseases Associated with Autoimmune Chronic Active Hepatitis

Thyroiditis	Pernicious anemia
Rheumatoid arthritis	Urticaria
Sjogren's syndrome	Coomb's positive hemolytic anemia
Thrombocytopenic purpura pleuritis, pericarditis	Membranoproliferative glomerulonephritis

ulin, the LE cell phenomenon, and a variety of non-organ-specific antibodies.[26] More recently, three other antibodies have been described.[20,26,27] Two of these antibodies are directed against components of the hepatocyte membrane: the liver-specific protein (LSP) and the liver membrane antigen (LMAg).[26] A third antibody is directed against a liver-soluble antigen (SLA).[27] None of these antibodies has been shown to be directly responsible for the hepatocellular injury.

Two HLA antigens, HLA B8 and DR3, have been shown to be more common in patients with autoimmune CAH compared with other patients with chronic liver disease.[16] Immunoglobulin allotype Gm ax is also found in a large number of patients with autoimmune CAH.[28,29] In fact, the combination of HLA B8 and Gm ax raised the risk of autoimmune CAH by 39-fold.[28] Other immunologic abnormalities have also been described in patients with autoimmune CAH. These include a decrease in the activity of suppressor T cells and an increased activity of cytotoxic T lymphocytes and B cells,[21,26,28] reflecting a defect in immunoregulation. The question as to what causes the immunologic response remains to be answered. A variety of possibilities, including drugs and viruses, in addition to environmental or genetic factors, have been considered. Better definition of non-A, non-B (NANB) hepatitis by identifying the virus(es) will help in further selecting the group of patients with autoimmune CAH.

5. NATURAL HISTORY

Early reports were characterized by patients with advanced liver disease[2–4]; most patients having cirrhosis on presentation with many having features of advanced liver disease, i.e., hyperbilirubinemia and coagulopathy. Mortality varied from 48% to 75% at 10 years.[3,30–32] These numbers, however, do not reflect the survival of patients with less advanced liver disease. Overall, approximately 50% of patients with autoimmune CAH will live for 15 years.[16] In two large series recently reported from England[14] and the United States,[15] most patients had mild to moderate disease. More data are needed to better understand the natural history of asymptomatic or mild autoimmune CAH.

6. TREATMENT

Compared with the other causes of CAH, the autoimmune form stands out because of its generally favorable response to corticosteroids.[31–34] Histologic remission and improved survival have been shown after treatment. Both 5- and 10-year survival improved to 87% and 63%, respectively.[30,31] Several issues concerning treatment, however, need to be addressed. The first is when to start therapy. Clinical, biochemical, and histologic factors have to be considered (Table VII). The

Table VII. Factors Favoring Treatment in Patients with Autoimmune Chronic Active Hepatitis

Clinical
Young female
Symptomatic patient
Laboratory
Elevated aminotransferase > 5 × normal
Elevated bilirubin
Elevated gammaglobulin
Bridging necrosis or active cirrhosis on liver biopsy

more of these factors the patient has, the more inclined the physician should be to treat. The second issue concerns the use of prednisone versus prednisolone. While prednisone is metabolized in the liver to prednisolone, studies have shown that prednisone is metabolized by the sick liver to prednisolone, with no significant difference in the therapeutic efficacy between the two.[36]

The issue of corticosteroid dosage is not resolved; probably there is no difference between starting with a high dose and decreasing it after biochemical resolution, or starting and maintaining the patient on a low dose (i.e., 10–20 mg). Everyday steroids are preferred, since alternate-day regimens are associated with less histologic resolution.[11] Azathioprine has a steroid-sparing effect,[32] and combination therapy with prednisone is probably the ideal choice, especially in elderly patients requiring treatment.[12,32] Major and minor side effects related to the use of steroids are listed in Table VIII. The incidence of side effects varies among studies and is dependent on the dosage and length of treatment. Combination regimens tend to be associated with a lesser incidence of both major and minor side effects,[35] while the use of steroids in elderly female patients is associated with an increased risk of side effects.[12] Even though the use of azathioprine has been associated with the development of lymphomas in post-transplant patients,[36] no such clear-cut association has been demonstrated in patients with liver disease.[11,37]

End points for treatment include clinical, biochemical, and histologic remission. In most patients, biochemical remission is seen in the first few months after starting treatment,[11,28] with an improved sense of well-being. In young females, the return or appearance of their menses is a sign indicating good response to treatment. Histological remission, defined by the regression of CAH features to chronic persistent hepatitis or active cirrhosis to inactive cirrhosis, takes longer. Most patients who respond to therapy will reach that point by 18 months.[32] Remission rates decrease substantially after 3 years[32] and despite treatment, 46–50% of patients will develop cirrhosis[11,32,38] and some will develop esophageal varices.[39] Hepatocellular carcinoma has been reported in patients with autoimmune CAH.[40,41] Its occurrence is rare and seems to be related to the development of cirrhosis.

Relapse after treatment withdrawal is very common, ranging from 50% in the Mayo Clinic trial[42] to 87% in the Royal Free study.[43] Relapse in the Mayo Clinic trial[40] occurred more often in patients who had cirrhosis on entry (83%) and was far less frequent in patients who reverted to a normal histology after treatment (28%). Even withdrawal of azathioprine in one study[44] was associated with 32% relapse rate. Overall, in the management of patients who satisfy the criteria for treatment, it is recommended to start with 20 mg prednisone or a combination of 10 mg prednisone and 50 mg azathioprine. If progressive improvement in clinical and biochemical parameters is seen, a repeat biopsy may be obtained after 2–3 years of treatment to assess histologic response, but

Table VIII. Side Effects Associated with the Use of Steroids in Chronic Active Hepatitis

Mild
Obesity
Acne
Cushingoid facies
Hypertension
Severe
Osteoporosis and vertebral collapse
Aseptic necrosis
Cataracts
Mycotic infections
Insulin-dependent diabetes

repeating the liver biopsy earlier is probably not indicated. If features of chronic persistent hepatitis or inactive cirrhosis are seen on repeat liver biopsy an attempt should be made to decrease corticosteroids slowly and later to discontinue them completely. Most patients, however, will need to be maintained on steroids and will relapse off treatment.

7. CONCLUSIONS

Autoimmune chronic active hepatitis is best regarded as a heterogeneous entity in which multiple etiologies associated with a variable genetic predisposition may lead to similar lesions in the liver because of the limited fashion by which the liver can respond. In addition, a better definition of what actually constitutes autoimmune CAH, as well as long-term studies looking at the natural history of asymptomatic and mildly symptomatic patients with CAH, are needed. Until that information is obtained, there will continue to be many questions about the diagnosis, management, and follow-up of these patients.

REFERENCES

1. Seeff LB, Wright EC: An overview and appraisal of the Mayo Clinic trial for chronic active hepatitis, in Czaja AJ, Dickson RE (eds): *Chronic Active Hepatitis. The Mayo Clinic Experience.* Dekker, New York, 1986, pp. 315–340.
2. Waldenstrom J: Leber Blutproteine und Nahrungseiweiss. *Dtsch Gesellsch Verdau Stoffwechselkr* **15**:113–119, 1950.
3. Bearn AG, Kunkel HG, Slater RJ: The problem of chronic liver disease in young women. *Am J Med* **21**:3–15, 1956.
4. MacLachlan MJ, Rodnan GP, Cooper WM, et al: Chronic active (lupoid) hepatitis: A clinical, serological and pathological study of 20 patients. *Ann Intern Med* **62**:425–462, 1965.
5. Joske RA, King WE. The "LE cell" phenomenon in active chronic viral hepatitis. *Lancet* **2**:477–480, 1955.
6. MacKay IR, Taft LT, Cowling DC: Lupoid hepatitis. *Lancet* **2**:1323–3126, 1956.
7. Soloway RD, Summerskill WHJ, Baggenstoss AH, et al: "Lupoid" hepatitis, a non-entity in the spectrum of chronic active liver disease. *Gastroenterology* **63**:458–465, 1972.
8. Czaja AJ, Davis GL, Ludwig J, et al: Autoimmune features as determinants of prognosis in steroid-treated chronic active hepatitis of uncertain etiology. *Gastroenterology* **85**:713–718, 1983.
9. Mistilis SP, Blackburn CRB: Active chronic hepatitis. *Am J Med* **48**:484–495, 1970.
10. Sherlock S: Progress report. Chronic hepatitis. *Gut* **15**:581–597, 1974.
11. Czaja AJ: Natural history, clinical features and treatment of autoimmune chronic active hepatitis. *Semin Liver Dis* **4**:1–12, 1984.
12. Lebovics E, Schaffner F, Klion FM, et al: Autoimmune chronic active hepatitis in post menopausal women. *Dig Dis Sci* **30**:824–828, 1985.
13. Plotz PH: Asymptomatic chronic hepatitis. *Gastroenterology* **68**:1629–1630, 1975.
14. Hodges JR, Millward-Sadler GH, Wright R: Chronic active hepatitis: The spectrum of disease. *Lancet* **1**:550–552, 1982.
15. Koretz RL, Lewin KJ, Higgins J, et al: Chronic active hepatitis. Who meets treatment criteria? *Dig Dis Sci* **25**:695–699, 1980.
16. Schaffner F: Autoimmune chronic active hepatitis. Three decades of progress, in Popper H, Schaffner F (eds): *Progress in Liver Disease,* Vol. VIII. Grune & Stratton, Orlando, Florida, 1986, pp. 485–503.
17. Davis GL, Czaja AJ, Baggenstoss AH, et al: Prognostic and therapeutic implications of extreme serum aminotransferase elevation in chronic active hepatitis. *Mayo Clin Proc* **57**:303–309, 1982.
18. Shouval D, Levij IS, Eliakim M: Chronic active hepatitis with cholestatic features. I. A clinical and immunologic study. *Am J Gastroenterol* **72**:542–550, 1979.
19. Doniach D, Roitt IM, Walker JG, et al: Tissue antibodies in primary biliary cirrhosis, active chronic

(lupoid) hepatitis, cryptogenic cirrhosis and other liver diseases and their clinical implication. *Clin Exp Immunol* **1**:237–262, 1966.
20. Meyer Zum Buschenfeld KH, Manns M: Mechanisms of autoimmune liver disease. *Semin Liver Dis* **4**:26–35, 1984.
21. Thomas HC, Lok ASF: The immunopathology of autoimmune and hepatitis B virus-induced chronic hepatitis. *Semin Liver Dis* **4**:36–46, 1984.
22. Maddrey WC: Subdivisions of idopathic autoimmune chronic active hepatitis. *Hepatology* **7**:1372–1375, 1987.
23. Homberg JC, Abuaf N, Bernard O, et al: Chronic active hepatitis associated with anti liver/kidney microsome antibody type 1: A second type of autoimmune hepatitis. *Hepatology* **7**:1333–1339, 1987.
24. Galbraith RM, Smith M, MacKenzie RM, et al: High prevalence of seroimmunologic abnormalities in relatives of patients with active chronic hepatitis or primary biliary cirrhosis. *N Engl J Med* **290**:64–69, 1974.
25. Golding PL, Smith M, Williams R: Multisystem involvement in chronic liver disease. Studies on the incidence and pathogenesis. *Am J Med* **55**:772–782, 1973.
26. Mackay IR: Immunological aspects of chronic active hepatitis. *Hepatology* **3**:724–728, 1983.
27. Manns M, Gerken G, Kynatsoulis A, et al: Characterization of a new subgroup of autoimmune chronic active hepatitis by auto antibodies against a soluble liver antigen. *Lancet* **1**:292–294, 1987.
28. MacKay IR: Genetic aspects of immunologically mediated liver disease. *Semin Liver Dis* **4**:13–25, 1984.
29. Eddelston ALWF. Immunology of chronic active hepatitis. *Q J Med* **55**:191–195, 1985.
30. Cook GC, Mulligan R, Sherlock S: Controlled prospective trial of corticosteroid therapy in active chronic hepatitis. *Q J Med* **158**:159–185, 1971.
31. Kirk AP, Jain S, Pocock S, et al: Late results of the Royal Free Hospital prospective controlled trial of prednisolone therapy in hepatitis B surface antigen negative chronic active hepatitis. *Gut* **21**:78–83, 1980.
32. Soloway RD, Summerskill WHJ, Baggenstoss AH, et al: Clinical, biochemical and histological remission of severe chronic active liver disease: A controlled study of treatments and early prognosis. *Gastroenterology* **63**:820–833, 1972.
33. Murray-Lyon IM, Stern RB, Williams R: Controlled trial of prednisone and azathioprine in active chronic hepatitis. *Lancet* **1**:735–737, 1973.
34. Wright EC, Seeff LB, Berk PD, et al: Treatment of chronic active hepatitis. An analysis of three controlled trials. *Gastroenterology* **73**:1422–1430, 1977.
35. Schalm SW, Summerskill WHJ, Go VLW: Prednisone for chronic active liver disease. Pharmakokinetics, including conversion to prednisolone. *Gastroenterology* **72**:910–913, 1977.
36. Penn I, Hammond N, Brettschneider L, et al: Malignant lymphomas in transplant patients. *Transplant Proc* **1**:106–112, 1969.
37. Czaja AJ, Summerskill WHJ. Malignancy in chronic liver disease. *Gastroenterology* **73**:192–193, 1977.
38. DeGroote J, Fevery J, Lepoutre L: Long term followup of chronic active hepatitis of moderate severity. *Gut* **19**:510–513, 1978.
39. Czaja AJ, Wolf AM, Summerskill WHJ: Development and early prognosis of esophageal varices in severe chronic active liver disease (CALD) treated with prednisone. *Gastroenterology* **77**:629–633, 1979.
40. Jackobovits AW, Gibson PR, Duddley FJ: Primary liver cell carcinoma complicating autoimmune chronic active hepatitis. *Dig Dis Sci* **26**:694–699, 1981.
41. Burroughs AK, Bassendine MF, Thomas HC, et al: Primary liver cancer in autoimmune chronic liver disease. *Br Med J* **282**:273, 1981.
42. Czaja AJ, Davis GL, Ludwig J, et al: Complete resolution of inflammatory active following corticosteroid treatment of HBsAg negative chronic active hepatitis. *Hepatology* **4**:622–626, 1984.
43. Hegarty JE, Nouri Aria KT, Portmann B, et al: Relapse following treatment withdrawal in patients with autoimmune chronic active hepatitis. *Hepatology* **3**:685–689, 1983.
44. Stellon AJ, Portman B, Hegarty JE, Williams R: Randomized controlled trial of azathioprine withdrawal in autoimmune chronic active hepatitis. *Lancet* **1**:668–670, 1985.

13

Chronic Lupoid Hepatitis: Autoimmune Chronic Active Hepatitis

Roderick N. M. MacSween

1. INTRODUCTION

In 1950 Waldenstrom[1] described a group of young female patients with chronic liver disease and marked hyperglobulinemia. Zimmerman et al.[2] reported similar findings a year later. Similarly, 1 year after Joske and King[3] reported the lupus erythematosus (LE) cell phenomenon in active chronic viral hepatitis, Zimmerman and colleagues[4] confirmed that the LE cell phenomenon was a feature in some forms of chronic hepatic disease.

The concept of an autoimmune form of chronic hepatitis was first proposed by Mackay et al.,[5] in 1956 when the syndrome of active chronic hepatitis associated with LE cells was confirmed. In addition, these patients frequently had other diseases of presumed autoimmune basis, as well as marked hyperglobulinemia, a number of autoantibodies, and the presence of a destructive chronic inflammatory cell infiltrate in the liver; they often showed clinical improvement in response to corticosteroids, probably on the basis of immunosuppression. Mackay and colleagues postulated that liver cell components became antigenic and stimulated the production of antibodies that damaged the liver, leading to perpetuation of the hepatitis and eventual progression to cirrhosis. Since then, the concept of chronic autoimmune or lupoid hepatitis has become generally accepted and many advances have been made in our understanding of its features, pathogenesis, and clinical management.[6]

Chronic hepatitis is defined as "a chronic necroinflammatory, primarily hepatocytic, lesion with or without cirrhosis, in which the lymphocyte dominates the inflammation and in which viral, autoimmune, drug, metabolic, or unknown causes are involved."[7] The diagnosis of autoimmune chronic active hepatitis is sustained when virus-induced, drug-induced, or metabolic etiology have been excluded and when the presence of one or more autoantibodies are demonstrated in the serum. There is an apparent heterogeneity within the group of autoimmune chronic active hepatitis (CAH), as summarized in Table I. The subgroup in which smooth muscle antibody (SMA) and/or anti-nuclear antibodies (ANA) are found constitutes classic autoimmune or lupoid CAH. However, from a clinical and pathologic point of view, there does not appear to be any justification for sub-classification on the basis of the autoantibody profile.

Roderick N. M. MacSween • Department of Pathology, University of Glasgow and Western Infirmary, Glasgow G11 6NT, Scotland, United Kingdom.

Table I. Heterogeneity in Autoimmune Chronic Active Hepatitis

Smooth muscle antibody (SMA), antinuclear antibody (ANA), and liver membrane antibody positive[a]
Smooth muscle antibody positive
Microsomal antibody positive
Soluble liver protein antibody positive
Antimitochondrial antibody (AMA) positive[b]

[a]Classic autoimmune chronic active hepatitis.
[b]Mixed type with features of PBC.

2. MORPHOLOGIC ASPECTS

A liver biopsy is necessary to confirm the diagnosis of CAH and to ascertain the degree of activity and the extent of fibrosis. In addition, repeat biopsies are indicated to assess the response to therapy.

Piecemeal necrosis is the hallmark of CAH, irrespective of its etiology—viral, autoimmune, metabolic, or drug induced. Piecemeal necrosis is defined as "the destruction of liver cells at an interface between parenchyma and connective tissue, together with a predominantly lymphocytic or plasma cell infiltrate."[8] These features are illustrated in Fig. 1. The lymphocytes and plasma cells,

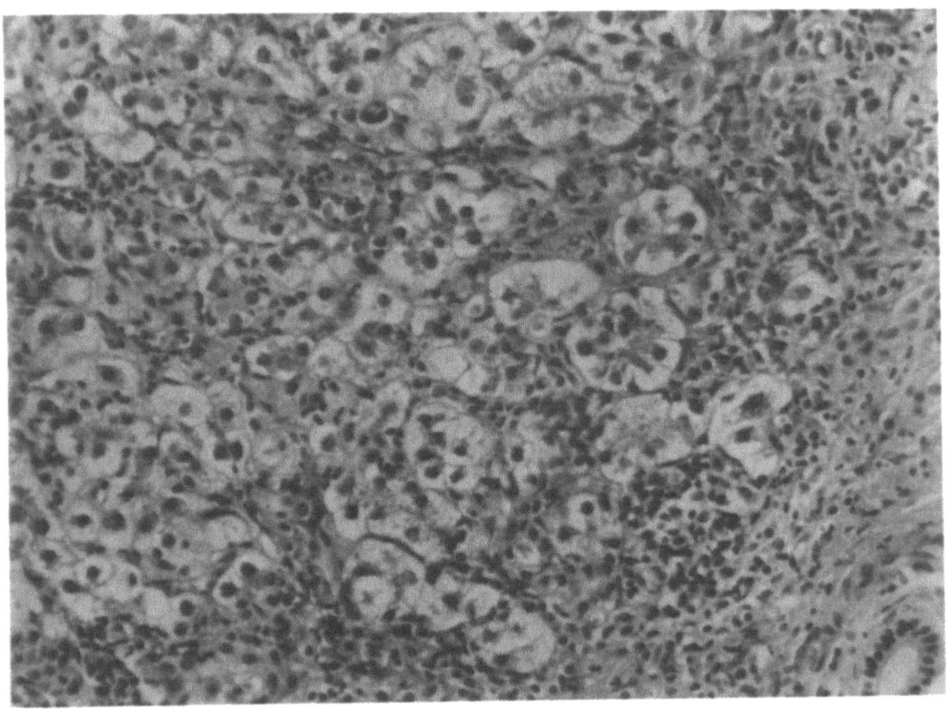

Figure 1. Chronic active hepatitis with periportal piecemeal necrosis. The limiting plate of the portal tract (lower right) is eroded, and a mixed mononuclear cell infiltrate extends into the periportal parenchyma separating and entrapping single liver cells and groups of cells, some of which form rosettes. (H&E, ×260)

accompanied by some neutrophils and eosinophils, infiltrate among and between the liver cells. Ultrastructural studies have shown close and intimate contact between lymphocytes and hepatocytes.[9] The term peripolesis[10] is applied to this close contact between cell membranes; sometimes the lymphocytes may invaginate, and indeed invade, the liver cell, a process known as emperipolesis.[7]

The liver cells show various degenerative changes, producing ballooning, cytolysis, and sometimes the formation of acidophil bodies. Active fibrogenesis occurs from an early stage and is in part responsible for the isolation and entrapment of single or small groups of liver cells. Collagen is laid down in the space of Disse, producing capillarization of hepatic sinusoids.[11] Liver cell regenerative activity occurs, and groups of hepatocytes surrounded by fibrous tissue may produce a striking pattern of pseudoglandular or rosette formation (Fig. 2). Laminin and type IV collagen are present, and it is thought that this basement membrane is produced by the hepatocytes in response to injury.[12] Initially considered to be confined to the periportal zones, it is now recognized that piecemeal necrosis may also occur at the interface between liver cells and the fibrous septa found as a consequence of bridging hepatic necrosis.

Two broad categories of CAH are recognized morphologically: (1) CAH without bridging hepatic necrosis, i.e., piecemeal necrosis alone; and (2) CAH with bridging necrosis. Bridging necrosis comprises confluent necrosis forming septa between either adjacent hepatic (central) veins or portal tracts, or both.[13] Thus, there may be central–central bridging, portal–portal bridging, central–portal bridging, and combinations of these. Evidence is now accumulating that piecemeal necrosis per se may be a benign lesion that may not necessarily progress to cirrhosis. By contrast, bridging necrosis is regarded as the intermediary lesion through which CAH progresses to cirrhosis.[14–18] However, this issue remains a topic of continuing controversy and, in particular, there

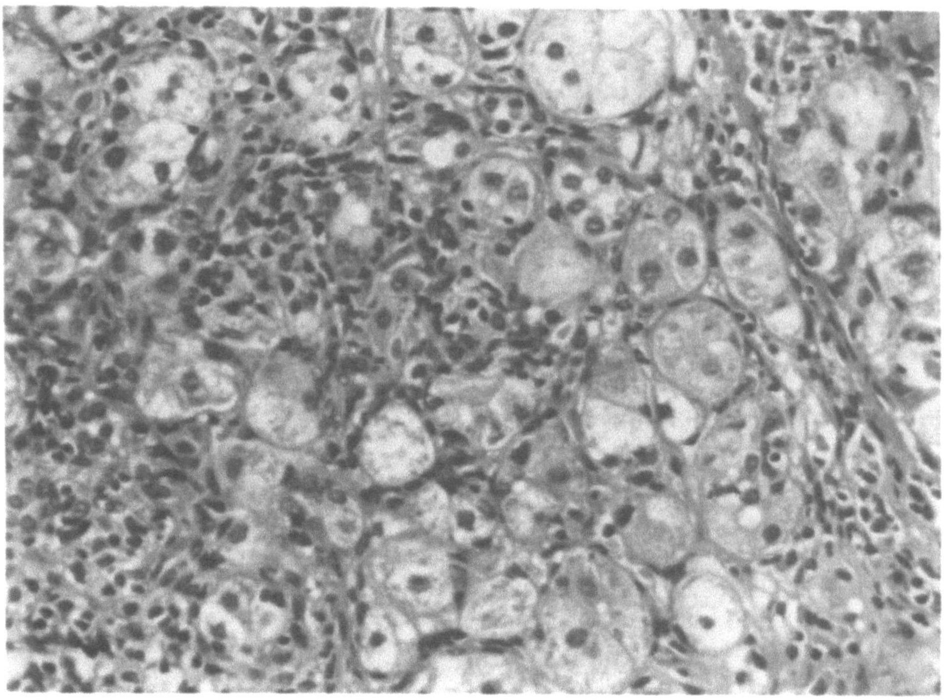

Figure 2. Another area in the same biopsy as Figure 1 shows similar features of piecemeal necrosis. Note the prominent rosette formation with pericellular fibrosis. (H&E, ×300)

is active debate as to whether there may be prognostic differences, depending on the pattern of bridging necrosis.[18]

It is important to remember that the histologic appearance in autoimmune CAH may show considerable variation. In earlier studies, emphasis was placed on the presence of many plasma cells, and the lesion was referred to as plasma cell hepatitis.[19] The foci of piecemeal necrosis are distributed irregularly throughout the liver so that in one biopsy one portal tract may show only a mild chronic inflammatory cell infiltrate, whereas adjacent tracts may show extensive disruption of their limiting plates. Similarly, the extent of periseptal piecemeal necrosis may vary. Some cases may not come to a physician's attention until cirrhosis is already present, and on biopsy there may or may not be evidence of continuing activity manifest by the presence of piecemeal necrosis.

The intensity of the chronic inflammatory cell infiltrate, the presence of spotty necrosis, the extent of periportal and periseptal piecemeal necrosis, and the extent of disruption of the liver cell plates are the morphologic indices of the degree of activity. Histologic activity is usually marked, and the extent of rosette formation and the abundance of plasma cells tend to contrast with the findings in virus-induced CAH.[7] However, it should be strongly emphasized that there are no distinctive features that permit a diagnosis of chronic lupoid hepatitis to be made purely on a morphologic basis.

3. PHENOTYPIC CHARACTERIZATION OF THE CELLULAR INFILTRATE IN THE LIVER

Several studies have been carried out in which the cellular subtypes of the mononuclear infiltrate in the liver in chronic hepatitis have been analyzed using immunohistochemical techniques with monoclonal and polyclonal antibodies of known specificity.[20–27] These have produced generally consistent findings: the infiltrate is composed predominantly of T cells; in portal tracts and fibrous septa, T-helper/inducer cells predominate; in areas of piecemeal necrosis, T-suppressor/cytotoxic cells are more numerous than in portal tracts, but helper/inducer cells remain predominant; within acini, T-suppressor/cytotoxic cells are more common; B cells are virtually absent; and natural killer (NK) cells are only occasionally identified.

These findings are not substantially different from those in other forms of CAH, including hepatitis B infection. Thus, irrespective of the initiating agent in chronic hepatitis, the immune effector mechanisms responsible for perpetuation of the liver cell injury may be similar. However, the different helper/inducer to cytotoxic/suppressor cell ratios between foci of intra-acinar liver cell necrosis and areas of piecemeal necrosis suggest that the immune effector mechanisms are different in these two lesions. However, more detailed phenotypic analyses at the ultrastructural level are required to clarify the precise mechanisms involved.

It is worth noting that electron microscopic examination has shown that interdigitating and dendritic reticulum cells are present in areas of piecemeal necrosis,[28] suggesting that the immunologic reactions occurring there are similar to those demonstrable in normal lymphoid tissues.

4. SIGNIFICANCE OF AUTOANTIBODIES

Some of the serum autoantibodies reported in autoimmune CAH have been listed in Table 1. Antinuclear antibodies, usually of immunoglobin G (IgG) class and in high titer occur in more than 50% of cases.[29] DNA-binding antibodies, most commonly associated with systemic lupus erythematosus (SLE), are present in a small proportion of patients.[30] SMA at high titer occur in 60% of patients and are directed against actin and other components of the cytoskeleton.[31–33] The demonstration of these antibodies is diagnostically useful, but they are neither disease specific nor organ specific.

Some of the various other autoantibodies reported in CAH are of similar limited clinical value.

These include antibodies against microsomes,[34] ribosomes,[35] and other intracellular components. High-titer antibodies to a variety of bacterial and viral antigens, including enterobacteria, measles, and rubella, also have been noted in autoimmune CAH.[36–38] Although there is an overall correlation between the presence of the antiviral antibodies and the presence of ANA and SMA, there is no evidence of cross-reactivity. A recent report of persistence of part of the measles genome in lymphocytes of patients with autoimmune CAH is of considerable interest; this may afford an explanation for the high antibody levels and may be relevant to the etiology of autoimmune CAH.[39]

There have been extensive studies in an effort to demonstrate a liver-specific autoantibody, pathogenetically reactive with hepatocytes and producing direct hepatocyte injury or mediating antibody-dependent mechanisms. Antibodies directed against a subcellular component of liver cells, liver-specific protein (LSP), have been found in various forms of acute and chronic liver diseases[40,41]; but their presence is not specific for autoimmune CAH.[42] Furthermore, LSP has been shown to be a heterogeneous complex of antigens containing not only surface membrane determinants but also a number of cytoplasmic components, including mitochondrial proteins[43,44]; nor is it certain that the antigen is liver specific.[45,46]

Using an immunofluorescence method and intact hepatocytes, antibodies to liver membrane antigen (LMA) have also been reported, chiefly in patients with autoimmune CAH.[47] However, using an immunoradiometric method, Weidmann and colleagues[48] reported that, whereas antibodies to LMA were found in the highest titer in patients with autoimmune CAH, they were also present in 32% of patients with PBC and were also occasionally present in hepatitis B-associated chronic hepatitis. The liver biopsies of all patients who had significant titers of liver membrane antibodies showed piecemeal necrosis, suggesting a correlation between the presence of the antibody and this histologic lesion.[48]

Using sophisticated immunoblotting techniques and liver plasma membrane preparations, Frazer et al.[43] were not able to define a liver-specific antigen exclusively reactive with autoimmune CAH sera. The current position, therefore, is that while sensitization to liver-derived antigens has been demonstrated in autoimmune CAH, reactivity with these antigens is not disease specific, nor has sensitization to a wholly liver-specific antigen been demonstrated.

5. CONCLUSIONS

From a pathologic viewpoint, numerous unanswered questions remain as far as chronic lupoid (autoimmune) hepatitis is concerned. There are no distinctive histologic or ultrastructural features that distinguish the disease. The significance, if any, of the non-organ-specific autoantibodies that enable the diagnosis to be made remain uncertain. Characterization of the mononuclear cell subsets present in the portal tract and in areas of piecemeal necrosis have not clearly established what effector mechanisms are responsible for the liver cell injury. The findings do not point to any pathologic process uniquely responsible for the pattern of hepatocyte damage. Similarly, sensitization to a wholly liver-specific antigen has not been shown in those patients. The continuing failure to identify the etiologic agents responsible for non-A non-B (NANB) hepatitis cannot be disregarded, and a viral etiology for presumed autoimmune chronic active hepatitis is not excluded.

REFERENCES

1. Waldenstrom J: Bluproteine und Nahrungeiweiss. *Dtsch Z Verdau Stoffwechselkr* **2**:113–119, 1950.
2. Zimmerman HJ, Heller P, Hill RP: Extreme hyperglobulinemia in subacute hepatic necrosis. *N Engl J Med* **244**:245–249, 1951.
3. Joske RA, King WE: The L.E.-cell phenomenon in active chronic viral hepatitis. *Lancet* **2**:477–480, 1955.
4. Heller P, Zimmerman HJ, Rozengvaig MD, et al: The L.E.-cell phenomenon in chronic hepatic disease. *N Engl J Med* **254**:1160–1165, 1956.

5. Mackay IR, Taft LI, Cowling DC: Lupoid hepatitis. *Lancet* **2:**1323–1126, 1956.
6. Schaffner F: Autoimmune chronic active hepatitis: Three decades of progress. In Popper H, Schaffner F (eds): *Progress in Liver Disease*. Vol. VIII. Grune & Stratton, Orlando, Florida, 1986, pp. 485–503.
7. Bianchi L, Spichtin HP, Gudat F: Chronic hepatitis. In MacSween RNM, Anthony PP, Scheuer PJ (eds): *Pathology of the Liver*, 2nd ed. Churchill Livingstone, Edinburgh, 1987, pp. 310–341.
8. Bianchi L, De Groote J, Desmet VJ, et al: Acute and chronic hepatitis revisited. *Lancet* **2:**914–919, 1977.
9. Kawanishi J: Morphologic association of lymphocytes with hepatocytes in chronic liver disease. *Arch Pathol Lab Med* **101:**286–290, 1977.
10. Kerr JFR, Cooksley WGE, Searle J, et al: The nature of piecemeal necrosis in chronic active hepatitis. *Lancet* **2:**827–828, 1979.
11. Schaffner F, Popper H: Capillarization of hepatic sinusoids in man. *Gastroenterology* **44:**239–242, 1963.
12. Bianchi FB, Biagini G, Ballardomo G, et al: Basement membrane production by hepatocytes in chronic liver disease. *Hepatology* **4:**1167–1172, 1984.
13. Boyer JL, Klatsin G: Pattern of necrosis in acute viral hepatitis: Prognostic value of bridging (subacute hepatic necrosis). *N Engl J Med* **283:**1063–171, 1970.
14. Baggenstoss AH, Soloway RD, Summerskill WHJ, et al: Chronic active liver disease. The range of histologic lesions, their response to treatment, and evolution. *Hum Pathol* **3:**183–198, 1972.
15. Schalm SW, Summerskill WHJ, Gitnick GL, et al: Contrasting features and responses to treatment of severe chronic active liver disease with and without hepatitis B s antigen. *Gut* **17:**781–786, 1976.
16. Okuno T, Okanoue T, Takino T, et al: Prognostic significance of bridging necrosis in chronic active hepatitis. *Gastroenterol Jpn* **18:**577–584, 1983.
17. Cooksley WGE, Bradbear RA, Robinson W, et al: The prognosis of chronic active hepatitis without cirrhosis in relation to bridging necrosis. *Hepatology* **6:**345–348, 1986.
18. Combes B: The initial morphologic lesion in chronic hepatitis, important or unimportant? *Hepatology* **6:**518–522, 1986.
19. Good RA: Plasma-cell hepatitis and extreme hyperglobulinemia in adolescent females. *Am J Dis Child* **92:**508–509, 1956.
20. Eggink HF, Houthoff HJ, Huitema S, et al: Cellular and humoral immune reactions in chronic active liver disease. I. Lymphocyte subsets in liver biopsies of patients with untreated idiopathic autoimmune hepatitis, chronic active hepatitis B and primary biliary cirrhosis. *Clin Exp Immunol* **50:**17–24, 1982.
21. Husby G, Blomhoff JP, Elgio K, et al: Immunohistochemical characterization of hepatic tissue lymphocyte subpopulations in liver disease. *Scand J Gastroenterol* **17:**855–860, 1982.
22. Colucci G, Colombo M, Del Ninno E, et al: In situ characterization by monoclonal antibodies of the mononuclear cell infiltrate in chronic active hepatitis. *Gastroenterology* **85:**1138–1145, 1983.
23. Pape GR, Rieber EP, Eisenburg J, et al: Involvement of the cytotoxic/suppressor T-cell subset in liver tissue injury of patients with acute and chronic liver diseases. *Gastroenterology* **85:**657–662, 1983.
24. Mariani E, Facchini A, Mighio F, et al: Analysis with OKT monoclonal antibodies of T-lymphocyte subsets present in blood and liver of patients with chronic active hepatitis. *Liver* **4:**22–28, 1984.
25. Montano L, Aranguibel F, Boffill M, et al: An analysis of the composition of the inflammatory infiltrate in autoimmune and hepatitis B virus induced chronic liver disease. *Hepatology* **3:**292–296, 1984.
26. Si L, Whiteside TL, Van Thiel DH, et al: Lymphocyte subpopulations at the site of "piecemeal" necrosis in end stage chronic liver diseases and rejecting liver allografts in cyclosporine-treated patients. *Lab Invest* **50:**341–347, 1984.
27. Frazer IH, MacKay IR, Bell J, et al: The cellular infiltrate in the liver in auto-immune chronic active hepatitis: Analysis with monoclonal antibodies. *Liver* **5:**162–172, 1985.
28. Baradin KA, Desmet VJ: Interdigitating and dendritic reticulum cells in chronic active hepatitis. *Histopathology* **8:**657–667, 1984.
29. Kurki P, Gripenberg M, Teppo AM, et al: Profiles of anti-nuclear antibodies in chronic active hepatitis, biliary cirrhosis and alcoholic liver disease. *Liver* **4:**134–138, 1984.
30. Davis P, Read AE: Antibodies to double stranded (native) DNA in active chronic hepatitis. *Gut* **16:**413–415, 1975.
31. Lidman K, Biberfeld G, Fagraeus A, et al: Anti-actin specificity of human smooth muscle antibodies in chronic active hepatitis. *Clin Exp Immunol* **24:**266–272, 1976.
32. Bretherton L, Brown C, Pedersen JS, et al: ELISA assay for IgG autoantibody to G-actin: Comparison of chronic active hepatitis and acute viral hepatitis. *Clin Exp Immunol* **51:**611–616, 1983.
33. Kurki P, Miettinen A, Salaspuro, et al: Cytoskeleton antibodies in chronic active hepatitis, primary biliary cirrhosis and alcoholic liver disease. *Liver* **3:**297, 1983.

34. Rizzetto M, Swana G, Doniach D: Microsomal antibodies in active chronic hepatitis and other disorders. *Clin Exp Immunol* **15:**331–344, 1973.
35. Gerber MA, Shapiro JM, Smith H Jr, et al: Antibodies to ribosomes in chronic active hepatitis. *Gastroenterology* **76:**139–43, 1979.
36. Triger DR, Alp MH, Wright R: Bacterial and dietary antibodies in liver disease. *Lancet* **1:**60–63, 1972.
37. Triger DR, Jurtz JB, Wright R: Viral antibodies in chronic liver disease. *Gut* **15:**94–98, 1974.
38. Christie KE, Endresen C, Haukenes G: IgM antibodies in sera from patients with chronic active hepatitis with the measles virus matrix protein and nucleo-protein. *J Med Virol* **14:**149–157, 1984.
39. Roberson DAF, Zhang SL, Guy EC, et al: Persistent measles virus genome in autoimmune chronic active hepatitis. *Lancet* **2:**9–11, 1987.
40. Jensen DM, McFarlane IG, Portman BS, et al: Detection of antibodies directed against a liver-specific membrane lipoprotein in patients with acute and chronic active hepatitis. *N Engl J Med* **299:**1–7, 1978.
41. Manns M, Meyer zum Buschenfelde K-H, Hess G: Autoantibodies against liver-specific membrane lipoprotein in acute and chronic liver diseases: Studies on organ-, species-, and disease specificity. *Gut* **21:**955–961, 1980.
42. Frazer IH, Mackay IR: Immune responses to liver-specific lipoprotein and liver membrane antigen: A tabular interpretative review. *J Clin Lab Immunol* **14:**165–167, 1984.
43. Frazer IH, Jordan W, Collins EC, et al: Antibody to liver membrane antigens in chronic active hepatitis. IV. Exclusion of specific reactivity to polypeptides and glycolipids by immunoblotting. *Hepatology* **7:**4–10, 1987.
44. Jensen DM, Hall C, Majewski T: The plasma membrane origin of liver-specific protein (LSP). *Liver* **3:**213–219, 1983.
45. Riisom K, Diederichsen H: Demonstration of organ-nonspecific antigens in liver-specific lipoprotein. *Gastroenterology* **85:**1271–1276, 1983.
46. Murakami H, Kukiki J, Kakumu S, et al: The specificity of human liver membrane lipoprotein: Studies with monoclonal antibodies. *Hepatology* **4:**192, 1984.
47. Hopf U, Meyer zum Buschenfelde KH, Arnold W: Detection of a liver-membrane autoantibody in HBsAg-negative chronic active hepatitis. *N Engl J Med* **294:**578–582, 1976.
48. Wiedmann KH, Bartholomew TC, Brown DJC, et al: Liver membrane antibody detected by immunoradiometric assay in acute and chronic virus-induced and autoimmune liver diseases. *Hepatology* **4:**199–204, 1984.

14

Primary Biliary Cirrhosis: Clinical Aspects

Marshall M. Kaplan

1. INTRODUCTION

Primary biliary cirrhosis, a chronic, progressive, and often fatal cholestatic liver disease, is characterized by the destruction of intrahepatic bile ducts, portal inflammation and scarring, and the eventual development of cirrhosis and liver failure. The diagnosis is usually made in a middle-aged woman (although the age range is 20–80 years) who initially has fatigue or itching or who is asymptomatic and has been found to have unexplained hepatomegaly or an elevated serum alkaline phosphatase level. Biochemical tests of liver function typically reveal a cholestatic pattern; i.e., the alkaline phosphatase and γ-glutamyltranspeptidase are disproportionately elevated compared with other biochemical tests. A positive antimitochondrial antibody test, present in 95% of patients with primary biliary cirrhosis, makes the diagnosis very likely. It is still important to ascertain that the bile ducts are patent. This can usually be done with ultrasonography or computed tomography (CT) scanning. If the results of these tests are equivocal, endoscopic retrograde cholangiopancreatography should be done. Percutaneous needle biopsy of the liver will provide confirmatory information and permit histologic staging of the disease. This is helpful in assessing prognosis.

There is no proven effective treatment for the underlying disease, although preliminary studies suggest that several immunosuppressive and/or anti-inflammatory agents may be helpful. A more complete discussion of therapy is given in Section 6. Current therapy is directed at relief of symptoms and the prevention of a deficiency of fat soluble vitamins. Cholestyramine or colestipal hydrochloride will usually relieve pruritus, the most common symptom. Vitamin nutriture with regard to the fat-soluble vitamins (vitamins A, D, E, and K) can be evaluated by appropriate blood tests and supplemental oral vitamins prescribed if necessary.

Primary biliary cirrhosis has been found in all races and is estimated to account for 0.6–2% of deaths from cirrhosis worldwide.[1] Estimates of prevalence range from 3.7 to 14.4 cases per 100,000 population,[2] whereas estimated incidence ranges from 5.8 to 15 cases per million population per year.[3,4] Genetic factors appear to play a role in the development of primary biliary cirrhosis, although the disorder is not inherited in any simple recessive or dominant pattern. There are familial occurrences of primary biliary cirrhosis,[5] and unaffected family members are more likely than normal individuals to have associated immunologic abnormalities such as circulating autoantibodies and impaired in vitro suppressor cell function.[6,7] A recent preliminary report suggests an association

Marshall M. Kaplan • Division of Gastroenterology, Tufts University School of Medicine, New England Medical Center Hospitals, Boston, Massachusetts 02111.

between primary biliary cirrhosis and haplotype HLA-DR8.[8] Earlier reports did not find such associations, but reliable antisera to detect HLA-DR8 were not available at the time these studies were performed.[9,10]

2. IMMUNOLOGIC ABNORMALITIES

The immunologic features and pathogenesis of primary biliary cirrhosis have recently been reviewed in detail.[11–14] The large number of immunologic abnormalities in patients with the disease suggests that it is caused by some abnormality of immune regulation. However, there is no direct proof of this. A partial list of immunologic abnormalities that may be present includes increased levels of serum immunoglobulins, particularly IgM; circulating autoantibodies; skin anergy; granulomas in the liver or lymph nodes draining the liver; increased turnover of complement; decreased in vitro suppressor cell function; histologic liver lesions that resemble those in graft-versus-host disease (GVHD) and in rejection of hepatic allografts; and an association with other diseases considered to have an autoimmune basis.[11] In one study, 84% of patients with primary biliary cirrhosis had at least one other disorder with a presumed autoimmune cause, and 41% had two or more such disorders.[14] These included autoimmune thyroiditis, scleroderma, rheumatoid arthritis, and Sjögren's syndrome.[11,15]

There are well-documented abnormalities of both humoral and cellular immunity in primary biliary cirrhosis. Many patients with primary biliary cirrhosis have increased levels of a serum IgM that is highly immunoreactive and highly cryoprecipitable, binds to conglutinin, and spontaneously converts complement factor C3 to C3b and C3c via the classic pathway.[16–18] This peculiarly immunoreactive IgM behaves like immune complexes with some immune complex assays[16] and may produce spuriously high serum IgM levels if the IgM levels are measured by radioimmunodiffusion.[19] These increased levels may be due to a defect in T suppressor cell function that permits a small subpopulation ($<1\%$) of circulating B cells to secrete large quantities of IgM.[20,21]

The list of circulating autoantibodies in primary biliary cirrhosis is long and includes antinuclear antibodies (ANA), one of which has recently been recognized and is specific for nuclear membranes,[22] antithyroid antibodies,[23] lymphocytotoxic antibodies,[23] antiacetylcholine-receptor (anti-ACLR) antibodies,[25] platelet-bound antiplatelet antibodies,[26] antiribonucleoprotein antigen Ro antibodies,[27] and antimitochondrial antibodies.[28] Antimitochondrial antibody is the most common autoantibody in primary biliary cirrhosis, occurring in 90–95% of such patients. It has no known inhibitory effect on mitochondrial function, nor does it affect the course of the disease. Antimitochondrial antibody is not one antibody; rather, it is a family of antibodies that react with different antigens within the mitochondria and give different immunofluorescent patterns with a variety of human and rat tissues.[28] The antimitochondrial antibody found most commonly in primary biliary cirrhosis has been labeled M2 and reacts with several antigens on the inner mitochondrial membrane that range in size from 45 kDa to 80 kDa.[29–31] Two other antibodies that are also associated with primary biliary cirrhosis—anti-M4 and anti-M8—react with antigens on the outer mitochondrial membrane. Anti-M8 is found only in patients who have anti-M2, and its presence may be associated with a more rapidly progressive course.[32] Other antimitochondrial antibodies are found in syphilis (anti-M1), drug-induced disorders (anti-M3 and M6), collagen vascular diseases (anti-M5), and some forms of heart disease (anti-M7).[28,29,33] Earlier suggestions that a subunit of ATPase was part of the M2 antigen have not been confirmed,[28,29] but anti-M2 will recognize antigens on normal colonic flora.[29] Newer techniques now available are more sensitive than immunofluorescent microscopy in detecting antimitocondrial antibody. These include radioimmunoassays (RIA),[33] enzyme-linked immunosorbent assay (ELISA) techniques,[34] and, most recently, immunoblotting techniques.[29]

The complement system appears to be in a chronically activated state in primary biliary cirrhosis, and complement component C3 turns over rapidly.[18,35,36] Complement hypercatabolism is due to activation of the classical complement pathway.[18,36] Patients with primary biliary cirrhosis have decreased Kupffer-cell-mediated clearance of C3b-coated erythrocytes.[35] This may be due to blockade of C3b receptors on circulating monocytes by IgM.[37,38]

Several groups of investigators have reported a high prevalence of circulating immune complexes in primary biliary cirrhosis.[39,40] Preliminary evidence suggested that these putative immune complexes might contain antimitocondrial antibody and biliary antigens and might have a role in the pathogenesis of the disease.[41,42] However, these results have not been confirmed by subsequent studies, in which only a few primary biliary cirrhosis patients were found to have immune complex-like reactive material in serum.[16,43] On the basis of current information, it is unlikely that immune complexes play a pathogenetic role in primary biliary cirrhosis.

There are decreased numbers of circulating T lymphocytes (both helper and suppressor cells) in the serum of patients with primary biliary cirrhosis, as well as abnormalities of the regulation and function of these cells.[44–48] The decreased number of T cells in peripheral blood may be an effect of the disease rather than a cause, since there are normal numbers of circulating T lymphocytes early in the course of primary biliary cirrhosis, but the numbers decline as the disease progresses.[45] The numbers of peripheral T lymphocytes in patients with stage 4 disease are similar to those in patients with other types of cirrhosis.[45]

The decreased in vitro T-suppressor cell function observed in patients with primary biliary cirrhosis also appears to have no role in pathogenesis; 25% of healthy first-degree relatives of patients with primary biliary cirrhosis have equally depressed in vitro suppression.[7] This abnormality may be one of several genetic markers that in combination lead to the development of primary biliary cirrhosis. However, depressed in vitro suppression alone does not cause the disease.

It seems likely that the initial destructive bile duct lesion in primary biliary cirrhosis is caused by cytotoxic T lymphocytes. Bile duct cells in patients with the disease express increased amounts of the class I histocompatibility complex antigens, HLA-A, -B, and -C, and they also express the class II HLA-DR antigens, in contrast to normal individuals.[49] Thus, bile duct cells are good targets for activated T cells.[50] Indeed, the bile duct lesion in primary biliary cirrhosis resembles that in GVHD and rejection of hepatic allografts,[51,52] disorders known to be mediated by cytotoxic lymphocytes. It is not known how or why the bile duct cells may be affected in this way. Lymphocytes from some patients with primary biliary cirrhosis do circulate in an activated state.[53] However, no conclusive evidence implicates any of the known mechanisms by which circulating lymphocytes may kill target cells, i.e., natural killer (NK) cell cytotoxicity,[54] antibody-dependent cellular cytotoxicity (ADCC),[55] or T-cell-mediated cytotoxicity.[56]

3. LABORATORY TESTS

Laboratory tests in patients with primary biliary cirrhosis demonstrate a cholestatic pattern. The serum alkaline phosphatase is invariably elevated, often to striking levels, and is of hepatic origin. The level tends to reach a plateau early in the course of the disease and usually fluctuates within 20% of this value thereafter.[57] Changes in the level of alkaline phosphatase are not of prognostic importance. The values of 5′-nucleotidase and γ-glutamyltranspeptidase parallel those for alkaline phosphatase. The serum levels of aminotransferases (transaminases) may be normal or slightly elevated, tend to fluctuate within a relatively narrow range, and are of no prognostic importance. Serum albumin and globulin levels and the prothrombin time are characteristically normal early in the course of disease, although immunoelectrophoresis will frequently indicate a selective elevation of IgM. A low serum albumin level or prolonged prothrombin time that fails to correct with parenteral vitamin K indicates advanced disease; both are poor prognostic signs.

The serum bilirubin level is usually normal early in the course of the disease but becomes elevated in 60% of patients as the disease progresses. Both the direct and indirect fractions are increased. An elevated serum bilirubin is a poor prognostic sign.[58,59]

Serum lipids may be strikingly elevated in primary biliary cirrhosis. Two distinct lipoprotein patterns are seen; these depend on the stage of the disease.[60] Patients with early primary biliary cirrhosis tend to have mild elevations of low-density and very-low-density lipoproteins (LDL and VLDL, respectively) and striking elevations of high-density lipoproteins (HDL), some of which are abnormally large.[61] Patients with advanced disease (histologic stage 4) have marked elevations in LDL, decreased HDL and the presence of lipoprotein X, an abnormal lipoprotein seen in chronic cholestasis. These changes in serum lipoprotein composition appear to be due to inhibition of hepatic lipase activity in early primary biliary cirrhosis and to decreased cholesterol esterification in advanced disease.[60] The fact that HDL cholesterol is elevated until late in the course of primary biliary cirrhosis probably accounts for the finding that atherosclerosis is rare in patients with this disease, despite their exceedingly high serum cholesterol values. Serum ceruloplasmin is characteristically elevated in primary biliary cirrhosis in contrast to Wilson disease, another disorder in which increased concentrations of hepatic copper are present.[5]

4. CLINICAL MANIFESTATIONS AND ASSOCIATED DISORDERS

Ninety to 95% of patients with primary biliary cirrhosis are women. Onset is typically between ages 30 to 65.[5,57,62] Before 1960, the diagnosis was usually made late in the course of disease, and symptoms such as jaundice, liver failure, and portal hypertension were common. The increased awareness of primary biliary cirrhosis in combination with improved diagnostic tests has enabled diagnoses to be made at earlier stages. As a result, the initial symptoms and physical findings are quite different. Fatigue and pruritus are the usual presenting symptoms. At diagnosis, pruritus occurs without jaundice in 50–60% of primary biliary cirrhosis patients, with jaundice in 20% and follows it in 8% of cases.[62] Pruritis may first occur during pregnancy and may be mistaken for the pruritus of pregnancy. However, the pruritis of pregnancy always resolves in the postpartum period, whereas that due to primary biliary cirrhosis persists. Once pruritus occurs in primary biliary cirrhosis, it is unusual for it to disappear spontaneously. The same is true with jaundice. The cause of the pruritis in primary biliary cirrhosis is uncertain and is probably not directly related to concentrations of the naturally occurring bile acids in skin. Itching does not correlate with either serum or skin concentrations of bile acids,[63] but it does respond to treatment with cholestyramine, a nonabsorbed ammonium resin that binds anions, including bile acids. A recent report indicates that rifampin, a potent inducer of hepatic drug-metabolizing enzymes, will also relieve itching,[64] as will large-volume plasmapheresis.[65]

Some patients with primary biliary cirrhosis may be asymptomatic. The prevalence of asymptomatic patients ranged from 13 to 48% in two recent series.[66,67] At the other extreme, patients may present initially with advanced disease that is manifested by hemorrhage from esophageal varices, ascites, or hepatic encephalopathy.[57,62] Findings on physical examination vary widely at presentation. Hepatomegaly occurs in 40–70% of patients and splenomegaly in up to 35% of cases.[68,69] Other common findings are increased skin pigmentation, excoriations, xanthelasma, and spider nevi. Gallstones are found more frequently in patients with primary biliary cirrhosis, but there are no data that demonstrate an increased incidence of symptomatic gallstone disease.

Steatorrhea is common in primary biliary cirrhosis. It is due to a decreased secretion of conjugated bile acids in patients with jaundice or cirrhosis and the resulting low concentration of bile acids within the small intestine.[70,71] In one study, steatorrhea was found in all patients with primary biliary cirrhosis whose aqueous concentrations of bile salts in the duodenum were below 3 mM.[70] In other reports, steatorrhea was present in 30% of patients with primary biliary cirrhosis who did not have bone disease[72] and in 60% of patients with symptomatic bone disease.[73] Steatorrhea may be clinically important and may reach levels as high as 40 g/day.[73] In patients with such levels, nocturnal diarrhea, weight loss, and muscle wasting may be prominent features of the disease. Pancreatic insufficiency may contribute to the steatorrhea[71] and is most likely to occur in patients with concomitant sicca syndrome.[74] Administration of medium-chain triglycerides and a diet low in neutral triglycerides are usually effective in improving the diarrhea and nutritional status in patients with steatorrhea.[70]

Hepatic osteodystrophy occurs frequently, most often in patients with steatorrhea. Since steatorrhea is often associated with vitamin D deficiency and calcium malabsorption, and since both problems may cause osteomalacia, it was long assumed that the bone disease in primary biliary cirrhosis was osteomalacia.[75–77] There appeared to be good circumstantial evidence for this assumption. Serum 25-hydroxyvitamin D concentrations are low in most patients with primary biliary cirrhosis.[72,73,76–78] The low levels are due to malabsorption of dietary vitamin D, binding of vitamin D to the cholestyramine used to treat pruritus, and increased urinary secretion of water-soluble vitamin D metabolites.[79,80] Contrary to expectation, there is not a significant impairment of the conversion of vitamin D to 25-hydroxyvitamin D in primary biliary cirrhosis patients,[79] nor does jaundice interfere noticeably with the endogenous synthesis of vitamin D_3 in skin.[81]

Although osteomalacia undoubtedly occurs in patients with primary biliary cirrhosis and has been stressed in some reports,[76,77] recent data indicate that osteoporosis is the more common and clinically more important lesion.[72,73,82] Even in the series in which a high prevalence of osteomalacia was reported, more than 50% of patients with bone demineralization had osteoporosis.[76] The cause of osteoporosis in primary biliary cirrhosis is uncertain, but it may be due to decreased osteoblast function, and it is associated with a low serum concentration of bone Gla-protein, an indicator of bone turnover.[82] There was a good correlation between the severity of bone demineralization and the rate of calcium absorption in one study.[73] Biochemical and bone biopsy data suggest that vitamin D deficiency is not the cause of hepatic osteodystrophy.[72,73,78,82,83] The values of total serum calcium, ionized calcium, phosphate, and 1,25-dihydroxy vitamin D were normal, as were the levels of parathyroid hormone. However, one study found an increase in the fractional resorptive surface of trabecular bone that was corrected after 6 months of parenteral vitamin D_2 therapy.[83]

The treatment of bone disease in patients with primary biliary cirrhosis is difficult and is directed toward the correction of any deficiencies of calcium or vitamin D that might be present. There is no evidence that this treatment will prevent or heal the osteoporosis.[72,73,75] Doses of 25-hydroxyvitamin D sufficient to raise serum levels of this vitamin to normal or above-normal values, together with supplemental oral calcium, do not consistently improve the bone wasting. In one study, trabecular bone volume fell by 25% after 1 year of treatment; in another, bone volume did not improve substantially.[72,73]

Low circulating levels of vitamin A are common in patients with primary biliary cirrhosis, but symptoms of vitamin A deficiency are uncommon.[84–86] Vitamin A levels correlate positively with serum retinol-binding protein and serum albumin levels and inversely with serum bilirubin values. Concomitant zinc deficiency has been reported in several patients with symptomatic vitamin A deficiency.[84] Vitamin E deficiency is rare.[86]

Liver failure and portal hypertension eventually develop in most patients with primary biliary cirrhosis. The manifestations of these disorders are similar to those in other patients with end-stage cirrhosis. However, patients with primary biliary cirrhosis who bleed from esophageal varices appear to be better candidates for portalsystemic anastomosis than are patients with other types of cirrhosis. Although survival after shunting is no longer than that in other patients with cirrhosis, the quality of life is better, and hepatic encephalopathy is uncommon.[87,88]

The association of scleroderma, Sjögren's syndrome, and arthropathy with primary biliary cirrhosis is well known. If specific testing for decreased lacrimation is performed, 72–100% of patients with primary biliary cirrhosis will be found to have either keratoconjunctivitis sicca, xerostomia, or a combination of both.[89,90] Arthropathy occurs in 4–42% of patients and has varying causes. Rheumatoid arthritis, psoriatic arthritis, chondrocalcinosis, hypertrophic osteodystrophy, and avascular necrosis have all been reported. The prevalence of frank arthritis has ranged from 5 to 24% in different series.[91,92]

The association between primary biliary cirrhosis and hypothyroidism has only been recently recognized. The hypothyroidism may predate the diagnosis of primary biliary cirrhosis, or it may occur during the course of the disease. Two recent studies report an 18%[23] and 22%[93] prevalence of hypothyroidism in patients with primary biliary cirrhosis.

Renal tubular acidosis occurs frequently but is usually subclinical. In one study, 33–53% of patients with primary biliary cirrhosis were found to have defective urinary acidification after administration of an acid load, although no patient had overt symptoms of acidosis.[94] Copper deposition in the kidney may cause the renal dysfunction. In one study, the plasma copper concentration and urinary copper excretion were significantly higher in patients with primary biliary cirrhosis and renal tubular acidosis than in patients without these disorders.[94] The decreased ability to acidify urine after an acid load correlated with both the plasma copper concentration and urinary copper excretion.

There appears to be an increased prevalence of hepatocellular and breast cancer among patients with primary biliary cirrhosis. In one study, 5 of 130 white patients with the disease were found to have hepatocellular carcinoma, an increase in prevalence similar to that in other types of cirrhosis.[95] In one recent report, 6 of 208 women with primary biliary cirrhosis were found to have breast cancer, more than a fourfold increase in expected prevalence,[96] and another study found a significant increase in the prevalence of breast cancer, $p < 0.0015$.[97]

An increased susceptibility to urinary tract infections (UTI) has also been observed in women with primary biliary cirrhosis. Bacteriuria was found in 19% of such women ($N = 87$) during a 1-year period, as compared with 7% of women with other chronic liver diseases and 8% of women with rheumatoid arthritis.[98] The incidence of bacteriuria increased to 35% when 144 consecutive women with primary biliary cirrhosis were evaluated during a 2-year period. The bacteriuria was associated with histologically advanced disease. The types of bacteria isolated and the antibiotic sensitivity patterns and cure rates were similar to those in women without underlying liver disease. However, the reinfection rate was 34%, double that reported in other women known to have recurrent bacteriuria. The cause of this susceptibility is unknown.

5. NATURAL HISTORY OF PRIMARY BILIARY CIRRHOSIS

Although primary biliary cirrhosis is a progressive disease, the rate of progression varies greatly among individual patients. Five-year survival rates range from a low of 30% in a multicenter study recently reported by Christensen et al.[99] to as high as 75% in a study reported by Roll et al.[66] The median 5-year survival in several large series was 63%.[66,68,99–101]

Patients who are asymptomatic at presentation may have normal life expectancies.[66] One such group of patients has now been followed for a median period of 11.4 years, and the survival curves remain similar to those in a normal population matched for age and sex.[102] Other than the fact that these patients were asymptomatic, the only other finding that correlated with a normal survival was portal granulomas on the initial liver biopsy. This result confirms earlier reports indicating that hepatic granulomas correlate with prolonged survival.[103] This finding may be related to the observation that granulomas are most often found in patients with stage 1 disease.[102] However, the correlation between hepatic granulomas and prolonged survival is not always found.[104] Associated autoimmune disorders such as thyroiditis, sicca syndrome, calcinosis cutis–Raynaud phenomenon–sclerodactyly–telangiectasia (CRST) syndrome, and Raynaud phenomenon are associated with decreased survival in asymptomatic patients.[102] In symptomatic patients, advanced age, hepatomegaly, elevated serum bilirubin, decreased serum albumin, and cirrhosis each correlate with shortened survival.[66,99]

6. TREATMENT

There is still no satisfactory treatment for primary biliary cirrhosis. Results with drugs used to treat most autoimmune cases have been disappointing. Although there has never been a prospective controlled trial of corticosteroids in primary biliary cirrhosis, most hepatologists have found that corticosteroids do not favorably influence the course of the disease but do accelerate the progression of osteoporosis, an already serious problem.

Azathioprine (in doses ranging from 1 to 2 mg/kg body weight per day) was initially shown to be of no therapeutic value in primary biliary cirrhosis in two prospective controlled trials.[105,106] Biochemical tests, the progression to cirrhosis, and survival were not improved by azathioprine. However, one of these studies was continued, and its most recent results suggest that azathioprine may prolong survival and retard the rate of clinical deterioration.[99] In this multinational double-blind trial, 127 patients received azathioprine and 121 patients received placebo.[99] Although survival curves suggested that azathioprine had no beneficial effect on outcome, Cox multiple-regression analysis indicated that the patients in the azathioprine group had more advanced disease when they entered the study. When this imbalance was corrected, azathioprine was found to have a significant beneficial effect on survival ($p = 0.01$).[99] Azathioprine appeared to improve survival by 20 months and to slow the rate of incapacitation. The effects of azathioprine on biochemical tests and liver histology were not described. The side effects in the patients receiving azathioprine were minor and similar to those observed in the placebo-treated group.

There have now been seven prospective controlled trials of D-penicillamine in primary biliary cirrhosis.[68,100,101,107–110] Penicillamine was tried because of its ability to remove body copper. Patients with primary biliary cirrhosis accumulate as much hepatic copper as do patients with Wilson disease,[5] and removal of body copper is curative in Wilson disease. Despite preliminary reports suggesting that penicillamine improved liver function, decreased Ig levels, and improved survival,[107] final analyses of all these studies indicate that penicillamine is not effective.[68,100,101,107–110] A total of 767 patients have now been studied in penicillamine trials, a number large enough to eliminate the likelihood of an important type II error.[100] The usual dose ranged from 600 to 1000 mg/day. Penicillamine had no beneficial effect on survival, histologic progression of disease, or improvement in any of the prognostically important laboratory tests. Of note, penicillamine was associated with a high incidence of serious side effects in primary biliary cirrhosis patients, up to 30% in some studies. In addition, several deaths have been attributed to penicillamine.

Recent data explain why penicillamine may not work as a treatment for primary biliary cirrhosis. First, liver copper is probably not hepatotoxic in this disease.[101] In one study, no correlation was found between hepatic copper concentration and the extent of liver cell damage assessed either biochemically or histologically.[111] In addition, hepatic copper appeared to be localized to different organelles in primary biliary cirrhosis than in Wilson disease. This finding suggests that there may be differences in the way the liver handles copper in these two diseases. Second, D-penicillamine did not decrease serum markers of hepatic collagen synthesis, prolylhydroxylase, and galactosylhydroxylysyl glucosyltransferase; also, serum levels of the aminoterminal propeptide of type 3 procollagen were not lowered in 21 patients with primary biliary cirrhosis treated with the drug.[112]

Recent data indicate that two other drugs may slow the progression of primary biliary cirrhosis. Colchicine, an anti-inflammatory agent, was reported to have halved the elevated serum alkaline phosphatase in five women with primary biliary cirrhosis after 2 years of treatment.[113] Because of this finding and the fact that there was no other treatment, three prospective double-blind trials of colchicine in the treatment of primary biliary cirrhosis were performed.[114–116] One study included 60 patients with primary biliary cirrhosis, 30 patients with early disease (stages 1 and 2), and 30 with histologically advanced disease (stages 3 and 4).[114] Colchicine appeared to decrease mortality from liver disease after 4 years and improved serum levels of bilirubin, albumin, alkaline phosphatase, aminotransferases, and cholesterol after 2 years. However, there was no improvement in histology, symptoms, or physical findings. Except for diarrhea in several patients, there was no toxicity. The results of the two other studies also showed favorable effects on survival and laboratory values.[115,116] In one of these investigations, there was a statistically significant improvement in alkaline phosphatase and alanine aminotransferase in patients receiving colchicine, and the improvement in serum bilirubin almost reached significance, at $p = 0.06$.

Chlorambucil has recently been evaluated prospectively in 24 patients with primary biliary cirrhosis.[117] Serum levels of bilirubin, albumin, IgM, IgG, and hepatic inflammation all improved significantly after 2 years, but there was no decrease in hepatic fibrosis or stage of disease. The small number of patients in the study and its relatively short duration did not permit analysis of survival. There was appreciable bone marrow toxicity despite the fact that only small doses of chlorambucil were administered (10 mg/day for 10 days and then ≤2 mg/day) in order to keep the lymphocyte counts at approximately 50% of pretreatment levels. Two of 13 patients had to stop chlorambucil during the first year, and two had to stop during the fourth year. The concern about the long-term toxicity of chlorambucil has prevented the start of a proposed larger prospective randomized trial.

Cyclosporine is also being evaluated in the treatment of primary biliary cirrhosis. In a study of six patients, cyclosporine lowered the serum alkaline phosphatase and aminotransferases but did not improve the serum bilirubin or Ig values.[118] Nephrotoxicity, as indicated by a rising level of serum creatinine in each patient, precluded long-term use of the drug. Prospective controlled trials of cyclosporine are now under way.

Despite attempts to find therapeutic agents that will prevent the progression of primary biliary cirrhosis or even cure the disease, it is clear that none of the agents discussed above is totally effective. The mortality rate among patients with primary biliary cirrhosis treated with any of these drugs is still considerably higher than that in a healthy age- and sex-matched population. Liver transplantation is now considered appropriate treatment in patients in whom liver failure or recurrent bleeding from esophageal varices has developed. One-year survival in patients with primary biliary cirrhosis who undergo liver transplantation is approximately 60–70%[119,120] and more than 80% of patients who survive liver transplantation are able to return to full-time employment.[120] An early report that primary biliary cirrhosis may recur in patients in whom transplantation is successful[52] has not yet been confirmed.

ACKNOWLEDGMENT. This chapter is based on a recent article printed in the *New England Journal of Medicine*[121] and is written with the permission of the *New England Journal of Medicine*.

REFERENCES

1. Hamlyn AN, Sherlock S: The epidemiology of primary biliary cirrhosis: A survey of mortality in England and Wales. *Gut* **15**:473–479, 1974.
2. Hamlyn AN, Macklan AF, James O: Primary biliary cirrhosis: Geographical clustering and symptomatic onset seasonality. *Gut* **29**:970–975, 1983.
3. Triger DR, Berg PA, Rodes J: Epidemiology of primary biliary cirrhosis. *Liver* **4**:195–200, 1984.
4. Lofgren J, Jarnerot G, Danielson D, Herndal I: Incidence and prevalence of primary biliary cirrhosis in a defined population of Sweden. *Scand J Gastroenterol* **20**:647–650, 1985.
5. Dickson ER, Fleming CR, Ludwig J: Primary biliary cirrhosis, in Popper H, Schaffner F (eds): *Progress in Liver Diseases*. Vol. 6. Grune & Stratton, Orlando, Florida, 1978, pp. 487–502.
6. Galbraith RM, Smith M, MacKenzie RM, et al: High prevalence of serioimmunologic abnormalities in relatives of patients with active chronic hepatitis or primary biliary cirrhosis. *N Engl J Med* **290**:63–69, 1974.

7. Miller KB, Sepersky RA, Brown KM, et al: Genetic abnormalities of immunoregulation in primary biliary cirrhosis. *Am J Med* **65**:75–80, 1983.
8. Gores GJ, Moore SB, Fisher LD, et al: Primary biliary cirrhosis: Associations with major histocompatibility complex class II antigens. *Gastroenterology* **90**:1728, 1986 (abst).
9. Bassendine MF, Dewar PJ, James DFW: HLA-DR antigens in primary biliary cirrhosis: Lack of association. *Gut* **26**:625–628, 1985.
10. Johnston DE, Kaplan MM, Miller KB, et al: Histocompatibility antigens in primary biliary cirrhosis, *Am J Gastroenterol* **82**:1127–1129, 1987.
11. James SP, Hoofnagle JH, Strober W, Jones EA: Primary biliary cirrhosis: A model autoimmune disease. *Ann Intern Med* **99**:500–512, 1983.
12. Epstein O: The pathogenesis of primary biliary cirrhosis. *Mol Aspects Med* **3**:293–305, 1985.
13. MacSween RN, Burt AD: The cellular pathology of primary biliary cirrhosis. *Mol Aspects Med* **3**:269–291, 1985.
14. McFarlane IG: Autoreactivity against biliary tract antigens in primary biliary cirrhosis. *Mol Aspects Med* **3**:249–267, 1985.
15. Culp KS, Fleming CR, Duffy J, et al: Autoimmune associations in primary biliary cirrhosis. *Mayo Clin Proc* **57**:365–370, 1982.
16. Lindgren S, Eriksson S: IgM in primary biliary cirrhosis. Physicochemical and complement activating properties. *J Lab Clin Med* **99**:636–645, 1982.
17. Taal BG, Schalm SW: Cryoglobulins in primary biliary cirrhosis: prevalence and modulation by immunosuppressive therapy. *Z Gastroenterol* **23**:228–234, 1985.
18. Lindgren S, Johnson U: Complement activation in primary biliary cirrhosis: An in vitro model. *J Lab Clin Med* **105**:432–435, 1985.
19. Fakunle YM, Aranguibel F, DeVilliers D, et al: Monomeric IgM in chronic liver disease. *Clin Exp Immunol* **38**:204–210, 1979.
20. Nouria-Aria KT, Hegarty JE, Neuberger J, et al: In vitro studies on the mechanism of increased serum IgM levels in primary biliary cirrhosis. *Clin Exp Immunol* **61**:297–304, 1985.
21. James SP, Jones EA, Hoffnagle JH, Strober W: Circulating activated B cells in primary biliary cirrhosis. *J Clin Immunol* **5**:254–260, 1985.
22. Ruffati A, Arslan P, Floreani A, et al: Nuclear membrane-staining antinuclear antibody in patients with primary biliary cirrhosis. *J Clin Immunol* **5**:357–361, 1985.
23. Elta GH, Sepersky RA, Connors CM, et al: Increased incidence of hypothyroidism in primary biliary cirrhosis. *Dig Dis Sci* **28**:971–975, 1983.
24. Pares A, Martorell J, Caballeria J, et al: Lymphocytotoxic antibodies in primary biliary cirrhosis. *Dig Dis Sci* **30**:829–833, 1985.
25. Sundewall AC, Lefvert AK, Olsson R: Anti-acetylcholine receptor antibodies in primary biliary cirrhosis. *Acta Med Scand* **217**:519–525, 1985.
26. Bassendine MF, Collins JD, Stephenson J, et al: Platelet associated immunoglobulins in primary biliary cirrhosis: A cause of thrombocytopenia? *Gut* **26**:1074–1079, 1985.
27. Penner E: Demonstration of immune complexes containing the ribonucleoprotein antigen Ro in primary biliary cirrhosis. *Gastroenterology* **90**:724–727, 1986.
28. Baum H, Berg PA: The complex nature of mitochondrial antibodies and their relation to primary biliary cirrhosis. *Semin Liver Dis* **4**:309–321, 1981.
29. Lindenborn-Fotinos J, Baum H, Berg PA: Mitochondrial antibodies in primary biliary cirrhosis: Species and nonspecies specific determinants of M2 antigen. *Hepatology* **5**:763–769, 1985.
30. Mendel-Hartvig I, Nelson BD, Loof L, Totterman TH: Primary biliary cirrhosis: Further biochemical and immunological characterization of mitochondrial antigens. *Clin Exp Immunol* **62**:371–379, 1985.
31. Frazer IH, MacKay IR, Jordan TW, et al: Reactivity of anti-mitochondrial autoantibodies in primary biliary cirrhosis: Definition of two novel mitochondrial polypeptide autoantigens. *J Immunol* **135**:1739–1745, 1985.
32. Weber P, Brenner J, Strechemesser E, et al: Characterization and clinical relevance of a new complement-fixing antibody-anti-M8 in patients with primary biliary cirrhosis. *Hepatology* **6**:553–559, 1986.
33. Manns M, Meyer Zum Buschenfelde K-H: A mitochondrial antigen–antibody system in cholestatic liver disease detected by radioimmunoassay. *Hepatology* **5**:763–769, 1985.
34. Kaplan MM, Gandolfo JV, Quaroni EG: An enzyme-linked immunoabsorbent assay (ELISA) for detecting antimitochondrial antibody. *Hepatology* **4**:727–730, 1984.

35. Jones EA, Frank MM, Jaffe CJ, Vierling JM: Primary biliary cirrhosis and the complement system. *Ann Intern Med* **90**:72–84, 1979.
36. Lindgren S, Laurell A-B, Eriksson S: Complement components and activation in primary biliary cirrhosis. *Hepatology* **4**:9–14, 1984.
37. Al-Agbar MN, Neuberger J, Williams R, Eddleston AL: Mononuclear cell complement receptor blockade in primary biliary cirrhosis. *Gut* **26**:20–25, 1985.
38. Minuk GY, Vergalla J, Hanson RG, et al: Anticomplement receptor activity in the serum of patients with primary biliary cirrhosis. *Gut* **27**:324–328, 1986.
39. Wands JR, Dienstag JL, Bhan AK, et al: Circulating immune complexes and complement activation in primary biliary cirrhosis. *N Engl J Med* **298**:223–237, 1978.
40. Gupta RC, Dickson ER, McDuffie FC, Baggenstoss AH: Circulating IgG complexes in primary biliary cirrhosis: A serial study in forty patients followed for two years. *Clin Exp Immunol* **34**:19–27, 1978.
41. Amoroso P, Vergani D, Wojicika BM, et al: Identification of biliary antigens in circulating immune complexes in primary biliary cirrhosis. *Clin Exp Immunol* **42**:95–98, 1980.
42. Penner EH, Goldenberg H, Albini B, et al: Immune complexes in primary biliary cirrhosis contain mitochondrial antigens. *Clin Immun Immunopathol* **22**:394–399, 1982.
43. Goldberg MJ, Kaplan MM, Mitamura T, et al: Evidence against an immune complex pathogenesis of primary biliary cirrhosis. *Gastroenterology* **83**:677–683, 1982.
44. Bahn AK, Dienstag JL, Wands JR, et al: Alterations of T-cell subsets in primary biliary cirrhosis. *Clin Exp Immunol* **47**:351–358, 1982.
45. Miller KB, Elta GH, Rudders RA, Kaplan MM: Lymphocyte subsets in primary biliary cirrhosis. *Ann Intern Med* **100**:385–387, 1984.
46. James SP, Elson CO, Jones EA, Strober W: Abnormal regulation of immunoglobulin synthesis in vitro in primary biliary cirrhosis. *Gastroenterology* **79**:242–244, 1980.
47. Zetterman RK, Woltjen JA: Supressor cell activity in primary biliary cirrhosis. *Dig Dis Sci* **25**:104–107, 1980.
48. James SP, Elson CO, Waggoner JG, et al: Deficiency of the autologous mixed lymphocyte reaction in patients with primary biliary cirrhosis. *J Clin Invest* **66**:1305–1310, 1980.
49. Ballardini G, Mirakian R, Bianchi FB, et al: Aberrant expression of HLA-DR antigens on bile duct epithelium in primary biliary cirrhosis: Relevance to pathogenesis. *Lancet* **2**:1009–1013, 1984.
50. Zinkernagel RM, Doherty PC: MCH-restricted cytotoxic cells: Studies on the biological role of polymorphic major transplantation antigens determine T cell restriction-specificity, functions, and responsiveness. *Adv Immunol* **27**:51–177, 1979.
51. Bernau D, Feldmann G, Degott MD, Gisselbrecht C: Ultrastructural lesions and bile ducts in primary biliary cirrhosis. A comparison with the lesions observed in graft versus host disease. *Hum Pathol* **12**:782–793, 1981.
52. Neuberger J, Portmann B, MacDougall BRD, et al: Recurrence of primary biliary cirrhosis after liver transplantation. *N Engl J Med* **306**:1–4, 1982.
53. McFarlane IG, Wojcicka BM, Isantoulas DC, et al: Leukocyte migration inhibition in response to biliary antigens in primary biliary cirrhosis, sclerosing cholangitis, and other liver diseases. *Gastroenterology* **76**:1333–1340, 1979.
54. James SP, Jones EA: Abnormal natural killer cytotoxicity in primary biliary cirrhosis: Evidence for a functional deficiency of cytolytic effector cells. *Gastroenterology* **89**:165–171, 1985.
55. Vierling JM, Nelson DL, Strober W, et al: In vitro cell-mediated cytotoxicity in primary biliary cirrhosis and chronic hepatitis: Dysfunction of spontaneous cell-mediated cytotoxicity in primary biliary cirrhosis. *J Clin Invest* **60**:1116–1128, 1977.
56. Geubel AP, Keller RH, Summerskill WHJ, et al: Lymphocyte cytotoxicity and inhibition studied with autologous liver cells: Observations in chronic active liver disease and the primary biliary cirrhosis syndrome. *Gastroenterology* **71**:450–456, 1976.
57. Christensen E, Crowe J, Doniach D, et al: Clinical pattern and course of disease in primary biliary cirrhosis based on an analysis of 236 patients. *Gastroenterology* **78**:236–246, 1980.
58. Shapiro JM, Smith H, Schaffner F: Serum bilirubin, a prognostic factor in primary biliary cirrhosis. *Gut* **20**:137–140, 1979.
59. Sasaki H, Inoue K, Higuchi K, et al: Primary biliary cirrhosis in Japan: National survey by the subcommittee on autoimmune hepatitis. *Gastroenterology* Jpn **5**:476–485, 1985.
60. Jahn CE, Schaeffer EJ, Taam LA, et al: Lipoprotein abnormalities in primary biliary cirrhosis. *Gastroenterology* **89**:1266–1278, 1985.

61. Teramoto T, Kato H, Hashimoto Y, et al: Abnormal high density lipoprotein of primary biliary cirrhosis analyzed by high performance chromatography. *Clin Chim Acta* **149**:135–148, 1985.
62. Sherlock S, Scheuer PJ: The presentation and diagnosis of 100 patients with primary biliary cirrhosis. *N Engl J Med* **289**:674–678, 1973.
63. Ghent CN, Bloomer JR, Klatskin G: Elevations in skin tissue levels of bile acids in human cholestasis: Relation to serum levels and to pruritus. *Gastroenterology* **73**:1125–1130, 1977.
64. Haensch HP, Balzer K, Kylewizc P, et al: Effect of rifampicin treatment on hepatic drug metabolism and serum bile acids in patients with primary biliary cirrhosis. *Eur J Clin Pharmacol* **28**:475–477, 1985.
65. Ambinder EP, Cohen LB, Wolke AM, et al: The clinical effectiveness and safety of chronic plasmapheresis in patients with primary biliary cirrhosis. *J Clin Apheresis* **2**:219–223, 1985.
66. Roll J, Boyer JL, Barry D, Klatskin G: The prognostic importance of clinical and histologic features in asymptomatic and symptomatic primary biliary cirrhosis. *N Engl J Med* **308**:1–7, 1983.
67. James O, Macklin AF, Watson AJ: Primary biliary cirrhosis—A revised clinical spectrum. *Lancet* **1**:1278–1281, 1981.
68. Dickson ER, Fleming TR, Wiesner RH, et al: Trial of penicillamine in advanced primary biliary cirrhosis. *N Engl J Med* **312**:1011–1015, 1985.
69. Long RG, Scheuer PJ, Sherlock S: Presentation and course of asymptomatic primary biliary cirrhosis. *Gastroenterology* **72**:1204–1207, 1977.
70. Ros E, Garcia-Puges A, Reixach M, et al: Fat digestion and exocrine pancreatic function in primary biliary cirrhosis. *Gastroenterology* **87**:180–187, 1984.
71. Lanspa SJ, Chan AT, Bell JS III, et al: Pathogenesis of steatorrhea in primary biliary cirrhosis . *Hepatology* **5**:837–842, 1985.
72. Herlong HF, Recker RR, Maddrey WC: Bone disease in primary biliary cirrhosis: Histologic features and response to 25-hydroxyvitamin D. *Gastroenterology* **83**:103–108, 1982.
73. Matloff DS, Kaplan MM, Neer RM, et al: Osteoporosis in primary biliary cirrhosis: Effects of 25-hydroxyvitamin D_3 treatment. *Gastroenterology* **83**:97–102, 1982.
74. Epstein O, Chapman RWG, Lake-Bakaar G, et al: The pancreas in primary biliary cirrhosis and primary sclerosing cholangitis. *Gastroenterology* **83**:1177–1182, 1982.
75. Kehayoglou AK, Holdsworth CD, Agnew JE, et al: Bone disease and calcium absorption in primary biliary cirrhosis—With special reference to vitamin D therapy. *Lancet* **1**:715–719, 1968.
76. Reed JS, Meredith SC, Nemchausky BA, et al: Bone disease in primary biliary cirrhosis: Reversal of osteomalacia with oral 25-hydroxyvitamin D. *Gastroenterology* **78**:512–517, 1980.
77. Long RG: Hepatic osteodystrophy: Outlook good but some problems unsolved. *Gastroenterology* **78**:644–647, 1980.
78. Kaplan MM, Goldberg MJ, Matloff DS, et al: Effect of 25-hydroxyvitamin D_3 metabolites in primary biliary cirrhosis. *Gastroenterology* **81**:681–685, 1981.
79. Krawitt EL, Grundman MJ, Mawer EB: Absorption, hydroxylation, and excretion of vitamin D_3 in primary biliary cirrhosis. *Lancet* **2**:1246–1249, 1977.
80. Mawer EB, Klass HJ, Warnes TW, Berry JL: Metabolism of vitamin D in patients with primary biliary cirrhosis and alcoholic liver disease. *Clin Sci* **69**:561–570, 1985.
81. Jung RT, Davie M, Siklos P, et al: Vitamin D metabolism in acute and chronic cholestasis. *Gut* **20**:840–847, 1979.
82. Hodgson SF, Dickson ER, Wahner HW, et al: Bone loss and reduced osteoblastic function in primary biliary cirrhosis. *Ann Intern Med* **103**:855–860, 1985.
83. Cuthbert JA, Pak CYC, Zerwekh JE, et al: Bone disease in primary biliary cirrhosis: Increased bone resorption and turnover in the absence of osteoporosis or osteomalacia. *Hepatology* **1**:1–8, 1981.
84. Herlong HF, Russell RM, Maddrey WC: Vitamin A and zinc therapy in primary biliary cirrhosis. *Hepatology* **1**:348–381, 1981.
85. Shepherd AN, Bedford GJ, Hill A, Bouchier IA: Primary biliary cirrhosis. Dark adaptometry, electro-oculography and vitamin A state. *Br Med J* **289**:1484–1485, 1984.
86. Elta GH, Furie BC, Furie B, et al: Fat soluble vitamins in primary biliary cirrhosis. *Hepatology* **2**:703 1982 (abst).
87. Spinsi R, Smith-Laing G, Epstein O, Sherlock S: Results of portal decompression in patients with primary biliary cirrhosis. *Gut* **22**:345–349, 1981.
88. Sepersky R, Callow A, Kanel G, Kaplan MM: Portasystemic shunts in primary biliary cirrhosis: Survival is the same as in patients with Laennec's cirrhosis and postnecrotic cirrhosis. *Dig Dis Sci* **27**:507–512, 1982.

89. Alarcon-Segovia D, Diaz-Jouanen E, Fishbein E: Features of Sjögren's syndrome in primary biliary cirrhosis. *Ann Intern Med* **79:**31–36, 1973.
90. Giovannini A, Ballardini G, Bonazzoli P, Bianchi FB: Patterns of lacrimal dysfunction in primary biliary cirrhosis. *Br J Ophthalmol* **69:**832–835, 1985.
91. Clark AK, Galbraith RM, Hamilton EBD, et al: Rheumatic disorders in primary biliary cirrhosis. *Ann Rheum Dis* **37:**42–47, 1978.
92. Crowe JP, Malloy MG, Wells I, et al: Increased Clq binding and arthritis in primary biliary cirrhosis. *Gut* **21:**418–422, 1980.
93. Crowe JP, Christensen E, Butler J, et al: Primary biliary cirrhosis and the prevalence of hypothyroidism and its relationship to thyroid autoantibodies and sicca syndrome. *Gastroenterology* **78:**1437–1441, 1980.
94. Pares A, Rimola A, Bruguera M, et al: Renal tubular acidosis in primary biliary cirrhosis. *Gastroenterology* **80:**681–686, 1981.
95. Melia WM, Johnson PJ, Neuberger J, et al: Hepatocellular carcinoma in primary biliary cirrhosis: Detection by alpha-fetoprotein estimation. *Gastroenterology* **87:**660–663, 1984.
96. Wolke AM, Schaffner F, Kopelman B, Sacks HS: Malignancy in primary biliary cirrhosis. High incidence of breast cancer in affected women. *Am J Med* **76:**1075–1078, 1984.
97. Goudie BM, Burt AD, Boyle P, et al: Breast cancer in women with primary biliary cirrhosis. *Br Med J* **291:**1597–1598, 1985.
98. Burroughs AK, Rosenstein IJ, Epstein O, et al: Bacteriuria and primary biliary cirrhosis. *Gut* **25:**133–137, 1984.
99. Christensen E, Neuberger J, Crowe J, et al: Beneficial effect of azathioprine and prediction of prognosis in primary biliary cirrhosis. *Gastroenterology* **89:**1084–1091, 1985.
100. James OFW: D-Penicillamine for primary biliary cirrhosis. *Gut* **26:**109–113, 1985.
101. Neuberger J, Christensen E, Portmann B, et al: Double blind controlled trial of D-penicillamine in patients with primary biliary cirrhosis. *Gut* **26:**114–119, 1985.
102. Beswick DR, Klatskin G, Boyer JL: Asymptomatic primary biliary cirrhosis. *Gastroenterology* **89:**267–271, 1985.
103. Lee RG, Epstein O, Jauregi H, et al: Granulomas in primary biliary cirrhosis: A prognostic feature. *Gastroenterology* **81:**983–986, 1981.
104. Portmann B, Popper H, Neuberger J, Williams R: Sequential and diagnostic features in primary biliary cirrhosis based on serial histologic study in 209 patients. *Gastroenterology* **88:**1777–1790, 1985.
105. Heathcote J, Ross A, Sherlock S: A prospective controlled trial of azathioprine in primary biliary cirrhosis. *Gastroenterology* **70:**656–660, 1976.
106. Crowe J, Christensen E, Smith M, et al: Azathioprine in primary biliary cirrhosis: A preliminary report of an international trial. *Gastroenterology* **78:**1005–1010, 1980.
107. Epstein O, Jain S, Lee RG, et al: D-Penicillamine treatment improves survival in primary biliary cirrhosis. *Lancet* **1:**1275–1277, 1981.
108. Matloff DS, Alpert E, Resnick RH, Kaplan MM: A prospective trial of D-penicillamine in primary biliary cirrhosis. *N Engl J Med* **306:**319–326, 1982.
109. Epstein O, Cook DG, Jain S, et al: D-Penicillamine and clinical trials in primary biliary cirrhosis. *Hepatology* **4:**1032, 1984 (abst).
110. Bodenheimer HC Jr, Schaffner F, Sternlieb I, et al: A prospective clinical trial of D-penicillamine in the treatment of primary biliary cirrhosis. *Hepatology* **5:**1139–1142, 1985.
111. Epstein O, Arborgh B, Sagiv M, et al: Is copper hepatotoxic in primary biliary cirrhosis? *J Clin Pathol* **34:**1071–1075, 1981.
112. Savolainen E-R, Miettinen TA, Pikkarainen P, et al: Enzymes of collagen synthesis and type III procollagen aminopropeptide in the evaluation of D-penicillamine and medroxyprogesterone treatments of primary biliary cirrhosis. *Gut* **24:**136–142, 1983.
113. Koldinger RE: Treatment of primary biliary cirrhosis with colchicine. *Gastroenterology* **78:**1309, 1980 (abst).
114. Kaplan MM, Alling DW, Zimmerman HJ, et al: A prospective trial of colchicine for primary biliary cirrhosis. *N Engl J Med* **315:**1448–1454, 1986.
115. Warnes TW, Smith A, Lee F, et al: A controlled trial of colchicine in primary biliary cirrhosis. *Hepatology* **4:**1022, 1984 (abst).
116. Bodenheimer H Jr, Schaffner F, Pezzullo J: Colchicine therapy in primary biliary cirrhosis. *Hepatology* **6:**1172, 1986.

117. Hoofnagle JH, David GL, Schafer DF, et al: Randomized trial of chlorambucil for primary biliary cirrhosis. *Gastroenterology* **91**:1327–1334, 1986.
118. Routhier G, Epstein O, Janossy G, et al: The effects of cyclosporin A on suppresion and inducer T-lymphocytes in primary biliary cirrhosis. *Lancet* **3**:1223–1226, 1980.
119. Scharschmidt BF: Human liver transplantation: Analysis of data on 540 patients from four centers. *Hepatology* **4**:955–1015, 1984.
120. Van Thiel DH, Tarter R, Gavaler JS, et al: Liver transplantation in adults. An analysis of costs and benefits at the University of Pittsburgh. *Gastroenterology* **90**:211–216, 1986.

15

Primary Biliary Cirrhosis: Pathology

Roderick N. M. MacSween

1. INTRODUCTION

The essential morphologic feature of primary biliary cirrhosis (PBC) comprises a chronic nonsuppurative destructive cholangitis.[1] This is the primary lesion and results in a progressive disappearing bile duct syndrome. Although there is clinical and/or biochemical evidence of a cholestatic syndrome from the time of diagnosis, morphologic evidence of cholestasis does not appear until there has been extensive loss of intrahepatic bile ducts; jaundice with bilirubinostasis is often a still later feature and of poor prognostic import.[2] In my view, the progress of the liver injury in PBC is secondary to cholestasis resulting from the loss of bile ducts and is, in effect, a secondary biliary cirrhosis. This chapter describes the morphologic features of PBC, discusses some of the immunological aspects, speculates as to pathogenetic mechanisms, and poses some unanswered questions relating to this enigmatic disease.

2. HISTOPATHOLOGIC FEATURES

These have been described in a number of recent reviews.[3–8]

3. BILE DUCT LESION

The initial lesions are focal within the liver, and there is segmental involvement of the bile ducts. The involved bile ducts are surrounded by a chronic inflammatory cell infiltrate (Fig. 1) in which plasma cells are often conspicuous and in which eosinophils are present as well. The bile duct epithelium becomes focally hyperplastic; there is a characteristic loss of the periodic acid-Schiff (PAS)-positive supranuclear cytoplasmic granules, and the cytoplasm becomes more eosinophilic. Some individual epithelial cells may show acidophilic degeneration–apoptosis; others show cytoplasmic vacuolation, usually when lymphocytes penetrate the basement membrane and become intraepithelial (Figs. 2 and 3). The basement membrane becomes fragmented, and there is focal degeneration and ulceration of the epithelium.

Roderick N. M. MacSween • Department of Pathology, University of Glasgow and Western Infirmary, Glasgow G11 6NT, Scotland, United Kingdom.

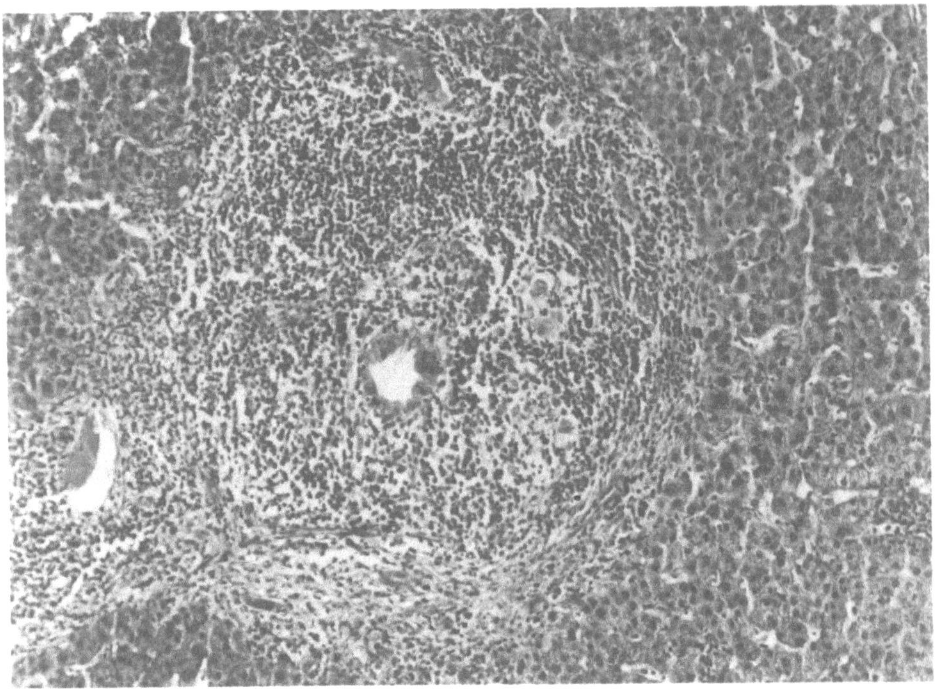

Figure 1. Portal tract containing a dense chronic inflammatory cell infiltrate in which a damaged bile duct is entrapped. (H&E, ×110)

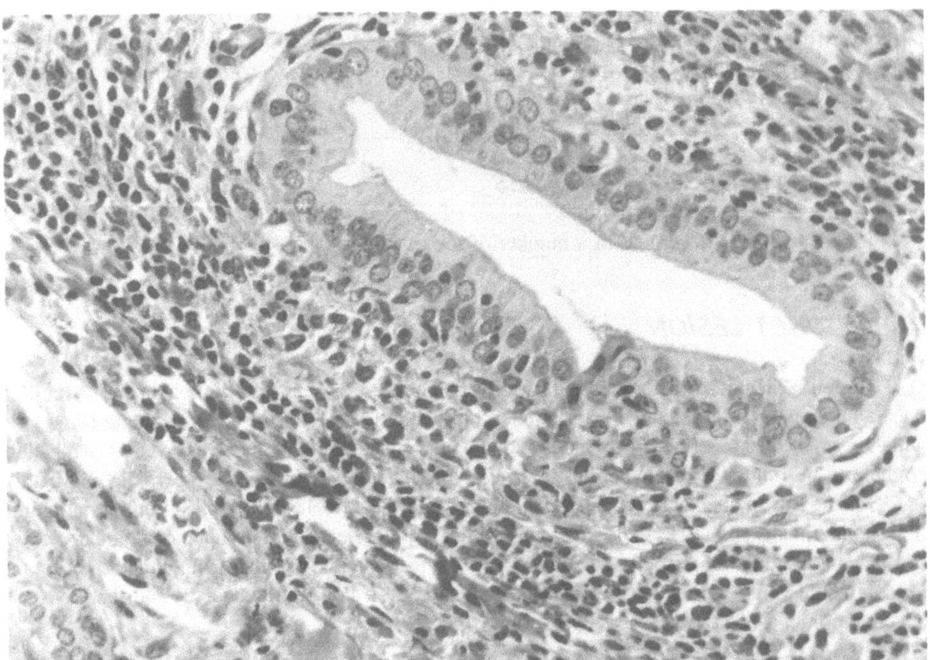

Figure 2. Bile duct lesion. The duct is surrounded by a granulomatous infiltrate; the duct epithelium is focally hyperplastic (lower aspect) and intraepithelial lymphocytes are evident. (H&E, ×310)

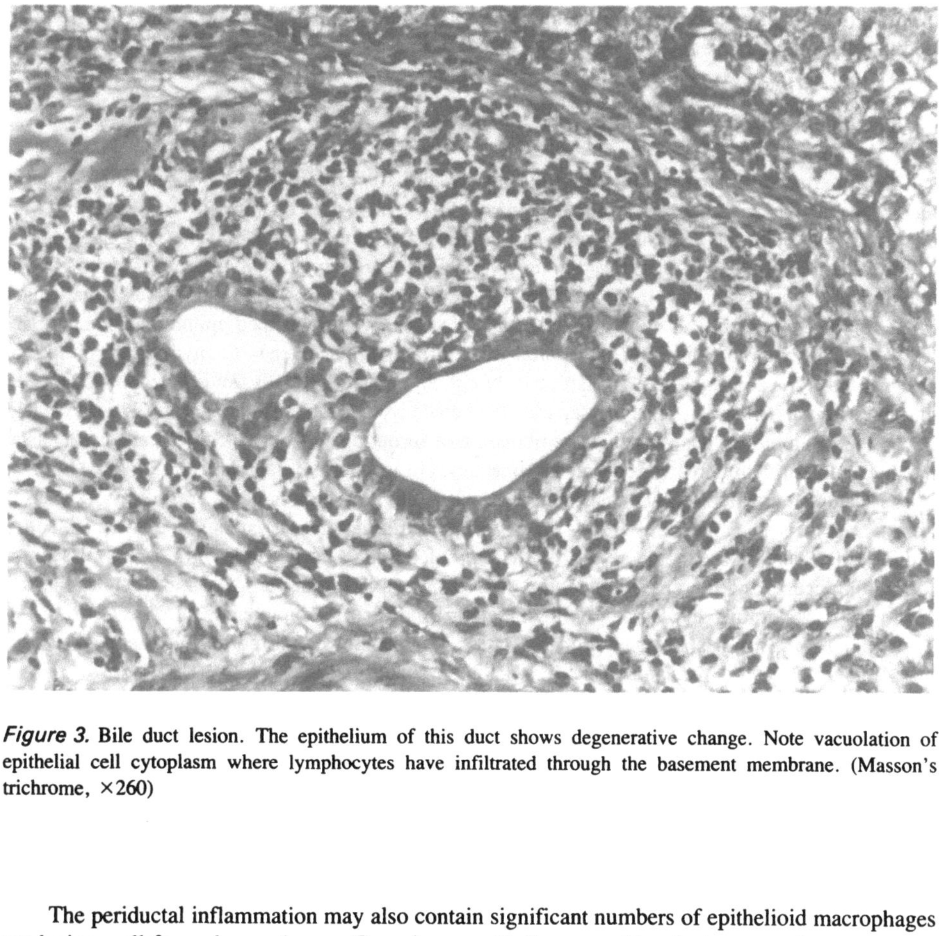

Figure 3. Bile duct lesion. The epithelium of this duct shows degenerative change. Note vacuolation of epithelial cell cytoplasm where lymphocytes have infiltrated through the basement membrane. (Masson's trichrome, ×260)

The periductal inflammation may also contain significant numbers of epithelioid macrophages producing well-formed granulomas. Granulomas with foamy multinucleate macrophages are conspicuous in some portal tracts and are probably a reaction to bile leakage from damaged ducts. It should be emphasized that there is considerable heterogeneity in the periductal and portal tract appearances; lymphocytes, plasma cells, plasmacytoid cells, eosinophils, macrophages, and epithelioid cells are present in various proportions. Thus, in some portal tracts, the appearances are of a well-developed periductal granulomatous reaction, whereas in others the duct remnants are surrounded by a predominantly lymphocytic reaction in which germinal centers may be formed. Furthermore, the proportions of the various cell types may vary in serial sections of the same bile duct lesion. These observations are no different from what one sees in a variety of chronic inflammatory processes. It is important to remember this, however, within the context of interpreting the data accumulated in phenotyping the chronic inflammatory cells present at various sites in the portal and periportal areas.

The earliest lesions are thought to involve the interlobular and septal bile ducts, although it is difficult to be absolutely certain of this. The smallest bile ducts are also progressively lost from an early stage.[9,10] Three types of periductal lesion, preceding the disappearance of the duct, were identified by Nakanuma and colleagues[9,10]: a periductal chronic inflammatory reaction, periductal edema, and periductal fibrosis. The simultaneous presence of these three types of lesions suggested that they were caused by the same etiologic factor, although it was noted that the fibrotic lesions were the most commonly found. This observation suggested that they might constitute the initial lesion, the edema and inflammation being a secondary reaction to the epithelial injury. It is also possible that the loss of the small ducts may be simply related to the destruction of the larger ducts, with a consequent upstream disuse atrophy of the draining biliary radicles.

4. PROGRESS OF THE LIVER INJURY

In some portal tracts, the bile duct disappears virtually without trace, a few chronic inflammatory cells marking the site previously occupied by the duct; in others a focal lymphocytic aggregate marks the site (Fig. 4). Fibrous scars, commonly found in primary sclerosing cholangitis, are not a residual feature in PBC. Within the liver acinus, early abnormalities comprise Kupffer cell hyperplasia, sometimes a prominent accumulation of mononuclear cells in sinusoids, small macrophage aggregates, and, in approximately 25% of cases, well-developed epithelioid granulomas.

With the evolution of PBC, the portal tract inflammation extends to involve the periportal parenchyma. The limiting plate is disrupted; lymphocytes, plasma cells, and macrophages extend into the parenchyma and disrupt and separate the hepatocytes; edematous loose fibrous tissue is laid down; there is liver cell necrosis and a combination of sprouting by small bile ducts, and metaplastic ductular transformation of liver cell plates contributes to a pattern of ductular proliferation (Fig. 4). These features constitute biliary piecemeal necrosis,[6] and they are regularly present in obstructive biliary tract disease of whatever etiology. The periportal inflammation extends to involve the entire limiting plate and also extends along the margins of terminal portal tracts. Portal–portal septum formation occurs, and there is architectural disturbance and eventual progression to an established cirrhosis. Regenerative hyperplasia with nodularity may be a prominent feature, antedating the development of cirrhosis,[8,11] and probably being responsible for the portal hypertension, which may sometimes be a conspicuous feature at an early stage of PBC.[8–12]

Cholestasis develops peripherally affecting periportal and periseptal hepatocytes. They become swollen and vacuolated, often producing a distinctive halo appearance (Fig. 5); Mallory bodies may be present, and substantial accumulations of copper-associated protein are demonstrable as black/brown granules with the orcein stain (Fig. 6).

The evolution of PBC has been divided into various stages by different investigators[3,13–15]: duct lesions and portal tract involvement, periportal extension, precirrhotic fibrous scarring, and cirrhosis. However, this has little to commend it. Because of the focal involvement of the initial bile duct injury, there is considerable overlap between the stages and duct lesions may be present in an end-stage cirrhotic liver. Furthermore, there is considerable variation in the progression of the liver disease; in some patients, progression is arrested, and they may remain at the same stage for years. Finally, there is frequently a poor correlation between the clinical state of the patient and the apparent histologic staging. Thus, histologic staging cannot be used to prognosticate on the clinical outcome.

5. ULTRASTRUCTURAL FEATURES

Electron microscopic studies have failed to demonstrate any lesions peculiar to PBC.[16–18] There is thickening, with reduplication and rarefaction of the bile duct basement membrane; intraepithelial lymphocytes are present in dilated intercellular spaces and adjacent to necrotic or partially necrotic epithelial cells; the lymphocytes have prominent pseudopods in intimate contact with the duct epithelium, but no fusion of cell membranes is apparent (Fig. 7). The epithelial cells become detached from the basement membrane and show various patterns of necrosis—coagulative, lytic, and sometimes apoptotic; this may occur apparently in the absence of intraepithelial and periductal lymphocytes. The heterogeneous nature of the periductal inflammatory cell infiltrate is confirmed on electron microscopy; in addition, fibroblasts, myofibroblasts, and collagen are also identified. Bernuau et al.[17] noted similarities between the changes in PBC and those seen in graft versus host disease, in which there is also loss and disappearance of bile ducts.

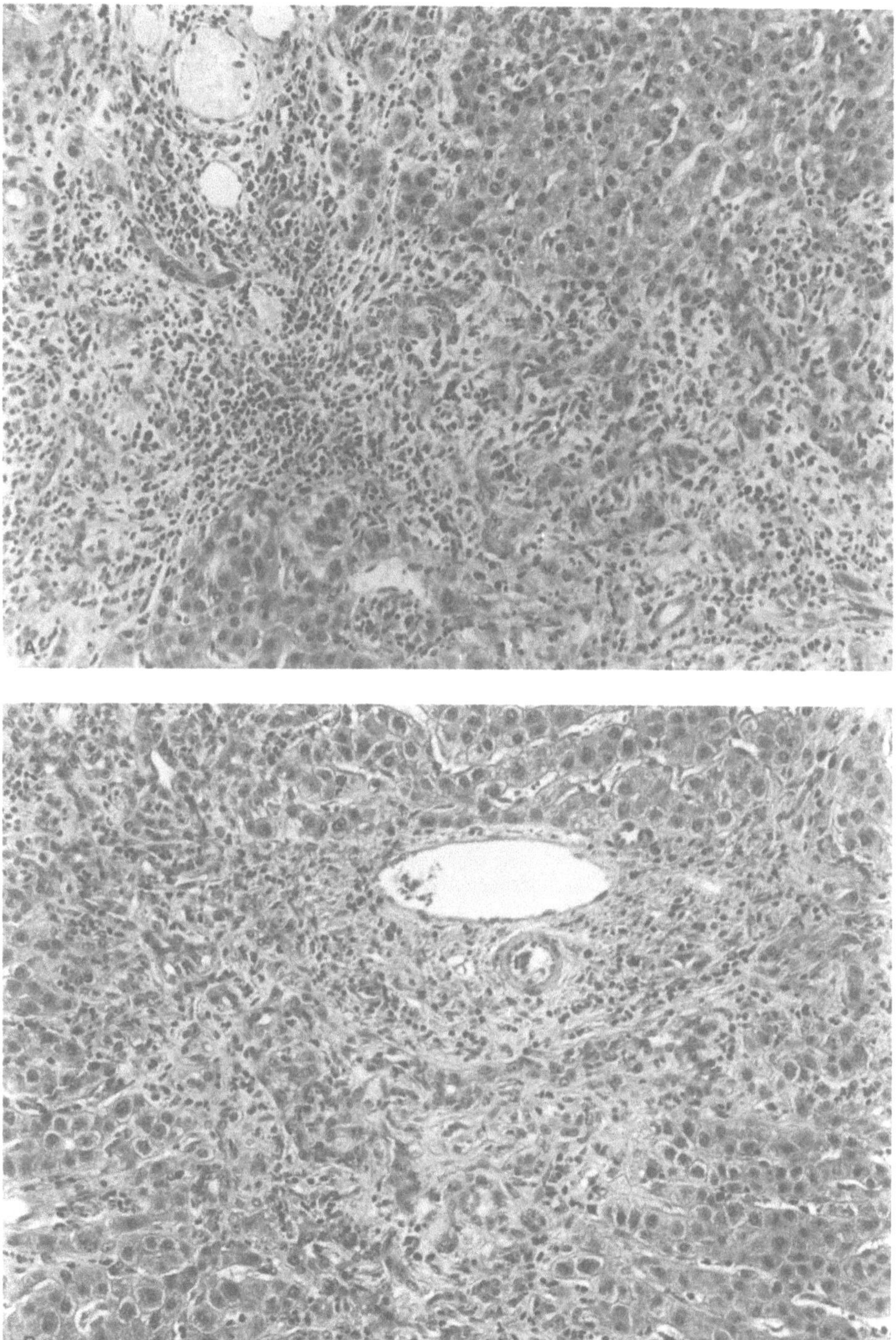

Figure 4. (A) In the portal tract on upper left, no bile duct is identified, and there is a focal lymphocytic aggregate at the site. (H&E, ×160) (B) In this portal tract, the bile duct has disappeared, and a light chronic inflammatory cell infiltrate is present. (H&E, ×150) (A,B) Note the periportal extension of the inflammatory process with a pattern of biliary piecemeal necrosis in which ductular proliferation is prominent.

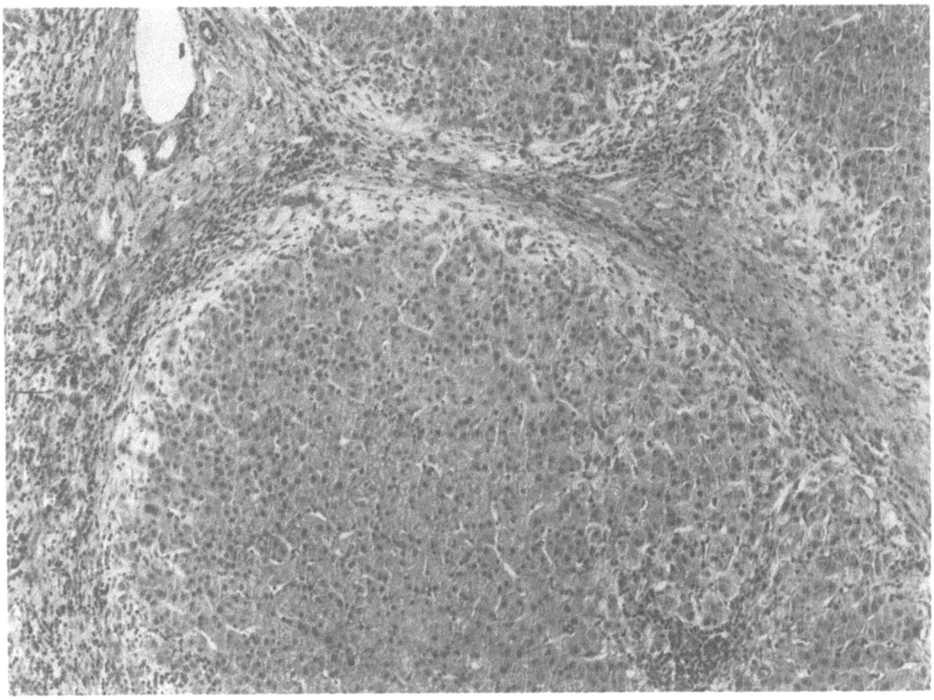

Figure 5. Cirrhotic stage of PBC. Note the perinodular halo due to the presence of peripheral cholestasis. (H&E, ×75)

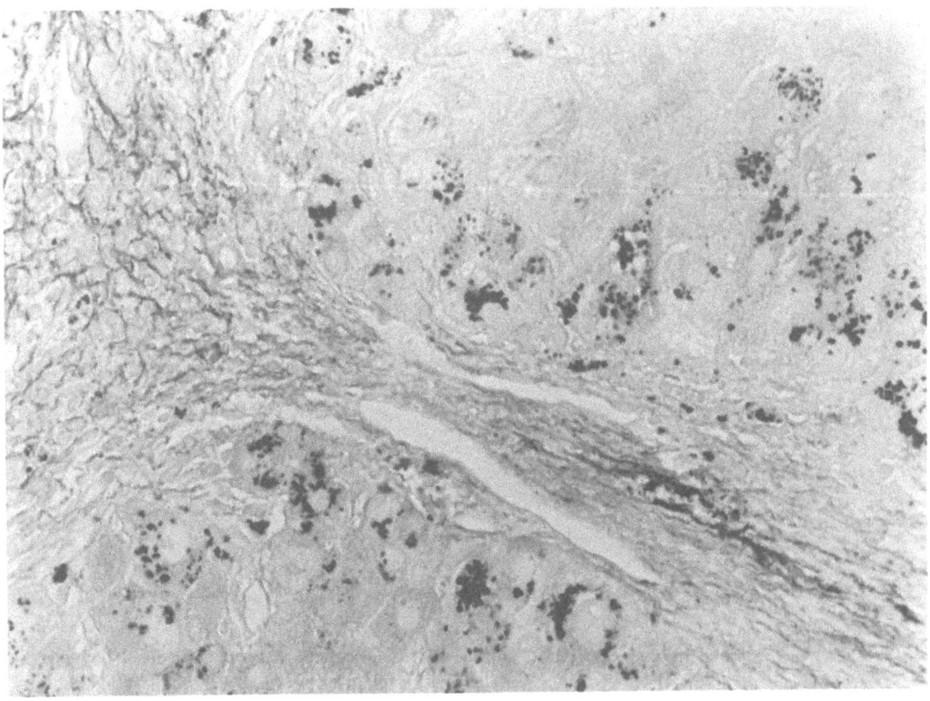

Figure 6. Periportal and periseptal granular accumulation of copper-associated protein. (Orcein, ×370)

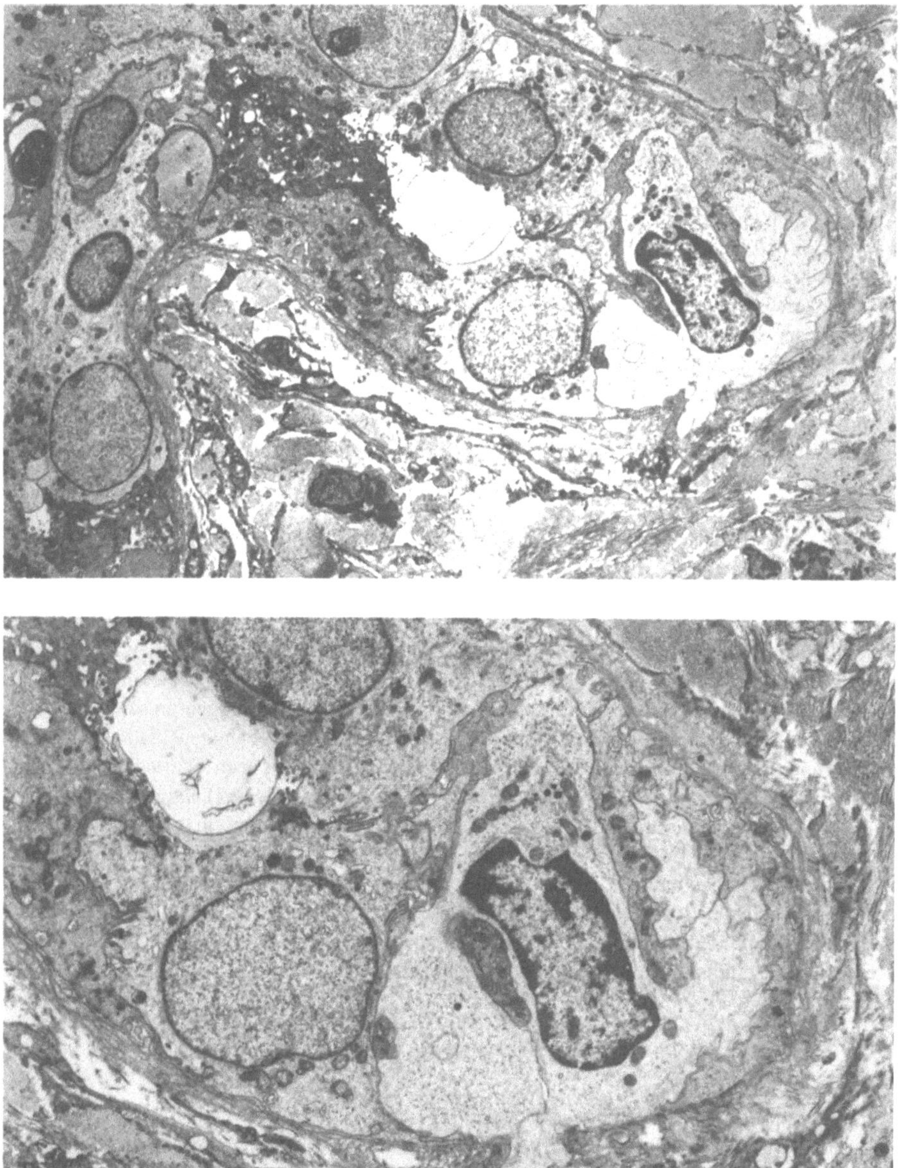

Figure 7. (A) Electron micrographs showing an early bile duct lesion. Note the dark degenerating epithelial cells (left) and an intraepithelial lymphocyte (right). (×4000) (B) At a higher magnification, note the increased thickness of the basement membrane and the close contact between the invaginating lymphocyte and the epithelial cells. (×8100)

6. PHENOTYPIC CHARACTERIZATION OF THE PORTAL AND PERIPORTAL INFLAMMATORY CELL INFILTRATE

Increasingly sophisticated immunohistochemical and enzyme labeling methods combined with polyclonal and monoclonal antibodies have been used to characterize the subtypes present in the portal and periportal cellular infiltrate. The results obtained have sometimes been contradictory. In part, this is related to the histologic stage examined and, as has been emphasized, to the heterogeneous nature of the portal tract inflammation. The findings can be summarized as follows: (1) immunoglobulin M (IgM) plasma cells and both helper/inducer and cytotoxic/suppressor T cells have been found to be intraepithelial; (2) T cells predominate in both the portal and periportal inflammation, but monocytes/macrophages are also present in considerable numbers; (3) the periductal infiltrate in early lesions is predominantly helper/inducer T cells with some IgM plasma cells; (4) in areas of ductular proliferation, B cells and helper/inducer T cells are present; and (5) in areas of biliary piecemeal necrosis, cytotoxic/suppressor T cells predominate, but helper/inducer T cells are also present in considerable numbers. These observations do not immediately afford an explanation for the cellular mechanisms involved in either the bile duct or liver cell injury, but they do suggest that different immune mechanisms are involved. Furthermore, it is noteworthy that in advanced stages of PBC, the composition of the inflammatory cell infiltrate in the portal tracts and parenchyma is not distinctly different from that found in the end stage of other chronic cholestatic syndromes and of chronic active hepatitides.[22,26–28]

7. PHENOTYPIC ALTERATIONS IN BILE DUCT EPITHELIUM

The major histocompatibility complex (MHC) class I antigens (HLA-A, -B, -C) are normally found on all nucleated cells. The class II antigens (HLA-DR, -DP, -DQ) are expressed by macrophages, B lymphocytes, vascular endothelium, dendritic and other antigen-presenting cells, and activated T cells. Normal bile duct epithelium does not express class II antigens. However, in PBC, enhanced expression of class I antigens and aberrant class II display has been reported[24,29] (A. D. Burt and R. N. M. MacSween, personal observations). The expression of class II antigens was multifocal in the early stage of the disease but universally affected any surviving ducts in the late stages.[24] Class II antigen expression by bile duct epithelium has also been found in hepatic graft-versus-host disease (GVHD)[30] and in the hepatitic lesions of chronic viral hepatitis.[29] These phenotypic changes, possibly induced by the local release of lymphokines, such as γ-interferon (IFN_{γ}), could enhance the local immune response by attracting major histocompatibility complex restricted cytotoxic T cells or by rendering the epithelial cells capable of antigen presentation.

8. POSSIBLE PATHOGENETIC MECHANISMS IN PBC

In addition to the immunologic abnormalities found within the liver, numerous other immunologic abnormalities have been described in PBC and are comprehensively summarized in Chapter 14. The presence of antimitochondrial antibodies (AMA) is characteristic of PBC, anti-M2 being virtually a universal finding, while the presence of anti-M4 and anti-M8 may distinguish subgroups of PBC with a more rapidly progressive clinical course.[31,32] The precise relationship of AMA to PBC remains uncertain, but it is difficult to escape the conclusion that such a marked disease specificity is important. There are considerable similarities between bacterial and mitocondrial membranes.[31,32] In addition, AMA of certain specificities may be found in the serum from spouses and relatives of PBC patients.[32] It has been suggested, therefore, that PBC may be due to persistence of an infectious agent.[31]

Studies of peripheral blood lymphocyte subsets in PBC have produced contradictory results, and the findings have varied depending on the stage of the disease.[33-35] Functional studies, however, have consistently shown impaired T-suppressor cell activity,[36,37] and it has been postulated that this disturbance in immunoregulation could facilitate the autoaggressive hyperresponsiveness demonstrated in PBC patients. However, this abnormality of T cells is not disease specific, occurring also in patients with systemic lupus erythematosus and in a proportion of healthy first-degree relatives of patients with PBC.[37]

Morphologic evidence that PBC may recur in hepatic allografts of transplant-treated patients remains equivocal.[38,39] In graft rejection, irrespective of the indicator disease in the recipient, there is a loss of intrahepatic bile ducts.[8] Thus, it is difficult to be certain that in the PBC recipient the bile duct loss is due to graft rejection rather than being a manifestation of the host abnormalities that had predisposed to the disease. Loss of intrahepatic bile ducts also occurs in GVHD,[8,30] and so there is strong circumstantial evidence that bile duct elimination may be immunologically mediated.

Changes in AMA titers have also been monitored in graft-treated PBC patients.[38,39] The titer falls after transplantation but then rises; the subtypes of AMA also reappear in the grafted patients. These observations indicate that the production of AMA is not dependent on the presence of a diseased PBC liver and that the primary disease process is probably a disturbance of the immune system rather than due to immunopathologic mechanisms primarily located in the liver.

The etiology and pathogenesis of PBC thus remain uncertain. There is evidence to suggest that there is an immune diathesis that predisposes to the disease process. Any unifying theory, however, must afford an explanation for the following questions:

Why is there such a marked female preponderance?
What initiates the early bile duct damage?
Why are the early lesions focal within the liver?
What are the mechanisms involved in the destruction of the bile ducts?
Is the liver cell involvement in the progress of the disease simply secondary to cholestasis, or is it part of the same postulated autoimmune process that affects the bile ducts?

REFERENCES

1. Rubin E, Schaffner F, Popper H: Primary biliary cirrhosis. Chronic non-suppurative destructive cholangitis. *Am J Pathol* **46**:387–407, 1965.
2. Shapiro JM, Smith H, Schaffner F: Serum bilirubin: A prognostic factor in primary biliary cirrhosis. *Gut* **20**:137–140, 1979.
3. Ludwig J, Dickson ER, McDonald GSA: Staging of chronic nonsuppurative destructive cholangitis (syndrome of primary biliary cirrhosis). *Virchows Arch Pathol Anat* **379**:103–112, 1978.
4. Schaffner F, Popper H: Clinical–pathologic relations in primary biliary cirrhosis, in Popper H, Schaffner F (eds): *Progress in Liver Diseases,* Vol. VII. Grune & Stratton, Orlando, Florida, 1982, pp. 529–554.
5. Scheuer PJ: Primary biliary cirrhosis: Diagnosis, pathology and pathogenesis. *Postgrad Med J* **59**(suppl 4):106–115, 1983.
6. Portmann B, Popper H, Neuberger J, et al: Sequential and diagnostic features in primary biliary cirrhosis, based on serial histologic study in 209 patients. *Gastroenterology* **88**:1777–1790, 1985.
7. MacSween RNM, Burt AD: The cellular pathology of primary biliary cirrhosis. *Mol Aspects Med* **8**:269–291, 1986.
8. Portmann B, MacSween RNM: Diseases of the intrahepatic bile ducts, in MacSween RNM, Anthony PP, Scheuer PJ (eds): *Pathology of the Liver,* 2nd ed. Churchill Livingstone, Edinburgh, 1987, pp. 424–453.
9. Nakanuma Y, Ohta G: Histometric and serial section observations of the intrahepatic bile ducts in primary biliary cirrhosis. *Gastroenterology* **76**:1326–1332, 1979.
10. Nakanuma Y, Miyamura H, Ohta G: Correlation between disappearance of the intrahepatic bile ducts and histologic changes in primary biliary cirrhosis. *Am J Gastroenterol* **76**:506–510, 1981.
11. Nakanuma Y, Ohta G: Nodular hyperplasia of the liver in primary biliary cirrhosis of early histological stages. *Am J Gastroenterol* **82**:8–10, 1987.

12. Kew MC, Varma RR, Dos Santos HA, et al: Portal hypertension in primary biliary cirrhosis. *Gut* **12:**830–834, 1971.
13. Scheuer PJ: Primary biliary cirrhosis. *Proc Soc Med* **60:**1257–1260, 1967.
14. Popper H, Schaffner F: Non-suppurative destructive chronic cholangitis and chronic hepatitis, in Popper H, Schaffner F (eds): *Progress in Liver Diseases,* Vol. III. Grune & Stratton, Orlando, Florida, 1970, pp. 336–354.
15. Popper H: The problem of histologic evaluation of primary biliary cirrhosis. *Virchows Arch Pathol Anat* **379:**99–102, 1978.
16. Chedid A, Spellberg MA, DeBeer RA: Ultrastructural aspects of primary biliary cirrhosis and other types of cholestatic liver disease. *Gastroenterology* **67:**858–869, 1974.
17. Bernuau D, Feldmann G, Degott C, et al: Ultrastructural lesions of bile ducts in primary biliary cirrhosis. A comparison with the lesions observed in graft-versus-host disease. *Hum Pathol* **12:**782–793, 1981.
18. Nakanuma N, Ohta G, Kono K, et al: Electron microscopic observation of destruction of biliary epithelium in primary biliary cirrhosis. *Liver* **3:**238–248, 1983.
19. Eggink HF, Houthoff HJ, Huitema S, et al: Cellular and humoral immune reactions in chronic active liver disease I. Lymphocyte subsets in liver biopsies of patients with untreated idiopathic autoimmune hepatitis, chronic active hepatitis B and primary biliary cirrhosis. *Clin Exp Immunol* **50:**17–24, 1982.
20. Montano L, Bofill M, Janossy G: An analysis of the inflammatory infiltrate in autoimmune and hepatitis B virus induced chronic liver disease. *Hepatology* **2:**748, 1982 (abst).
21. Pape GR, Rieber EP, Eisenburg R, et al: Involvement of the cytotoxic/suppressor T-cell subset in liver tissue injury of patients with acute and chronic liver diseases. *Gastroenterology* **85:**657–662, 1983.
22. Si L, Whsiteside TL, Van Thiel DH, et al: Lymphocyte subpopulations at the site of "piecemeal" necrosis in end stage chronic liver diseases and rejecting liver allografts in cyclosporine-treated patients. *Lab Invest* **50:**341–347, 1984.
23. Van den Oord JJ, Fevery J, De Groote J, et al: Immunohistochemical characterization of inflammatory infiltrates in primary biliary cirrhosis. *Liver* **4:**264–274, 1984.
24. Ballardini G, Bianchi FB, Doniah D, et al: Aberrant expression of HLA-Dr antigens on bile duct epithelium in primary biliary cirrhosis: Relevance to pathogenesis. *Lancet* **2:**1009–1013, 1984.
25. Saita N: Lymphocyte subsets in the liver of patients with primary biliary cirrhosis. *Acta Hepatol Jpn* **26:**1062–1071, 1985.
26. Colucci G, Colombo M, Del Ninno E, et al: In situ characterization by monoclonal antibodies of the mononuclear cell infiltrate in chronic active hepatitis. *Gastroenterology* **85:**1138–1145, 1983.
27. Frazer IH, Mackay IR, Bell J, et al: The cellular infiltrate in the liver in auto-immune chronic active hepatitis: Analysis with monoclonal antibodies. *Liver* **5:**162–172, 1985.
28. Whiteside TL, Lasky S, Si L, et al: Immunologic analysis of mononuclear cells in liver tissues and blood of patients with primary sclerosing cholangitis. *Hepatology* **5:**468–474, 1985.
29. Van den Oord JJ, Sciot R, Desmet VJ: Expression of MHC products by normal and abnormal bile duct epithelium. *J Hepatol* **3:**310–317, 1986.
30. Dilly SA, Sloane JP: An immunohistological study of human hepatic graft-versus-host disease. *Clin Exp. Immunol* **62:**545–553, 1985.
31. Berg PA, Klein R: Clinical and prognostic relevance of different mitochondrial antibody profiles in primary biliary cirrhosis (PBC). *Molec Aspects Med* **8:**235–247, 1986.
32. Berg PA, Klein R: Mitochondrial antigens and auto antibodies: From anti-M1 to anti-M9. *Klin Wochenschr* **64:**897–909, 1986.
33. Sandilands GP, MacSween RNM, Gray KG, et al: Reduction in peripheral blood K cells and activated T cells in primary biliary cirrhosis. *Gut* **18:**1017–1020, 1977.
34. Bhan AK, Dienstag JL, Wands JR: Alterations of T-cell sub-sets in primary biliary cirrhosis. *Clin Exp Immunol* **47:**351–358, 1982.
35. Miller KB, Elta GH, Rudders RA, et al: Lymphocyte subsets in primary biliary cirrhosis. *Ann Intern Med* **100:**385–387, 1984.
36. Jones EA: Primary biliary cirrhosis: Potential pathogenic mechanisms and the effects of therapies on the disease process, in Thomas HC, MacSween RNM (eds): *Recent Advances in Hepatology.* Vol. I. Churchill Livingstone, Edinburgh, 1983, pp. 131–151.
37. Miller KB, Sepersky RA, Brown KM, et al: Genetic abnormalities of immunoregulation in primary biliary cirrhosis. *Am J Med* **75:**75–80, 1983.

38. Neuberger J, Portmann B, MacDougall BRD, et al: Recurrence of primary biliary cirrhosis after transplantation. *N Engl J Med* **306**:1–4, 1982.
39. Hoagsma EB, Manns M, Klcin R, et al: Subtypes of antimitochondrial antibodies in primary biliary cirrhosis before and after orthotopic liver transplantation. *Hepatology* **7**:129–133, 1987.

16

Primary Sclerosing Cholangitis: Clinical Aspects

Stanley B. Benjamin

1. INTRODUCTION

Primary sclerosing cholangitis (PSC) is an obliterative inflammatory fibrosis of the extrahepatic bile ducts, with or without involvement of the intrahepatic ducts.[1–4] The etiology of PSC is unknown. It is a disease without specific, independently diagnostic, pathologic features, requiring appropriate clinical and radiographic criteria for its diagnosis.[5,6]

At one time, PSC was regarded as a rare or uncommon disease,[7–9] but since the advent of endoscopic cholangiography, the diagnosis is made with increasing frequency.[6] This is most clearly demonstrated in association with idiopathic ulcerative colitis where aggressive evaluation in a large group of such patients will lead to its discovery in up to 4% of patients.[10]

2. CLINICAL FEATURES

Primary sclerosing cholangitis is a disease of adult males (60–70%) typically occurring in the third to fifth decades.[5,6] Symptoms at presentation are those typical of a cholestatic process, i.e., jaundice and pruritis. Abdominal pain, fever, and weight loss are also commonly seen (Table I). In early series, only a small percentage of patients (7 and 10%) were completely asymptomatic.[11,12] More recently, however, a larger percentage of patients being diagnosed with PSC are asymptomatic and may remain so for extended periods of time. This seeming change in the character of the disease more accurately reflects the aggressiveness with which the diagnosis is pursued in a population at risk (i.e., idiopathic ulcerative colitis). If elevations in alkaline phosphatase are evaluated in these patients, the percentage of completely asymptomatic individuals will continue to increase analogous to the increased number of patients with primary biliary cirrhosis since the advent of automatic serum chemistry analysis.[13]

The physical examination in patients with PSC may be quite variable (Table II). It may be completely normal in up to 50% of patients, with a normal examination being directly related to the number of asymptomatic patients in these series. Conversely, in a symptomatic population, changes

Stanley B. Benjamin • Division of Gastroenterology, Georgetown University School of Medicine, Washington, D.C. 20007.

Table I. Symptoms in Primary Sclerosing Cholangitis

Symptom	La Russo et al.[4] (%)	(%)	Chapman et al.[5] (%)
Jaundice	68	—	72
Pruritis	62	—	69
Pain	50	—	72
Fever	28	—	45
Weight loss	28	—	79
Varceal bleeding		14	—
Malaise		3	—
Asymptomatic		7–10	—

of chronic cholestasis (jaundice, excoriations, and weight loss) and portal hypertension (hepatomegaly, splenomegaly, and ascites) can be foun l.

One of the most intriguing and clinically relevant observations relative to PSC is its association, either synchronously or metachronously, with other disease states. Since the original association of inflammatory bowel disease, primarily idiopathic ulcerative colitis,[10,14,15] this observation has been repeatedly confirmed, accounting for 54–72% of recent large series.[4,5] An incidence as high as 4% has been found in a series of consecutive patients with ulcerative colitis.[10] Although there are a few reported patients with Crohn disease and PSC, the incidence is very low in this form of inflammatory bowel disease and may simply represent a chance occurrence of the two conditions.[16,17]

A variety of other disease states occur in association with a cholangragraphic pattern of sclerosing cholangitis (Table III). The syndrome of mediastinal and retroperitoneal fibrosis, Reidel thyroiditis, pseudotumor cerebri, and sclerosing cholangitis (familial multifocal fibrosclerosis) has been well documented.[18–23] Sclerosing cholangitis has been reported in association with immune deficiency syndromes both idiopathic and acquired.[24–26] A chronic infection of the biliary system, e.g., cryptosporidiosis or cytomegalovirus (CMV), is thought to be responsible for this pattern of changes in many of these patients, especially those with acquired immune deficiency syndrome.[25–28] In addition, a cholangiographic picture resembling PSC has been seen in patients undergoing intrahepatic infusion of 5-fluorouracil (5-FU) or following an episode of acute cholangitis.[29]

Table II. Physical Signs in Primary Sclerosing Cholangitis[a]

Sign	Percent
Jaundice	44
Hepatomegaly	38
Splenomegaly	29
Spider angiomata	17
Ascites	4
Clubbing	4

[a]After La Russo et al.[4] and Chapman et al.[5]

Table III. Diseases Associated with Primary Sclerosing Cholangitis

Chronic ulcerative colitis/proctitis
Crohn disease
Familial multifocal fibrosclerosis (retroperitoneal fibrosis, mediastinal fibrosis, Riedel thyroiditis, pseudotumor of orbit and PSC)
Pancreatitis
Peyronie disease
Immunedeficiency disease

3. LABORATORY FEATURES

The biochemical alterations in PSC reflect the cholestatic nature of the disease.[4,5] As expected, the alkaline phosphatase is almost universally abnormal; in most cases, it is 3–10 times the upper limit of normal and may fluctuate (Table IV). A small, but unknown, number of patients may have completely normal values.[30] Hepatic transaminase values are usually elevated, but typically the elevations are modest. Progressive elevations of bilirubin, as well as decreasing levels of albumin and prolongation of the prothrombin time are manifestations of progression of disease with the development of cirrhosis and subsequent hepatic insufficiency.

Conspicuous by their absence in PSC are serologic markers of autoimmunity, including antimitochondrial antibody (AMA), antinuclear antibody (ANA), antismooth muscle antibody (ASMA), lupus erythematosus (LE) test, and viral hepatitis markers. Low titers of ANA, ASMA, and AMA have been reported in a small number of these patients but are thought to be nonspecifically present.[4,5] The AMA is crucial in distinguishing primary biliary cirrhosis from other cholestatic diseases, including PSC.

Tests reflecting copper metabolism are predictably abnormal in PSC.[31] Most patients will have elevations in both hepatic and urinary copper determinations. Levels of hepatic copper are elevated to those found in Wilson disease, primary biliary cirrhosis, and Indian childhood cirrhosis. These changes in copper metabolism are associated with elevations in the serum ceruloplasmin levels. The accumulation of copper in PSC is thought to reflect an inability to excrete copper, a feature of chronic cholestatic hepatic diseases.

Table IV. Laboratory Features of Primary Sclerosing Cholangitis

Laboratory feature	Percent abnormal
Alkaline phosphatase	97–100
(% >3 × ULN)[a]	76–85
Total bilirubin	67–83
Aminotransferases	85–97
Albumin	17–29
Gamma globulin	30–45
Prothrombin time	6

[a]ULN, upper limit of normal.

4. RADIOLOGIC FEATURES

In practice, the diagnosis of PSC is a radiographic specifically cholangiographic one.[4,5,32–34] Histology can be diagnostic in a limited number of patients, but it is usually consistent with a generic diagnosis of cholestasis (intrahepatic or extrahepatic injury) and these are best separated by cholangiography. The characteristic changes are described as diffuse narrowing and/or irregularity (often referred to as beading) of the extrahepatic biliary ducts with or without involvement of the intrahepatic ducts in the absence of predisposing cause, such as previous surgery or cholangitis.[4,6]

The general availability of endoscopic retrograde cholangiography (ERCP) has enabled clinicians to easily make the diagnosis of PSC and dramatically increased the frequency with which the diagnosis is made.[5,10,30,33] Intravenous cholangiography appears to have little value in the diagnosis of this or any other cholestatic disease.[5,35] Percutaneous cholangiography (PTC) can be used to visualize the biliary tree but, because of the nature of the ductal disease in PSC, the success rate is not high and poor filling of the intrahepatic ducts may cause considerable confusion. A similar problem can occur during ERCP if complete filling of the intrahepatic ducts is not accomplished (Fig. 1A,B).

Four patterns of ductal involvement have been described in PSC:

1. Involvement of both the intrahepatic and extrahepatic biliary system: This is the most common pattern (Fig. 2A,B).
2. Involvement of the extrahepatic biliary system alone: a pattern potentially amenable to dilation or stenting.
3. Involvement of the intrahepatic system alone (Fig. 3A,B): This pattern of intrahepatic ductal involvement alone has been reported to occur frequently in patients with ulcerative colitis and the histologic finding of "pericholangitis."[11] The diagnosis of pericholangitis in a patient with ulcerative colitis should not be made as a distinct entity in the absence of a well-filled retrograde cholangiogram.
4. Involvement of a small segment of the biliary system, particularly when involvement occurs at the bifurcation of the common hepatic duct[36,37]: This is the most unusual and clinically troublesome radiographic pattern of PSC (Fig. 4). When encountered, this pattern must be

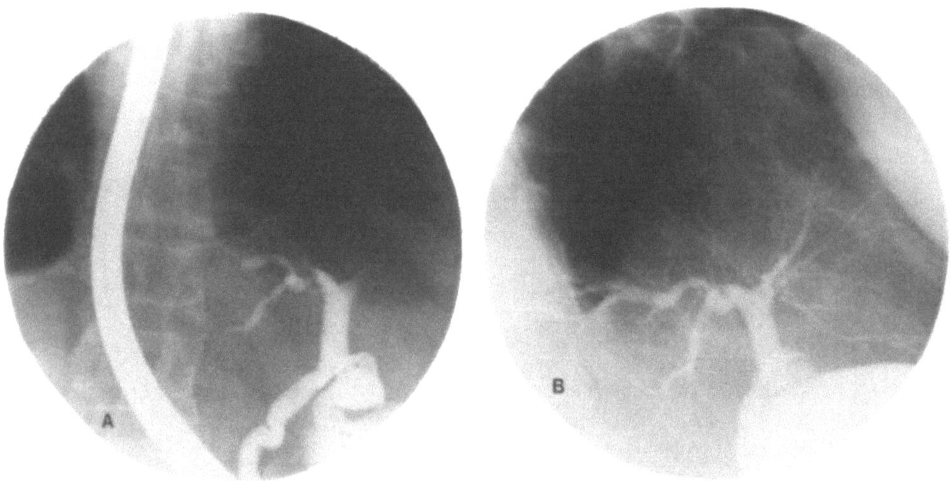

Figure 1. (A) Apparent narrowing and irregularity of intraheptic biliary system noted during ERCP. (B) After complete filling of the gallbladder, the intrahepatic biliary system is completely filled and is normal in appearance.

distinguished from cholangiocarcinoma.[38] Since patients with ulcerative colitis and/or PSC are at increased risk for this form of carcinoma, this pattern must be evaluated very carefully and followed very closely; it will often require surgery in an attempt to determine its precise nature (Fig. 5).

5. PATHOGENESIS

The etiology of PSC is unknown, although both genetic and acquired factors appear to be important. Clustering of cases of PSC and ulcerative colitis has been reported, and HLA associations have been observed (e.g., increased HLA B-8). Speculation regarding the effects of endogenous toxins associated with portal bacturemia have led to a variety of therapies, especially the removal of the colon to prevent progression of PSC. The failure of this therapy and the metachronous nature of PSC and ulcerative colitis have led to a discontinuation of colectomy as a recommendation in these patients.[39] The role of autoimmunity and copper in the pathogenesis of PSC has also resulted in the use of prednisone and D-penicillamine, both appearing to have little clinical value in this disease.[31,40–42]

6. CLINICAL DIAGNOSTIC EVALUATION

In clinical practice, a wide variety of diseases present with cholestatic features. In recent years, our ability to determine the precise nature of the diseases responsible has improved dramatically. In the symptomatic patient, well-defined algorithms for the evaluation of cholestasis are available.[43] As in other clinical situations, the physical examination is the cornerstone of this evaluation. The presence of an elevated alkaline phosphatase in association with proper associated diseases (e.g., ulcerative colitis, retroperitoneal fibrous) makes PSC very likely but is certainly not diagnostic; ultrasonography, cholangiography (preferably ERCP), and possibly liver biopsy are indicated. It is in the asymptomatic patient that a decision to proceed with evaluation may be more difficult. In an asymptomatic patient with ulcerative colitis, persistent elevation of alkaline phosphatase may be met with an ambivalent response. In the absence of our ability to treat PSC, why should the diagnosis be pursued? The clinician must decide that knowing the precise nature of the underlying process is necessary and appropriate. As important as the diagnosis of PSC should be the exclusion of other associated diseases, e.g., gallstone disease, cholangiocarcinoma, or metastatic colon carcinoma. Since PSC can be diagnosed with little risk to the patient, the diagnosis should certainly be pursued.

7. NATURAL HISTORY OF SCLEROSING CHOLANGITIS

The natural history of PSC in most patients is a slow progression to secondary biliary cirrhosis and death, primarily from liver failure (Table V). We know, however, that patients may remain asymptomatic for long periods of time.[10,13,15] This is especially true in light of our earlier diagnosis of these patients when cholangiography is performed based on altered biochemical parameters. In series with long-term follow-up, 38% and 33% of the patient groups were dead at a mean time of 34 and 57 months, respectively, from the time of original diagnosis.[4,5] Liver failure was the primary cause of death in both series, with bile duct and colon carcinoma the next two leading causes of death (Table V). In these series, most surviving patients had advanced liver disease at the time of publication.

It is likely that the general availability of ERCP will increase the number of patients with earlier, often asymptomatic, disease in a manner reminiscent of primary biliary cirrhosis, where an elevated alkaline phosphatase and presence of antimitochondral antibody led to the earlier, pre-

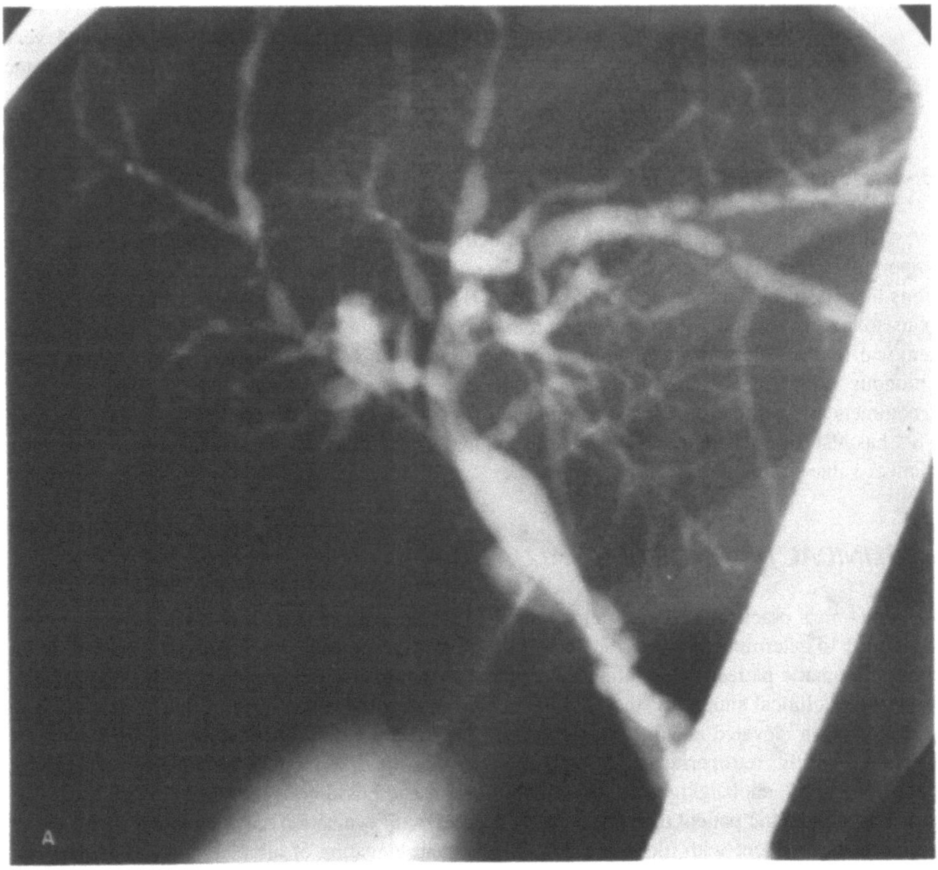

Figure 2. (A) Patient with a 7-year history of ulcerative colitis. Diffuse intraductal involvement diagnostic of PSC noted. (B) Oblique view of same patient demonstrate extrahepatic ductal stricturing (arrow).

symptomatic, diagnosis and "changed" the natural history of this disease.[13,44,45] The early diagnosis of PSC is currently of no particular benefit to the patient; however, it is of paramount importance to exclude disease states that might be treatable. It is hoped that the current interest in drug therapy for PSC with a variety of agents will change this and allow us to have a less than nihilistic approach to PSC.

8. THERAPY OF PSC

Until quite recently, because of the infrequent nature of patients with PSC, very few controlled data were available to guide the approach to PSC. In the future, the results of a wide array of therapies being systematically evaluated in these patients may lead to specific guidelines for therapy, but in the interim, specific generally effective therapy is not available.

The earliest attempts at intervention in this disease were surgical. These were typically patients with associated ulcerative colitis for which therapy was directed at the biliary tree and/or the colon. Palliation of pruritis and jaundice was often attempted and sometimes accomplished using T-tube

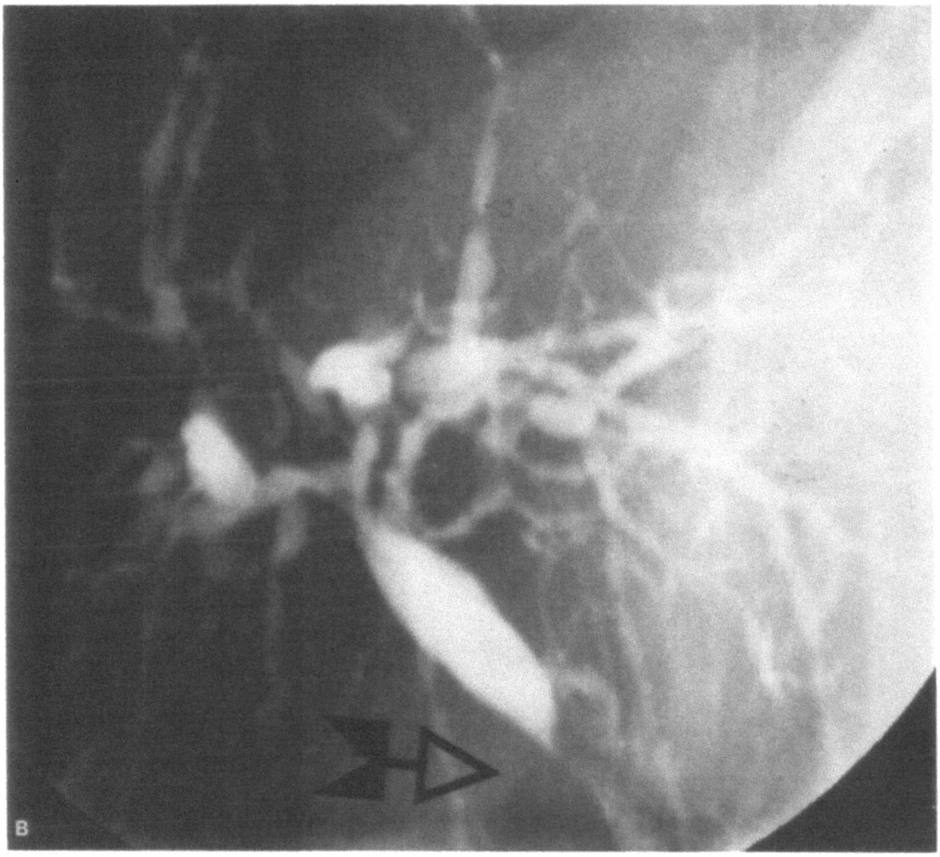

Figure 2. (*Continued*)

drainage; however, this did not appear to alter the natural history of the disease and was associated with an increased risk of cholangitis.[5] Other investigators have reported benefit by surgically inserting biliary stents and instilling antibiotic solutions.[39] Colectomy had been considered as a means of arresting the progression of PSC in patients with ulcerative colitis, but the failure of this intervention and the occurrence and progression of PSC years after colectomy in some patients did not support this concept and have led to the general discontinuation of this approach.[5,10] The newest and most helpful surgical intervention in PSC is hepatic transplantation. Initial data demonstrating 5-year survival of approximately 60% offer new hope for a number of these patients.[46,47]

Directed dilation of dominant strictures by endoscopic, transhepatic, or surgically constructed Roux loop has been used with increasing frequency. Although this approach is not likely to alter the natural history of the disease, it has proved an effective pallation for pruritis and recurrent cholangitis in selected patients.[48]

To date, medical therapy of PSC has not resulted in the emergence of any drug regimen that reproducibly benefits these patients. Drug therapy aimed at immunosuppression, copper depletion, and antifibrogenesis has been tried. No controlled published data are yet available to evaluate clearly the results of these treatments.

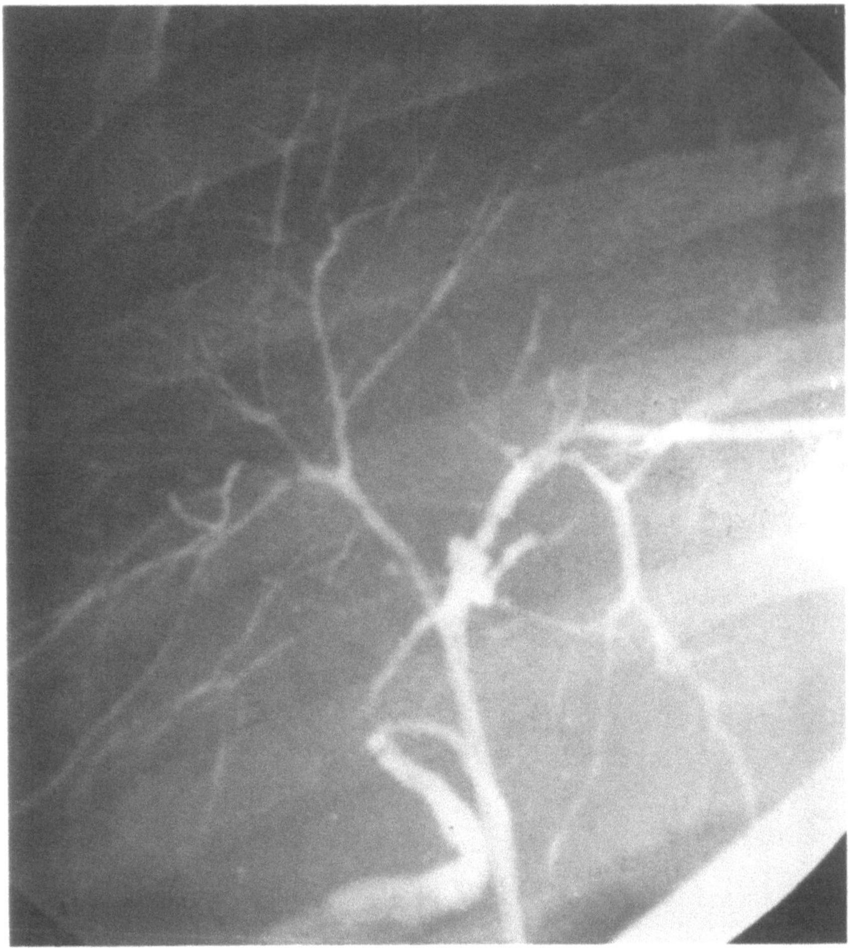

Figure 3. (A) Patient with ulcerative colitis and persistent elevation of alkaline phosphatase. Note diffuse narrowing of intrahepatic biliary tree. (B) Same patient, demonstrating normal extrahepatic duct.

As with most diseases associated with inflammation, corticosteroids have been tried empirically in a variety of patients. Although occasionally a beneficial result is documented (Fig. 6A,B), the consensus of opinion based on broad clinical experience and the few controlled data available suggest that corticosteroids do not appear to benefit these patients. Similar observations have been recorded with azathioprine. Recent publications on the use of methotrexate in two patients with PSC have raised considerable interest in this agent and may lead to larger trials with this agent.[49] Cyclosporine, one of the newest immunosuppressive agents, is currently being evaluated in a trial at the Mayo Clinic.

In light of the elevated copper levels found in patients with PSC, attempts at cupruresis with D-penicillamine were undertaken in patients with PSC. Despite the predicted depletion of copper, there were no improvements in clinical biochemical, radiographic, or histologic features or in survival.[50] In addition, the predictable occurrence of major side effects in one of five patients clearly establishes that D-penicillamine has no role in the treatment of PSC.

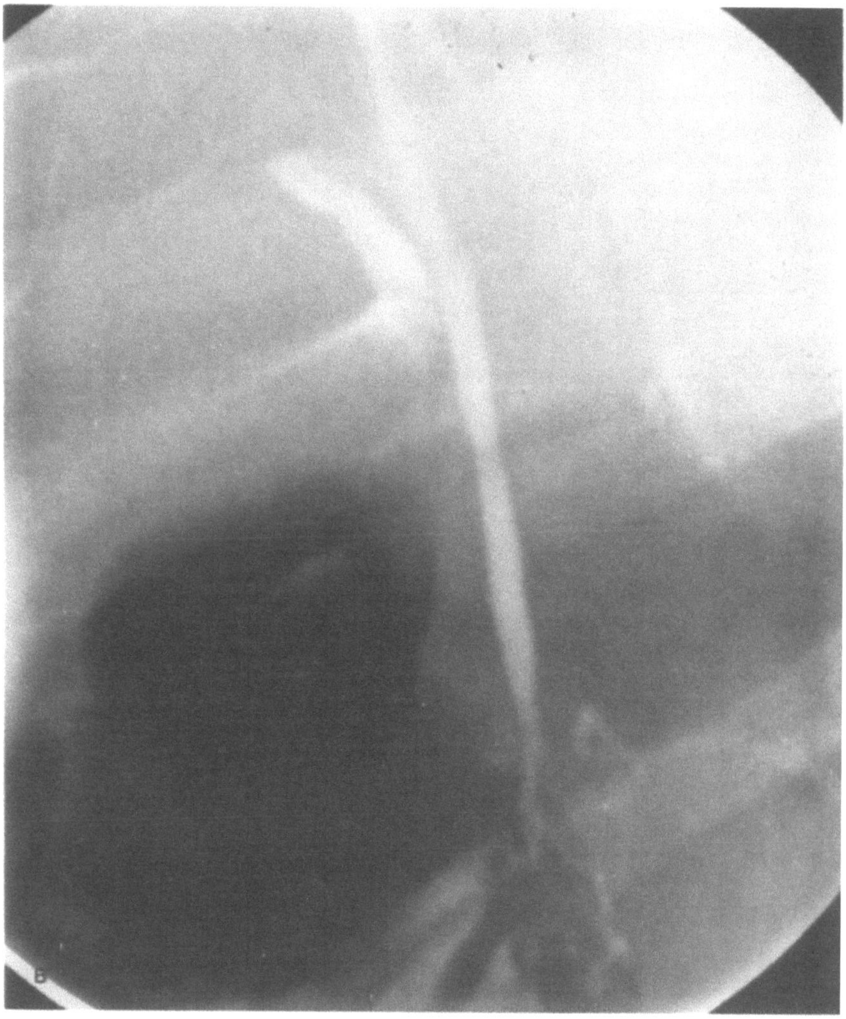

Figure 3. (*Continued*)

Recent information relating to collagen synthesis and deposition has led to the use of colchicine in a variety of chronic liver diseases. In a single patient with PSC, colchicine was used with beneficial effects in laboratory and histologic parameters at 12 months.[51] Additional study with this agent, therefore, may be warranted.

It should be emphasized that at this time no drug or combination of drugs can be recommended outside the setting of a controlled trial in patients with PSC. Given the toxicity of each of these potentially beneficial treatment regimens and the potential for long periods of asymptomatic disease, the decision to intervene with drug therapy should be made only after clear-cut information on beneficial effects is obtained. In the interim, emphasis should be given to the referral of patients with PSC to institutions with ongoing controlled trials.

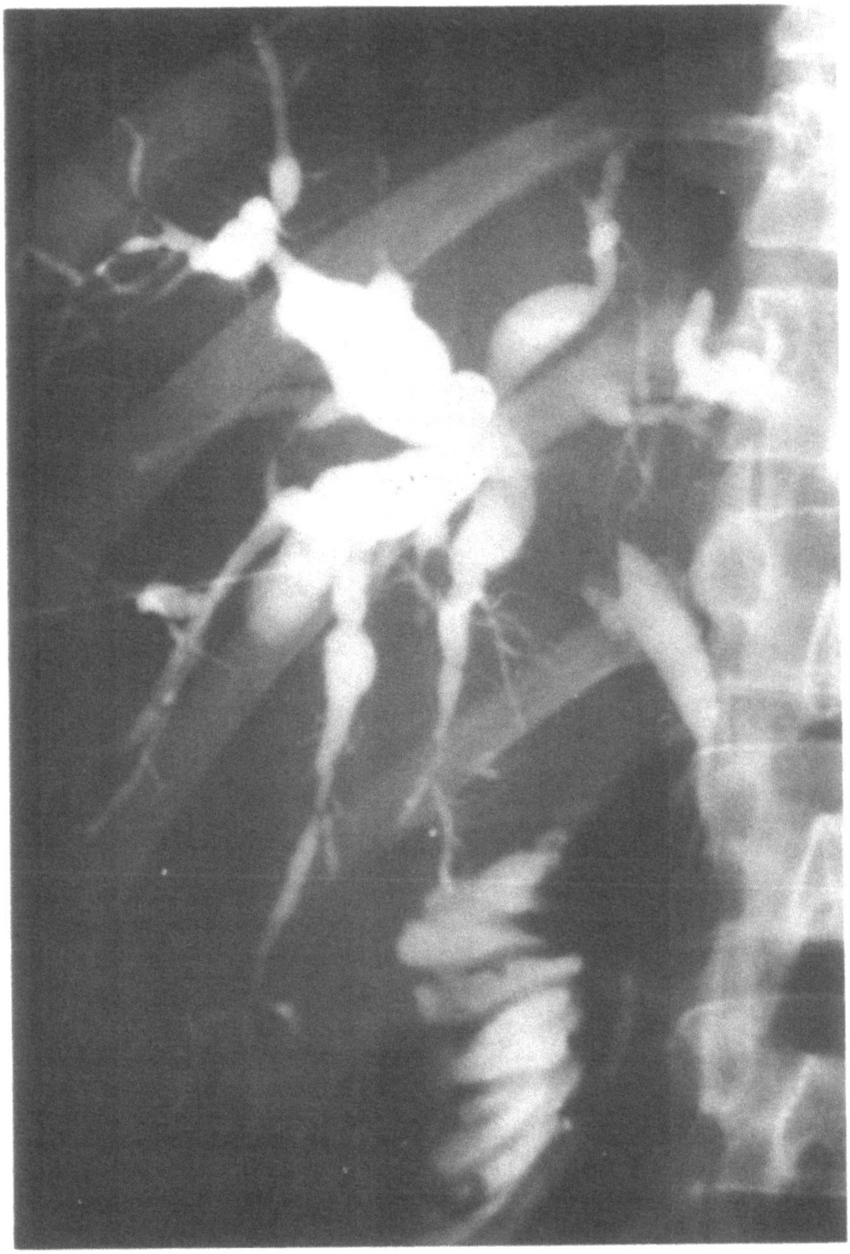

Figure 4. Percutaneous cholangiogram in a patient with dominant stricture at bifurcation of common hepatic duct, proximal ductal dilation, and changes of sclerosing cholangitis in peripheral ducts. (From Zeman and Burell,[37a] by permission.)

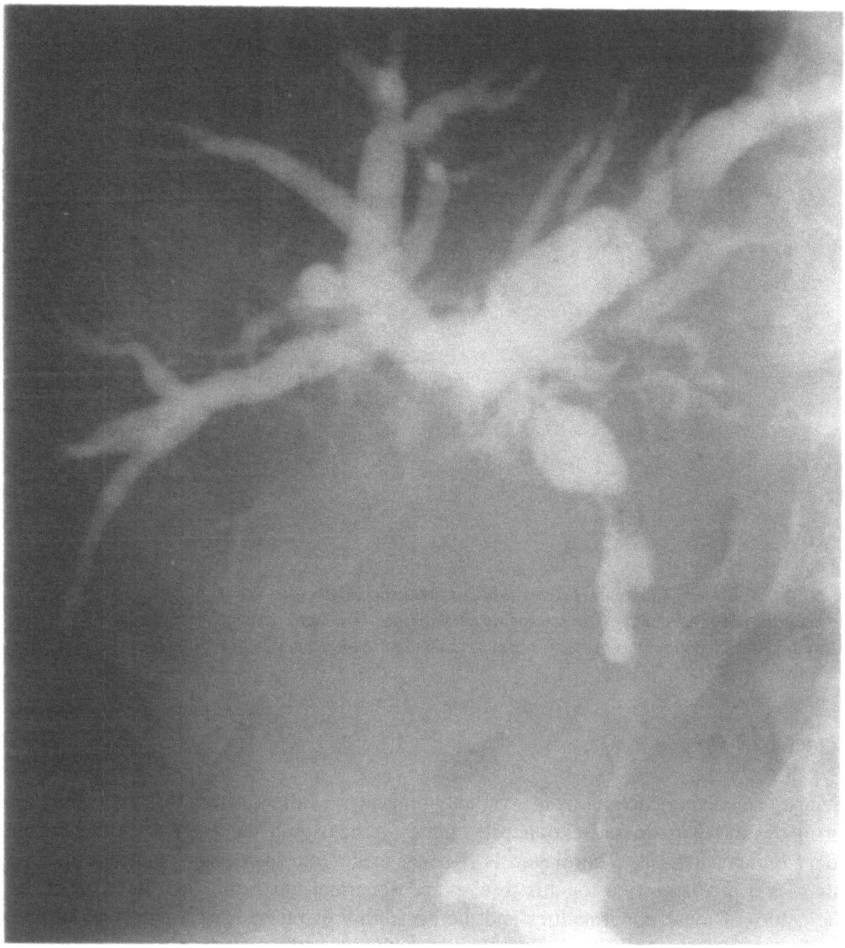

Figure 5. Dominant stricture of common bile duct with "pseudoulceration" in patient with ulcerative cholangitis. Confirmation that malignancy was not the etiology required surgery. (From Zeman and Burell,[37a] by permission.)

Table V. Natural History of Primary Sclerosing Cholangitis

Cause of death	La Russo et al.[4]	Chapman et al.[5]
Liver failure	11/13	8/11
Bile duct carcinoma	1/13	2/11
Colon carcinoma	1/13	1/11
Patients with ulcerative colitis	7/13	10/11
Status of survivors		
Cirrhosis/portal hypertension	12/26	3/18
Cirrhosis	6/20	
Recurrent acute cholangitis	—	11/18
Asymptomatic	—	4/18

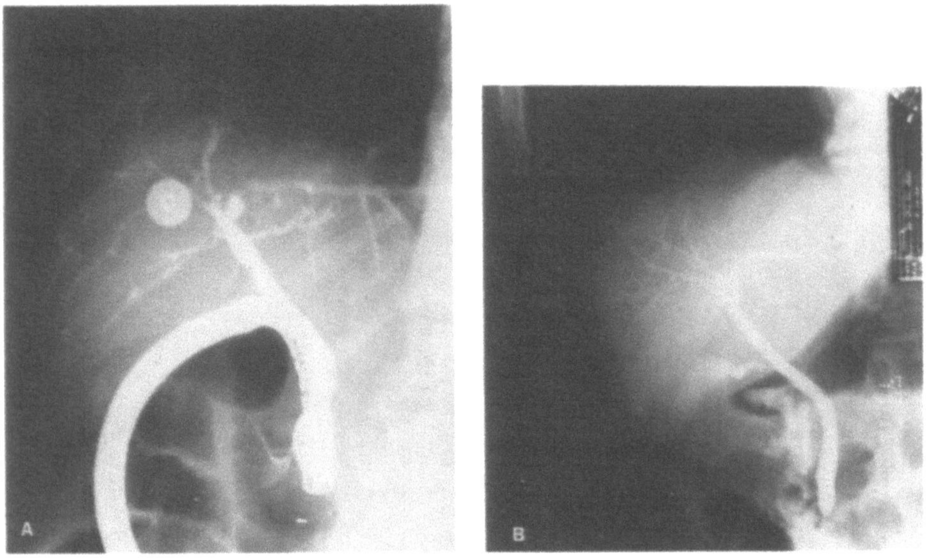

Figure 6. (A) A 65-year-old male patient with retroperitoneal fibrosis and new onset of jaundice. ERCP demonstrates intrahepatic changes of sclerosing cholangitis. (B) Same patient after 1 year of corticosteroid administration. Intrahepatic ducts are now normal, coincident with normalization of biochemical abnormalities.

9. SUMMARY

Primary sclerosing cholangitis is a variably progressive inflammatory disease leading to obliteration of the intrahepatic and extrahepatic biliary system with the subsequent development of secondary biliary cirrhosis. The diagnosis is being made with increasing frequency in groups of patients with a predisposition for this disease and abnormal biochemistries. Because of the nonspecific nature of these abnormalities and the possibility of other disease processes occurring in these patients, a definitive diagnosis should be made. This usually requires retrograde cholangiography. Once the diagnosis is made, decisions regarding therapy must be individualized. Patients with early disease (cholangographic changes without symptoms or cirrhosis) require no therapy but, if treated, should be entered in controlled trials of medical therapy. Patients with more advanced disease may require palliation by means of surgical or endoscopic dilation of dominant biliary structures. The development of liver failure or cholangiocarcinoma should prompt consideration of liver transplant. Our ability to interdict the progression of disease in these patients will require carefully done long-term trials to assess the risks and benefits of these therapies.

ACKNOWLEDGMENTS. The author would like to thank Dr. Robert Zeman, Professor of Radiology at Georgetown University, for providing some of the radiographs used in this publication, and Mrs. Erna Lee Benjamin for her expert editorial and secretarial support in the preparation of this manuscript.

REFERENCES

1. Smith LP, Loe RH: Sclerosing cholangitis. *Am J Surg* **110:**239–246, 1965.
2. Manesis TG, Sullivan RF: Primary sclerosing cholangitis. *Arch Intern Med* **115:**137–139, 1965.

3. Glenn F, Whitsel JC: Primary sclerosing cholangitis. *Surg Gynecol Obstet* **123:**1037–1046, 1966.
4. La Russo NF, Wiesner RH, Ludwig J, et al: Primary sclerosing cholangitis. *N Engl J Med* **310:**899–903, 1984.
5. Chapman RWG, Marborgh BA, Rhodes JM, et al: Primary sclerosing cholangitis: A review of its clinical features, cholangiographic and hepatic histology. *Gut* **21:**870–877, 1980.
6. Wiesner RH, La Russo NA: Clinicopathologic features of the syndrome of primary sclerosing cholangitis. *Gastroenterology* **79:**200–206, 1980.
7. Delbet P: Retrecissement du choledogue: Cholecystoduodenostomie. *Bull Mem Soc Nat Chir* 1924:1144.
8. Danzi JT, Makipur H, Farmer RG: Primary sclerosing cholangitis: A report of nine cases and clinical review. *Am J Gastroenterol* **65:**589–593, 1976.
9. Fee HJ, Gerwitz H, Schiller J, et al: Sclerosing cholangitis and primary biliary cirrhosis—A disease spectrum: *Ann Surg* **186:**589–593, 1977.
10. Schrumpt E, Elgio K, Favsa O, et al: Sclerosing cholangitis in ulcerative colitis. *Scan J Gastroent* **15:**689–697, 1980.
11. Blackstone MD, Nemchavsky BA: Cholangiographic abnormalities in ulcerative colitus associated pericholangitis which resemble sclerosing cholangitis. *Dig Dis Sci* **23:**579–585, 1978.
12. Chapman RWG, Burroughs AK, Bass NM, et al: Long-standing asymptomatic primary sclerosing cholangitis. *Gut* **26:**778–782, 1981.
13. James O, Macklon AF, Watson AJ: Primary biliary cirrhosis. A revised clinical spectrum. *Lancet* **1:**1278–1281, 1981.
14. Warren KW, Arthanassiales S, Marge JI: Primary sclerosing cholangitis. *Am J Surg* **11:**23–28, 1966.
15. Thrope ME, Schever PJ, Sherlock S: Primary sclerosing cholangitis, the biliary tree and ulcerative colitis. *Gut* **8:**435–448, 1967.
16. Segal I, Tim LO, Rubin A, et al: Rare and unusual manifestations of Crohn's disease with pyoderma gangrenosum and sclerosing cholangitis. *S Afr Med J* **55:**596–599, 1979.
17. Brantigan CD, Brantigan OC: Primary sclerosing cholangitis: Case report and review of the literature. *Am Surg* **39:**191–198, 1973.
18. Comings DE, Skubi KB, Van Eyes J, et al: Familial multifocal fibrosclerosis. Findings suggesting that retropertoneal fibrosis, mediastinal fibrosis, sclerosing cholangitis, Riedel's thyroiditis and pseudotumor of the orbit may be different manifestations of a single disease. *Ann Intern Med* **66:**884–892, 1967.
19. Hellstrom HR, Perezstable EC: Retro-peritoneal fibrosis with disseminated vasculitis and intrahepatic sclerosing cholangitis. *Am J Med* **40:**184–187, 1966.
20. Thompson BW, Read RC: Sclerosing cholangitis and other intra-abdominal fibroses. *Am J Surg* **128:**777–781, 1974.
21. Waldrom R, Kopelman H, Tsantoulas P, et al: Chronic pancreatitis, sclerosing cholangitis and sicca complex in two siblings. *Lancet* **1:**550–552, 1975.
22. Sjogren I, Wengle B, Lorsgren M: Primary sclerosing cholangitis associated with fibrosis of the submandibular glands and the pancreas. *Acta Med Scand* **205:**139–141, 1979.
23. Viteri AL, Hardin WJ, Dyck WP: Peyronie's disease and sclerosing cholangitis in a patient with ulcerative colitis. *Dig Dis Sci* **24:**490–491, 1979.
24. Record CO, Shilkin KB, Eddleson AC, et al: Intrahepatic sclerosing cholangitis associated with a familial immunodeficiency syndrome. *Lancet* **2:**18–20, 1973.
25. Pitlik SD, Fainstein V, Garza D, et al: Human cryptosporidiosis: spectrum of disease. Report of six cases and review of the literature. *Arch Intern Med* **143:**2269–2275, 1983.
26. Margulis SI, Honig CL, Soave R, et al: Biliary tract obstruction in the acquired immunodeficiency syndrome. *Ann Intern Med* **105:**207–210, 1986.
27. Agha FP, Nostrant TT, Abrams GD, et al: Cytomegalic cholangitis in a homosexual man with acquired immune deficiency syndrome. *Am J Gastroenterol* **81:**1068–1072, 1986.
28. Scheinderman DJ, Cello JP, Laing FC: Papillary stenosis and sclerosing cholangitis in the acquired immunodeficiency syndrome. *Ann Intern Med* **106:**546–549, 1987.
29. Pien EH, Zeman RK, Benjamin SB: Iatrogenic sclerosing cholangitis following intermittent continuous hepatic arterial chemotherapy infusion. *Radiology* **156:**329–330, 1985.
30. Balasubromaniam K, Wiesner RH, LaRusso NF: Can serum alkaline phosphatase levels be normal in primary sclerosing cholangitis? *Gastroenterology* **92:**1303, 1987 (abst).
31. Gross JB, Ludwig J, Wiesner RH, et al: Abnormalities in tests of copper metabolism in primary sclerosing cholangitis. *Gastroenterology* **89:**272–278, 1985.

32. Elias E, Summerfield JA, Dick R et al: Endoscopic retrograde cholangio-pancreatography in the diagnosis of jaundice associated with ulcerative colitis. *Gastroenterology* **67:**907–911, 1974.
33. Abbruzzese AA: Retrograde cholangiography and sclerosing cholangitis. *Am J Dig Dis* **19:**571–574, 1974.
34. MacCarty RL, LaRusso NF, Wiesner RH, et al: Primary sclerosing cholangitis: Findings on cholangiography and pancreatography. *Radiology* **149:**39–44, 1983.
35. Goodman MW, Ansel HJ, Vennes TA, et al: Is intravenous cholangiography still useful? *Gastroenterology* **79:**642–645, 1980.
36. Golematis B, Papchristou DN, Drieling DA: Sclerosing cholangitis of the bifurcation of the common hepatic duct. *Am J Gastroenterology* **75:**370–372, 1981.
37. Case records of the Massachusetts General Hospital: *N Engl J Med* **306:**349–358, 1982.
37a. Zeman RK, Burell MI (eds): *Gall Bladder and Bile Duct Imaging,* Churchill Livingston, New York, 1987, pp. 513–519.
38. MacCarty RL, LaRusso NF, May GR, et al: Cholangiocarcinoma ccomplicating primary sclerosing cholangitis: Cholangiographic features. *Radiology* **156:**43–46, 1985.
39. Wood RAB, Cuschiere A: Is sclerosing cholangitis complicating ulcerative colitis a reversible condition? *Lancet* **2:**716–718, 1980.
40. Lindor KD, Wiesner RH, Katzmann JA, et al: Lymphocyte subsets in primary sclerosing cholangitis. *Dig Dis Sci* **32:**720–725, 1987.
41. Lindor KD, Wiesner RH, LaRusso NR, et al: Enhanced autoreactivity of T-lymphocytes in primary sclerosing cholangitis. *Hepatology* **7:**884–888, 1987.
42. Chapman RW, Cottone M, Selby WS, et al: Serum autoantibodies, ulcerative colitis and primary sclerosing cholangitis. *Gut* **27:**86–91, 1986.
43. Lumeng L, Snodgrass PJ, Swonder JE, et al: Final report of a blinded prospective study comparing non-invasive approaches in the differential diagnosis of medical and surgical jaundice. *Gastroenterology* **78:**1312, 1980 (abst).
44. Lebovics E, Palmer M, Woo J, et al: Outcome of primary sclerosing cholangitis. Analysis of long-term observation of 38 patients. *Arch Intern Med* **147:**729–731, 1987.
45. Helzberg JH, Petersen JM, Boyer JL: Improved survival with primary sclerosing cholangitis. A review of clinicopathologic features and comparison of symptomatic and asymptomatic patients. *Gastroenterology* **92:**1869–1875, 1987.
46. Scharschmidt BF: Human liver transplantation: Analysis of data on 540 patients with four centers. *Hepatology* **4:**955–1015, 1984.
47. Marsh JW, Iwatsuki S, Makowka L, et al: Orthotopic liver transplantation for primary sclerosing cholangitis. *Ann Surg* **207:**21–25, 1988.
48. May GR, Bender CE, LaRusso NF, et al: Nonoperative dilatation of dominant strictures in primary sclerosing cholangitis. *Am J Radiol* **145:**1061–1064, 1985.
49. Kaplan MM, Arora S, Pincus SH. Primary sclerosing cholangitis and low-dose oral pulse methotrexate therapy. *Ann Intern Med* **106:**231–235, 1987.
50. LaRusso N, Wiesner R, Ludwig J, et al: Randomized trial of penicillamine in primary sclerosing cholangitis. *Hepatology* **6:**1205, 1986 (abst).
51. Leiser A, Kadish V: Beneficial effect of colchicine in a case of sclerosing cholangitis. *Am J Med Sci* **291:**416–418, 1986.

17

Primary Sclerosing Cholangitis: Histopathology

Jay H. Lefkowitch

1. INTRODUCTION

Primary sclerosing cholangitis (PSC) is a chronic idiopathic fibrosing and inflammatory disease affecting the intrahepatic and extrahepatic bile ducts.[1–7] Abundant data on liver pathology in PSC are now available because of the increased frequency of cholangiographic diagnosis and availability of livers for examination from PSC patients who have undergone transplantation.[8] This chapter reviews our current understanding of hepatic pathology in this condition, its differentiation from other cholestatic conditions, and the diagnostic terminology.

2. TERMINOLOGY

An appreciation of the diverse pathologic lesions in PSC requires clarification of a number of terms applied in this disorder:

Primary sclerosing cholangitis: idiopathic chronic fibrosis and inflammation involving intrahepatic and extrahepatic bile ducts with or without gallbladder and pancreatic duct involvement; associated with ulcerative colitis in one half to three fourths of patients

Secondary sclerosing cholangitis: chronic fibrosis and inflammation involving extrahepatic ducts primarily, in which a cause can be defined (biliary stricture, choledocholithiasis, pancreatitis, pancreatic carcinoma, bile duct carcinoma, or other anatomic lesions involving major bile ducts)

Pericholangitis: a term coined by Mistilis[9] to describe the periductal inflammatory infiltrates, fibrosis and bile ductular proliferation seen in livers of patients with chronic ulcerative colitis; the term has now dropped into disfavor; rather than a syndrome believed to be associated with ulcerative colitis, it most likely represents involvement of small, interlobular bile ducts by PSC in inflammatory bowel disease

Small duct PSC: changes of periduct fibrosis, inflammation, and obliteration involving in-

Jay H. Lefkowitch • Department of Pathology, College of Physicians and Surgeons, Columbia University, New York, New York 10032.

terlobular bile ducts <100 μm in diameter in PSC (commonly in patients with ulcerative colitis)[8]

Large duct PSC: periductal fibrosis, fibrous obliteration, and segmental dilatation of major extrahepatic bile ducts or intrahepatic, perihilar branches measuring 400–800 μm in diameter in PSC[8]

Cholangiectasis: focal saccular dilation of large bile duct developing between strictured areas in PSC[8]

Cholate stasis: a foamy, cytoplasmic rarefaction or pseudoxanthomatous change in periportal hepatocytes in chronic biliary tract disease

Copper-binding protein: a lysosomal metallothionein protein to which copper is bound in chronic hepatic copper toxicosis; characteristically prominent within periportal hepatocytes in various forms of late stage biliary tract disease; may be seen on routine hematoxylin and eosin (H&E) stains as slightly basophilic granules, while on periodic acid-Schiff (PAS) stain with diastase digestion, appears as purple-to-red granules, and on orcein or Victoria bile stains as brown-black or blue granules, respectively

Fibrous-obliterative cholangitis: replacement of bile duct lumens and epithelium by fibrous tissue scar in PSC (or in other cholestatic syndromes associated with loss of intrahepatic bile ducts)

Bile duct-to-hepatic artery ratio: normally ⩾0.9, this ratio implies that for each portal hepatic artery branch there should be an approximately equal-caliber bile duct; ratio decreased in conditions that cause loss of bile ducts (e.g., PSC, syndromatic and nonsyndromatic paucity of bile ducts, graft-versus-host liver disease, and liver transplant rejection)[10]

Bile ductular proliferation: a reactive proliferation of newly formed small ductular structures (neocholangioles) within portal connective tissue or at its edge, differing structurally from indigenous interlobular ducts in that proliferating ductules have absent or poorly defined lumens, variations in nuclear morphology, associated mild neutrophilic infiltrates, and inherent tortuosity; structures may be derived from portal interlobular bile ducts or from metaplasia of periportal hepatocytes.[11]

3. LIVER PATHOLOGY IN PSC

Hepatic morphology in PSC reflects both the size of bile ducts involved and whether involved ducts are present in the tissue sample examined. In approximately 85% of cases, both extrahepatic and intrahepatic ducts are involved.[2] In 15% the extrahepatic ducts alone are involved,[2] and small numbers of patients (usually with chronic ulcerative colitis) have involvement of only intrahepatic ducts.[2] Because the portal lesions in PSC are often similar if not identical, to those seen in other causes of large bile duct obstruction, a truly diagnostic lesion (e.g., the florid bile duct lesion of primary biliary cirrhosis) does not exist. However, certain characteristic or near-diagnostic lesions of PSC (Table I) must be recognized. The three general classes of hepatic lesions in PSC can be summarized as follows: (1) near-diagnostic lesions, (2) compatible lesions, and (3) misleading lesions (Table I).

3.1. Near-Diagnostic Lesions

Periductal, "onion-skin" concentric fibrosis (Figs. 1 and 2) may be the most diagnostic histopathologic finding in PSC. A collar of fibrous tissue surrounds bile ducts of varying sizes, may squeeze off duct epithelium (Fig. 3), or may actually obliterate the bile duct (Fig. 4). Once the ducts are obliterated, focal portal scars and hepatic arterioles without adjacent ducts are seen (Fig. 5). The

Table I. Histopathologic Features of Primary Sclerosing Cholangitis

Type of sample	Comment	Biopsy features
Near-diagnostic liver biopsy[a]	Ducts involved by PSC are in sample	Periductal, "onion-skin" fibrosis Fibrous cord or scar replaces duct Decreased bile duct: hepatic artery ratio
Compatible liver biopsy	Ducts involved by PSC are proximal to sample	Portal tract edema, neutrophils, bile ductular proliferation (portal changes of any large bile duct obstruction) Parenchymal cholestasis Lymphoid aggregates or follicles in portal tracts Mixed portal inflammatory cells
Misleading liver biopsy (other liver disease is diagnosed	Biopsy features are not diagnostic and suggest another disorder	Chronic active hepatitis Cryptogenic cirrhosis

[a]True diagnostic lesions do not exist in primary sclerosing cholangitis, in contrast to the diagnostic (pathognomonic) florid bile duct lesion of primary biliary cirrhosis. More appropriate terms may be near-diagnostic or characteristic lesions.

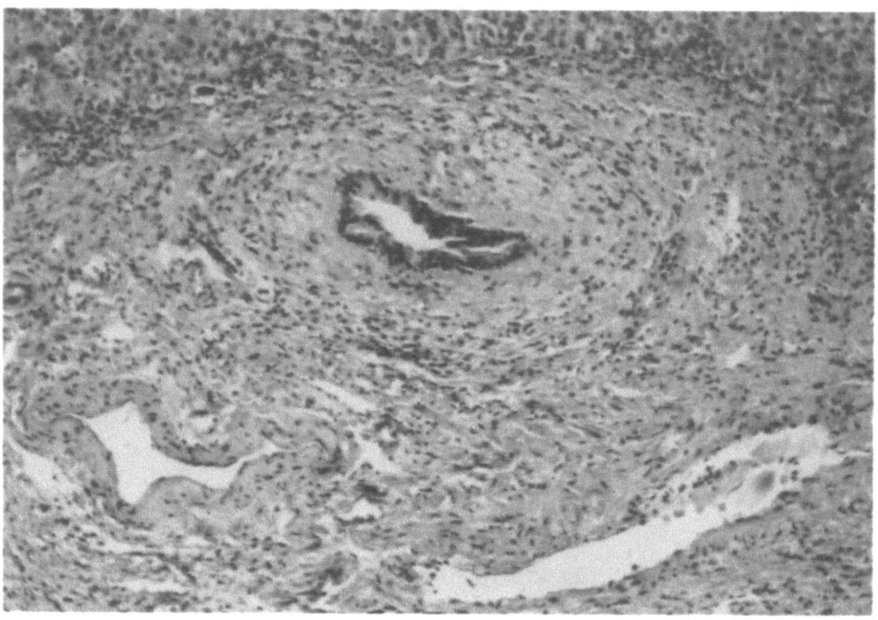

Figure 1. Large duct primary sclerosing cholangitis. A septal bile duct is surrounded by a concentric collar of fibrosis and inflammation. (H&E, ×100)

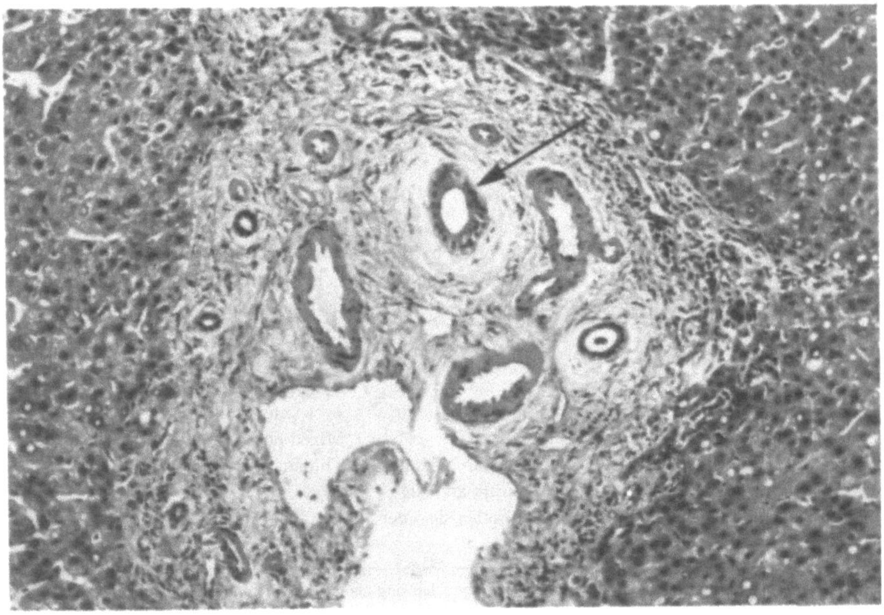

Figure 2. Periductal fibrosis in primary sclerosing cholangitis about interlobular bile duct (arrow). (H&E, ×160)

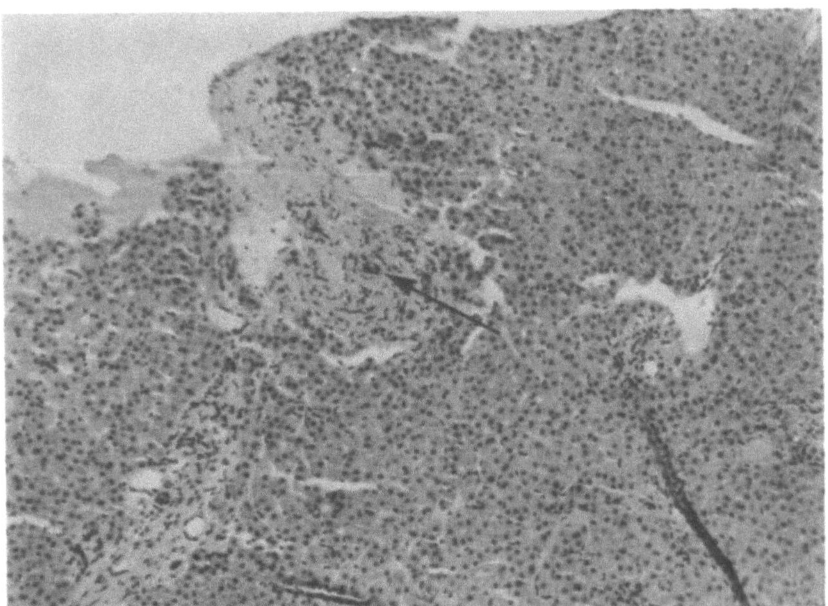

Figure 3. Small duct primary sclerosing cholangitis. A small interlobular duct (arrow) is atrophic and squeezed by periduct fibrosis and inflammation. (H&E, ×63)

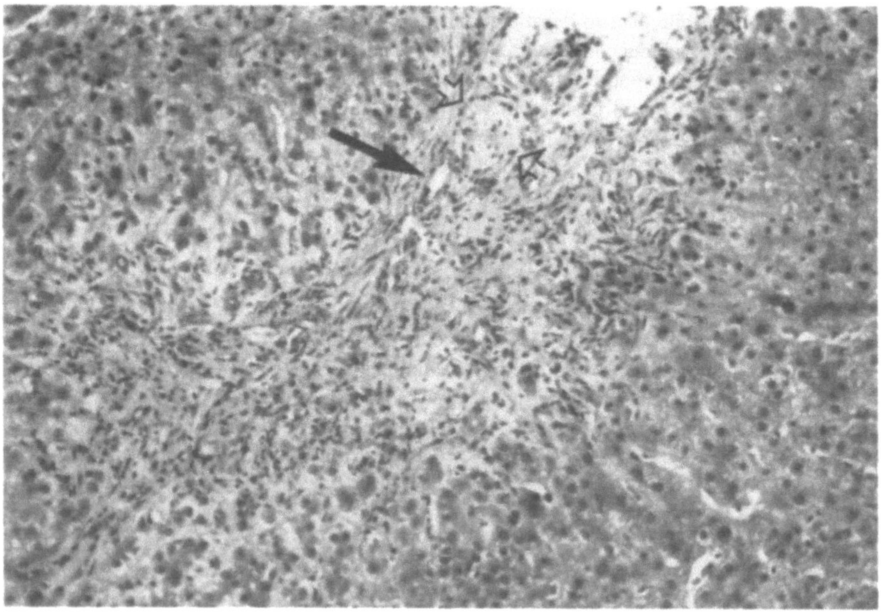

Figure 4. Fibrous–obliterative primary sclerosing cholangitis. An interlobular duct is replaced by fibrous scar (between open arrows), but the corresponding hepatic arteriole branch (solid arrow) is still visible. Note the general features of chronic biliary tract disease in the portal tract, including edema, ductular proliferation, inflammation, and pseudoxanthomatous change (cholate stasis) in periportal hepatocytes. (H&E, ×160)

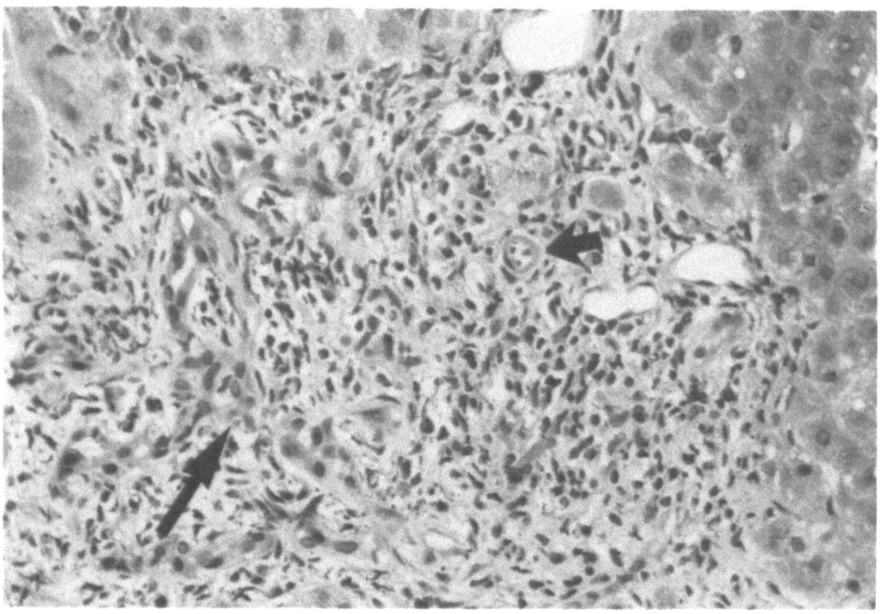

Figure 5. Loss of bile duct in primary sclerosing cholangitis. A small arteriole is visible (small arrow), but the interlobular duct has been replaced by an admixture of lymphocytes, histiocytes, and neutrophils. There is associated portal edema and bile ductular proliferation (large arrow). (H&E, ×250)

consequent decreased bile duct-to-hepatic artery ratio becomes a useful criterion of bile duct loss. Other diseases leading to duct loss must then enter the differential diagnosis, including primary biliary cirrhosis,[12] drug hepatitis, graft-versus-host disease (GVHD), and liver transplant rejection.[10] The background portal changes in which near-diagnostic lesions of PSC develop include portal edema, bile ductular proliferation, and mixed inflammatory cells (neutrophils), as well as lymphocytes, histiocytes, plasma cells, and occasional eosinophils. Periportal cholate stasis becomes prominent as later stages of PSC with portal fibrosis evolve.

3.2. Compatible Lesions

These lesions consist of portal edema, bile ductular proliferation, and mixed inflammatory cell infiltrates, which could also reflect large bile duct obstructive diseases other than PSC. Portal lymphoid aggregates or follicles (Fig. 6) may accumulate near bile ducts. Periductal inflammation, often featuring lymphocytes and/or plasma cells with piecemeal necrosis (Fig. 7) may simulate the picture of chronic active hepatitis (CAH) (see Section 3.3). These lesions in patients with ulcerative colitis probably represent small duct PSC (or what was formerly considered pericholangitis).[13]

3.3. Misleading Lesions

Problematic cases of PSC for pathologists are those in which the portal changes are so nonspecific as not to be indicative of biliary disease or those in which another diagnosis is suggested altogether (CAH, cryptogenic cirrhosis). For such cases particularly, cholangiography must play a definitive role and ancillary data such as liver tissue staining for copper and copper-binding protein or tissue copper quantitation[6] may be helpful.

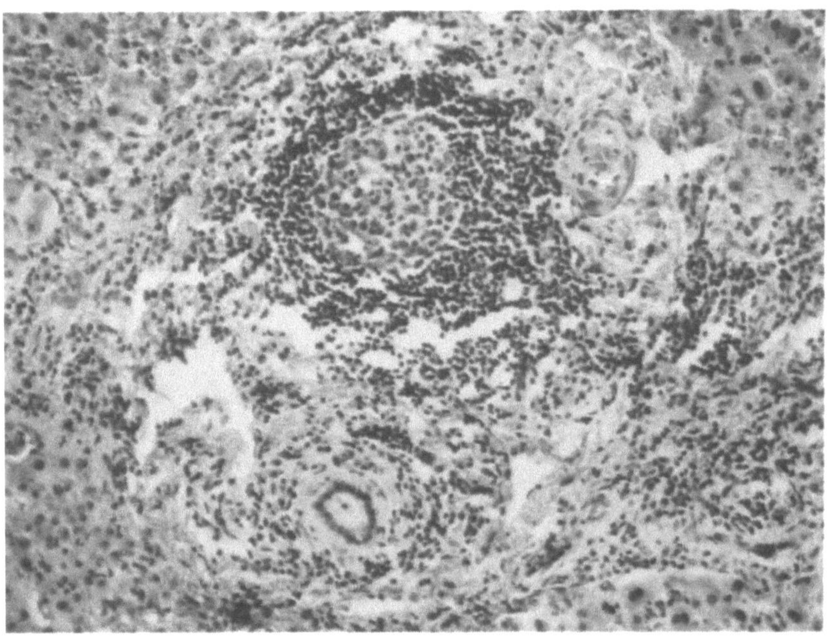

Figure 6. Lymphoid follicle with pale germinal center adjacent to interlobular duct with periduct fibrosis in primary sclerosing cholangitis. (H&E, ×160)

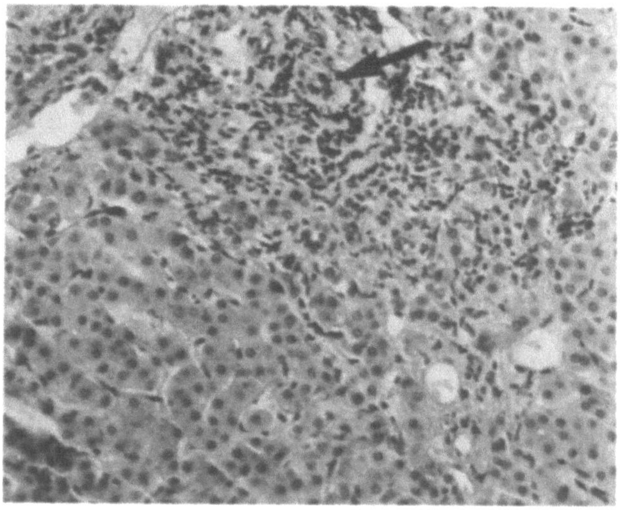

Figure 7. Small duct primary sclerosing cholangitis. An interlobular duct (arrow) is surrounded by chronic inflammatory cells (an appearance previously designated pericholangitis). Inflammation erodes the limiting plate (piecemeal necrosis). (H&E, ×192)

4. STAGING OF PSC

Using broad guidelines available from the staging of primary biliary cirrhosis (PBC) (see Chapter 15), investigators at the Mayo clinic have defined four stages: stage 1 (cholangitis or portal hepatitis), stage 2 (periportal fibrosis or periportal hepatitis), stage 3 (septal fibrosis, bridging necrosis, or both), and stage 4 (biliary cirrhosis).[3]

5. CHOLESTASIS, COPPER, DUCT EPITHELIAL CHANGES, AND ELECTRON MICROSCOPY

Parenchymal cholestasis is variable in PSC, estimated at 50% of biopsy specimens.[7] Cholestasis is not common in pediatric PSC, however.[14] Stainable copper and copper-binding protein (Fig. 8) are not usually present until more advanced stages of the disease with extensive fibrosis and developing biliary cirrhosis. Tissue copper levels in these stages are typically above 200 μg/g dry weight.[6]

Bile duct epithelium in PSC varies from normal to papillary hyperplasia,[8] to a spectrum of atrophic changes, including epithelial flattening, attenuation, and complete obliteration.[8,10,13] Electron microscopy has demonstrated fingerlike projections at the bases of duct cells with duplication of basement membranes at these sites.[15] Fibroblasts accumulate about the basal portion of the bile duct. Infiltrating lymphocytes showing point contact with duct epithelial cells have an uncertain role in the disease pathogenesis.[15]

6. DATA FROM LIVER TRANSPLANT PATIENTS WITH PSC

A recent elegant study of livers from PSC patients who underwent liver transplantation[8] demonstrated striking cholangiectatic duct lesions, segmental fibrous strictures and crests, and duct obliteration by fibrous cords (Fig. 9). Papillary hyperplasia of duct epithelium may be a premalignant change, particularly when located within a saccular cholangiectasis.[8]

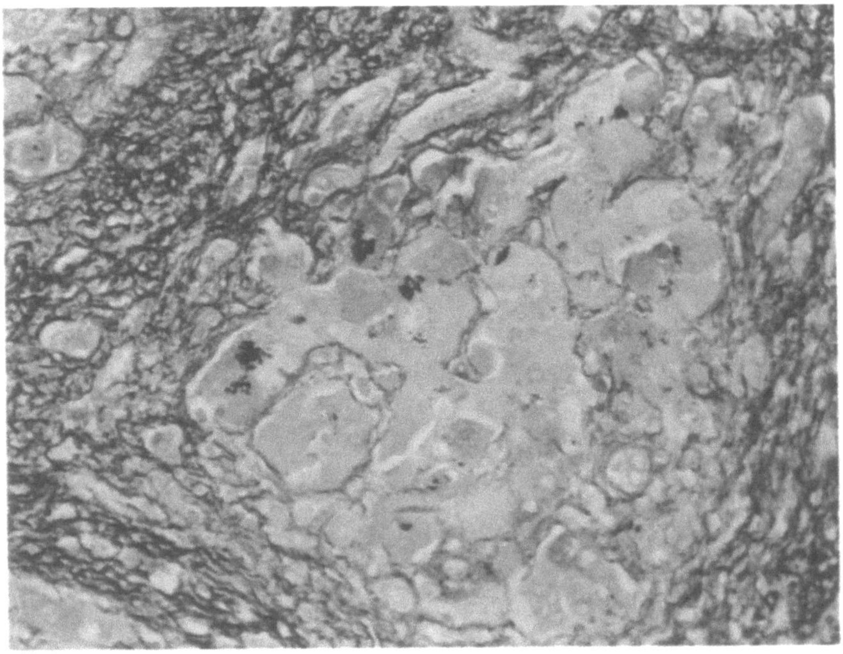

Figure 8. Copper-binding protein in periportal hepatocytes appears as dark brown-black granules on orcein stain. (Orcein stain, ×250)

7. PATHOLOGIC DISTINCTION OF PSC FROM PBC

Clinical and pathologic features may overlap in PSC and PBC, causing diagnostic confusion.[12] The following pathologic features are useful in distinguishing these conditions:

1. Granulomas are rare in PSC but may be present in up to 50% of patients with PBC (Fig. 10).
2. Cholestasis is often present in PSC but is uncommon in PBC until its late stages.
3. Periductal fibrosis is rare in PBC.
4. Bile ducts more often remain preserved in the later stages of PSC than in PBC.
5. Portal tracts in PBC show more chronic inflammatory cells and better developed piecemeal necrosis than in PSC.
6. Histologic changes among portal tracts vary considerably more in PBC than in PSC.

8. SUMMARY

The major histopathologic challenge in primary sclerosing cholangitis is to distinguish this idiopathic disease from other forms of large bile duct obstruction and from primary biliary cirrhosis. The least controversial cases are those in which periductal fibrosis or fibrous obliteration of bile ducts is present. Other portal lesions are often nonspecific. The existence of small duct and large duct varieties of PSC now clarifies the diffuse spectrum of duct disease in PSC as well as archaic

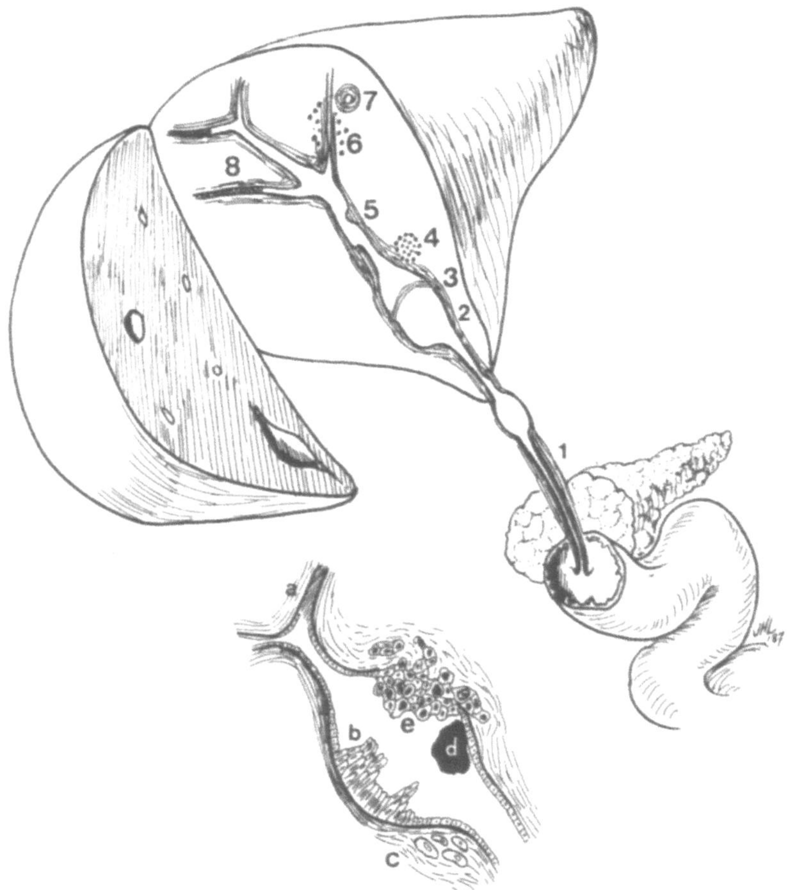

Figure 9. Schematic diagram of pathologic features of primary sclerosing cholangitis, as reconstructed from studies of livers from transplant patients by Ludwig et al.[8] Lesions include the following: 1, periduct fibrosis; 2, cholangiectasis; 3, fibrous stricture; 4, periductal lymphoid aggregates and follicles; 5, fibrous tissue crest; 6, periductal inflammation; 7, arteriosclerosis, a change adjacent to fibrosed and inflamed ducts; 8, fibrous obliteration of bile duct. At bottom, an enlarged saccular cholangiectasis with proximal and distal strictures shows details of potential epithelial and periductal changes in primary sclerosing cholangitis. a, fibrous–obliterative cholangitis; b, papillary hyperplasia of duct epithelium; c, accumulation of lipid-laden foamy histiocytes in duct walls; d, inspissated bile; e, in situ and invasive carcinoma.

concepts such as pericholangitis. In certain instances, when the morphologic changes suggest CAH or cryptogenic cirrhosis, the diagnosis of PSC may be missed entirely. Slowly evolving bile duct carcinomas may masquerade as PSC or may be a late complication of PSC.[16] The histopathologic features of PSC can be reproduced by chemotherapeutic intra-arterial infusions of fluoxuridine[17] or by cytomegalovirus (CMV) and cryptosporidial biliary infections in patients with acquired immune deficiency syndrome (AIDS).[18] Familiarity with the spectrum of hepatic morphology in PSC, combined with cholangiographic and clinical data, now affords improved accuracy in the diagnosis of this distinctive liver disease.

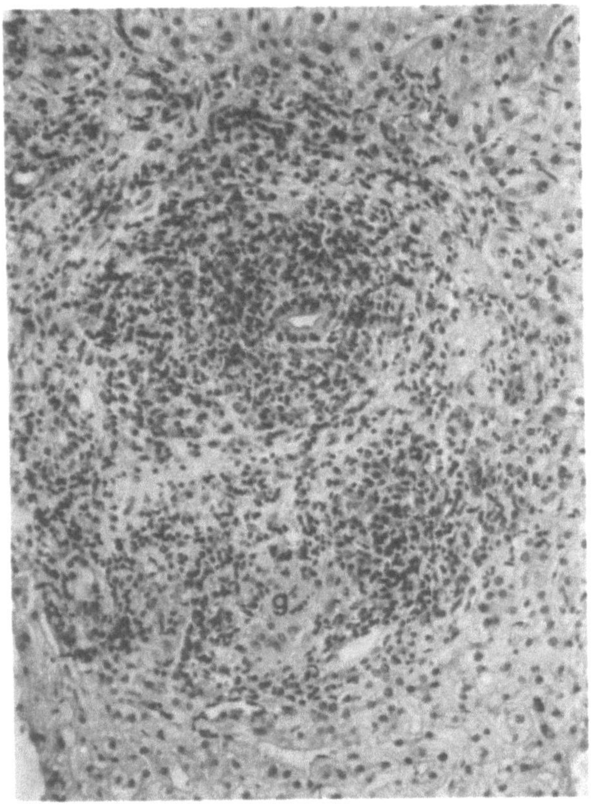

Figure 10. Damaged bile duct in primary biliary cirrhosis (PBC). The duct is surrounded and infiltrated by lymphocytes and plasma cells. A granulomatous infiltrate with giant cell (g) has formed at bottom. The nature of chronic nonsuppurative bile duct destruction with granuloma formation in PBC must be distinguished from periduct changes in primary sclerosing cholangitis. (H&E, ×160)

REFERENCES

1. Chapman RWG, Arborgh BAM, Rhodes JM, et al: Primary sclerosing cholangitis: A review of its clinical features, cholangiography, and hepatic histology. *Gut* **21:**870–877, 1980.
2. Wiesner RH, LaRusso NF: Clinicopathologic features of the syndrome of primary sclerosing cholangitis. *Gastroenterology* **79:**200–206, 1980.
3. LaRusso NF, Wiesner RH, Ludwig J, MacCarty RL: Primary sclerosing cholangitis. *N Engl J Med* **310:**899–903, 1984.
4. Lefkowitch JH: Primary sclerosing cholangitis. *Arch Intern Med* **142:**1157–1160, 1982.
5. Ludwig J, Czaja AJ, Dickson ER, et al: Manifestations of non-suppurative cholangitis in chronic hepatobiliary diseases: Morphologic spectrum, clinical correlations and terminology. *Liver* **4:**105–116, 1984.
6. Ludwig J, Barham SS, LaRusso NF, et al: Morphologic features of chronic hepatitis associated with primary sclerosing cholangitis and chronic ulcerative colitis. *Hepatology* **1:**632–640, 1981.
7. Summerfield JA: Primary sclerosing cholangitis. *Postgrad Med J* **59**(suppl):99–105, 1983.
8. Ludwig J, MacCarty RL, LaRusso NF, et al: Intrahepatic cholangiectases and large-duct obliteration in primary sclerosing cholangitis. *Hepatology* **6:**560–568, 1986.
9. Mistilis SP: Pericholangitis and ulcerative colitis. I. Pathology, etiology and pathogenesis. *Ann Intern Med* **63:**1–16, 1965.
10. Bianchi L: Intrahepatic bile duct damage in various forms of liver diseases, in Brunner H, Thaler H (eds): *Hepatology. A Festschrift for Hans Popper*. Raven, New York, 1985, pp. 295–310.
11. Desmet VJ: Current problems in diagnosis of biliary disease and cholestasis. *Semin Liver Dis* **6:**233–245, 1986.
12. Wiesner RH, LaRusso NF, Ludwig J, Dickson ER: Comparison of the clinicopathologic features of primary sclerosing cholangitis and primary biliary cirrhosis. *Gastroenterology* **88:**108–114, 1985.

13. Wee A, Ludwig J: Pericholangitis in chronic ulcerative colitis: Primary sclerosing cholangitis of the small ducts? *Ann Intern Med* **102**:581–587, 1985.
14. Johnson DA, Cattau EL, Hancock JE: Pediatric primary sclerosing cholangitis. *Dig Dis Sci* **31**:773–777, 1986.
15. Nakanuma Y, Hirai N, Kono N, Ohta G: Histological and ultrastructural examination of the intrahepatic biliary tree in primary sclerosing cholangitis. *Liver* **6**:317–325, 1986.
16. Mir-Madjlessi SH, Farmer RG, Sivak MV: Bile duct carcinoma in patients with ulcerative colitis. Relationship to sclerosing cholangitis: Report of six cases and review of the literature. *Dig Dis Sci* **32**:145–154, 1987.
17. Dikengil A, Siskind BN, Morse SS, et al: Sclerosing cholangitis from intraarterial floxuridine. *J Clin Gastroenterol* **8**:690–693, 1986.
18. Schneiderman DJ, Cello JP, Laing FC: Papillary stenosis and sclerosing cholangitis in the acquired immunodeficiency syndrome. *Ann Intern Med* **106**:546–549, 1987.

III

Toxic Liver Injury

18

Alcoholic Hepatitis Syndrome: Prognosis and Course

Harold O. Conn and R. Hallak

Long quaffing maketh a short lyfe.
John Lyly

1. INTRODUCTION

The *alcoholic hepatitis syndrome* is a disease that is relatively easy to define for groups of patients. It is much more difficult to define for individual patients. This acute disorder of the liver is characterized by a history of excessive alcohol intake, by jaundice and hepatomegaly, and by laboratory abnormalities that include increased serum aminotransferase and alkaline phosphatase activity and leukocytosis composed largely of neutrophils. Prolongation of prothrombin time is common. Fever, ascites, and splenomegaly are often present. Abdnominal pain and anorexia occur frequently.

Typically, patients with alcohol-associated fatty infiltration of the liver almost invariably have hepatomegaly; they may show little else. However, any or all of the findings of alcoholic hepatitis may be present.

Alcoholic cirrhosis has some or all of the findings of alcoholic hepatitis, and, in addition, may show evidence of the complications of portal hypertension—bleeding varices, intractable ascites, portal–systemic encephalopathy, bacterial peritonitis, and/or the hepatorenal syndrome.

2. DIAGNOSIS

Studies by Orrego-Matte and co-workers in Toronto,[1] Kryger and co-workers in Copenhagen,[2] and Poynard et al. in France[3] lead to the following conclusions. Clinical diagnosis of fatty liver are confirmed histologically in about one third, clinical diagnoses of alcoholic hepatitis in approximately two thirds, and the clinical diagnosis of alcoholic cirrhosis in 80–85% of patients. When the clinical picture is characteristic, the histologic diagnosis confirms it in the great majority of instances (75–80%). When the hepatic histology is equivocal, the diagnosis is uncertain. Neverthe-

Harold O. Conn and R. Hallak • Yale University School of Medicine; Liver Disease Unit, Veterans Administration Medical Center, West Haven, Connecticut 06516.

less, using the histologic diagnosis of alcoholic hepatitis as the gold standard, the best clinicolaboratory profiles are confirmed in only three fourths of the cases that satisfy the criteria (T. Poynard and H. O. Conn, unpublished observations).

This is an issue of some importance because the requirement of doing a biopsy to establish the diagnosis may introduce a selection bias. In order to be acceptable for a liver biopsy, patients must have a normal or near-normal prothrombin time, usually within 3 sec of the control time (thereby excluding the most severe stratum of patients in some cases). Similarly, those patients with massive ascites or overt encephalopathy are often not biopsied. This bias has affected randomized clinical trials of therapy such as that of Helman et al.[4] in which a histologic diagnosis of alcoholic hepatitis was required for inclusion in their study of steroid therapy. How it affected the results is not clear, but in this study virtually all the untreated control patients died and all the steroid-treated patients survived. Since the results of this investigation have not been confirmed in most other controlled trials, selection bias has been blamed for the results. Despite statistical significance small sample size is another possible explanation.

If one employs the alternative of basing the diagnosis of alcoholic liver disease on autopsy data, the interval between evaluation and death may obfuscate the results. Therefore, as most of us are forced to do, we make the best of what we have. Our conclusions are therefore approximate, never exact.

Is it necessary to perform a liver biopsy to make the diagnosis of alcoholic liver disease? There is no one answer to this question.

If the question is asked in regard to clinical investigations, it is desirable, whenever possible, to have histologic confirmation of the diagnosis to ensure the most accurate information and interpretation. When it is required by the investigation, however, the need to know may introduce bias by the systematic exclusion of some patients, e.g., those with gross ascites. If the aim of the study is to assess the effect of therapy on a specific pathologic lesion, however, histologic diagnosis is essential.

Aside from clinical investigations, liver biopsy is only necessary when the clinical picture is not clear. For example, alcoholic liver disease is frequently cholestatic and may therefore simulate biliary obstructing lesions.[5] Similarly, the pattern of liver "function" tests in alcoholic liver disease may mimic those of metastatic liver disease. It is necessary to identify and to treat patients with treatable cholestatic disease, such as extrahepatic obstructive jaundice and to establish the presence of neoplasia if it exists. If the diagnosis of obstructive jaundice or malignancy cannot be excluded by imaging or endoscopic techniques, biopsy can establish the diagnosis.[6]

If one assumes that alcoholic liver disease represents a spectrum of disorders for which there is no specific effective therapy, then biopsy is neither logical, cost effective, nor necessary. One of our most effective therapeutic adjuncts is watchful waiting, known in the old days as "tincture of time." The cholestasis of alcoholic hepatitis will almost always subside. It is important to realize that modest delay rarely causes serious consequences, even in extrahepatic obstructive jaundice.

For this presentation we analyzed the clinical and laboratory data of 50 patients with alcoholic hepatitis. These cases are part of an investigation designed to establish the temporal patterns of the conventional liver function tests during alcoholic liver disease. The patients were retrospectively selected from our hospital records with the following criteria: a clinical diagnosis of alcoholic hepatitis, abuse of alcohol, no other explanation for the liver disease, and admission to the hospital directly, i.e., the patients had not been transferred from some other hospital after a period of withdrawal from alcohol and/or treatment.

These clinical criteria for alcoholic hepatitis seem to be effective diagnostically. Approximately 20% of the 50 patients had liver biopsies and all showed alcoholic hepatitis. We recognize, of course, that the selection of patients for liver biopsy represents a subtle type of bias which may determine many facets of the patients under analysis. Each of the components of the alcoholic hepatitis syndrome requires definition and qualification.

Alcohol abuse has been defined as >20 g, >40 g, >80 g, >160 g, or >200 g alcohol consumption per day. The higher the threshold, the more common the alcohol hepatitis and the more reproducible the syndrome. The threshold for women is much lower than for men.[7] The nature of the increased susceptibility of women to alcohol remains a mystery. Perhaps, one of the undesirable aspects of women's liberation may be the emergence of alcoholic liver disease as a preferentially female disorder rather than a bastion of male machoism.

All our patients had consumed >100 g alcohol per day for at least 10 years. More than one half had consumed >200 g for even longer periods. These are major league drinkers.

Hepatomegaly per se is not necessarily a sign of alcoholic hepatitis since this syndrome is almost always accompanied by fatty infiltration of the liver, which is often the cause of the increased hepatic volume. The increased size of hepatocytes in alcoholic hepatitis may contribute, however.[8] Furthermore, the estimation of liver size by physical examination is quite variable. In the presence of ascites, the mere detection of the liver on physical examination may be difficult. Under some circumstances, however, physical examination can give accurate assessment of liver size.[9] Physical examination for the signs of alcoholic liver disease is not easy. Studies of interobserver variability indicate that any one examination may be unreliable, and that the actual measurement of liver size is especially variable.[10] Approximation of size based on hepatic scintigraphy or other imaging techniques is more objective and more precise,[11] but such quantification is rarely performed clinically.

In our series hepatomegaly, i.e., a span of >10 cm determined by percussion or palpation, a fast-disappearing art form, is present in 85% of the patients. Only two patients (4%) had livers with spans of only 8–10 cm.

Jaundice is visible when the total serum bilirubin concentration approaches 2.5 mg/dl and can usually be detected when it exceeds 3.0 mg/dl. Its perception may depend to some degree on the nature of the jaundice, on the serum albumin concentration, and on the duration of the jaundice.[12] Often serum bilirubin concentrations in alcoholic hepatitis are <3 mg/dl and, therefore, jaundice is not a sine qua non of the syndrome. In several recent randomized investigations of the therapy of alcoholic hepatitis, the mean serum bilirubin was <2.5 mg%.[13,14] Various observers agree about the presence or absence of jaundice in about two thirds of patients. This percentage could be made to vary by the type of patients selected and the severity of their disease. In our series of 50 patients, almost one half had total serum bilirubin levels of <3.0 mg/dl, i.e., twice the upper limit of normal.

It is well known that in alcoholic hepatitis, serum bilirubin levels increase for 1–2 weeks after patients are admitted to the hospital. Data to support this observation are difficult to locate in the literature. Our preliminary observations, however, do not confirm this phenomenon.

Among our 50 patients, one third showed an increase and the remainder a decrease in total serum bilirubin levels during the first week in hospital. The mean serum bilirubin concentration remained at approximately the same level at the end of the first week as on admission. There was a trend for those with higher serum bilirubin levels, e.g., >5 mg%, to increase during the first week, while those with lower bilirubin levels almost all decreased. During the second week, bilirubin levels fell in 95% of the patients, and the mean bilirubin had fallen by one third to one half its initial value (Fig. 1). During the third week, serum bilirubin levels tended to remain unchanged.

Transaminase elevations are almost always present in alcoholic hepatitis, although there are wide variations in degree that do not necessarily correlate with clinical features, other laboratory measurements or histologic criteria. In our 50 patients, 94% had elevated SGOT activity, and in two thirds, the level was more than twice the upper limit of normal (50 IU/ml), i.e., >100 units. SGOT levels tend to decrease during the first week after admission to the hospital and then to decrease gradually thereafter (Fig. 1).

As noted by Zimmerman and Seeff[15] 20 years ago, SGOT is elevated more than SGPT in alcoholic liver disease. These observations have been confirmed and extended.[16] Recently, mitochondrial SGOT has been shown to be more specific and more sensitive than total SGOT for alcoholic liver disease.[17]

By contrast, SGPT activity was abnormally elevated in <40% of our patients. Only 10% had

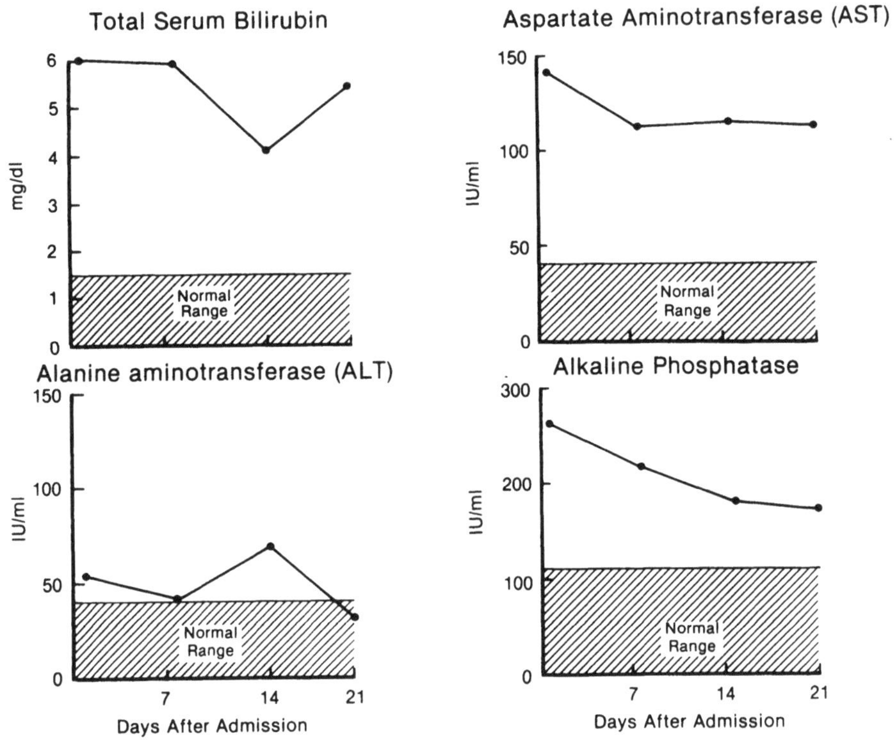

Figure 1. Patterns of liver function tests after admission to the hospital. Mean total serum bilirubin levels remained constant during the first week in the hospital and then fell to about two thirds of admission values. SGOT and SGPT activity decreased significantly during the first week and then leveled off. Serum alkaline phosphatase activity decreased gradually and progressively after admission.

levels more than twice the upper limit of normal, however. They, too, tended to fall during the first week after hospitalization (Fig. 1).

Serum alkaline phosphatase elevations occurred in almost all patients with alcoholic hepatitis syndrome. These elevations also occur in cholestatic conditions, infiltrative disorders, and granulomatous and congestive conditions. There is no clear-cut correlation between the severity of the alcoholic hepatitis and the degree of elevation of the alkaline phosphatase, however.

In our 50 patients, 96% showed elevations of serum alkaline phosphatase. Thus, it appeared to be the single most sensitive test for alcoholic hepatitis (and, probably, the least specific). About one third had mild elevations, i.e., within twice the upper limit of normal; the remainder had much greater elevations. After admission alkaline phosphatase activity tended to fall slowly and progressively (Fig. 1).

Prothrombin time is a relatively insensitive test for alcoholic hepatitis. It is usually abnormal, but the degree of abnormality is generally small. In our 50 patients, 20% had prolongations of less than 1 sec, and in more than one half it was less than 3 sec prolonged. In most institutions, elective liver biopsics are routinely performed in patients within this prothrombin range. When it is grossly prolonged, i.e., more than 3 sec, the alcoholic hepatitis is usually severe and the prognosis poor. The prothrombin time does not change rapidly and tends to improve as other evidence of alcoholic hepatitis diminishes.

Leukocytosis, too, is a variable abnormality. The white blood cell (WBC) count may range from sub- to supranormal. In some patients, hypersplenism may cause leukopenia. In our series of patients, 5% were leukopenic (<4000 WBC/mm^3), and almost 60% were normal (4000–10,000). About 40% had leukocytosis (>10,000). The WBC counts did not change greatly or rapidly during the first 2 weeks of hospitalization.

Serum albumin levels are usually decreased in alcoholic hepatitis. Hypoalbuminemia represents a combination of factors: poor nutrition, the nonspecific effects of chronic illness, and alcohol-induced injury that inhibits hepatic synthesis of albumin. About 20% of our patients had serum albumin levels >4 g/dl. Sixty percent had levels <3 g/dl.

3. PROGNOSIS

One of the problems in managing alcoholic liver disease is the difficulty in estimating its prognosis. It seems evident that in patients without or with barely detectable clinical or laboratory evidence of liver disease, the prognosis is excellent and is extremely poor in those with fulminant alcohol-induced injury. Orrego et al.[18] proposed an index based on a large variety of clinical and laboratory features that is cumbersome but reasonably accurate. Maddrey et al.[19,20] proposed two different, but related, indices (discriminant factors) based on retrospective analyses of serum bilirubin levels and prothrombin times in two groups of patients. Several years ago, one of us (HOC) pointed out that the mean total serum bilirubin concentration of the patients in the control groups of randomized trials of therapy of alcoholic hepatitis at the time of randomization correlated closely with the mortality percentage during that hospitalization.[21] Further analysis has shown that this relationship is highly significant[22] (Fig. 2). It must be emphasized that this correlation is based on the mean serum bilirubin concentration and that the clinical value of this relationship in individual patients is unknown. It would be lovely if such a simple, ubiquitous index were of true prognostic value.

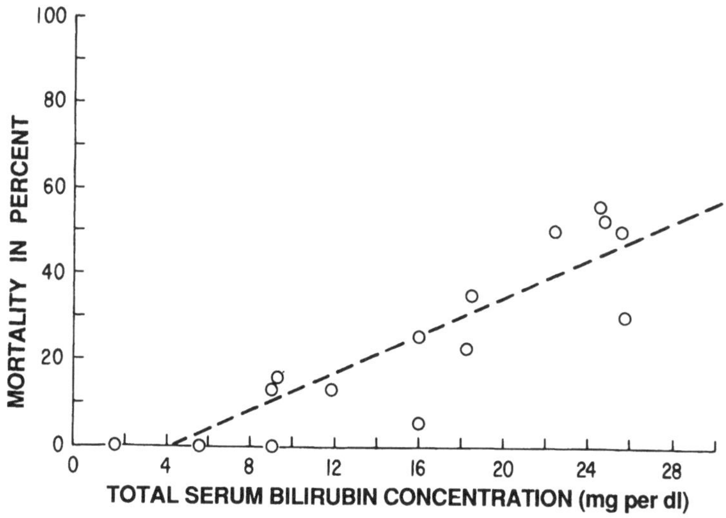

Figure 2. Correlation of serum bilirubin concentration with mortality. Mean total serum bilirubin levels for the *control* groups of 15 randomized clinical trials correlate closely with the percentage who died in each group. It must be emphasized that each point is the mean of 9–88 individual values. Bilirubin concentrations were determined on the day of randomization, which was on average about 1 week after admission.

4. THERAPY

There is no effective therapy for alcoholic hepatitis at the present time. Adrenocorticosteroids have been studied in a number of randomized clinical trials.[4,19,20,23–29] In three studies, steroids have shown statistically significant improvement in survival.[4,20,26] In other trials, no statistically significant effects have been noted. The recent investigation conducted by Maddrey et al.[20] is the most convincing of these studies, but one cannot ignore the majority of studies in which steroids do not improve survival.

Two randomized clinical trials (RCTs) have evaluated the effects of anabolic steroids in alcoholic hepatitis. One by Mendenhall et al.[29] has found a marked but delayed beneficial effect of oxandrolone on survival. In the other trials, testosterone had no such beneficial effect.[30]

One controlled investigation of the intravenous administration of a conventional mixture of amino acids has shown improvement in clinical and laboratory manifestations of alcoholic hepatitis and in survival.[31] Another similar study did not show such benefits.[32] The combination of intravenous infusions of insulin and glucagon, which had been demonstrated to improve the survival of mice with murine viral hepatitis, did not show significant benefits in human alcoholic hepatitis.[33]

Antithyroid therapy, with propylthiouracil, which was touted as being useful in uncontrolled trials,[18] has not been shown to be beneficial in a randomized trial in patients with alcoholic hepatitis.[34] (+)-Cyanidanol-3, a free radical scavenger, did not show survival benefits in a small study of mild alcoholic hepatitis.[13] Penicillamine, too, showed no survival advantage.[35]

Thus, the effect of therapy on alcoholic hepatitis is not impressive. Of the 15 investigations under discussion (i.e., all the published randomized clinical trials in which the requisite information is available), nine were trials of adrenocorticosteroid therapy, two of amino acids,[31,32] and one each of penicillamine,[35] prophylthiouracil,[34] (+)-cyanidanol-3,[13] and insulin plus glucagon.[33] Of these, three showed a statistically significant decrease in mortality with steroid therapy[4,20,26] and one with amino acid infusions.[31] Several others show statistically significant trends in favor of the therapy group. The relative lack of effect of therapy is shown in Fig. 3, which demonstrates graphically that

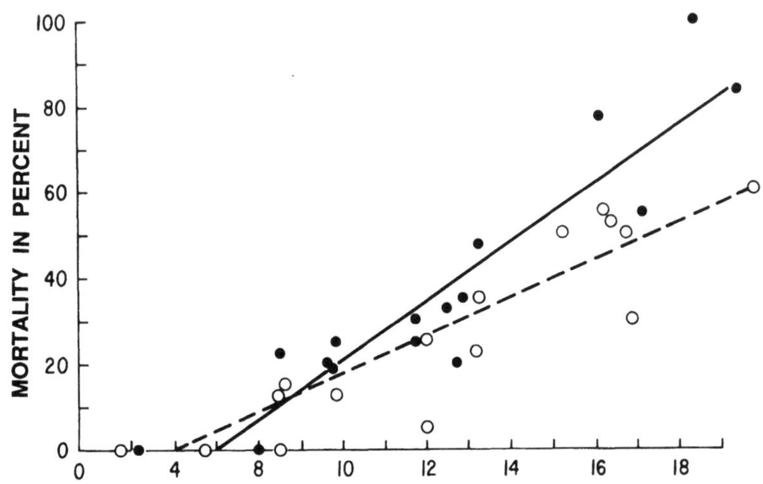

Figure 3. Correlation of serum bilirubin concentrations with mortality for the control and treatment groups. Mean total serum bilirubin levels in the control groups are depicted as closed circles and in the treatment groups as open circles. The similarity of the slopes suggests that the relationship between bilirubin concentration and outcome is not altered by therapy.

the relationship between bilirubin concentration and outcome is not greatly altered by treatment.

Fortunately, alcoholic beverages will be with us forever; unfortunately, alcoholic liver disease will be, too. Despite the prevalence of these disorders, the recognition of their importance as a disruptive social disease and the enormous amount of investigative effort devoted to them, we do not understand their pathogenesis, how to diagnose them precisely, or how to predict their outcome or how to treat them. Presumably, the chapters presented in this volume, and many others, will contribute to further attempts to control this serious problem.

REFERENCES

1. Rankin JGD, Orrego-Matte H, Deschenes J, et al: Alcoholic liver disease: The problem of diagnosis. *Alcoholism: Clin Exp Res* **2**:327–328, 1978.
2. Kryger P, Schlichting O, Dietrichson O, et al: The accuracy of the clinical diagnosis in acute hepatitis and alcoholic liver disease. Clinical versus morphological diagnosis. *Scand J Gastroenterol* **18**:691–696, 1983.
3. Poynard T, Degott C, Munoz C, et al: Relationship between degree of portal hypertension and liver histologic lesions in patients with alcoholic cirrhosis. Effect of acute alcoholic hepatitis on portal hypertension. *Dig Dis Sci* **32**:337–343, 1987.
4. Helman RA, Temko MH, Nye SW, et al: Alcoholic hepatitis. Natural history and evaluation of prednisolone therapy. *Ann Intern Med* **74**:311–321, 1987.
5. Conn HO, Blei AT, Chojkier M, et al: The naked physician: The blind interpretation of liver function tests in the differential diagnosis of jaundice, in Preisig R, Bircher J (eds): *The Liver: Quantitative Aspects of Structure and Function.* Third International Gstaad Symposium, Gstaad, 1978, pp. 386–394.
6. Morris JS, Gallo GA, Scheuer PJ, et al: Percutaneous liver biopsy in patients with large bile duct obstruction. *Gastroenterology* **68**:750–754, 1975.
7. Morgan MY, Sherlock S: Sex-related differences among 100 patients with alcoholic liver disease. *Br Med J* **1**:939–941, 1977.
8. Orrego H, Blendis LM, Crossley IR, et al: Correlation of intrahepatic pressure with collagen in the Disse space and hepatomegaly in humans and in the rat. *Gastroenterology* **80**:546–556, 1981.
9. Skrainka B, Stahlhut J, Fulbeck CL, et al: Measuring liver span. Bedside examination versus ultrasound and scintiscan. *J Clin Gastroenterol* **8**:267–270, 1986.
10. Espinoza P, Ducot B, Pelletier G, et al: Interobserver agreement in the physical diagnosis of alcoholic liver disease. *Dig Dis Sci* **32**:244–247, 1987.
11. Rasmussen SN: Liver volume by ultrasonic scanning. *Br J Radiol* **45**:579, 1972.
12. Weiss JS, Gautam A, Lauff JJ, et al: The clinical importance of a protein-bound fraction of serum bilirubin in patients with hyperbilirubinemia. *N Engl J Med* **309**:147–150, 1983.
13. Sanchez-Tapias JM, Fiol B, Rodes J: (+)-Cyanidanol-3 in mild alcoholic hepatitis, in Conn HO (ed): *International Workshop on (+)-Cyanidanol-3 in Diseases of the Liver.* Royal Society of Medicine, Academic Press, London and Grune and Stratton, New York, 1981, pp. 173–175.
14. Palmas S: Treatment of alcoholic cirrhosis with (+)-Cyanidanol-3, in Conn HO (ed): *International Workshop on (+)-Cyanidanol-3 in Diseases of the Liver.* Royal Society of Medicine, Academic Press, London and Grune and Stratton, New York, 1981, pp. 167–171.
15. Zimmerman HJ, Seeff LB: Enzymes in hepatic disease, in Coodley EL (ed): *Diagnostic Enzymology.* Philadelphia, Lea & Febiger, 1970, pp. 1–38.
16. Cohen JA, Kaplan MM: The SGOT/SGPT Ratio—An indicator of alcoholic liver disease. *Dig Dis Sci* **24**:835–838, 1979.
17. Nalpas B, Vassault A, Charpin S, et al: Serum mitochondrial asparate aminotransferase as a marker of chronic alcoholism: Diagnostic value and interpretation in a liver unit. *Hepatology* **6**:608–614, 1986.
18. Orrego H, Kalant H, Israel Y, et al: Effect of short-term therapy with propylthiouracil in patients with alcoholic liver disease. *Gastroenterology* **76**:105–115, 1979.
19. Maddrey WC, Boitnott JK, Bedine MS, et al: Adrenocosteroid therapy of alcoholic hepatitis. *Gastroenterology* **75**:193–199, 1978.
20. Maddrey WC, Carithers Jr RL, Herlong HF, et al: Prednisolone therapy in patients with severe alcoholic hepatitis. Results of a multicenter trial. Hepatology **6**:1202, 1986 (abst).
21. Conn HO: The management of alcoholic hepatitis, in Conn HO (ed): *International Workshop on (+)-*

Cyanidanol-3 in Diseases of the Liver. Royal Society of Medicine, Academic Press, London and Grune and Stratton, New York, 1981, pp. 147–156.

22. Hallak A, Conn HO: Prognostic value of blood tests in alcoholic hepatitis (AH). Analysis of the randomized clinical trials (RCT). (in preparation)
23. Porter HP, Simon FR, Pope CE, et al: Corticosteroid therapy in severe alcoholic hepatitis: A double-blind drug trial. *N Engl J Med* **284:**1350–1355, 1971.
24. Campra JL, Hamlin EM, Kirshbaum RJ, et al: Prednisone therapy of acute alcoholic hepatitis: Report of a controlled trial. *Ann Intern Med* **79:**625–631, 1973.
25. Blitzer BL, Mutchnick MG, Joshi PH, et al: Adrenocorticosteroid therapy in alcoholic hepatitis: A prospective, double-blind randomized study. *Am J Dig Dis* **22:**477–484, 1977.
26. Lesesne HR, Bozymski EM, Fallon HJ: Treatment of alcoholic hepatitis with encephalopathy: Comparison of prednisolone with caloric supplements. *Gastroenterology* **74:**169–173, 1978.
27. Shumaker JB, Resnick RH, Galambos JT, et al: A controlled trial of 6-methylprednisolone in acute alcoholic hepatitis. *Am J Gastroenterol* **69:**443–449, 1978.
28. Depew W, Boyer T, Omata M, et al: Double-blind controlled trial of prednisolone therapy in patients with severe acute alcoholic hepatitis and spontaneous encephalopathy. *Gastroenterology* **78:**524–529, 1980.
29. Mendenhall CL, Anderson S, Garcia-Pont P, et al: Short-term and long-term survival in patients with alcoholic hepatitis treated with oxandrolone and prednisolone. *N Engl J Med* **23:**1464–1470, 1984.
30. The Copenhagen Study Group for Liver Diseases: Testosterone treatment of men with alcoholic cirrhosis. A double-blind study. *Hepatology* **6:**807–813, 1986.
31. Nasrallah SM, Galambos JT: Aminoacid therapy of alcoholic hepatitis. *Lancet* **2:**1276–1277, 1980.
32. Diehl AM, Boitnott JK, Herlong F, et al: Effect of parenteral amino acid supplementation in alcoholic hepatitis. *Hepatology* **5:**57–63, 1985.
33. Baker AL, Jaspan JB, Haines NW, et al: A randomized clinical trial of insulin and glucagon infusion for treatment of alcoholic hepatitis: Progress report in 50 patients. *Gastroenterology* **80:**1410–1414, 1981.
34. Halle P, Pare P, Kaptein E, et al: Double-blind, controlled trial of propylthiouracil in patients with severe acute alcoholic hepatitis. *Gastroenterology* **82:**925–931, 1982.
35. Resnick RH, Boitnott J, Iber FL, et al: Preliminary observations of d-penicillamine therapy in acute alcoholic liver disease. *Digestion* **11:**257–265, 1974.

19

Acute Drug-Induced Hepatic Injury

James H. Lewis

1. INTRODUCTION

The field of hepatotoxicity owes much to the contributions of Dr. Hyman J. Zimmerman. The publication of his monograph, *Hepatotoxicity: The Adverse Effects of Drugs and Other Chemicals on the Liver* in 1978 was eagerly awaited. Affectionately known as the Bible of hepatotoxicity, it represented nearly three decades of study and observations on every clinical and experimental aspect of drug-induced hepatic injury. Virtually all classes of medicinal agents and a multitude of chemicals and environmental toxins are capable of causing acute injury to the liver. The spectrum of hepatic lesions produced by these drugs and chemicals is diverse, mimicking most infectious, inflammatory, vascular, and neoplastic disorders. While a discussion of the hepatotoxicity of each agent is beyond the scope of this chapter, I nevertheless endeavor to provide an overview of various aspects of acute drug-induced liver disease. For information on particular agents, the reader is urged to consult Dr. Zimmerman's textbook[1] or any number of reference works.[2-4]

2. HISTORICAL PERSPECTIVES

In describing alcoholic cirrhosis during the 1500s, Vesalius may have been the first to associate a chemical agent with hepatic injury.[1] However, not until 1774, when Bang suggested an association between arsenic and chronic liver disease, was an explicit reference to chemical hepatic injury first recorded.[5] Nearly 75 years would pass before active efforts were made to link hepatic injury to toxic chemical exposure. Fatal chloroform poisoning with jaundice was recognized in 1847 by Simpson, who first employed the anesthetic agent, but the liver-failure basis of death was overlooked for nearly a half-century.[6] In 1860, Hauff reported severe fatty liver as a result of phosphorus intoxication.[1]

The year 1866 marked the first demonstration of experimental hepatotoxicity, with Nothnagel's observation of hepatic injury in dogs that received chloroform. During the latter part of the nineteenth century, the effects of elemental phosphorus and inorganic arsenicals also were studied in dog livers. During the early twentieth century, senecio alkaloids were discovered to afflict both domesticated animals as well as humans in bush teas and other folk medicines.[1]

James H. Lewis • Georgetown University School of Medicine; Division of Gastroenterology, Georgetown University Hospital, Washington, D.C. 20007.

The modern era of hepatotoxicity caused by drugs can be said to have begun in 1923, with the first reports of liver injury induced by cinchophen.[7] Shortly after the introduction of sulfonamides, gold salts, and diethylstilbestrol (DES) in the 1930s came reports linking each of these agents with hepatic injury. Similarly, anabolic steroids, organic arsenicals, and the antithyroid agent, thiouracil—all developed in the 1940s—also were linked to instances of hepatic injury soon after their release.[1] Table I lists the chronologic appearance of hepatic injury with modern-day medicinal agents. The selected references[1-78] reflect Dr. Zimmerman's widespread contributions to the field.

The veritable explosion of new drugs introduced since the 1950s has emphasized the importance of the liver as a target organ of drug toxicity. Although the detection of hepatic injury has been simplified with today's automated serum chemistry analyses and the ample availability of endoscopic, radiographic, and isotopic tests to delineate the structure and function of the hepatobiliary system, the recognition of hepatic injury has not always been so easy or as readily accepted. For example, the fatal cause of delayed chloroform poisoning was not recognized to be due to hepatic failure for almost 50 years.[6] The time from the first recognition of salicylate hepatitis to its widespread acceptance spanned nearly 75 years.[44] Similarly, several decades elapsed between the time that reports of hepatic injury due to several other drugs first appeared and full recognition of their hepatotoxic potential (Table II). Some agents, such as the halogenated anesthetics, halothane and enflurane, while clearly regarded as hepatotoxic by most,[1,27,50] remain controversial in the opinion of others.[79,80]

Some two dozen drugs have been withdrawn from clinical use, and many more potentially

Table I. Chronology of Drug-Induced Liver Disease during the Twentieth Century[a,b]

Year	Drug
1900	Senecio alkaloids[1]
1920s	Cinchophen[7]
1930s	Sulfonamides,[8] gold salts,[9,10] DES[11]
1940s	Organic arsenicals,[12] anabolic steroids,[1,13] thiouracil,[14] carbamazepine[15]
1950s	PAS,[16] iproniazid,[17,18] PBZ,[19] 6-MP,[20] antidepressants,[21] tetracycline,[22] penicillin,[22,23] dapsone,[24] methotrexate[1,20]
1960s	INH,[25,26] halothane,[1,27] E. estolate,[1,28] nitrofurantoin,[29] chlorpropamide,[30] chlorzoxazone,[31] OCS,[32,33] methyldopa,[34] CPZ,[35,36] TAO,[37] PTU,[38] procainamide,[39] papaverine,[41] ethionamide[42]
1970s	DPH,[42] oxyphenisatin,[43] salicylates,[44] methoxyflurane,[45] acetaminophen,[46,47] cimetidine,[48] VPA,[49] enflurane,[50] allopurinol,[51] perhexiline maleate,[52] oxacillin,[53] sulfasalazine,[54] dantrolene,[55,56] danazol,[57] propoxyphene,[58] ibuprofen,[59] sulindac,[60] rifampicin,[61] penicillamine,[62] dihydralazine,[63] hydralazine,[64] flurazepam,[65] paraquat[66]
1980s	Benoxaprofen,[10,59] oxmetidine,[48,67] captopril,[68] ranitidine,[48] amiodarone,[69] ticrynafen,[70,71] ketoconazole,[72] cyclosporin A,[73] chenodeoxycholate,[74] lovastatin,[75] nifedipine,[76] warfarin,[77] verapamil[78]

[a]CPZ, chlorpromazine; DES, diethylstilbestrol; DPH, diphenylhydantoin; E. estolate, erythromycin estolate; INH, isoniazid; 6-MP, 6-mercaptoprine; OCS, oral contraceptive steroids; PAS, Para-aminosalicylate; PBZ, phenylbutazone; PTU, propylthiouracil; TAO, triacetyloleardomycin; VPA, valproic acid.
[b]References are cited as superscript numbers.

Table II. Delayed Recognition of Drug-Induced Liver Injury

Agent	Years
Chloroform	50
Salicylates	75
Oxyphenisatin	40
Quinidine	50
Papaverine	50
Thorotrast	25
Cinchophen	12

useful compounds have been abandoned in premarketing phases because of severe hepatotoxicity (Table III). A number of these agents, such as chloroform, were used for decades before being withdrawn,[1] while others were abandoned shortly after their commercial release, e.g., benoxaprofen,[10,59] ticrynafen,[71] and, in some instances, just before marketing because of severe hepatotoxic potential, e.g., oxmetidine.[48] Several medicinal agents currently in use have an appreciable incidence of subclinical and overt hepatic injury associated with their use. Aspirin, for example, might not be approved by the Food and Drug Administration (FDA) if it were being considered in 1987!

3. PREVALENCE OF ACUTE DRUG-INDUCED HEPATIC INJURY

The frequency of acute drug-induced liver disease has been difficult to quantify. Cases spontaneously reported to the adverse drug reactions branch of the FDA as well as published case reports tend to underestimate the prevalence of an adverse reaction by a factor of up to 100-fold. Even large

Table III. Medicinal Agents Withdrawn or Abandoned Due to Hepatotoxicity

Anti-inflammatory	Antimicrobial agents
Benoxaprofen	Organic arsenicals
Fenclozic acid	Triacetyloleandomycin
Ibufenac	Novobiocin
Fluproquazone	Carbon tetrachloride
Sudoxicam	Anesthetics
Cinchophen	Chloroform
Laxatives	Anticonvulsants
Oxyphenisatin	Phenurone
Antiulcer	Beta Blockers
Oxmetidine	Practolol
Anticoagulants	Muscle relaxants
Phenindione	Zoxazolamine
Antidepressants	Hypoglycemics
Iproniazid	Carbutamide
Radiographic dyes	Metahexamide
Thorotrast	Miscellaneous
Diuretics	Tannic acid
Ticrynafen	

postmarketing surveillance studies tend to miss rare adverse events, such as unpredictable acute drug-induced hepatitis.[81] Rossi et al.[82] in 1983 and Faich et al.[83] in 1987 both reported that adverse drug effects on the gastrointestinal (GI) and hepatobiliary tracts together accounted for only a small percentage of all adverse reactions reported to the FDA. In Denmark, 6% of all adverse reaction reports specifically involved hepatotoxicity.[84] A study of patients admitted with jaundice to several hospitals in Boston in 1970 gave the incidence of drug-induced jaundice as only 2%.[85] The Boston Collaborative Drug Surveillance Program found a total of 13 instances of drug-induced hepatitis or jaundice among 260 patients requiring admission for an adverse drug reaction, for an incidence of 5%.[86] However, as Zimmerman has frequently pointed out, the relative importance of drug-induced hepatic injury assumes a far greater significance among special populations. For example, Eastwood[87] reported a 20% incidence of jaundice from drugs in a geriatric population. Similarly high percentages have also been noted for patients receiving psychoactive or antituberculous therapies.[88,89] Among the causes of fulminant hepatic failure recorded in various series, medicinal agents have accounted for 20%–50% of cases.[90-94]

While precise figures on the incidence of hepatic injury for most individual agents are not available, reasonable estimates, based on case reports and the results of serial monitoring and other surveillance studies, where available, can be made for many drugs (Tables IV and V). The diagnosis of drug-induced liver injury is generally one of clinical awareness and suspicion. Viral hepatitis, ischemic injury, congestive heart failure (CHF), and other disease processes that may mimic drug-induced injury must be excluded. In these times of polypharmacy, it is often difficult to ascribe causality to one agent amid a myriad of others. Alcohol consumption is prevalent in many populations and often constitutes another confounding variable in the diagnosis of drug-induced injury. Histologic changes on liver biopsy may be suggestive but are rarely diagnostic. Even subcellular changes seen electron microscopically rarely offer completely pathognomonic clues. As a result, the clinician must look to the circumstances surrounding the injury and be reasonably confident in the exclusion of other causes. A clinical diagnosis is usually confirmed after observing an appropriate response to removing the offending agent (dechallenge) or to rechallenge with the suspected drug (*vide infra*).

Table IV. Estimated Prevalence of Subclinical Hepatic Enzyme Elevations with Various Drugs[a]

Agent	Percent
CPZ, TAO, DPH, amiodarone, perhexiline, papaverine, cisplatin, nicotinic acid, VPA, heparin, nafcillin, 6-MP	20–50%
INH, ketoconazole, androgens, erythromycin estolate, etretinate	10–20%
Penicillamine, chenodeoxycholate, flucytosine, disulfiram	5–10%
Salicylates, gold salts, sulfonamides, dantrolene, sulfonylureas, quinidine, thiabendazole, ticarcillin, tricyclic antidepressants, ethionamide	<5%

[a]Percentages listed are generally the highest reported in the literature.

Table V. Estimated Frequency of Overt Hepatitis or Jaundice from Medicinal Agents

Agent	Percent
PAS, TAO, dapsone, chenodexoy-cholate	>2
Lovastatin, cyclosporine, dantrolene	1–2
INH, PAS, amidarone	1
Phenytoin, sulfonamides, chlorpromazine	0.5–1
Gold salts, salicylates, methyldopa, chlorpropamide, E. estolate	0.1–0.5
Ketoconazole, contraceptive steroids	<0.01
Penicillin, hydralazine, halothane, enflurane, cimetidine, ranitidine	<0.0001

4. SPECTRUM OF INJURY

Medicinal and chemical agents may mimic many clinical syndromes (Table VI). A variety of extrahepatic manifestations are recognized.[1] Traditional hallmarks of hypersensitivity, such as fever, rash, and eosinophilia, are characteristic of reactions due to chlorpromazine, dapsone, phenytoin, sulfanamides, erthromycin estolate, and halothane—drugs that act through drug allergy mechanisms. Phenytoin may produce a syndrome that resembles infectious mononucleosis complete with lymphadenopathy and atypical lymphocytosis. Curiously, penicillin and procainimide, drugs associated with a high incidence of hypersensitivity reactions, rarely lead to hepatic injury. Many drugs (e.g., INH, valproate, amiodarone, and acetaminophen) produce hepatic injury in the absence

Table VI. Clinical Syndromes Caused by Acute Hepatotoxins

Syndrome	Agent
Fever, rash, eosinophilia	CPZ, PBZ, halogenated anesthetics
Acute viral hepatitis	INH, halothane
Acute extrahepatic obstruction	CPZ, erythromycin estolate
Pseudomononucleosis	DPH
Serum sickness syndrome	PAS, DPH, sulfonamides
Autoimmune hemolysis	Methyldopa, oxyphenisatin
Muscular syndrome[a]	Clofibrate
Antinuclear antibodies	Procainamide
Associated marrow injury	Anticonvulsants, gold salts, propylthiouracil, PBZ, chloramphenicol
Associated pulmonary injury	Amiodarone, nitrofurantoin
Associated renal injury	Methoxyflurane, gold salts, penicillamine
Fatty liver of pregnancy	Tetracycline
Bland jaundice	C_{17}-steroids, rifampicin

[a]Myalgia, stiffness, weakness, ↑ CPK.

of associated hallmarks of hypersensitivity or other organ injury. In these cases, the mechanism of injury is presumed to be the production of hepatotoxic metabolites rather than drug allergy as will be discussed.

As diverse as the clinical syndromes of hepatotoxicity are, so, too, is the histopathologic spectrum of injury they cause. Morphologic patterns of acute drug-induced injury are divided into cytotoxic (hepatocellular necrosis, steatosis), cholestatic (canalicular, hepatocanalicular, ductular), mixed cytotoxic–cholestatic, granulomatous, and vascular types. In general, one morphologic pattern of injury tends to predominate in each therapeutic class of agents (Table VII). Categories with numerous types of drugs, such as the various antimicrobial and cardiovascular agents, are reflected by a wide array of morphologic injury patterns (see Chapter 21).

Cytotoxic injury refers to hepatocellular degeneration or necrosis or to the development of toxic steatosis. Cholestatic agents may produce injury with (hepatocanalicular) or without (canalicular) associated parenchymal involvement or bile duct injury. Agents producing mixed injury have morphologic features of both cytotoxicity and cholestasis. Hepatic necrosis often leads to a syndrome resembling that of acute viral hepatitis. Values for aspartate aminotransferase (AST) and alanine aminotransferase (ALT) may be elevated to at least 10–100 times the upper limit of normal. Values for alkaline phosphatase are generally only modestly elevated (i.e., less than threefold). The most important clinical aspect of acute hepatocellular jaundice is the development of fulminant hepatic failure, which carries a case fatality rate of up to 50%. Acute drug-induced toxic steatosis, such as that produced by tetracycline or valproic acid, leads to clinical and biochemical features resembling Reye syndrome or acute fatty liver of pregnancy. Aminotransferase levels are usually only moderately elevated and deep jaundice is rare, but case fatality rates for this form of injury are also high.

It has become useful to categorize cytoxic drug injury according to the zonality of the injury pattern.[1] Most agents that produce cytotoxic injury lead to diffuse rather than zonal injury. However, zonal injury is characteristic of a number of agents and is a useful diagnostic feature (Table VIII). In general, intrinsic (predictable) hepatotoxins produce zonal injury, while idiosyncratic (unpredictable) hepatotoxins lead to diffuse or massive injury. Notable exceptions include the

Table VII. Relationship between Therapeutic Category and Type of Injury[a,b]

Agent	Injury
Anesthetics	H-cell
Tranquilizers	H-can
Antidepressants	H-cell
Anticonvulsants	H-cell, mixed
Antiinflammatory	H-cell, H-can
Antirheumatic, antigout	H-cell
Muscle relaxants	H-cell
Antineoplastics	H-cell, steat
Antimicrobials	Variable
Oral hypoglycemics	Variable
Cardiovascular	Variable
Anabolic, contraceptive steroids	H-can
Antithyroid	H-can, H-cell

[a]After Zimmerman.[1]
[b]H-cell, hepatocellular; H-can, hepatocanalicular; mixed, hepatocellular–cholestatic; steat, steatosis; variable, multiple injury types, depending on the agent.

Table VIII. Acute Drug-Induced Cytotoxic Hepatic Injury

Necrosis	
Zonal	
Central	(acetaminophen, halothane, carbon tetrachloride, bromobenzene)
Mid	(Ngaione, beryllium)
Periportal	(allyl alcohol, ferrous sulfate, phosphorus)
Massive	(INH, sulfonamides, phenytoin)
Diffuse, focal	(phenylbutazone, phenytoin, propylthiomacil, salicylates, sulfonamides, methyldopa, acetohexamide, galactosamine)
Degeneration	(many agents)
Mallory bodies	(ethanol, griseofulvin amiodarone, perhexiline maleate, Coralgil, diethylstilbestrol)

centrizonal necrosis due to several halogenated anesthetic agents[27] that produce injury as a result of host idiosyncracy. The experimental hepatotoxin, galactosamine,[95] is an intrinsic toxin that produces diffuse rather than zonal injury. The zonality of hepatocellular necrosis appears to be related to the mechanism of the injury for some intrinsic toxins.[1] For example, the centrizonal necrosis induced by carbon tetrachloride and bromobenzene has been attributed to the centrizonal concentration of the enzyme system responsible for the conversion of these agents to hepatotoxic metabolites. Likewise, the peripheral zone necrosis produced by allyl formate has been attributed to a similar mechanism.

Cholestatic injury may mimic one of several clinical syndromes, depending on the nature and location of the anatomic and physiologic defect (Table IX). Hepatocanalicular cholestasis, exemplified by chlorpromazine and erythromycin estolate, resembles extrahepatic obstructive jaundice with abdominal pain and a severalfold elevation of alkaline phosphatase, aminotransferase, and bilirubin levels. Indeed, patients with unsuspected injury due to these cholestatic agents have been subjected to needless laparotomy to explore the biliary tree.[10] Canalicular cholestasis, produced by the C_{17}-alkylated anabolic and contraceptive steroids, results in a more bland form of extrahepatic-like jaundice. In contrast to hepatocanalicular cholestasis, there is little or no portal inflammation or histologic evidence of parenchymal injury. Such drugs as phenylbutazone and phenytoin often lead to prominent hepatocellular injury accompanied by prominent cholestasis. This form of injury is referred to as cholestatic hepatitis, which may accompany some cases of acute viral hepatitis. Finally, ductal cholestasis refers to those syndromes that result from depletion of or injury to interlobular bile ducts. This may take the form of acute cholangitis or chronic injury resembling primary biliary cirrhosis or sclerosing cholangitis.

Among the various agents that interfere with the movement of lipid within, or the exit of lipid from, the cell leading to steatosis, two forms of fatty change can be recognized.Microvesicular steatosis, in which many tiny fat droplets fill the hepatocyte without displacing the nucleus, is characteristic of tetracycline, valproic acid, and aspirin. Macrovesicular steatosis, in which the hepatocytes contain a large droplet of fat that displaces the nucleus toward the periphery, is characteristic of alcohol, methotrexate, and glucocorticoids.

Phospholipidosis is another form of lipid accumulation within hepatocytes. First described in

Table IX. Site-Specific Physiologic Lesions in Drug-Induced Cholestasis

Physiologic lesion	Specific site	Drug examples
Defects in anatomic pathway of bile formation and flow	Basolateral membrane	EE, CPZ, phalloidin, LCA, cytochalasin B, endotoxin
	Canalicular membrane	LCA, norethandrolone, cytochalasin B, phalloidin
	Microfibrillar network	Cytochalasin B, phalloidin, CPZ, norenthandrolone
	Tight junction	EE, ANIT, phalloidin, CPZ, LCA
	Microtubules	Colchincine, vinblastin
	Cholangioles	Benoxaprofen
	Portal area ducts (interlobular)	Paraquat, ANIT, rapeseed (Margosa) oil, chlorpropamide, erythromycin
	Extrahepatic ducts	5-fluorouridine (5-Fu)
Change in character of bile	↑ Viscosity	CPZ, LCA, EE, norethandrolone
	↑ Solubility–precipitation	CPZ, LCA
	Abnormal micelles	LCA, CPZ, C_{17}-alkylated steroids
Functional defect	↓ Uptake bile acids	EE, CPZ
BADF	↓ Processing in hepatocyte	Estrogens
	↓ ATP formation	Dinitrophenol
	Anion competition	LCA, foreign dyes, rifampicin
	↓ Transport to canaliulus	Colchicine, vinblastin
BAIF	Tight junction defect	EE, ANIT, CPZ, LCA
	↑ Na-K-ATPase	EE, CPZ
	↑ Mg-ATPase	Many agents (except EE)

[a]ANIT, α-naphthylisocyanate; BADF, bile acid-dependent flow; BAIF, bile acid-independent flow; CPZ, chlorpromazine; EE, ethinyl estradiol; LCA, lithocholate.

Japan following the administration of the coronary vasodilator, 4,4′-diethylaminoethoxyhexestrol (Coralgil), more than 30 drugs are capable of producing this change[96] (Table X). All share a common structural similarity, having a hydrophilic cationic side chain juxtaposed to a hydrophobic lipophilic apolar ring system, rendering these compounds amphiphilic.[96] Morphologically phospholipidosis is characterized by enlarged foamy hepatocytes that resemble the inborn lipidoses, such as Gaucher and Niemann–Pick disease. Whorled lamellated lysosomal inclusions are characteristically present on electron microscopy. The mechanism by which these compounds induce phospholipidosis changes within the cells is thought to be through inhibition of lysosomal phospholipases. This is postulated to be a pH-mediated effect by which phospholipid degradation is impaired. While the binding of amphiphilic compounds to phospholipids within lysosomes is a potentially reversible process, drugs such as amiodarone may persist within the liver for several months.[97] Evidence of functional impairment due to phospholipidosis comes from clinical and experimental observations with 4,4-DH, perhexiline maleate, and, most recently, amiodarone. Morphologic changes resembling alcoholic liver disease with Mallory bodies, steatosis, fibrosis, and occasionally cirrhosis, characterize the injury seen with these drugs.[52,69,97,98]

Table X. Selected Drugs Causing Hepatic Phospholipidosis[a]

Coronary vasodilators
4,4′-diethylaminoethoxyhexestrol, perhexiline maleate, amiodarone
Anorectics
Chlorophentermine
Inhibitors of cholesterol synthesis
Triparanol, azacosterol
Antimalarials
Chloroquine, mepacrine
Antidepressants
Amitriptyline, ipridole, imipramine, noxiptiline
Neuroleptics
Chlorpromazine, thioridazine
Antihistamines
Chlorcyclizine, tripelennamine
Miscellaneous
Amantadine, propranolol, contraceptive steroids

[a]After Lullmann et al.[96]

5. MECHANISMS OF ACUTE DRUG-INDUCED LIVER INJURY

The Zimmerman classification[1] of hepatotoxic agents takes into account both the mechanism of injury and the type of lesion produced (Table XI). Two major categories of hepatotoxins are recognized: intrinsic and idiosyncratic. Intrinsic (true or predictable) hepatotoxins are agents that lead to a high incidence of hepatic injury in exposed persons. They produce similar lesions in experimental animals, and the development and degree of injury are dose related. The interval between their administration and the onset of hepatic injury is consistent for each drug and is generally of short duration (hours–days). Idiosyncratic (nonpredictable) hepatotoxins produce injury only in highly susceptible persons. As a result, the incidence of injury is very low; the development of injury in humans is independent of the dose, and these agents do not produce hepatic lesions in experimental animals. The latent period between the first dose and the onset of injury is quite variable and generally longer compared with that seen with intrinsic hepatotoxins (weeks–months).

Intrinsic hepatotoxins can be divided into direct hepatotoxins, which produce direct physicochemical distortion and destruction of the hepatocyte, and indirect hepatotoxins, which interfere with specific metabolic pathways, leading to structural injury or interference with hepatic excretory pathways. Carbon tetrachloride is a useful prototype of the direct hepatotoxins. Acting through a reactive metabolite, it leads to peroxidation and denaturation of the cell and its components.[1] No intrinsic direct hepatotoxic drugs are currently in use, although tannic acid was given to burn victims into the 1940s, carbon tetrachloride was employed as an antihelminthic as late as 1954, and chloroform was used as an anesthetic into the 1960s.[99]

Indirect intrinsic hepatotoxins leading to cytotoxic injury include several cancer chemotherapeutic agents such as 6-MP and mithramycin, as well as acetaminophen and inorganic iron, which are hepatotoxic in the setting of an acute overdose. Toxic steatosis is seen with tetracycline, methotrexate, valproic acid, L-asparaginase, as well as alcohol. Indirect hepatoxins that interfere with specific hepatic excretory pathways are classified as cholestatic agents. Examples include the contraceptive and anabolic C_{17}-alkylated steroids, chlorpromazine, erythromycin estolate, and benoxaprofen (Tables IX and XI).

Table XI. Zimmerman Classification of Hepatotoxic Agents

Category	Mechanism	Biochemical abnormality[a]			Clinical aspects	Examples
		AST/ALT	Alk Phos	Histology		
Intrinsic toxicity						
Direct	Direct physicochemical destruction or distortion of cells	8–500	1–2	Necrosis and/or steatosis	Hepatic, renal failure	CCl_4, $CHCl_3$, phosphorus
Indirect						
Cytotoxic	Interference with specific metabolic pathways, leading to structural injury	8–500	1–2	Necrosis	Severe viral hepatitis-like illness	Bromobenzene, ACM, 6-MP, mycotoxins
		5–20	1–2	Steatosis (microvesicular)	Fatty liver of pregnancy, Reye syndrome	Valproate, ethionine, tetracycline
		1–3	1–2	Steatosis (macrovesicular)	Few manifestations	MTX, ethanol
Cholestatic	Interference with hepatic excretory pathways					
	Canalicular	1–5	1–3	Bile casts	Bland jaundice	Anabolic, contraceptive steroids

	Hepatocanalicular	1–8	3–10	Portal infiltrates	Resembles extrahepatic obstruction	CPZ, E. estolate
	Ductal	1–5	3–10			
	Ductules			Inspissated bile	Jaundice	Benoxaprofen
	Intertubular ducts			Destruction of portal area ducts	Primary biliary cirrhosis	Paraquat, Margosa oil
	Septal ducts			Fibrosis of septal ducts	Sclerosing cholangitis	5-FUDR
Mixed injury	Variable	Variable	Variable	Variable cholestatic and hepatacellular injury	May resemble viral hepatitis or obstructive jaundice	PBZ, PAS, sulfonamides
Host idiosyncracy						
Hypersensitivity	Drug allergy	Variable	Variable	Necrosis or cholestasis	Variable	Phenytoin, PAS, CPZ, sulfonamides, E. estolate
Metabolic abnormality	Production of hepatotoxic metabolites	Variable	Variable	Necrosis or cholestasis	Variable	INH, halothane, ACM, hydralazine, valproate, ticrynafen, ketoconazole, methyldopa

[a]Times (fold) increased above normal.

The vast majority of drugs currently in use that lead to hepatic injury do so on an idiosyncratic basis. Idiosyncratic hepatotoxins are subdivided into those associated with hypersensitivity (drug allergy) and those thought to produce injury through the production of hepatotoxic metabolites (so-called metabolic idiosyncracy) (Table XI). Injury attributed to hypersensitivity generally develops after a period of sensitization of 1–5 weeks and is often associated with clinical hallmarks of hypersensitivity, as well as histologic evidence of drug allergy (eosinophilia or granulomatous inflammation). Reproduction of the patient's clinical symptoms or enzyme abnormalities after a challenge dose is characteristic.

The development of hepatic injury after weeks or months of exposure to a particular agent, without associated hallmarks of hypersensitivity, is often presumed to be the result of a metabolic aberration leading to production of a hepatotoxic metabolite(s). In keeping with metabolic idiosyncracy as the cause, response to a challenge dose is often delayed for many days and even weeks and may result in only modest biochemical abnormalities or clinical symptoms. For a number of agents, hypersensitivity appears to lead to overt hepatic injury only when the particular drug has some intrinsic hepatotoxic potential. This appears to be the case with chlorpromazine, ethinyl estradiol, and phenylbutazone. A number of drugs that frequently lead to hypersensitivity reactions, such as penicillin, hydralazine, and procainamide, are apparently devoid of any intrinsic hepatotoxic potential and lead to hepatic injury very rarely.[1]

6. SUSCEPTIBILITY TO HEPATIC INJURY

Numerous factors affect host susceptibility with respect to the development of hepatic injury (Table XII). With regard to age, it has been Dr. Zimmerman's clinical impression that most forms of drug-induced hepatic injury tend to spare children. A few notable exceptions appear to be valproic acid[49] and aspirin[44]—the latter especially among youngsters with underlying rheumatic diseases. The greater vulnerability of adults to hepatic injury may bear some relationship to the decrease in activity and inducibility of the hepatic mixed-function oxidase (MFO) enzyme system that occurs with increasing age. One of the most striking examples of age-related injury is seen with isoniazid, in which susceptibility increases progressively with age.[1] Similarly, halothane injury is seen predominantly in adults. No consistent differences between the genders or races have been shown for most hepatotoxins. Only in mice and rats can the sexes be regularly separated according to susceptibility to some hepatotoxins.

The underlying nutritional state of the host may be important but remains controversial. Low-protein diets lead to reduced activity of MFO enzymes and of the glutathione content of the liver cells. This may result in reduced toxicity from agents that are less injurious than their metabolites but may enhance injury due to agents acting through toxic metabolites, such as acetaminophen. Protein-deficient and choline-deficient diets also lead to fatty infiltration that can contribute to hepatotoxicity in their own right. Fasting potentiates the experimental hepatoxicity of some agents (e.g., CC14, CHC13, and bromobenzene in animals) probably through a reduction of endigenous glutathione.[1]

Heritable influences on host susceptibility may relate to species-specific or individual differences in drug metabolism and disposition. In humans, hydroxylation and acetylation are both under genetic control. The rapid acetylator status identified in many patients with INH-induced injury has been cited as a predisposing factor,[100] although this is controversial.[22] The gene responsible for the metabolism of the antihypertensive drug, debrisoquine, appears to regulate several other drug oxidations.[101] For example, an impaired debrisoquine metabolizer phenotype has been linked to injury from perhexiline maleate.[102] Poor debrisoquine metabolizers are also defective oxidizers of the agents antipyrine, phenytoin, tolbutamide, nifedipine, and phenacetin, among others.[101] As with acetylator status, there are wide interethnic differences in the frequency of occurrence of the poor debrisoquine metabolizer phenotype. A possible familial tendency toward halothane hepatitis

Table XII. Factors Increasing Susceptibility to Drug-Induced Hepatic Injury

Factor	Drug at risk
Age	
Older	INH, cinchophen, phenytoin, halothane, benoxaprofen, ticrynafen
Younger	Valproate, salicylates
Gender	
Female	Halothane?, methyldopa, ketoconazole, ticrynafen
Race	
Black	Phenytoin
Oriental	INH
Underlying disease state	
Alcoholism	CCl_4, INH, acetaminophen, MTX?
JRA, SLE	Salicylates
Obesity	Halothane, MTX?
Diabetes	MTX?
Liver disease	Anabolic steroids, INH?, MTX
Renal failure	Benoxaprofen, penicillamine, allopurinol
Intrauterine radiotherapy	Halothane
Malnutrition	Dapsone
Penicillin allergy	Penicillamine
Genetic predisposition	
Rapid acelylator phenotype	INH
Slow acelylator phenotype	Sulfonamides, dapsone, hydralazine
Impaired debrisoquine oxidation	Perhexiline maleate, phenytoin?
HLA haplotype	
B8	Nitrofurantoin
A1-B8, A3	MTX?
DR3	Gold
Family history of drug injury	Chlorpromazine, halothane

has been reported in a few kindreds,[103,104] suggesting a genetic vulnerability to injury for this and possibly other drugs. Histocompatability antigen phenotype may bear some relationship to drug-induced hepatic injury through its influence on immune responsiveness.[105] A possible association between the development of chronic liver injury from nitrofurantoin and the presence of HLA-B8 antigen has been reported,[106] As has HLA-A1 and B8 with susceptibility to methotrexate injury[4] and DR3 with gold salts.[107] For most hepatotoxins, however, HLA associations have not been established.

The underlying disease state for which a medication is being taken may also influence the potential for hepatotoxicity. For example, the risk of hepatic injury due to aspirin appears to be increased in patients with juvenile rheumatoid arthritis, systemic lupus erythematosus (SLE), and rheumatic fever.[44,46] Finally, some agents appear to have their hepatic potential for injury enhanced when given with other drugs. This is apparent with therapeutic doses of acetaminophen taken in the setting of chronic alcohol ingestion [that depletes glutathione (GSH)] or with enzyme-inducing agents, such as phenobarbital (PB) or diphenylhydantoin (DPH), that may lead to the increased production of its toxic metabolite.[47] Similarly, most cases of valproic acid injury have been associated with the concomitant use of PB or DPH.[illegible] The combination of INH and rifampicin leads to hepatic injury more often than with either agent alone.[1] Besides INH, alcohol is thought to enhance the toxicity associated with several other agents.[108] Trimethoprim is not thought to be hepatotoxic by itself but in combination with sulfamethoxazole becomes a potential cholestatic hepatotoxin.[22]

The role of exposure to various hepatic enzyme inducers in the environment and in the workplace is of significant theoretical, if not practical, concern.[1,109] A partial list of drugs and chemicals capable of inducing hepatic enzymes in humans is given in Table XIII.

7. MECHANISMS OF CELL INJURY

Substances that are toxic to the liver may exert their adverse effects by one or more diverse mechanisms of injury: (1) direct physicochemical effects on vital cell structures or interference with specific metabolic pathways by reactive metabolites, (2) induction of various immunogenic reactions, (3) impairment of hepatic blood supply, (4) carcinogenic actions, and (5) aggravation of underlying liver disease.

Two major types of toxic metabolites are involved in drug-induced hepatotoxicity[110]: electrophiles and free radicals. Electrophiles, produced by the oxidation of certain drugs, bind covalently to nucleophilic sites, such as the thiol group of cysteine that exists in most cells as glutathione. Glutathione normally serves a major protective function by binding to potentially toxic metabolites. Electrophilic metabolites interact preferentially with glutathione rather than with cellular proteins. In the case of an acetaminophen overdose, depletion of cytoplasmic glutathione leaves the electrophilic metabolite no choice but to bind to cellular proteins, leading to cell death.

Free radicals are metabolites formed as a result of reductive reactions of P450 cytochromes. They undergo one of several additional reactions, including binding covalently to proteins or to unsaturated lipids or forming fatty acid radicals that combine with oxygen, leading to lipid peroxidation and cellular damage.[111] Free radical metabolites lead to cell death through impairment of vital cell functions, such as calcium homeostasis, membrane pumps, and mitochondrial function.[110]

Immune reactions that may lead to drug hepatotoxicity include the formation of haptens (e.g.,

Table XIII. Medicinal and Chemical Enzyme Inducers of Drug Metabolism[a]

Antipyrine
Chloral hydrate
Chlordiazepoxide
DDT
Diphenylhydantoin
Ethanol
Glutethimide
Griseofulvin
Halothane
Lindane
Meprobamate
Phenobarbital
Phenylbutazone
Prednisone
Promethazine
Rifampicin
Secobarbital

[a]After Zimmerman.[1]

halothane, chlorpromazine, INH), immune complexes (e.g., DPH, INH), and autoantibodies (e.g., procainamide, hydralazine) (Table XIV). Immunologic mechanisms appear to be particularly important in the development of hepatic injury due to halothane when the formation of a reactive metabolite(s) may be the cause of the mild direct hepatotoxicity seen in approximately 20% patients receiving this anesthetic. Severe hepatic injury leading to fulminant hepatitis and death in up to 50% of cases usually follows sensitization to halothane after multiple exposures and appears to be immune mediated.[112,113] One possible explanation for the apparent rarity of severe hepatocellular necrosis after halothane anesthesia (estimated to occur in only 1 in 10,000–30,000) centers on the assumptions that (1) only persons with a genetic predisposition to organ-specific autoimmunity are at risk, and (2) such a defect in immune regulation must be superimposed on the production of hepatotoxic metabolites before the complication of hepatic injury can develop.[114]

Agents that produce cholestasis may do so by interference with any number of cellular processes involved in the formation and flow of bile. Table IX lists the site-specific morphologic defects that may lead to cholestatis, as well as the various drugs responsible. A more complete discussion of drug-induced cholestasis is found in a recent review by Zimmerman and Lewis.[10]

8. DIAGNOSIS OF DRUG-INDUCED HEPATIC INJURY

The diagnosis of drug-induced hepatic injury is generally one of exclusion. Recent or ongoing exposure to the suspected drug, biochemical or histologic evidence of the injury pattern most often associated with that drug, and the presence or absence of associated signs and symptoms that may or may not accompany injury with the particular drug generally permit a presumptive diagnosis. When the injury is hepatocellular, exclusion of viral hepatitis is necessary, although the lack of a serologic test for the non-A non-B virus(s) continues to hamper our ability to exclude this entity. In the case of cholestatic injury, extrahepatic biliary obstruction due to gallstones, benign or malignant strictures, sclerosing cholangitis, and carcinoma of the pancreas, among others, should be ruled out using ultrasonography, computed tomographic (CT) scan, endoscopic retrograde cholangio-pancreatography (ERCP), or percutaneous transhepatic cholangiography (PTC), alone or in combination. Intrahepatic cholestasis requires the exclusion of pregnancy, sepsis, postoperative state, and transfusion reaction, among other causes. Histologic confirmation may become necessary to exclude primary biliary cirrhosis, sarcoidosis, and other chronic intrahepatic cholestatic conditions.

Perhaps the most definitive means of diagnosing drug injury is with a challenge dose. An appropriate response to removal of the offending drug (dechallenge) often falls short of being conclusive. Once the decision to discontinue a medication has been made, biochemical and clinical

Table XIV. Immunologic Basis of Drug Hepatotoxicity

Mechanism	Examples
Hapten formation	Halothane, thiabendazole, chlopromazine, INH, aspirin, oxyphenisatin, thiabendazole
Immune complexes (serum sickness)	DPH, INH, azulfadine
Autoantibody formation	
Antinuclear	Procainamide, CPZ, hydralazine, methyldopa
Liver/kidney microsomal	Halothane
Antismooth muscle (ASM)	Methyldopa, nitrofurantoin
IgE mast cell activation (eosinophilia)	Halothane, CPZ
Positive lymphocyte stimulation test	Halothane, oxacillin, PAS, INH, allopurinol, E. estolate, TAO, CPZ, sulfonamides

resolution is expected within 1–2 weeks of discontinuation. Occasionally, drugs that produce severe portal inflammation may go on to a chronic active-like hepatitis and take a longer time to resolve. Certain other drugs (e.g., chlorpromazine) may lead to a chronic PBC-like syndrome, discussed in Chapter 20. Although inadvertent challenges with particular agents do occur, purposefully rechallenging a patient with a drug is generally not performed because of the risk of producing subsequent injury that is more severe than the initial insult. Rechallenge is often unnecessary if an alternative therapeutic agent is available for the clinical situation. Nevertheless, rechallenge testing may be warranted in situations in which no equally efficacious substitute agent is available when ongoing therapy is mandatory. In general, it is considered much safer to rechallenge with agents that produce cholestatic injury than with drugs that produce hepatocellular injury. Agents associated with hypersensitivity reactions will often exhibit a flamboyant response to a challenge dose. By contrast, drugs acting through metabolic idiosyncracy may fail to react promptly to a challenge dose, and the response may be relatively meager.

Although some investigators have identified serum markers that may predict injury (e.g., the cholestatic factor identified by Mizoguchi et al.,[115] increased release of glutathione transferase,[116] and the presence of liver–kidney microsonal antibodies[117] with halothane), the diagnosis of drug-induced hepatic injury remains largely one of clinical suspicion. While morphologic patterns of injury have been identified for most agents, histologic changes for many drugs and chemical agents are nonspecific, and biopsies are generally performed only to provide information about the severity of the injury and to provide additional clues as to etiology.

9. PROGNOSIS AND TREATMENT OF ACUTE DRUG-INDUCED HEPATIC INJURY

Treatment of acute drug-induced liver injury is generally one of supportive care. The use of *N*-acetylcysteine to prevent or ameliorate hepatic injury due to acetaminophen overdose is well known. Unfortunately, such specific therapy exists only for a handful of other hepatotoxic drugs. Corticosteroids are often used, especially in cases of severe injury, although their benefit is of questionable value. Most authorities see little rationale for the use of cortosteroids, even in the face of fulminant injury.[1,110]

The decision to discontinue a potential hepatotoxin must also take into account the risk of continuing the medication. In the case of isoniazid, for example, approximately 10% of recipients will show the development of aminotransferase elevations that do not progress.[25,26] In only 1% of recipients will overt hepatitis develop, with the remainder developing tolerance to the effects of the medication. In some cases, the enzyme abnormality resolves despite continuation of therapy. Amiodarone produces enzyme elevations in approximately 25% of recipients, but overt injury in only approximately 1% of cases.[118] However, when amiodarone is discontinued because of organ toxicity, the possibility of sudden death due to a cardiac event is a legitimate concern.

The case fatality rate for acute drug-induced hepatocellular injury with jaundice ranges from 10 to 50%, depending on the agent (Table XV). Death is generally the result of acute or subacute hepatic necrosis leading to liver failure. Nonfatal cases often show regression of jaundice and biochemical abnormalities in a fashion similar to that observed for viral hepatitis (i.e., values decline to approximately 25% of their peak after 3 weeks).[1] Recovery is complete in most patients who survive, although the development of chronic active hepatitis (CAH)-like injury may occur with a few agents, and recovery from cholestasis injury may be prolonged (see Chapter 20). Case fatality rates for agents causing microvesicular steatosis (e.g., tetracycline, valproic acid) are also in the range of that for hepatocellular injury.[1] Acute cholestatic hepatitis rarely results in fatal injury. The one notable exception would appear to be the injury associated with benoxaprofen (Oraflex).[59] The paradoxically high case fatality rate for this cholestatic compound was surprising and led to the suggestion that death was not due to liver failure but to associated renal failure and other generalized effects of the agent.[10]

Table XV. Mortality from Acute Drug-Induced Hepatotoxicity

Type of injury	Mortality
Hepatocellular jaundice (INH, halothane, DPH ketoconazole, methyldopa, ticrynafen)	10–50%
Toxic steatosis (tetracycline, VPA)	Increased
Subclinical (trivial) enzyme elevations (many agents)	Nil
Cholestatic hepatitis (CPZ, E. estolate, benoxoprofen[a])	<1%
Pure cholestasis (C_{17}-alkylated, steroids)	Nil
Mixed injury	Variable

[a]Mortality likely due to other factors.

10. MONITORING FOR HEPATOTOXICITY

Monitoring for drug-induced hepatic injury may take one of several forms (Table XVI). Instructing the patient to be aware of symptoms of possible hepatic injury, such as anorexia, nausea, vomiting, fatigue, dark urine, or jaundice, is an insensitive approach to detect early hepatic injury.[1] Generally, by the time that such symptoms are present, significant injury will already have occurred. Nevertheless, in the case of INH prophylaxis, in patients <35 years the American Thoracic Society (ATS) and the Centers for Disease Control (CDC) call only for the monitoring of symptoms.[119] Although it is assumed that monitoring for ALT elevations might detect injury at an earlier date (depending on the frequency of monitoring), biochemical monitoring for younger INH recipients is not encouraged by the ATS and other responsible organizations due in part to the lack of cost–benefit data. However, whenever symptoms suggest INH toxicity, the drug is stopped and hepatic enzymes are obtained for confirmation. ALT values that exceed 100 IU/liter in an asymptomatic patient seem useful to call for a reevaluation of the need for INH therapy, especially in cases in which it is being used prophylactically. If it is elected to continue INH, biochemical monitoring should be performed more frequently and the drug stopped if the enzyme elevation progresses.

While not the endorsed standard of practice for all INH recipients, biochemical monitoring is nonetheless recommended for a number of other medications as outlined in their respective package inserts[120] (Table XVI). Monitoring AST levels is not thought to be as useful as ALT in most situations, owing to the high prevalence of concomitant alcohol ingestion in many segments of the population, and the fact that alcohol frequently leads to increased AST values. By contrast, ALT is generally unaffected by alcohol use.[121,122]

The frequency with which liver-associated enzymes are obtained is often rather arbitrarily determined. In the case of lovastatin, which has been associated with persistent elevations in aminotransferase values more than threefold the upper limit of normal in 2% of adult patients, the manufacturer recommends that aminotransferase values be performed every 4–6 weeks during the first 15 months of therapy and periodically thereafter in all patients. The drug should be discontinued if elevations exceed three times the upper limits of normal, and liver biopsy should be considered if elevations persist after the drug is discontinued. The manufacturer also suggests that active liver disease or unexplained aminotransferase elevations contraindicate the use of lovastatin, and it should be used with caution in patients who are alcoholic.

Aminotransferase elevations should be measured before initiating therapy with ketoconazole; the manufacturer recommends monitoring at monthly (or even more frequent) intervals during

Table XVI. Monitoring Recommendations for Selected Potential Hepatotoxic Drugs[a]

Agent	Recommendation
INH	Monitor for prodromal symptoms of hepatitis[b] (if present, proceed with biochemical testing)
Chlorpromazine	
Allopurinol	
Phenytoin	
	Biochemical testing[c]
Lovastatin	q4–6wk × 15 mo
Ketoconazole	q4–6wk during Tx
Valproic acid	Frequently × 6 mo at appropriate interval
Dantrolene	
Rifampicin	Mandatory periodically
Amiodarone	On a regular basis
Cyclosporin	Assessed repeatedly
Methyldopa	During first 6–12 wk
Tetracycline	Periodically during long-term use
Nitrofurantoin	Periodically
Chenodeoxycholate	Periodically
Dapsone	Periodically
Methotrexate	Periodic liver biopsy (as indicated)

[a]Manufacturer's recommendations as given in 1987 *PDR*.
[b]Weakness, malaise, anorexia, nausea, vomting, fatigue (lymphadenopathy, fever, rash for DPH; FUO for methyldopa).
[c]Generally includes serum aminotransferases with or without alkaline phosphatase, bilirubin.

treatment. The drug should be discontinued if enzyme abnormalities persist or worsen and certainly if they are accompanied by symptoms suggestive of acute hepatic injury. Similarly, enzymes should be monitored on a regular basis for patients receiving ≥400 mg of amiodarone daily. The manufacturer recommends considering dosage reduction or discontinuing amiodarone entirely if serum aminotransferase values rise more than threefold or more than twofold in a patient with elevated baseline values. For many other drugs, monitoring at periodic intervals is the only guidance provided.

The third form of monitoring involves the periodic use of liver biopsy to predict, and ultimately to prevent, irreversible liver injury from agents such as methotrexate (MTX). When used chronically, MTX may lead to overt injury without accompanying aminotransferase or clinical abnormalities. As a result, intermittent low-dose treatment regimens have been devised to minimize toxicity, although pre- and post-treatment biopsies remain the best monitoring tool.[123]

11. HEPATOPROTECTION

A number of agents have been termed hepatoprotective for their protective effects against various hepatotoxins[124] (Table XVII). Perhaps the best known is *N*-acetylcysteine (Mucomyst), used in the prevention or amelioration of severe liver injury from acetaminophen overdose. In animal models, pretreatment with cimetidine has protected against injury from acetaminophen by a mechanism assumed to be inhibition by cimetidine of cytochrome P450 oxidation.[48,125] As a result, it is assumed that the production of reactive acetaminophen metabolites is inhibited, or at least

Table XVII. Potential Hepatoprotective Agents[a]

Protector	Mechanism	Hepatotoxin
N-Acetylcysteine	GSH	ACM
Cimetidine	Inhibits P450 oxidation	ACM, INH, CCl_4 halothane, cocaine
Prostaglandin E_2	Membrane stabilizer; maintain Ca^{2+} homeo.; enhanced regeneration; inc. GSH synthesis?	BMBZ, ANIT, CCl_4, ACM, galactosamine
Tocopherol	Radical scavenger?	CCl_4, galactosamine
Threonine	Promotes repair processes?	Valproate
Propylthiouracil	Acts as nucleophile	CCl_4, ACM, ETOH?
BHA	Induces GSH S-transferases	CCl_4, carcinogens

[a]ACM, acetaminophen; BHA, 2(3)-*t*-butyl-4-hydroxyanisole; BMBZ, bromobenzene; ETOH, ethanol.

reduced. However, in human volunteers given therapeutic doses of acetaminophen, cimetidine[126] (like ranitidine[127]), has had little or no effect on acetaminophen metabolism, and no controlled trials have been attempted to assess the clinical efficacy of cimetidine in an actual acetaminophen overdose in human subjects.[48] Cimetidine cannot be recommended for use by itself, given the wide availability and proven efficacy of *N*-acetylcysteine. Whether cimetidine can be used adjunctively remains to be determined. In one experimental animal study, the combination of *N*-acetylcysteine plus cimetidine was more protective than either drug alone.[128]

Other potential hepatoprotective agents include prostaglandins that act as membrane stabilizers, maintain calcium homeostasis within the cell, enhance cellular regeneration, and possibly increase glutathione synthesis.[129] Free radical scavengers, such as tocopherol, are also being studied. Propylthiouracil (PTU) acts as a protective nucleophile in cases of experimental carbon tetrachloride and acetaminophen hepatotoxicity.[124] Its role in alcoholic hepatitis remains controversial.[130,131] BHA (2,3-*t*-butyl-4-hydroxyanisole) induces glutathione *S*-transferases and DT-diaphorase in mice and has been used to protect against various carcinogens and carbon tetrachloride experimentally.[124] A number of amino acids are thought to promote repair processes within the cell. Threonine, for example, has been shown to reduce the hepatotoxicity of valproic acid in a rat model.[132] The potential clinical value of any of these investigative hepatoprotective substances in the clinical setting remains to be established.

REFERENCES

1. Zimmerman HJ: Hepatotoxicity. The Adverse Effects of Drugs and Other Chemicals on the Liver. Appleton-Century-Crofts, New York, 1978.
2. Zimmerman HJ, Maddrey WC: Toxic and drug-induced hepatitis, in Schiff L, Schiff ER (eds): *Diseases of the Liver,* 6th ed. JB Lippincott, Philadelphia, 1987, pp. 591–668.
3. Zimmerman HJ, Ishak KG: Hepatic injury due to drugs and toxins, in MacSween RNM, Anthony PP, Scheuer PJ (eds): *Pathology of the Liver.* Churchill Livingstone, Edinburgh, 1979, pp. 335–386.
4. Stricker BHC, Spoelstra P: *Drug-Induced Hepatic Injury.* Elsevier, Amsterdam, 1985.
5. Wade HJ, Frazer ES: Toxipathic hepatitis due to Fowler's solution: A case treated with dimercaprol. *Lancet* **1**:269–271, 1953.
6. Defalque RJ: The first delayed chloroform poisoning. *Anesth Analg* **47**:374–382, 1968.
7. Zimmerman HJ: Clinical and laboratory manifestations of hepatotoxicity. *Ann NY Acad Sci* **104**:954–987, 1963.

8. Dujovne CA, Chan CH, Zimmerman HJ: Sulfonamide hepatic injury. Review of the literature and report of a case due to sulfamethoxazole. *N Engl J Med* **277**:785–788, 1967.
9. Favreau M, Tannenbaum H, Lough J: Hepatotoxicity associated with gold therapy. *Ann Intern Med* **87**:717–719, 1977.
10. Zimmerman HJ, Lewis JH: Drug-induced cholestasis. *Med Tox* **2**:112–160, 1987.
11. Selye H: On the toxicity of estrogens with special reference to diethylstilbestrol. *Can Med Assoc J* **41**:48–49, 1939.
12. Hanger FM Jr, Gutman AB: Post-arsphenamine jaundice. *JAMA* **115**:263–271, 1940.
13. Bassan H, Kendler J, Harinasuta U, Zimmerman HJ: Effects of an anabolic steroid (Norbolethone) on the function of the isolated perfused rat liver. *Biochem Pharmacol* **20**:1429–1435, 1971.
14. Gargill SL, Lesses MF: Toxic reactions to thiouracil. Report of cases with one fatality. *JAMA* **127**:890–891, 1945.
15. Hopen G, Nesthuss I, Laerum OD: Fatal carbamazepine-associated hepatitis. Report of two cases. *Acta Med Scand* **210**:333–335, 1981.
16. Simpson DG, Walker JH: Hypersensitivity to para-aminosalicylic acid. *Am J Med* **29**:297–306, 1960.
17. Zetzel L, Kaplan H: Liver damage concurrent with iproniazid administration. *N Engl J Med* **258**:1209–1212, 1958.
18. Rosenblum LE, Korn RJ, Zimmerman HJ: Hepatocellular jaundice as a complication of iproniazid therapy. *Arch Intern Med* **105**:583–593, 1960.
19. Benjamin SB, Ishak KG, Zimmerman HJ, Grushka A: Phenylbutazone liver injury: A clinical-pathologic survey of 23 cases and review of the literature. *Hepatology* **1**:255–263, 1981.
20. Zimmerman HJ: Hepatotoxic effects of oncotherapeutic agents. *Prog Liver Dis* **8**:621–642, 1986.
21. Abernathy CO, Lukacs L, Zimmerman HJ: Toxicity of tricyclic antidepressants to isolated rat hepatocytes. *Biochem Pharmacol* **24**:347–350, 1975.
22. Zimmerman HJ, Lewis JH: Hepatic toxicity of antimicrobial agents, in Root RK, Sande MA (eds): *New Dimensions in Antimicrobial Therapy*. Churchill Livingstone, New York, 1984, pp. 153–202.
23. Goldstein LI, Ishak KG: Hepatic injury associated with penicillin therapy. *Arch Pathol Lab Med* **98**:114–117, 1974.
24. Johnson DA, Cattau EL Jr, Kuritsky JN, Zimmerman HJ: Liver involvement in the sulfone syndrome. *Arch Intern Med* **148**:875–877, 1986.
25. Black M, Mitchell JR, Zimmerman HJ, et al: Isoniazid-associated hepatitis in 114 patients. *Gastroenterology* **69**:289–302, 1975.
26. Mitchell JR, Zimmerman HJ, Ishak KG, et al: Isoniazid liver injury; clinical spectrum, pathology, and probable pathogenesis. *Ann Intern Med* **84**:181–192, 1976.
27. Benjamin SB, Goodman ZD, Ishak KS, et al: The morphologic spectrum of halothane-induced hepatic injury: Analysis of 77 cases. *Hepatology* **5**:1163–1171, 1985.
28. Zimmerman HJ, Kendler J, Libber S: Studies on the in vitro cytotoxicity of erythromycin estolate. *Proc Soc Exp Biol Med* **144**:759–761, 1973.
29. Sharp JR, Ishak KG, Zimmerman HJ: Chronic active hepatitis and severe hepatic necrosis associated with nitrofurantoin. *Ann Intern Med* **92**:14–19, 1980.
30. Brown G, Zoidis J, Spring M: Hepatic damage during chlorpropamide therapy. *JAMA* **170**:2085–2088, 1959.
31. Powers BJ, Cattau EL Jr, Zimmerman HJ: Chlorzoxazone hepatotoxic reactions. An analysis of 21 identified or presumed cases. *Arch Intern Med* **146**:1183–1186, 1986.
32. Ishak KG: Hepatic lesions caused by anabolic and contraceptive steroids. *Semin Liver Dis* **1**:116–128, 1981.
33. Lewis JH, Tice HL, Zimmerman HJ: Budd–Chiari syndrome associated with oral contraceptive steroids. Review of treatment of 47 cases. *Dig Dis Sci* **28**:673–683, 1983.
34. Rodman JS, Deutch DJ, Gutman SI. Methyldopa hepatitis: A report of six cases and review of the literature. *Am J Med* **60**:941–948, 1976.
35. Abernathy CO, Lukacs L, Zimmerman HJ: Adverse effects of chlorpromazine metabolites on isolated hepatocytes. *Proc Soc Exp Biol Med* **155**:474–478, 1977.
36. Kendler J, Bowry S, Seeff LB, Zimmerman HJ: Effect of chlorpromazine on the function of the perfused isolated liver. *Biochem Pharmacol* **20**:2439–2445, 1971.
37. Ticktin HE, Zimmerman HJ: Hepatic dysfunction and jaundice in patients receiving triacetyloleandomycin. *N Engl J Med* **267**:964–968, 1962.

38. Mihas AA, Holley P, Koff RS, Hirschowitz BI: Fulminant hepatitis and lymphocyte sensitization due to propylthiouricil. *Gastroenterology* **70:**770–774, 1976.
39. Rotmensch HH, Yust I, Siegman-Igra Y, et al: Granulomatous hepatitis: A hypersensitivity response to procainamide. *Ann Intern Med* **89:**646–647, 1978.
40. Zimmerman HJ: Papaverine revisited as a hepatotoxin. *N* Engl J Med **281:**1364–1365, 1969.
41. Conn HO, Binder HJ, Orr HD: Ethionamide-induced hepatitis. A review with a report of an additional case. *Am Rev Respir Dis* **90:**542–552, 1964.
42. Harinasuta U, Zimmerman HJ: Diphenylhydantoin sodium hepatitis. *JAMA* **203:**1015–1018, 1968.
43. Reynolds TB, Peters RL, Yamada S: Chronic active and lupoid hepatitis caused by a laxative, oxyphenisatin. *N Engl J Med* **285:**813–820, 1971.
44. Zimmerman HJ: Aspirin-induced hepatic injury. *Ann Intern Med* **80:**74–76, 1974.
45. Joshi PH, Conn HO: The syndrome of methoxyflurane-associated hepatitis. *Ann Intern Med* **80:**395–401, 1974.
46. Zimmerman HJ: Effects of aspirin and acetaminophen on the liver. *Arch Intern Med* **141**(3 spec no): 333–342, 1981.
47. Seeff LB, Boccherini BA, Zimmerman HJ, et al: Acetaminophen hepatotoxicity in alcoholics. A therapeutic misadventure. *Ann Intern Med* **104:**399–404, 1986.
48. Lewis JH: Hepatic effects of drugs used in the treatment of peptic ulcer disease. *Am J Gastroenterol* **82:**987–1003, 1987.
49. Zimmerman HJ; Ishak KG: Valproate-induced hepatic injury: Analyses of 23 fatal cases. *Hepatology* **2:**591–597, 1982.
50. Lewis JH, Zimmerman HJ, Ishak KS, Mullick FG: Enflurane hepatotoxicity. A clinicopathologic study of 24 cases. *Ann Intern Med* **98:**984–992, 1983.
51. Al-Kawas FH, Seeff LB, Berendson RA, et al: Allopurinol hepatotoxicity. Report of two cases and review of the literature. *Ann Intern Med* **95:**588–590, 1981.
52. Pessary RED, Bichara M, Feldmann G, et al: Perhexaline maleate-induced cirrhosis. *Gastroenterology* **76:**170–177, 1979.
53. Bruckstein AH, Attia AA: Oxacillin hepatitis. Two patients with liver biopsy and review of the literature. *Am J Med* **64:**519–522, 1978.
54. Sotolongo RP, Neefe LI, Rudzki C, Ishak KG: Hypersensitivity reaction to sulfazalazine with severe hepatotoxicity. *Gastroenterology* **75:**95–99, 1978.
55. Utili R, Boitnott JK, Zimmerman HJ: Dantrolene-associated hepatic injury. Incidence and character. *Gastroenterology* **72:**810–816, 1977.
56. Abernathy CO, Utili R, Zimmerman HJ, Ezekiel M: The effects of dantrolene sodium on excretory function in the isolated perfused rat liver. *Toxicol Appl Pharmacol* **44:**441–453, 1978.
57. Pearson K, Zimmerman HJ: Danazol and liver damage. *Lancet* **1:**845–846, 1980.
58. Klein NC, Magida MG: Propoxyphene (Darvon) hepatotoxicity. *Am J Dig Dis* **16:**467–469, 1971.
59. Lewis JH: Hepatoxicity of non-steroidal anti-inflammatory drugs. *Clin Pharm* **3:**128–138, 1984.
60. Wood LJ, Mundo F, Searl J, Powell LW: Sulindac hepatotoxicity: Effects of acute and chronic exposure. *Aust NZ J Med* **15:**397–401, 1985.
61. Scheuer P, Summerfield JA, Lal S, Sherlock S: Rifampicin hepatitis: A clinical histological study. *Lancet* **1:**421–425, 1974.
62. Langan MN, Thomas P: Penicillamine-induced liver disease. *Am J Gastroenterol* **82:**130–131, 1987.
63. Knoblauch M, Cueni B, Spycher M, et al: Dehydralazin-induzurte, akute Hepatitis bei IgM-Mangel. *Schweiz Med Wochenschr* **107:**651–656, 1977.
64. Itoh S. Yamaba Y, Ichinoe A, Tsukuda Y: Hydralazine-induced liver injury. *Dig Dis Sci* **25:**884–887, 1980.
65. Fang MH, Ginsberg AL, Dobbins WO III: Cholestatic jaundice associated with flurazepam hydrochloride. *Ann Intern Med* **89:**363–364, 1978.
66. Mullick FG, Ishak KG, Mahabier R, et al: Hepatic injury associated with paraquat toxicity in humans. *Liver* **1:**209–221, 1981.
67. Zimmerman HJ, Jacob L, Bassan H, et al: Effects of H2-blocking agents on hepatocytes in vitro; correlation with potential for causing hepatic disease in patients. *Proc Soc Exp Biol Med* **182:**511–514, 1986.
68. Rahmat J, Gelfand RL, Gelfand MC, et al: Captopril-associated cholestatic jaundice. *Ann Intern Med* **102:**56–58, 1985.

69. Poucell S, Ireton J, Valencia-Mayoral P, et al: Amiodarone-associated phospholipidosis and fibrosis of the liver. Light, immunohistochemical, an electron microscopic studies. *Gastroenterology* **86:**926–936, 1984.
70. Zimmerman HJ, Abernathy CO, Lukacs L, Ezekiel M: Effects of ticrynasfen on hepatic excretory function in the isolated perfused rat liver. *Hepatology* **2:**255–257, 1982.
71. Zimmerman HJ, Lewis JH, Ishak KG, Maddrey WC: Ticrynafen-associated hepatic injury. Analysis of 340 cases. *Hepatology* **4:**315–323, 1984.
72. Lewis JH, Zimmerman HJ, Benson GD, Ishak KG: Hepatic injury associated with ketoconazole therapy. Analysis of 33 cases. *Gastroenterology* **86:**503–513, 1984.
73. Cohen DJ, Loertscher R, Rubin MF, et al: Cyclosporine: A new immunosuppressive agent for organ transplantation. *Ann Intern Med* **101:**667–682, 1984.
74. Zimmerman HJ. Chenodeoxycholic acid and the liver: good news–bad news. (Editorial.) *Hepatology* **2:**288–289, 1982.
75. Lovastatin for hypercholesterolemia. *Med Lett* **29:**99–101, 1987.
76. Richter WO, Schwandt P: Serious side effect of nifedipine. *Arch Intern Med* **147:**1852, 1987.
77. Adler E, Benjamin SB, Zimmerman HJ: Cholestatic hepatic injury related to warfarin exposure. *Arch Intern Med* **145:**1837–1839, 1986.
78. Brodsky SJ, Cutler SS, Weiner DA, Klein MD: Hepatotoxicity due to treatment with verapamil. *Ann Intern Med* **94:**490–491, 1981.
79. Simpson BR, Strunin L, Walton B: The halothane dilemma: A case for the defense. *Br Med J* **9:**96–100, 1971.
80. Eger EI II, Smuckler EA, Ferrell LD, et al: Is enflurane hepatoxic? *Anesth Analg* **65:**21–30, 1986.
81. Humphries TJ, Myerson RM, Gifford LM, et al: A unique postmarket out-patient surveillance program of cimetidine: report on phase II and final summary. *Am J Gastroenterol* **79:**593–596, 1984.
82. Rossi AC, Knapp DE, Anello C, et al: Discovery of adverse drug reactions: A comparison of selective phase IV studies with spontaneous reporting methods. *JAMA* **249:**2226–2228, 1983.
83. Faich GA, Knapp D, Dreis M, Turner W: National Adverse Drug Reaction Surveillance: 1985. *JAMA* **257:**2068–2070, 1987.
84. Dossing M, Buch Andreasen P: Drug-induced liver disease in Denmark. An analysis of 572 cases of hepatoxicity reported to the Danish Board of Adverse Reactions to Drugs. *Scand J Gastroenterol* **17:**205–211, 1982.
85. Koff RS, Gardner R, Harinasuta U, et al: Profile of hyperbilirubinemia in three hospital populations. *Clin Res.* **18:**680, 1970.
86. Miller RR: Hospital admissions due to adverse drug reactions. A report from the Boston Collaborative Drug Surveillance Program. *Arch Intern Med* **134:**219–223, 1974.
87. Eastwood HOH: Causes of jaundice in the elderly: A survey of diagnosis and investigation. *Geront Clin* **13:**69, 1971.
88. Graham GS: Chlorpromazine jaundice in a general hospital. *Br Med J* **2:**1080, 1957.
89. Shimano K: Drug-induced hepatic injury with special reference to antitubercular agents. *Acta Hepatol Jpn* **6**(suppl 74), 1965.
90. Trey C, Davidson CS: The management of fulminant hepatic failure, in Hopper H, Schaffner F (eds): *Progress in Liver Disease,* Vol. 3. Grune & Stratton, Orlando, Florida, 1970, pp. 282.
91. Caravati CM, Hooker TH: Acute massive hepatic necrosis with fatal hepatic failure. *Am J Dig Dis* **16:**803, 1971.
92. Rakela J, Lang SM, Ludwig J, Baldus WP: Fulminant hepatitis: Mayo Clinic experience with 34 cases. *Mayo Clin Proc* **60:**289–292, 1985.
93. Williams R, Gimson AES: An assessment of orthotopic liver transplantation in acute liver failure. *Hepatology* **4**(suppl)**:**22S–24S, 1984.
94. Bottiger LE, Furhoff AK, Holmberg L: Fatal reactions to drugs. A 10-year material from the Swedish Adverse Drug Reaction Committee. *Acta Med Scand* **205:**451–456, 1979.
95. Koff RS, Fitts JJ, Sabesin SM, Zimmerman HJ: D-galactosamine hepatotoxicity. II. Mechanism of fatty liver production. *Proc Soc Exp Biol Med* **138:**89–92, 1971.
96. Lullmann H, Lullmann-Rauch R, Wassermann O: Drug-induced phospholipidoses. *CRC Crit Rev Toxicol* **4:**185–218, 1975.
97. Simon JB, Manley PN, Brien JF, Armstrong PW: Amiodarone hepatotoxicity simulating alcoholic liver disease. *N Engl J Med* **311:**167–172, 1984.

98. Ranard RC, Lewis JH, Ragsdale BD, et al: Amiodarone hepatotoxicity: Histopathologic correlations. *Gastroenterology* **92:**1766, 1987.
99. Zimmerman HJ: Drug-induced liver disease. *Drugs* **16:**25–45, 1978.
100. Mitchell JR, Thorgeirsson UP, Black M, et al: Increased incidence of isoniazid hepatitis in rapid acetalators: Possible relation to hydrazine metabolites. *Clin Pharmacol Ther* **18:**70–79, 1975.
101. Jacqz E, Hall SD, Branch RA: Genetically determined polymorphisms in drug oxidation. *Hepatology* **6:**1020–1032, 1986.
102. Morgan NY, Reshef R, Shah RR, et al: Impaired oxidation of debrisoquine in patients with perhexiline liver injury. *Gut* **25:**1057–1064, 1984.
103. Hoft RH, Bunker JP, Goodman HI, Gregory PB: Halothane hepatitis in three pairs of closely related women. *N Engl J Med* **304:**123–124, 1981.
104. Farrell G, Prendergast D, Murray M: Halothane hepatitis. Detection of a constitutional susceptibility factor. *N Engl J Med* **313:**1310–1314, 1985.
105. Welch KI, Batchelor JR: HLA and drug reactions, in David M, Tredger JN, Williams R (eds): *Drug Reactions and the Liver.* Pittman Medical, London, 1981, pp. 111–117.
106. Hatoff DE, Cohen M, Schweigert BF, Talbert WM: Nitrofurantoin: Another cause of drug-induced chronic active hepatitis? *Am J Med* **67:**117–121, 1979.
107. Gran JT, Husby G, Thorsby E: HLA DR antigens and gold toxicity. *Ann Rheum Dis* **42:**63–66, 1983.
108. Zimmerman HJ: Effects of alcohol on other hepatotoxins. Alcoholism. *Clin Exp Res* **10:**3–15, 1986.
109. Aw TY, Hanna P, Petrini J, Kaplowitz N: Hepatic drug metabolism and drug-induced liver injury, in Gitnick G (ed): *Current Hepatology,* Vol. 5. Year Book, Chicago, 1985, pp. 113–196.
110. Kaplowitz N, Aw TY, Simon FR, Stolz A: Drug-induced hepatotoxicity. *Ann Intern Med* **104:**826–839, 1986.
111. Tribble DL, Aw TY, Jones DP: The pathophysiological significance of lipid peroxidation in oxidative cell injury. *Hepatology* **7:**377–387, 1987.
112. Davis M, Vergani D, Eddleston ALWF, Williams R: Halothane hepatitis-toxicity and immunity, in Eddleston ALWF, Weber JCP, Williams R (eds): *Immune Reactions in Liver Disease.* Pitman Medical, London, 1979, pp. 235–296.
113. Dienstag JL: Halothane hepatitis. Allergy or idiosyncracy? *N Engl J Med* **303:**102–104, 1980.
114. Vergani D, Mieli-Vergani G, Alberti A, et al: Antibodies to the surface of halothane-altered rabbit hepatocytes in patients with severe halothane-associated hepatitis. *N Engl J Med* **303:**66–71, 1980.
115. Mizoguchi Y, Ohnishi F, Monna T, et al: Studies on intrahepatic cholestasis induced in the rat by culture supernatant of activated lymphocytes. *Hepatogastroenterology* **28:**147–151, 1981.
116. Allan LG, Hussey AJ, Howie J, et al: Hepatic glutathione *S*-transferase release after halothane anaesthesia: Open randomised comparison with isoflurane. *Lancet* **1:**771–774, 1987.
117. Walton B, Simpson BR, Stunin L, et al: Unexplained hepatitis following halothane. *Br Med J* **1:**1171–1176, 1976.
118. Caruso AC, Ranard RC, Lewis JH, et al: Multi-organ toxicity associated with amiodarone-induced hepatic dysfunction. *Gastroenterology* **92:**1724, 1987.
119. American Thoracic Society: Treatment of tuberculosis and tuberculosis infection in adults and children. *Am Rev Respir Dis* **134:**355–363, 1986.
120. *Physicians Desk Reference,* 41st ed. Medical Economics, Oradell, New Jersey, 1987.
121. Harinasuta U, Chomet B, Ishak K, Zimmerman HJ: Steatonecrosis—Mallory body type. *Medicine (Baltimore)* **46**(2)**:**141–162, 1967.
122. Cohen JA, Kaplan MM: The SGOT/SGPT ratio—An indicator of alcoholic liver disease. *Dig Dis Sci* **24:**835–838, 1979.
123. Lewis JH, Schiff E. Methotrexate-induced chronic liver injury: guidelines for detection and prevention. *Am J Gastroenterol* **83**(12), 1988.
124. Kaplowitz N. Drug-induced hepatotoxicity, in Gitnick G (ed): *Current Hepatology,* Vol. 6. Year Book, Chicago, 1986, pp. 239–268.
125. Speeg KV Jr, Patwardhan RV, Avant Gr, et al: Inhibition of microsomal drug metabolism by histamine H2-receptor antagonists studied in vivo and in vitro in rodents. *Gastroenterology* **82:**84–88, 1982.
126. Vendemiale G, Altomare E, Trizio T, et al: Effect of acute and chronic cimetidine administration on acetaminophen metabolism in humans. *Am J Gastroenterol* **82:**131–134, 1987.
127. Jack, D, Thomas M, Skidmore IF: Ranitidine and paracetamol metabolism. *Lancet* **2:**1067, 1985.
128. Speeg KV, Mitchell MC, Maldonado AL: Additive protection of cimetidine and N-acetylcystaime treat-

ment against acetaminophen-induced hepatic necrosis in the rat. *J Pharmacol Exp Ther* **234:**550–554, 1985.

129. Burk RF: Hepatocytoprotective substances. *Gastroenterology* **81:**397–398, 1981.
130. Orrego H, Kalant K, Israel Y, et al: Effect of short-term therapy with propylthiouracil in patients with alcoholic liver disease. *Gastroenterology* **76:**105–115, 1979.
131. Orrego H, Blake JE, Blendis LM, et al: Long-term treatment of alcoholic liver disease with propylthiouracil. *N Engl J Med* **317:**1421–1427, 1987.
132. Lewis JH, Zimmerman HJ, Garrett CT, Marcus JA: Threonine protects against hepatic injury due to valproic acid in rats. *Gastroenterology* **88:**1675, 1985.

20

Chronic Drug-Induced Hepatotoxicity: Clinical Aspects

Martin Black

1. INTRODUCTION

It is a special privilege to contribute a discussion of one aspect of drug hepatotoxicity that is well recognized as having been a major interest of Dr. Zimmerman for much of his professional life. Dr. Zimmerman suspected, and argued without much early success, in favor of the primacy of biochemical events in mediating certain forms of drug hepatotoxicity at a time when the prevailing wisdom focused on the importance of (largely unsubstantiated) immune mechanisms. While observations over the past decade have generally supported Dr. Zimmerman's views, the area of chronic drug-induced hepatotoxicity is one in which supporting data for the role of biochemical events in mediating such injury remain elusive.

The issue of chronic drug-induced hepatotoxicity embraces a wide spectrum of liver injury, including the disorders shown in Table I. This discussion concentrates on drug-induced chronic necroinflammatory disorders of the liver that are manifested clinically as instances of chronic active hepatitis (CAH) and/or cirrhosis. The subject is rich in anecdotal observations, yet soft on objective scientific data.

2. DRUGS CAUSING A LUPOID FORM OF CHRONIC HEPATITIS

2.1. Oxyphenisatin

The first medication suspected of causing chronic active hepatitis in humans was oxyphenisatin (Fig 1), a compound widely used for many years in laxative preparations in the United States and Europe. Two U.S. groups published reports simultaneously in 1970,[1,2] identifying a total of six female patients with a "moderately severe illness" characterized by fatigue, abdominal complaints, variable jaundice, marked abnormalities of liver-function tests [often including aspartate transaminase (AST) and alanine transaminase (ALT) values of greater than 100 IU/liter], hypergammaglobulinemia, and (in three patients) liver biopsy appearances of portal tract inflammation and hepatocellular necrosis. In each case, onset of disease followed 6–18 months ingestion of Dialose

Martin Black • Liver Unit, Temple University School of Medicine, Philadelphia, Pennsylvania 19140.

Table I. Partial Listing of Forms of Liver Disease Resulting from Long-Term Drug Therapy[a]

Veno-occlusive disease of the liver (e.g., pyrrolizidine alkaloids, azathioprine)
Oncogenic effects
Benign
Hepatic adenoma, FNH (e.g., estrogens)
Malignant
Hepatoma (e.g., androgenic/anabolic steroids, estrogens, thorotrast)
Hepatoblastoma (e.g., estrogens)
Angiosarcoma (e.g., thorotrast, arsenic, vinyl chloride)
Porphyrias (PCT and AIP) (e.g., hexachlorobenzene, estrogens)
Sclerosing cholangitis (e.g., FUDR via hepatic artery infusion)
Primary biliary cirrhosis (AMA negative, e.g., sulfonylureas)
Peliosis hepatis (e.g., androgenic/anabolic steroids)
Periportal sinusoidal dilation (e.g., estrogens)
Noncirrhotic portal hypertension (e.g., arsenic, vinyl chloride)

[a]Excluding chronic active hepatitis with or without cirrhosis.
[b]AIP, acute intermittent porphyria; AMA, antimitochondrial antibody; FNH, focal nodular hyperplasia; FUDR, floxuridine; PCT, porphyria cutanea tarda.

Plus, a popular laxative preparation containing oxyphenisatin. Discontinuation of laxative ingestion led to remission of liver disease, and restarting the medication in several of the patients resulted in temporary worsening of the disease.

Publication of these reports was not universally hailed. An accompanying editorial[3] by the AMA Department of Drugs "deplored the current tendency to deprive the medical profession and the public of useful chemicals, pharmaceuticals or otherwise, that is sometimes done for inadequate or even frivolous reasons "and indicated that the editorial had been prepared without relish." In making such ill-conceived and inappropriate comments, the editorialists sided with the halothane apologists[4] and with other groups anxious to minimize serious toxicities from popular medications.

Following publication of the reports by Reynolds et al.[1] and McHardy and Balart[2] additional cases were identified in the United States,[5] United Kingdom,[6] Australia,[7] and Norway.[8] Oxyphenisatin was withdrawn from Dialose Plus and from most other proprietary laxative preparations in the United States, Australia, and Europe. Nevertheless, the possibility needs to be entertained that preparations containing oxyphenisatin might still be commercially available in countries that do not have strict regulations on pharmaceuticals.

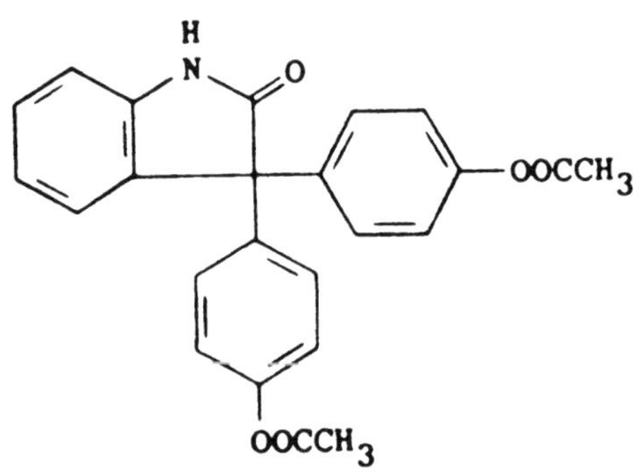

Figure 1. Structure of oxyphenisatin acetate.

2.2. α-Methyldopa

The next commonly used medication to become associated with CAH was α-methyldopa (Aldomet). Although sporadic reports of acute hepatotoxicity from α-methyldopa had appeared during the 1960s,[9,10] Goldstein et al.[11] in Australia and Hoyumpa and Connell[12] in the United States were among the first to associate prolonged use of this drug with instances of CAH. Duration of therapy prior to recognition of severe liver damage varied from several weeks to many months and years, and laboratory abnormalities were prominent with serum transaminases in the several hundreds to 1000 IU/liter. Substantial hyperglobulinemia was often present, and antinuclear antibodies (ANA) and smooth muscle antibodies (SMA) were often detected.[13] Liver biopsy appearances showed marked hepatocellular injury with prominent mononuclear inflammation of portal areas and moderate fibrosis. Biochemical improvement was rapid following termination of drug therapy, but hyperglobulinemia and the presence of circulating antibodies tended to resolve much more slowly.

2.3. Nitrofurantoin

A form of CAH closely simulating the spontaneously occurring lupoid form of chronic active hepatitis was identified during the 1970s in many patients on long-term therapy with nitrofurantoin.[14-17] The great majority of these patients were Scandinavian residents, but a small number of residents in the United States were also identified as having this problem.[18] Whether this disparity reflected a special susceptibility of Scandinavians to this complication of nitrofurantoin therapy or whether it reflected better recognition of the problem or even regional differences in the way nitrofurantoin was used is unknown. The exclusive predilection for females is likely to have reflected the more common occurrence of recurrent urinary tract infections (UTI) in female patients and their more frequent use of long-term nitrofurantoin.

Patients with nitrofurantoin-induced CAH typically presented after more than 6 months therapy and manifested characteristic clinical, laboratory, and histopathologic features of CAH. In addition, in many instances considerable hypergammaglobulinemia and high titers of serum ANA and/or SMA were noted. In this respect, the disease might have been interpreted as lupoid CAH were it not for the history of nitrofurantoin ingestion. Termination of drug therapy, without utilization of corticosteroids, customarily led to remission of the disease and long-term recovery.

Nitrofurantoin hepatotoxicity was occasionally associated with drug-related pulmonary injury. Some of the patients reported to have nitrofurantoin-induced CAH were noted to have radiologic evidence of (usually) bilateral pulmonary infiltrates without experiencing significant pulmonary symptoms.[14,15] Histopathologic examination of lung biopsy material[19,20] has revealed interstitial fibrosis and inflammation and alveolar epithelial changes. Discontinuation of nitrofurantoin therapy in these patients led to resolution of the pulmonary changes. In a few patients evidence of pulmonary involvement secondary to nitrofurantoin therapy was observed in the absence of signs of hepatotoxicity, but with equally high titers of ANA and SMA.[21]

A representative patient treated by the author is depicted in Table II. This 56-year-old woman was diagnosed as suffering from CAH 1 year after being placed on daily nitrofurantoin therapy for recurrent UTI. The possible etiologic role of nitrofurantoin was not considered, and the drug was continued. No other therapy was initiated for the CAH. One year later, a routine chest roetgenogram was obtained (in the absence of pulmonary symptoms), and a bilateral interstitial infiltrate was identified. The patient was admitted to hospital for further investigation and transbronchial biopsy. The latter test demonstrated a diffuse interstitial fibrosis with a prominent mononuclear infiltrate. Consideration was now given to the possible involvement of the nitrofurantoin in both the lung and liver processes, and the drug was discontinued. Improvement in both processes followed, without other drug intervention. This experience confirmed the validity of the Scandinavian reports and, incidentally, pointed out the lack of familiarity with this literature of otherwise knowledgeable U.S.

Table II. Clinical Features and Course of Patient

56-year-old woman with onset of fatigue and exhaustion 18 months after starting nitrofurantoin (100 mg day)
Abnormal liver-function tests led to liver biopsy, which showed typical chronic active hepatitis
No treatment offered, nitrofurantoin continued
One year later, reevaluated because of abnormal CXR
Lung biopsy: nonspecific interstitial fibrosis and chronic inflammation with alveolar lining hyperplasia
S. bilirubin 0.7 mg/dl, alk phos 4 fold incr, AST 79, ALT 49 alb. 4.3, gamma glob 3.1, SMA 1:40, ANA 1:640
Liver biopsy: chronic active hepatitis
Cessation of nitrofurantoin resulted in resolution of LFT abnormalities, CXR, and slow decline in ANA

internists. It also confirmed that protracted nitrofurantoin therapy is associated with unacceptable toxicity and should be avoided where possible or followed very closely (routine laboratory testing and chest roentgenograms) when absolutely required.

The mechanism of liver injury from nitrofurantoin is unknown. It is also uncertain as to whether the mechanism of acute liver injury differs from that involved in production of CAH. The relationship between either form of liver injury and pulmonary injury is equally obscure. While there is experimental evidence that furan compounds are capable of producing hepatic necrosis in mice[22] and are cytotoxic to mammalian cells,[23] the relevance of these observations to human events is unproved. The prominent hypergammaglobulinemia and high-titer circulating antibodies lent credence to the possible involvement of immunologic processes, as did an observation on positive lymphocyte transformation (in an in vitro assay employing the patients' lymphocytes, autologous plasma, and a range of concentrations of nitrofurantoin[18]) demonstrated early in the course (but not several months later) of one patient with nitrofurantoin-induced CAH. Although such a mechanism cannot presently be ruled out, it seems likely that the hypergammaglobulinemia and antibody formation represent epiphenomena and are not directly related to the liver cell necrosis.

3. DRUGS CAUSING A MILD FORM OF CAH

In light of the particular features of CAH resulting from oxyphenisatin, α-methyldopa, and nitrofurantoin, there may be merit in separating them from other causes of drug-induced chronic progressive parenchymal liver disease, such as that resulting from isoniazid, acetaminophen, and methotrexate (Table III). Oxyphenisatin, α-methyldopa, and nitrofurantoin cause a form of CAH that closely resembles the lupoid form, with its prominent laboratory abnormalities, hypergammaglobulinemia, high-titer ANA and SMA, and other features. Such drugs as isoniazid, acetaminophen, and methotrexate (MTX) cause CAH with few of these associated epiphenomena. An additional group of drugs produces a form of CAH that histopathologically resembles alcoholic liver disease (see discussion of perhexilene hepatotoxicity). Thus, it is convenient in the present state of knowledge to subdivide drug-induced chronic active hepatitis as shown in Table III. It should be recognized, however, that the mechanism of hepatotoxicity with most of the drugs listed remains unknown, and the particular listing should not be interpreted as implying anything regarding mechanism of injury.

Table III. Classification of Drug-Induced Chronic Active Hepatitis with or without Cirrhosis

CAH		Alcoholic hepatitis-like with or without cirrhosis (phospholipidosis)	Silent cirrhosis
Lupoid form	Mild form		
Gamma globulins, pos. ANA, SMA	Lesser increased AST, ALT, normal gamma globulins, neg. ANA, SMA		
Oxyphenisatin	INH	Amiodarone	Methotrexate
Aldomet	Acetaminophen	Perhexilene	
Nitrofurantoin	Halothane, sulfonamides, propylthiouracil		

3.1. Isoniazid

Isoniazid is typically regarded as a drug that causes acute hepatotoxicity rather than a CAH or cirrhosis. Nevertheless, in a study in which I was fortunate enough to work closely with Dr. Zimmerman,[24] we submitted to our colleague, Dr. Kamal Ishak, available biopsy material from 34 patients who were suspected of having acute isoniazid hepatotoxicity. In four of these patients, review of the biopsies revealed changes that were considered typical of CAH. Others[25] have also reported on similar findings.

3.2. Acetaminophen

Similarly, acetaminophen is better known for its acute hepatotoxicity than for chronic disorders. However, it, too, has been associated with induction of a chronic form of hepatitis in a handful of patients.[26] Of much greater concern is the accumulating evidence that its hepatotoxic properties are greatly potentiated by concomitant alcohol ingestion.[27] Patients have been described as having developed severe acute liver injury with minor doses of acetaminophen while simultaneously abusing alcohol. It is the author's opinion[28] that the reported cases represent the "tip of the iceberg" for such events in the United States. The probability must be considered, therefore, that less florid examples of liver injury that escape clinical recognition carry the potential of causing progressive liver damage in the alcoholic patient.

4. DRUGS CAUSING CIRRHOSIS

4.1. Methotrexate

Production of cirrhosis by the long-term administration of MTX has been recognized since the late 1960s[29,30] and led to the creation of an international group of scientists to evaluate the issue.[31,32] Patients with severe psoriasis comprised the major group considered at risk from this problem, reflecting the increasing use of long-term oral MTX therapy in management of such patients. The development of fibrosis and cirrhosis was typically unaccompanied by symptoms or laboratory abnormalities and pointed up the need for routine interval liver biopsies to identify liver damage. Factors found to be significantly associated with MTX-induced liver damage included increased alcohol intake, dose of drug given, frequency of administration, obesity, and diabetes mellitus. More recently, use of oral MTX to treat rheumatoid (and psoriatic) arthritis has expanded the patient groups at risk. It is recommended that any patient undergoing prolonged oral MTX therapy be considered at risk of developing severe hepatotoxicity and undergo interval liver biopsy to identify important injury before it evolves into a fully developed cirhosis.[33] The mechanism of the hepatotoxicity from MTX is unknown.

5. DRUGS CAUSING PHOSPHOLIPIDOSIS

A novel form of chronic liver disease resulting from drugs has been described in recent years. The histopathologic appearances of the liver closely simulate alcoholic hepatitis and cirrhosis, thereby representing an additional entity to be considered in the differential diagnosis of steatohepatitis syndrome.[34] The two drugs most often associated with this change have been perhexilene and amiodarone, but the author has also observed a case following allopurinol ingestion (M. Black and L. Rabin, unpublished observations).

Amiodarone is a new antiarrhythmic medication that has enjoyed more prolonged use in Europe, Canada, and elsewhere than the United States. Most North American reports on its hepatotoxicity, therefore, come from Canada,[35,36] although one group in the United States has recently published its experience with the entity.[37] The drug is characterized by unusual physicochemical properties that cause it to become deposited in certain tissues for prolonged periods of time and are asociated with an extraordinarily prolonged half-life.[38] It has shown a broad spectrum of toxicity,[39,40] including alterations in thyroid function, eye toxicity, skin rashes, pulmonary fibrosis, and neuromuscular abnormalities, in addition to its hepatotoxicity.

Amiodarone hepatotoxicity typically presents after more than 6 months therapy with evidence of progressive liver failure. Ascites and jaundice are common, and the liver is usually enlarged. Laboratory abnormalities are modest in nature, but significant hyperbilirubinemia may be documented relatively early in the course. Withdrawal of the drug does not lead to a rapid reversal of the hepatic disease (not surprising in view of the properties of amiodarone), and a significant mortality has been reported. The mechanism of injury is unknown and appears to be independent of the ability of the drug to cause a secondary phospholipidosis.

Hepatotoxicity from perhexilene resembles that of amiodarone but with an interesting aspect that Dr. Zimmerman would surely appreciate. It, too, is an antiarrhythmic agent that enjoys reasonable use in Europe but is not available in North America. Hepatotoxicity customarily occurs after greater than 6 months therapy, and presentation, laboratory features, and liver histology are similar to those reported with amiodarone. There is also a substantial mortality rate.[41]

The interest of perhexilene hepatotoxicity lies in regard to its pathogenesis. Recent studies[42] have shown a particular susceptibility to this side effect of perhexilene therapy in a group of patients characterized as being poor hydroxylators of the antihypertensive medication, debrisoquine. The debrisoquine polymorphism (which relates to the 4-hydroxylation of debrisoquine[43]) has been much investigated in Europe in the decade since its original description, but it is still something of a mystery to U.S. physicians (debrisoquine is not available in the United States). It has been found to affect 5–10% of the population[44] and influences the outcome of therapy with debrisoquine, nortryptiline, encainide, and so forth, as well as perhexilene. Investigators have identified the specific cytochrome P450 in human liver responsible for this metabolic event.[45] Success in tying perhexilene hepatotoxicity to an inherited alteration of drug metabolism clearly strengthens the likelihood that biochemical factors play a decisive role in predisposing patients to this form of drug hepatotoxicity. Nevertheless, the actual biochemical basis remains unknown.

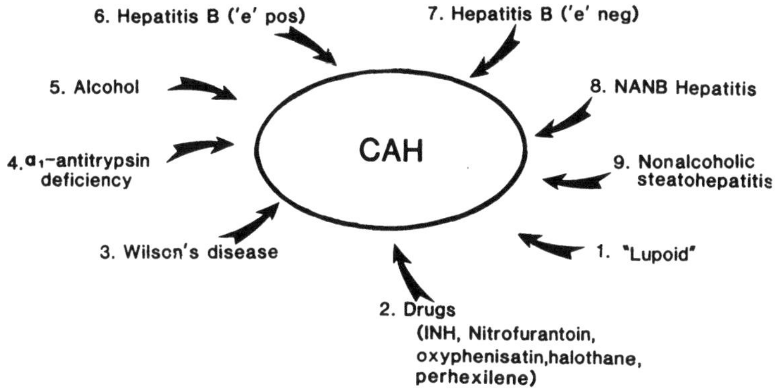

Figure 2. Etiology of chronic active hepatitis.

6. CONCLUSIONS

Increasing recognition of the ability of certain drugs to produce chronic forms of parenchymal liver disease greatly expands the spectrum of drug hepatotoxicity encountered with commonly used medications. Furthermore, appreciation of this phenomenon requires the practicing clinician to consider a possible drug etiology in patients identified with chronic active hepatitis and/or cirrhosis. As shown in Fig. 2, the etiologic basis for such forms of liver disease has become much more complex than was recognized just a decade ago.

REFERENCES

1. Reynolds TB, Lapin AC, Peters RL, Yamahiro HS: Puzzling jaundice. Probable relationship to laxative ingestion. *JAMA* **211**:86–90, 1970.
2. McHardy G, Balart LA: Jaundice and oxyphenisatin. *JAMA* **211**:83–85, 1970.
3. Anon: Jaundice from oxyphenisatin acetate. *JAMA* **211**:114, 1970.
4. Simpson BR, Strunin L, Walton B: Evidence for halothane hepatotoxicity is equivocal, in Ingelfinger FJ, Ebert RV, Finland M, Relman AS (eds): *Controversy in Internal Medicine*, Vol. 11. WB Saunders, Philadelphia, 1974, pp. 580–594.
5. Mallory A, Frank BW, Kern F Jr: Oxyphenisatin and chronic active hepatitis. *N Eng J Med* **285**:1266, 1971.
6. Pearson AJG, Grainger JM, Scheuer PJ, Mc Intyre N: Jaundice due to oxyphenisatin. *Lancet* **1**:994–996, 1971.
7. Willing RL, Hecker R: Oxyphenisatin and liver damage. *Med J Aust* **58**:1179–1182, 1971.
8. Gjone E. Blomhoff JP, Ritland S, Elgjo K, Husby G: Laxative-induced chronic liver disease. *Scand J Gastroenterol* **7**:395–402, 1971.
9. Zarday Z, Rosenthal WS, Wolff FW: Severe liver toxicity after methyldopa. *NY State J Med* **67**:1897–1899, 1967.
10. Elkington SG, Schreiber WM, Conn HO: Hepatic injury caused by L-alpha-methyldopa. *Circulation* **40**:589-595, 1967.
11. Goldstein GB, Lam KC, Mistilis SP: Drug-induced chronic active hepatitis. *Dig Dis* **18**:177–184, 1973.
12. Hoyumpa AM Jr, Connell AM: Methyldopa hepatitis: Report of three cases. *Dig Dis* **18**:213–222, 1973.
13. Maddrey WC, Boitnott JK: Severe hepatitis from methyldopa. *Gastroenterology* **68**:351–360, 1975.
14. Klemola H, Penttila O, Runeberg L, Tallqvist G: Anicteric liver damage during nitrofurantoin medication. *Scand J Gastroenterol* **10**:501–505, 1975.

15. Back O, Lundgren R, Wiman LG: Nitrofurantoin-induced pulmonary fibrosis and lupus syndrome. *Lancet* **1**:930, 1974.
16. Fagrell B, Strandberg I, Wengle B: A nitrofurantoin-induced disorder simulating chronic active hepatitis. *Acta Med Scand* **199**:237–239, 1976.
17. Stromberg A, Wangle B: Chronic active hepatitis induced by nitrofurantoin. *Br Med J* **3**:174–175, 1976.
18. Black M, Rabin L, Schatz N: Nitrofurantoin-induced chronic active hepatitis. *Ann Intern Med* **92**:62–64, 1980.
19. David RB, Andersen HA, Stickler GB: Nitrofurantoin sensitivity: Report of a child with chronic inflammatory lung disease. *Am J Dis Child* **116**:418–421, 1968.
20. Israel KS, Brashear RE, Sharma HM, et al: Pulmonary fibrosis and nitrofurantoin. *Am Rev Respir Dis* **108**:353–356, 1973.
21. Selroos O, Edgren J: Lupus-like syndrome associated with pulmonary reaction to nitrofurantoin. *Acta Med Scand* **197**:125–129, 1975.
22. Horiuchi T, Ohtsubo K, Saito M: Furylfuramide-induced hepatic necrosis in mice and its modification by phenobarbital. *Jpn J Exp Med* **42**:111–121, 1976.
23. Olive PL, McCalla DR: Cytotoxicity and DNA damage to mammalian cells by nitrofurans. *Chem Biol Interact* **16**:223–233, 1977.
24. Black M, Zimmerman H, Ishak I, et al: Isoniazid hepatitis in 114 patients. *Gastroenterology* **69**:289–302, 1975.
25. Graham WG, Dundas GR: Isoniazid-related liver disease: Occurrence with portal hypertension, hypoalbuminemia and hypersplenism. *JAMA* **242**:353–354, 1979.
26. Black M: Acetaminophen hepatotoxicity. *Annu Rev Med* **35**:577–593, 1984.
27. Seeff LB, Cuccherini BA, Zimmerman HJ, et al: Acetaminophen hepatotoxicity in alcoholics: A therapeutic misadventure. *Ann Intern Med* **104**:399–404, 1986.
28. Black M: Hepatotoxic and hepatoprotective potential of H_2-receptor antagonists. *Am J Med* **83**(Suppl. 6A): 68–75, 1987.
29. Coe RO, Bull FE: Cirrhosis associated with methotrexate treatment of psoriasis. *JAMA* **206**:1515–1520, 1968.
30. Dahl MGC, Gregory MM, Scheuer PJ: Liver damage due to methotrexate in patients with psoriasis. *Br Med J* **1**:625–630, 1971.
31. Roenigk HH Jr, Maibach HI, Weinstein GP: Methotrexate therapy for psoriasis: guideline revisions. *Arch Dermatol* **108**:35, 1973.
32. Weinstein GP, Roenigk H, Maibach HI, et al: Psoriasis–liver–methotrexate interactions. *Arch Dermatol* **108**:36–42, 1973.
33. Roenigk HH Jr, Auerbach R, Maibach HI, Weinstein GP: Methotrexate guidelines—Revised. *J Am Acad Dermatol* **6**:145–155, 1982.
34. Itoh S, Yougel T, Kawagoe K: Comparison between non-alcoholic steatohepatitis and alcoholic hepatitis. *Am J Gastroenterol* **82**:650–654, 1987.
35. Poucell S, Ireton J, Valencia-Mayoral P, et al: Amiodarone-associated phosphilipidosis and fibrosis of the liver: Light, immunohistochemical, and electron microscopic studies. *Gastroenterology* **86**:926–936, 1984.
36. Simon JB, Manley PN, Brien JF, Armstrong PW: Amiodarone hepatotoxicity simulating alcoholic liver disease. *N Engl J Med* **311**:167–172, 1984.
37. Rigas B, Rosenfeld LE, Barwick KW, et al: Amiodarone hepatotoxicity a clinicopathologic study of five patients. *Ann Intern Med* **104**:348–351, 1986.
38. Holt DW, Tucker GT, Jackson PR, Storey GCA: Amiodarone pharmacokinetics. *Am Heart J* **106**:840–846, 1983.
39. Harris L, McKenna WJ, Rowland E, et al: Side effects of long-term amiodarone therapy. *Circulation* **67**:45–51, 1983.
40. Mason JW: Amiodarone, *N Engl J Med* **316**:455–466, 1987.
41. Pessayre D, Bichara M, Feldmann G, et al: Perhexilene maleate-induced cirrhosis. *Gastroenterology* **76**:170–177, 1979.
42. Morgan MY, Reshef R, Shah RR, et al: Impaired oxidation of debrisoquine in patients with perhexilene liver injury. *Gut* **25**:1057–1064, 1984.
43. Mahgoub A, Idle JR, Dring LG, et al: Polymorphic hydroxylation of debrisoquine in man. *Lancet* **2**:584–586, 1977.

44. Price Evans DA, Mahgoub A, Sloan TP, et al: A family and population study of the genetic polymorphism of debrisoquine oxidation in a white British population. *J Med Genet* **17:**102–105, 1980.
45. Distlerath LM, Reilly PEB, Martin MV, et al: Purification and characterization of the human liver cytochromes P-450 involved in debrisoquine 4-hydroxylation and phenacetin O-deethylation, two prototypes for genetic polymorphism in oxidative drug metabolism. *J Biol Chem* **260:**9057–9067, 1985.

21

Acute and Chronic Hepatotoxicity: Pathologic Aspects

Florabel G. Mullick

1. INTRODUCTION

Almost the entire morphologic spectrum of hepatic disorders may be produced by drug administration. Thus, the clinical history is crucial, because the diagnosis can seldom be made on the basis of histologic criteria alone. The methodology used for evaluation and validation of cases in which there is an alleged drug reaction has been discussed at length.[1–4]

A number of acute hepatic lesions can result from adverse reactions to therapeutic drugs. The acute reactions include panlobular degeneration (hepatitis-like), submassive and massive necrosis, mononucleosis-like hepatitis, acute combined hepatocellular/cholestatic injury, acute intrahepatic cholestasis, microvesicular steatosis, vasculitis of the hypersensitivity type, and necrotizing angitis. A number of chronic hepatic lesions can result. Chronic reactions include chronic active hepatitis, chronic intrahepatic cholestasis, microvesicular steatosis, phospholipidosis, granulomatous reactions, fibrosis, cirrhosis, sinusoidal dilatation, peliosis hepatis, veno-occlusive disease, hepatic vein thrombosis, and benign and malignant neoplasms.

2. ACUTE REACTIONS

2.1. Hepatitis-like Degeneration

This lesion involves all zones of the lobule. It is characterized by ballooning degeneration of hepatocytes, acidophilic degeneration, sinusoidal acidophilic bodies, and small foci of necrosis (Fig. 1). The portal areas are usually free of any inflammatory response.

Examples of drugs leading to this type of injury include isoniazid,[5] *p*-aminosalicylic acid,[6] rifampin,[6] sulfonamides,[7] sulfasalazine,[8] methyldopa,[9] halothane,[10] phenylbutazone,[11] papaverine,[12] indomethacin,[13] and disulfiram.[14]

Florabel G. Mullick • Department of Environmental and Drug-Induced Pathology, Armed Forces Institute of Pathology, Washington, D.C. 20306. The opinions or assertions contained herein are the private views of the author and are not to be construed as official or as reflecting the views of the Department of the Army or the Department of Defense.

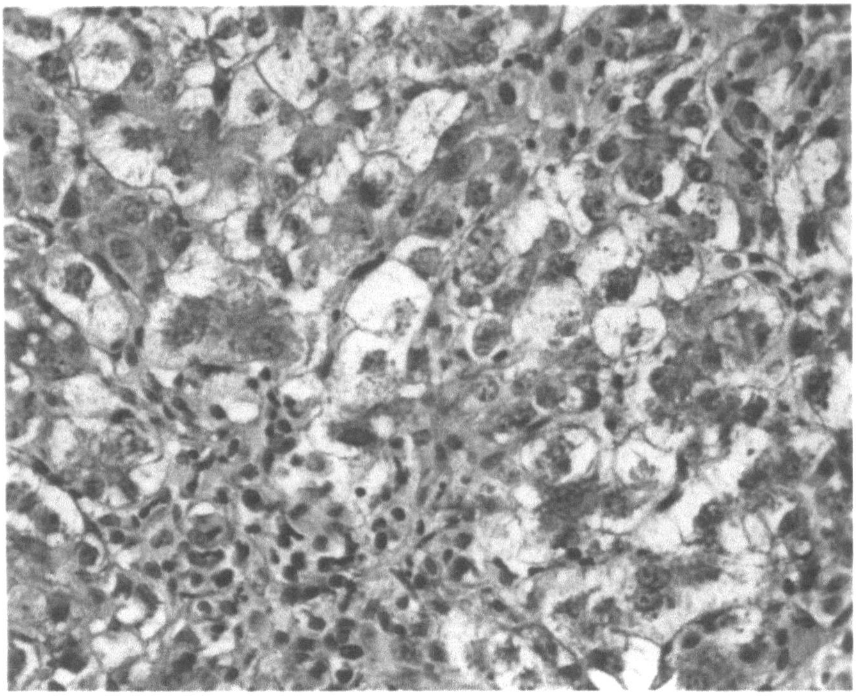

Figure 1. Acute hepatocellular injury associated with sulfasalazine. Note ballooning and acidophilic bodies. (H&E, ×625)

2.2. Mononucleosis-like Hepatitis

The liver shows increased cellularity of sinusoids in the so-called beading arrangement. There is marked infiltration of portal spaces with lymphocytes and eosinophils. Hepatocellular injury in the form of scattered acidophilic bodies and foci of necrosis is present. There are multiple mitotic figures.

Examples of drugs leading to this type of injury are diphenylhydantoin,[15] *p*-aminosalicylic acid,[16] sulfonamides,[17] and dapsone.[18]

2.3. Submassive Necrosis

Centrilobular (zone 3) necrosis is the one most commonly seen. This lesion consists of loss of hepatocytes from central zones (Fig. 2). Inflammatory cells are seen in the stroma. The portal areas might show inflammation as well.

Examples of drugs that can lead to this type of centrilobular necrosis are halothane,[10] enflurane,[19] acetaminophen,[20] methoxyflurane,[21] ketoconazole,[22] mithramycin,[23] tannic acid,[24] toxic mushrooms,[25] aflatoxin,[26] copper,[27] tetrachlorethylene,[28] and carbon tetrachloride.

Peripheral (zone 1) necrosis is associated with ferrous sulfate,[29] intoxication, and phosphorous[30] poisoning.

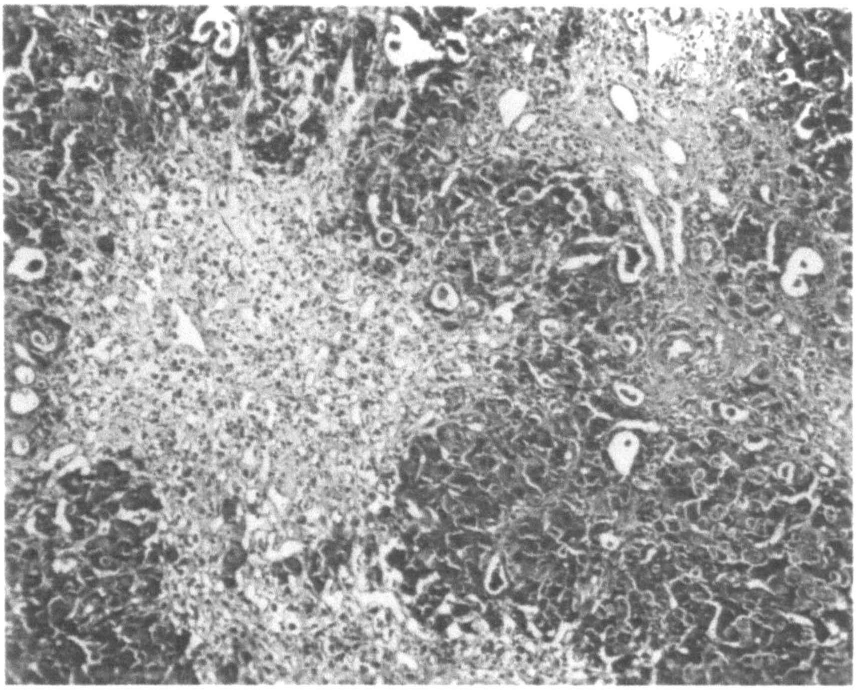

Figure 2. Submassive necrosis associated with halothane. Note necrosis of acinar zone 3. (H&E, ×90)

2.4. Massive Necrosis

In this type of injury, there is total loss of hepatocytes with collapse of the residual stroma (Fig. 3). There is prominent cholangiolar proliferation with infiltration by neutrophils (Fig. 4).

Examples of drugs that can lead to this type of injury are the same as those that cause centrilobular (zone 3) necrosis. The most frequent causes are halothane and isoniazid.

2.5. Acute Intrahepatic Cholestasis

This type of lesion is basically of four types. The first type consists of cholestasis without evidence of hepatocellular injury as associated with anabolic[31] or contraceptive steroids, or both.[32] The second type of lesion is characterized by cholestasis with minimal hepatocellular injury (Fig. 5), as in injuries associated with chlorpromazine,[33] chlordiazepoxide,[33] erythromycin estolate,[34] tolbutamide,[35] chlorpropamide,[36] oxyphenisatin,[37] and 6-mercaptopurine.[38] The third type of lesion is cholestasis accompanied by bile duct degeneration as seen in cases of paraquat[39] poisoning. Finally, the fourth type of lesion consists of cholestasis with cholangitis, as has been noted with such drugs as chlorpromazine,[40] allopurinol,[41] chlorpropamide,[42] and hydralazine.[43]

2.6. Acute Combined Hepatocellular/Cholestatic Injury

This type of injury leads to either hepatocellular degeneration or necrosis, or both, and a significant degree of intrahepatic cholestasis.

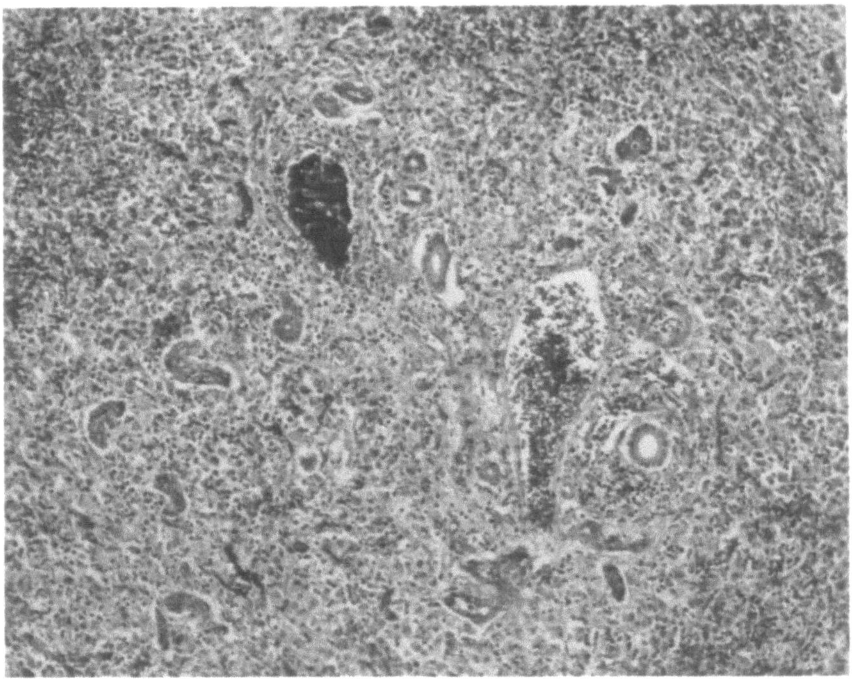

Figure 3. Massive necrosis associated with diphenylhydantoin. (H&E, ×114)

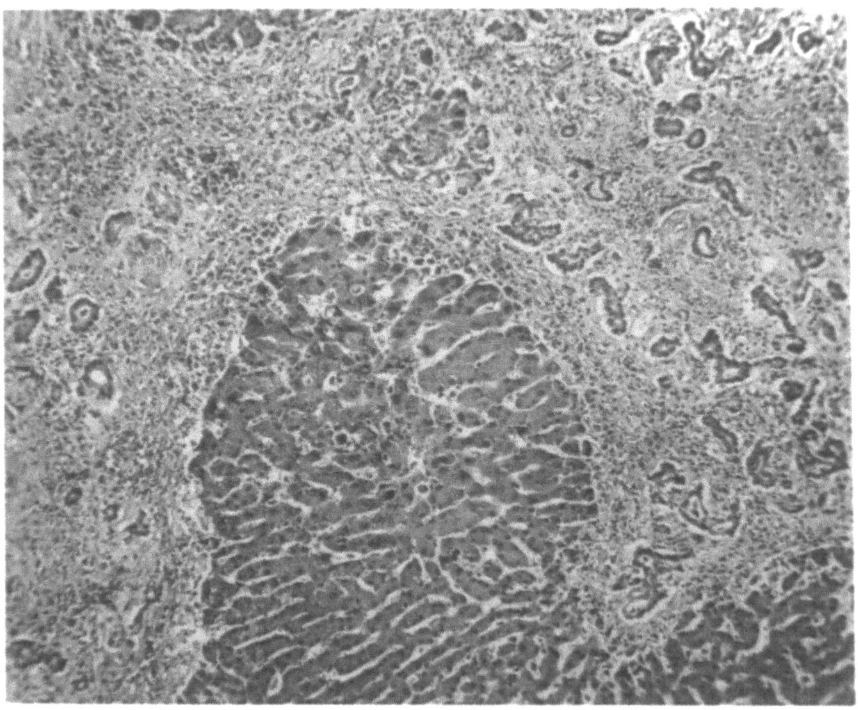

Figure 4. Cholangiolar proliferation and infiltration with neutrophils. (H&E, ×80)

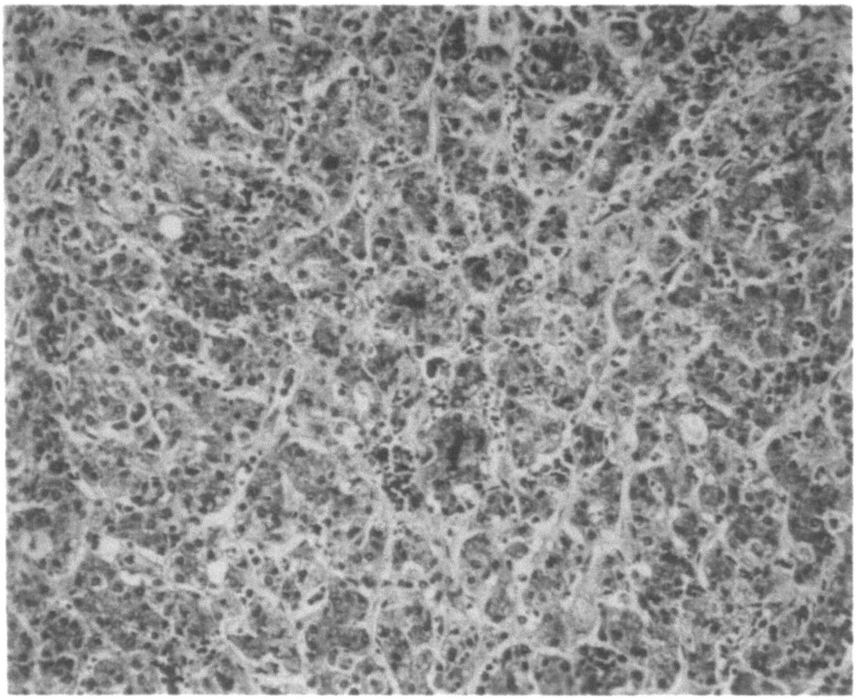

Figure 5. Intrahepatic cholestasis associated with total parenteral nutrition (TPN). Note several intracanalicular bile plugs (H&E, ×60)

Examples of drugs that can lead to this type of injury are isoniazid,[44] *p*-aminosalicylic acid, phenylbutazone,[45] carbamazepine,[46] and diphenylhydantoin.[15]

2.7. Microvesicular Steatosis

In this type of steatosis or fatty infiltration, the hepatocytes become enlarged and have one or two centrally placed nuclei. The cytoplasm is finely vacuolated (Fig. 6), the vacuoles varying from <1–8 μm in diameter. The presence of fat can be confirmed with a frozen oil Red O stain.

Examples of drugs that can lead to this type of injury are tetracycline, sodium valproate,[47] salicylate intoxication,[48] and aflatoxin intoxication. In addition to microvesicular steatosis, sodium valproate[47] also causes submassive (zone 3) necrosis.

2.8. Vascular Lesions

Drug-induced acute vascular lesions include vasculitis of both arteries and veins and necrotizing angiitis. Drug-induced vasculitis consists of mononuclear cells and eosinophils. There is no fibrinoid necrosis, and all lesions are of the same age.[49]

Examples of drugs that can induce this type of lesion include diphenylhydantoin, phenylbutazone, allopurinol, penicillin, and chlorothiazide.

Necrotizing vasculitis is characterized by fibrinoid necrosis of the vessel wall with inflammation and edema.

Examples of drugs that can induce this type of lesion are the sulfonamides,[50] penicillin,[51] and allopurinol.[52]

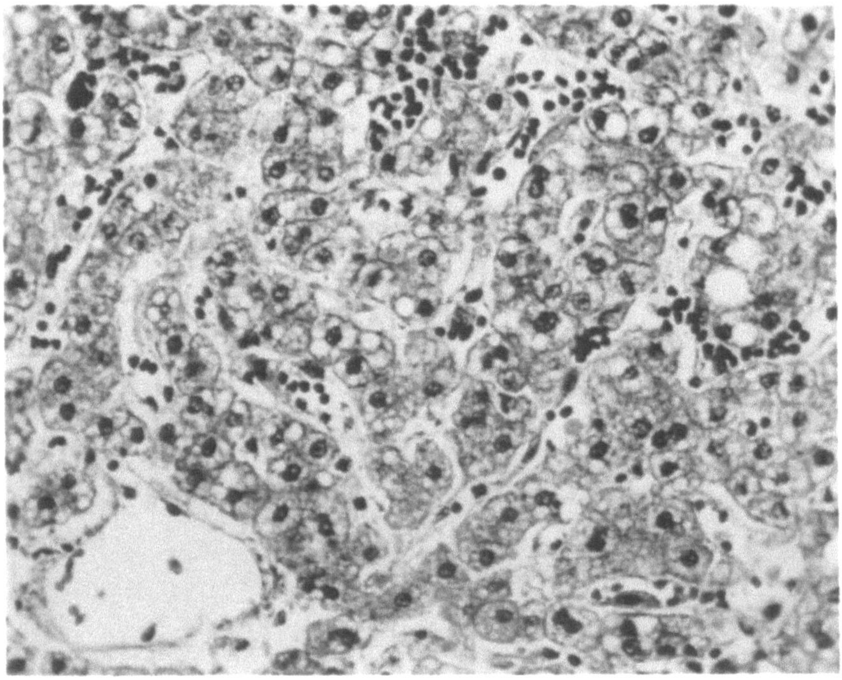

Figure 6. Microvesicular steatosis associated with tetracycline. (H&E, ×300)

3. CHRONIC REACTIONS

3.1. Chronic Active Hepatitis

The morphologic changes in this type of lesion are marked portal periportal inflammation composed mostly of mononuclear cells, fibrous expansion of the portal area, and extension of the inflammation into the periportal parenchyma, accompanied by individual cell necrosis (piecemeal necrosis).

Examples of drugs that can produce this type of injury are nitrofurantoin,[53] oxyphenisatin,[37] propylthiouracil, methyldopa,[54] ticrynafen, isoniazid, and aspirin.[55]

3.2. Chronic Intrahepatic Cholestasis

This lesion is characterized by periportal cholestasis, pseudoxanthomatous transformation of hepatocytes, and accumulation of copper in periportal liver cells. There is also degeneration and necrosis of periportal hepatocytes (piecemeal necrosis), minimal to moderate portal inflammation, and cholangiolar proliferation.

Examples of drugs that can lead to this type of injury include chlorpromazine, prochlorperazine, methyltestosterone,[56] imipramine, tolbutamide, haloperidol, and thiobendazole.

3.3. Macrovesicular Steatosis

In this type of injury, most of the liver cells contain one large droplet of fat that pushes the nucleus to the periphery.

Examples of drugs that can cause this lesion are alcohol, corticosteroids, methotrexate, L-asparaginase, and organ solvents.

3.4. Phospholipidosis

This lesion is characterized light microscopically by enlargement of hepatocytes and Kupffer cells having a foamy appearance (Fig. 7). Electron microscopically, the characteristic lamellar lysosomal inclusions can be seen.

Examples of drugs that can lead to this type of change are amiodarone,[57] 4,4-diethylaminoethoxyhexestrol (Coralgil),[58] perhexilene maleate,[59] and chloroquine.

3.5. Granulomatous Reactions

This type of lesion can be of three types. Granulomas can occur alone as simple or "bland" granulomas; they can be accompanied by hepatocellular injury (Fig. 8). The third type is characterized by granulomas with vasculitis (Fig. 9).

Examples of drugs associated with the aforementioned lesions are multiple, of which the most commonly encountered are sulfonamides, sulfonylurea compounds, diphenylhydantoin, quinidine, methyldopa, carbamazepine, phenylbutazone, and allopurinol.[60]

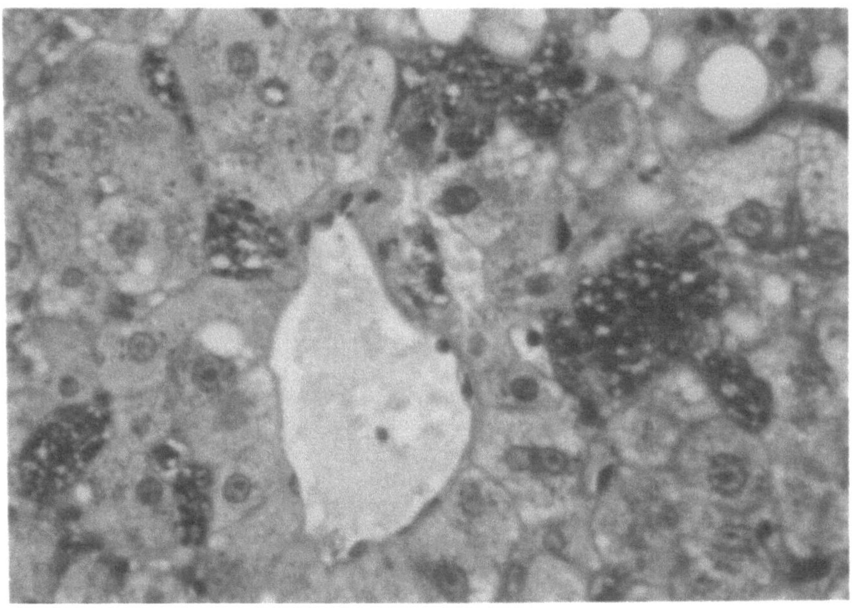

Figure 7. Phospholipidosis associated with amiodarone. Note the "foam" cells after diastase digestion. (Periodic acid-Schiff, ×300)

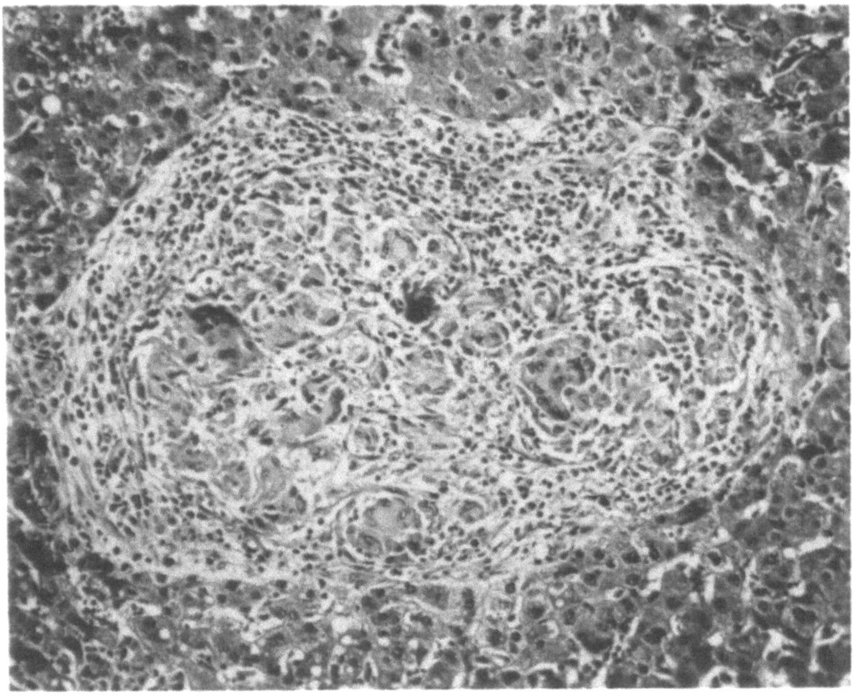

Figure 8. Noncaseating granuloma associated with phenylbutazone. (H&E, ×160)

3.6. Fibrosis

Irregular and patchy, portal, periportal, and subcapsular fibrosis is seen associated with Thorotrast and exposure to vinyl chloride. Periportal fibrosis is caused by methotrexate and after prolonged hyperalimentation therapy.

3.7. Cirrhosis

This type of lesion can be micronodular (Fig. 10) or macronodular. It can resemble cardiac or inverted cirrhosis.

Examples of drugs associated with cirrhosis are methotrexate,[61] amiodarone, iproniazid, isoniazid, ticrynafen, dantrolene, and total parental nutrition (TPN). Chronic intrahepatic cholestasis can lead to biliary cirrhosis after prolonged therapy with chlorpromazine.[62]

3.8. Vascular Lesions

The drug-induced chronic vascular lesions include sinusoidal dilatation, peliosis hepatis (Fig. 11), veno-occlusive disease (Fig. 12), and hepatic vein thrombosis (Fig. 13). Sinusoidal dilatation is characteristically periportal and is associated with the use of oral contraceptives.

Peliosis hepatis consists of cysts of various sizes that contain blood and do not have an endothelial lining.

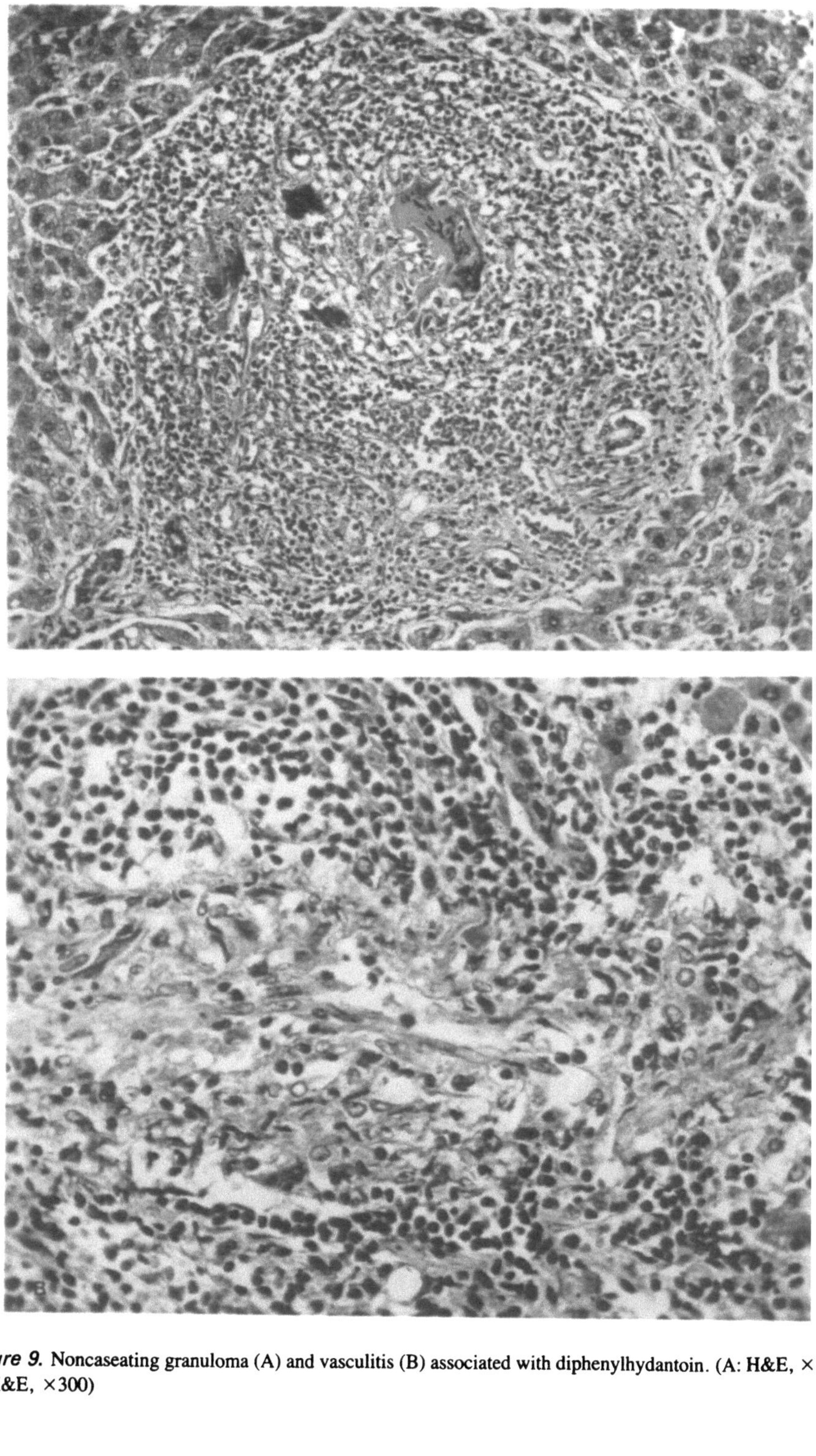

Figure 9. Noncaseating granuloma (A) and vasculitis (B) associated with diphenylhydantoin. (A: H&E, ×145; B: H&E, ×300)

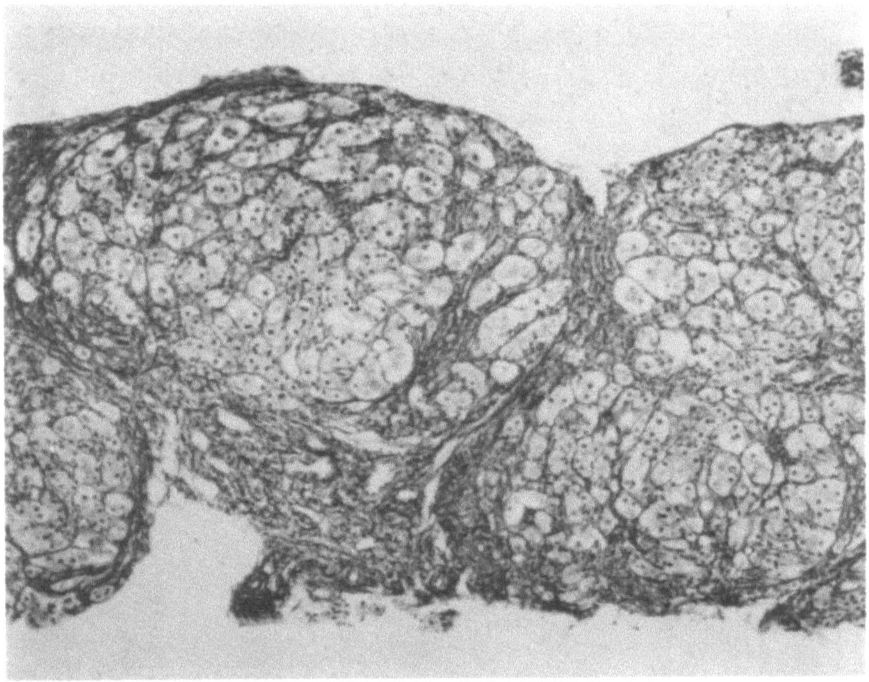

Figure 10. Micronodular cirrhosis associated with amiodarone. (H&E, ×60)

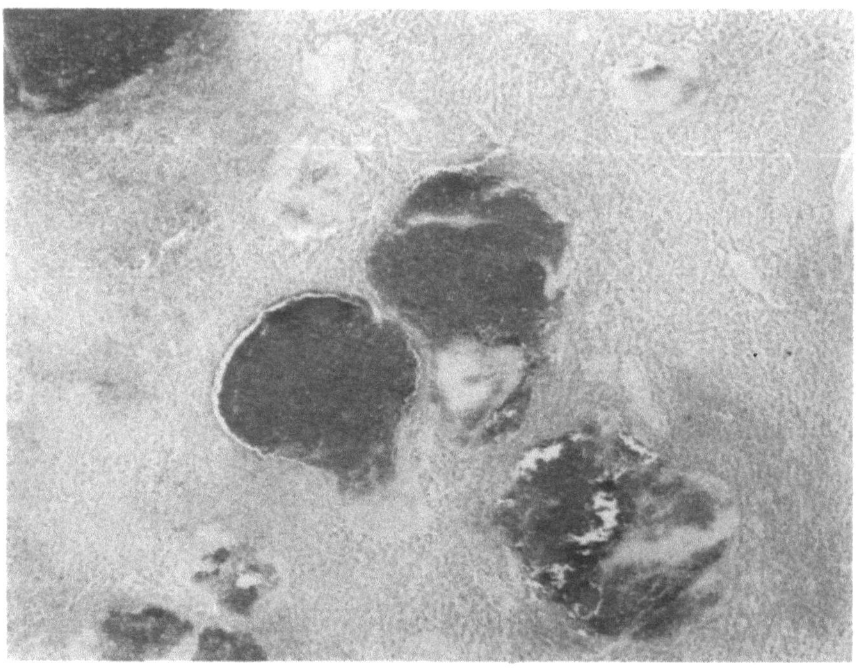

Figure 11. Peliosis hepatis associated with oxymetholone. (H&E, ×30)

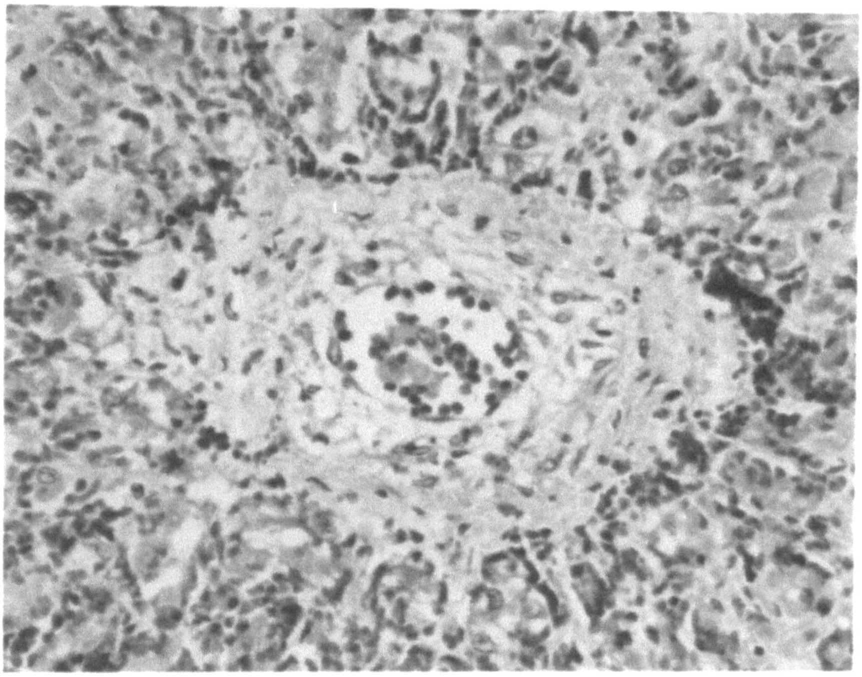

Figure 12. Veno-occlusive disease associated with pyrrolizidine alkaloids. (H&E, ×400)

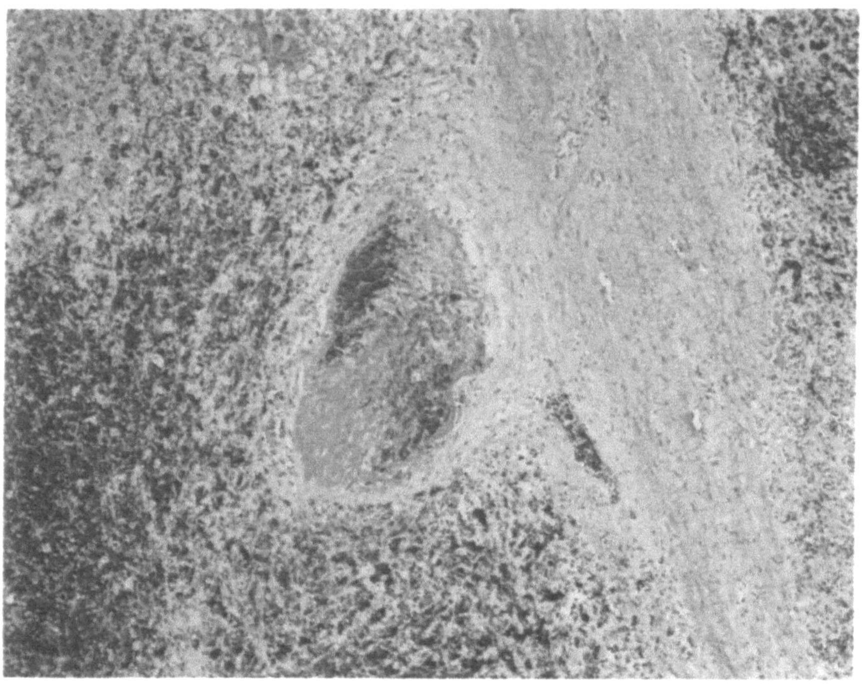

Figure 13. Hepatic vein thrombosis associated with oral contraceptives. (H&E, ×400)

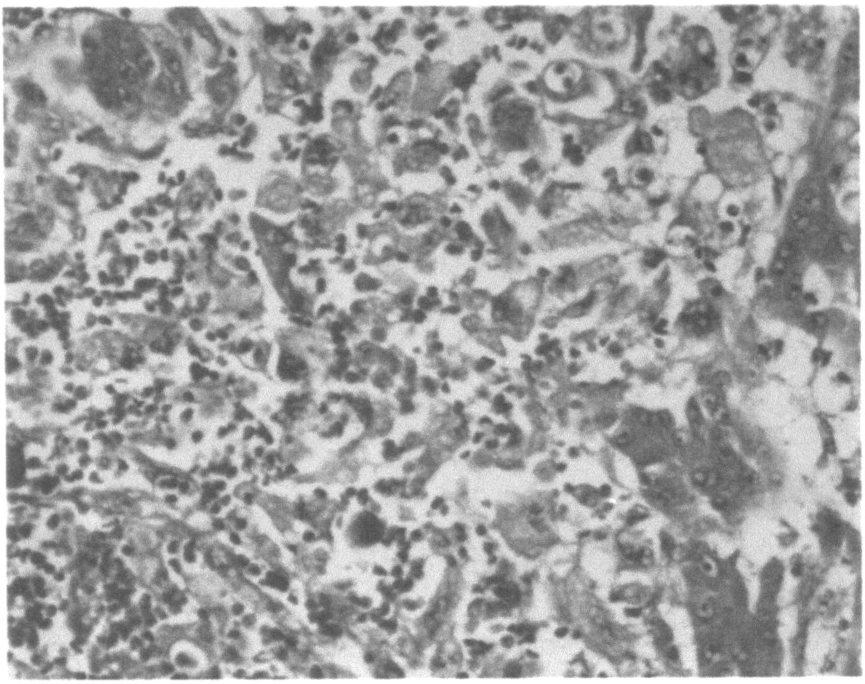

Figure 14. Angiosarcoma associated with thorotrast. (H&E, ×150)

Examples of drugs that cause peliosis hepatis are the androgenic/anabolic steroids,[63] danazol, tamoxifen, and Thorotrast.[64]

Veno-occlusive disease involves the terminal hepatic venules. There is intimal hyperplasia, accumulation of fluid, extravasation of erythrocytes, and collagen deposition, causing narrowing and occlusion of the vessels. The hepatic parenchyma shows coagulation necrosis.

Examples of drugs and chemicals associated with this type of lesion are the bush teas containing pyrrolizidine alkaloids.[65]

Other causes are alcohol, aflatoxin, hypervitaminosis A,[66] azathioprine in renal transplant recipients,[67] and mitomycin C.

Hepatic vein thrombosis can also be associated with coagulation necrosis. The tributaries of hepatic veins are involved by thrombi that may recanalize.

Examples of drugs that can lead to this type of lesion are the oral contraceptives.[68]

3.9. *Neoplasms*

A benign neoplasm associated with drug therapy is hepatocellular adenoma. This is associated with the use of contraceptive steroids. This is a well-established relationship, and there is no doubt that these benign tumors are caused by contraceptive steroids. The malignant neoplasms associated with chemicals are hepatocellular carcinoma associated with alcohol, as well as Thorotrast; cholangiocarcinoma and angiosarcoma (Fig. 14) associated Thorotrast[69] (Fig. 15A,B), and angiosarcoma associated with vinyl chloride, Thorotrast, and arsenic.[70]

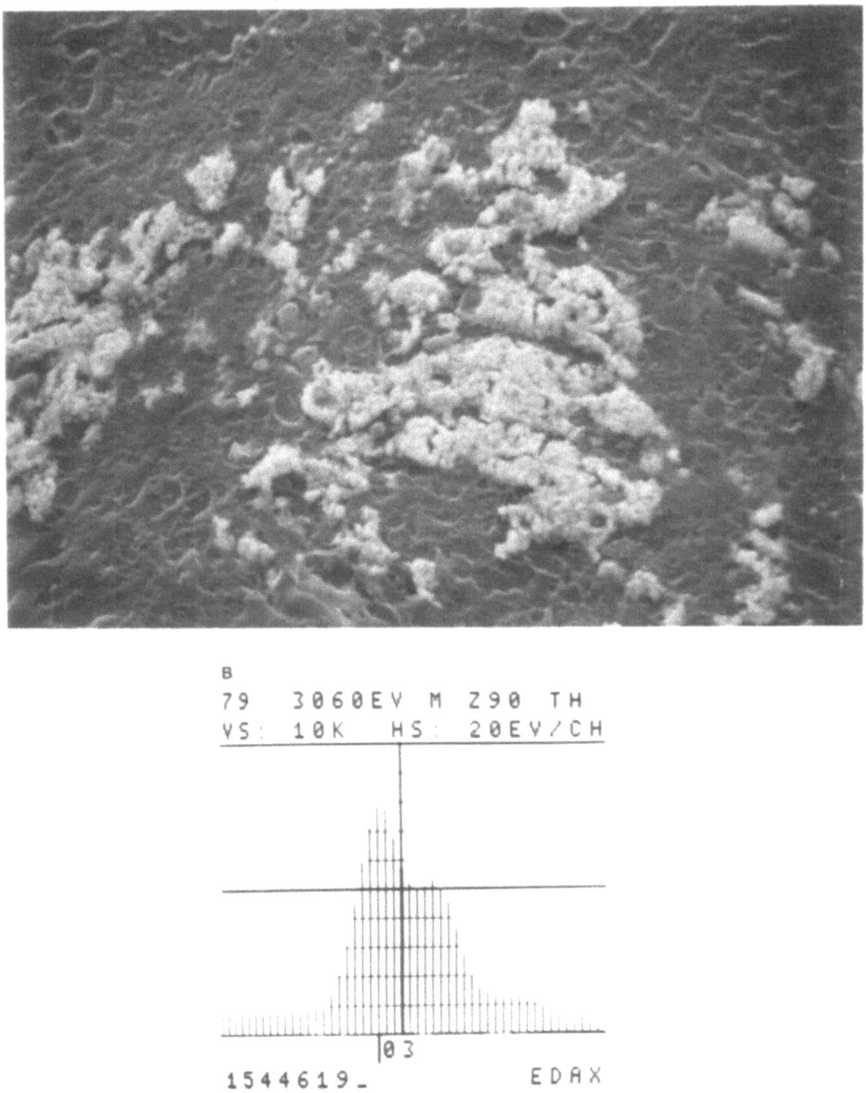

Figure 15. (A) Scanning electron micrograph showing Thorotrast deposits. (×1250). (B) Energy-dispersive X-ray microanalysis identifying thorium.

REFERENCES

1. Irey NS: Tissue reaction to drugs. *AM J Pathol* **82:**617–648, 1976.
2. Irey NS: Microscopic changes in adverse drug reactions, in Perper JA, Wecht CH (eds): *Microscopic Diagnosis in Forensic Pathology.* Charles C Thomas, Springfield, Illinois, 1980, pp. 67–148.
3. Irey NS; When is a disease drug-induced?, in Riddell RH (ed): *Pathology of Drug-Induced and Toxic Diseases.* Churchill Livingstone, New York, 1982, pp. 1–18.
4. Ishak KG, Mullick, FG: Drug-induced and toxic liver injury, in Peters RL, Craig JR (eds): *Liver Pathology.* Churchill Livingstone, New York, 1986, pp. 221–254.
5. Black M, Mitchell JR, Zimmerman HJ, et al: Isoniazid hepatitis in 114 patients. *Gastroenterology* **69:**289–301, 1975.
6. Scheuer PJ, Summerfield JA, Lal S, et al: Rifampicin hepatitis: A clinical and histological study. *Lancet* **1:** 421–425, 1974.
7. Dujovne CA, Chan CH, Zimmerman HJ: Sulfonamide hepatic injury: Review of the literature and report of a case due to sulfamethazole. *N Engl J Med* **277:**785–788, 1967.
8. Fich A, Schwartz J, Braveman D, et al: Sulfasalazine hepatotoxicity. *Am J Gastroenterol* **79:**401–402, 1984.
9. Hoyumpa AM Jr, Connell AM: Methyldopa hepatitis: Report of three cases. *Am J Dig Dis* **18:**213–222, 1973.
10. Peters RL, Edmondson HA, Reynolds TB, et al: Hepatic necrosis associated with halothane anesthesia. *Am J Med* **47:**748–764, 1969.
11. Benjamin SB, Ishak KG, Zimmerman HJ, et al: Phenylbutazone liver injury: A clinicopathologic survey of 23 cases and review of the literature. *Hepatology* **1:**255–263, 1981.
12. Kiaer HW, Olson S, Ronnov-Jessen V: Hepatotoxicity of papaverine. *Arch Pathol Lab Med* **98:**292–296, 1974.
13. Fenech PF, Bannister WH, Gretch JL: Hepatitis with biliverdinaemia in association with indomethacin therapy. *Br Med J* **3:**155–156, 1967.
14. Nässberger L: Disulfiram-induced hepatitis—Report of a case and review of the literature. *Postgrad Med J* **60:**639–641, 1984.
15. Mullick FG, Ishak KG: Hepatic injury associated with diphenylhydantoin therapy: A clinicopathologic study of 20 cases. *Am J Clin Pathol* **74:**442–452, 1980.
16. Lichtenstein MR, Cannemeyer W: Severe para-aminosalicylic acid hypersensitivity simulating mononucleosis or hepatitis. *JAMA* **152:**606–607, 1953.
17. Zimmerman HJ: *Hepatotoxicity:* The adverse effects of drugs and other chemicals on the liver. Appleton-Century-Crofts, New York, 1978, 481–482.
18. Gan TE, Van Der Weyden MB: Dapsone-induced infectious mononucleosis-like syndrome. *Med J Aust* **1:** 350–351, 1982.
19. Lewis JH, Zimmerman HJ, Ishak, KG, et al: Enflurane hepatoxicity: A clinicopathologic study of 24 cases. *Ann Intern Med* **98:**984–992, 1983.
20. Lesna M, Watson AJ, Douglas AP, et al: Evaluation of paracetamol-induced damage in liver biopsies: Acute changes and follow-up findings. *Virchows Arch* **370:**333–344, 1976.
21. Joshi PH, Conn HO: The syndrome of methoxyflurane-associated hepatitis. *Ann Intern Med* **80:**395–401, 1974.
22. Lewis JH, Zimmerman HJ, Benson GD, et al: Hepatic injury associated with ketoconazole therapy: Analysis of 33 cases. *Gastroenterology* **96:**503–513, 1984.
23. Kennedy BJ: Metabolic and toxic effect of mithramycin tumor therapy. *Am J Med* **49:**494–503, 1970.
24. Zimmerman HJ: *Hepatotoxicity:* The adverse effects of drugs and other chemicals on the liver. Appleton-Century-Crofts, New York, 1978, 238–239.
25. Wepler W, Opitz K: Histologic change in the liver biopsy in *Amanita phalloides* intoxication. *Hum Pathol* **3:**249–254, 1972.
26. Ngindu A, Johnson BK, Kenya PR, et al: Outbreak of acute hepatitis caused by aflatoxln poisoning in Kenya. *Lancet* **1:**1346–1348, 1982.
27. Chuttani HK, Gupta PS, Gulati S, et al: Acute copper sulfate poisoning. *Am J Med* **39:**849–852, 1964.
28. Baerg RD, Kimberg DV: Centrilobular hepatic necrosis and acute renal failure in "solvent sniffers." *Ann Intern Med* **73:**713–720, 1970.
29. Luongo MA, Bjornson SS: The liver in ferrous sulfate poisoning: A report of three fatal cases and an experimental study. *N Engl J Med* **251:**995–999, 1954.

30. Diaz-Rivera RS, Collazo PJ, Pons ER, et al: Acute phosphorous poisoning in man: A study of 56 cases. *Medicine (Baltimore)* **29:**269–298, 1950.
31. Zimmerman HJ, Ishak KG: Drug-induced and toxic liver injury, in MacSween RNM, Anthony PP, Scheuer P (eds): *Pathology of the Liver.* Churchill Livingstone, Edinburgh, 1979, pp. 335–386.
32. Ishak KG: The liver, in Riddell RH (ed): *Pathology of Drug-Induced and Toxic Diseases,* Churchill Livingstone, New York, 1982, pp. 457–513.
33. Ishak KG, Irey NS: Hepatic injury associated with phenothiazines. A clinicopathologic and follow-up study of 36 cases. *Arch Pathol Lab Med* **93:**283–304, 1972.
34. Zafrani ES, Ishak KG, Rudzki C: Cholestatic and hepatocellular injury associated with erythromycin esters: Report of 9 cases. *Am J Dig Dis* **24:**385–396, 1979.
35. Baird RW, Hull JG: Cholestatic jaundice from tolbutamlde. *Ann Intern Med* **53:**194–196, 1960.
36. Reichel J, Goldberg SB, Ellenberg M, et al: Intrahepatic cholestasis following administration of chlorpropamide: Report of a case with electron microscopic observations. *Am J Med* **28:**654–660, 1960.
37. Reynolds TB: Laxative liver disease. In Gerok W, Sickinger K (eds): *Drugs and the Liver.* Schattauer Verlag, Stuttgart, 1975, pp. 319–325.
38. Einhorn M, Davidsohn I: Hepatotoxicity of mercaptopurine. *JAMA* **188:**802–806, 1984.
39. Mullick FG, Ishak KG, Mahabir R, et al: Hepatic injury with paraquat toxicity in humans. *Liver* **1:**209–221, 1981.
40. Zelman S: Liver cell necrosis in chlorpromazine jaundice (allergic cholangiolitis). *Am J Med* **27:**708–729, 1959.
41. Al-Kawas FH, Seeff LB, Berendson RA, et al: Allopurinol hepatotoxicity: Report of two cases and review of the literature. *Ann Intern Med* **95:** 588–590, 1981.
42. Schneider HL, Hornbach KD, Kruaz JL, et al: Chlorpropamide hepatotoxicity: Report of a case and review of the literature. *Am J Gastroenterol* **79:**721–724, 1984.
43. Myers JL, Augur NA: Hydralazine-induced cholangitis. *Gastroenterology* **87:**1185–1188, 1984.
44. Mitchell JR, Zimmerman HJ, Ishak KG, et al: Isoniazid liver injury. Clinical spectrum, pathology and probable pathogenesis. *Ann Intern Med* **84:**181–192, 1976.
45. Benjamin SB, Ishak KG, Zimmerman HJ, et al: Phenylbutazone liver injury: A clinicopathologic survey of 23 cases and review of the literature. *Hepatology* **1:**255–263, 1981.
46. Davion T, Capron JP, Andrejak M, et al: Hepatite aigueë a la carbamezepine (Tegretol): Etude d'un case et revue de la litterature. *Gastroenterol Clin Biol* **8:**52, 1984.
47. Zimmerman HJ, Ishak KG: Valproate-induced hepatic injury: Analyses of 23 fatal cases. *Hepatology* **2:** 591–597, 1982.
48. Starko KM, Mullick FG: Hepatic and cerebral pathology findings in children with fatal salicylate intoxication: Further evidence for a causal relation between salicylates and Reye's syndrome. *Lancet* **1:**326–329, 1983.
49. Mullick FG, McAllister HA, Wagner BM, et al: Drug related vasculitis *Hum Pathol* **10:**313–325, 1979.
50. Lichtenstein L, Fox LJ: Necrotizing arterial lesions resembling those of periarteritis nodosa and focal necroses following administration of sulfathiazole. *Am J Pathol* **22:**665–677, 1946.
51. Waugh D: Myocarditis, arteritis and focal hepatic, splenic and renal granulomas due to penicillin sensitivity. *Am J Pathol* **24:**437–447, 1952.
52. Boyer TD, Sun N, Reynolds TB: Allopurinol—Hypersensitivity vasculitis and liver damage. *West J Med* **126:**143–147, 1977.
53. Sharp JR, Ishak KG, Zimmerman HJ: Chronic active hepatitis and severe hepatic necrosis associated with nitrofurantoin. *Ann Intern Med* **92:**14–19, 1980.
54. Goldstein GB, Lam KC, Mistilis SP: Drug-induced chronic active hepatitis. *Am J Dig Dis* **18:**177–184, 1973.
55. Seaman WE, Ishak KG, Plotz PH: Aspirin-induced hepatotoxicity in patients with lupus erythematosus. *Ann Intern Med* **80:**1–8, 1974.
56. Glober GA, Wilkerson JA: Biliary cirrhosis following the administration of methyltestosterone. *JAMA* **204:** 170–173, 1968.
57. Poucell S, Ireton J, Valencia-Mayoral P, et al: Amiodarone-associated phospholipidosis and fibrosis of the liver. Light, immunohistochemical and electron microscopic studies. *Gastroenterology* **86:**926–936, 1984.
58. Oda T, Shikata T, Naito C, et al: Phospholipid fatty liver: A report of three cases with a new type of fatty liver. *Jpn J Exp Med* **40:**127–140, 1970.
59. Paliard P, Vitrey D, Fournier G, et al: Perhexilene maleate-induced hepatitis. *Digestion* **17:**419–427, 1978.

60. Ishak KG: Granulomas of the liver, in Ioachim HL (ed): *Pathology of Granulomas*. Raven, New York, 1983, pp. 307–369.
61. Scheuer PJ: Hepatotoxicity of methotrexate and azathioprine, in Gerok W, Sickinger K (eds): *Drugs and the Liver*. Schattauer Verlag, Stuttgart, 1975, pp. 281–286.
62. Walker CO, Combes B: Biliary cirrhosis induced by chlorpromazine. *Gastroenterology* **51:**631–640, 1966.
63. Boyer JL: Androgenic-anabolic steroid associated peliosis hepatis in man: A review of 38 reported cases. *Adv Pharmacol Ther* **8:**175–185, 1979.
64. Okuda K, Omata M, Itoh Y, et al: Peliosis hepatis as a late and fatal complication of Thorotrast liver disease: Report of five cases. *Liver* **1:**110–122, 1981.
65. Stillman AE, Huxtable R, Consaoe P, et al: Hepatic veno-occlusive disease due to pyrrolizidine (senecio) poisoning in Arizona. *Gastroenterology* **73:**349–352, 1977.
66. Russell RM, Boyer JL, Bagheri SA, et al: Hepatic injury from chronic hypervitaminosis A resulting in portal hypertension and ascites. *N Engl J Med* **291:**435–440, 1974.
67. Marubbio AT, Danielson B: Hepatic veno-occlusive disease in a renal transplant patient receiving azathioprine. *Gastroenterology* **69:**739–743, 1975.
68. Lewis JH, Tice H, Zimmerman HJ: Budd-Chiari syndrome associated with oral contraceptive steroids: Review of treatment of 47 cases. *Dig Dis Sci* **38:**673–683, 1983.
69. Rubel LR, Ishak KG: Thorotrast-associated cholangiocarcinoma: An epidemiologic and clinicopathologic study. *Cancer* **50:**1408–1415, 1982.
70. Goodman ZD, Ishak KG: Non-parenchymal and metastatic malignant tumors of the liver, in Berk JE (ed): *Bockus Gastroenterology* 4th ed. WB Sanders Company, Philadelphia, 1985, pp. 3377–3386.

IV

Metabolic and Infectious Liver Diseases

22

α_1-Antitrypsin Deficiency and Neonatal Cholestasis

William F. Balistreri and J. Thomas Stocker

1. INTRODUCTION

Neonatal cholestasis, in its broadest definition, i.e., prolonged conjugated hyperbilirubinemia, regardless of the site of injury, offers an interesting exercise in differential diagnosis. There are multiple areas of overlap between discrete and apparently disparate disease categories. A simple conceptual approach is to categorize neonates presenting with cholestasis into those with predominant extrahepatic disease and those with predominant intrahepatic disease (Fig. 1).

The relative frequency of liver-based metabolic disease as a cause of neonatal cholestasis is low (8–10%) (Table I). However, the largest single category, i.e., idiopathic neonatal hepatitis, may well include liver-based metabolic diseases, which are currently undeciphered. For example, α_1-antitrypsin deficiency, previously lumped in the idiopathic neonatal hepatitis category, is now recognized as a specific cause of neonatal cholestasis. Future studies will lead to further refinement of the idiopathic category as other liver-based metabolic diseases are discovered.

2. EVALUATION OF THE NEONATE WITH CHOLESTASIS

Underlying suspicion of the possibility of liver-based metabolic diseases should characterize the approach to any infant presenting with cholestasis. The traditional sequential approach to an affected infant involves (1) identification, (2) early recognition of specific treatable/life-threatening entities, and (3) delineation of extrahepatic biliary atresia from idiopathic neonatal hepatitis.

2.1. Identification

The initial, primary step in the early stages of evaluation of a jaundiced infant is to fractionate the serum bilirubin; this seems self-evident but deserves repeating. Too often an erroneous assumption that "all babies get jaundice" is made. The commonly found benign physiologic hyper-

William F. Balistreri • Division of Pediatric Gastroenterology and Nutrition, Children's Hospital Medical Center, Cincinnati, Ohio 45229. *J. Thomas Stocker* • Armed Forces Institute of Pathology, Washington, D.C. 20306–6000.

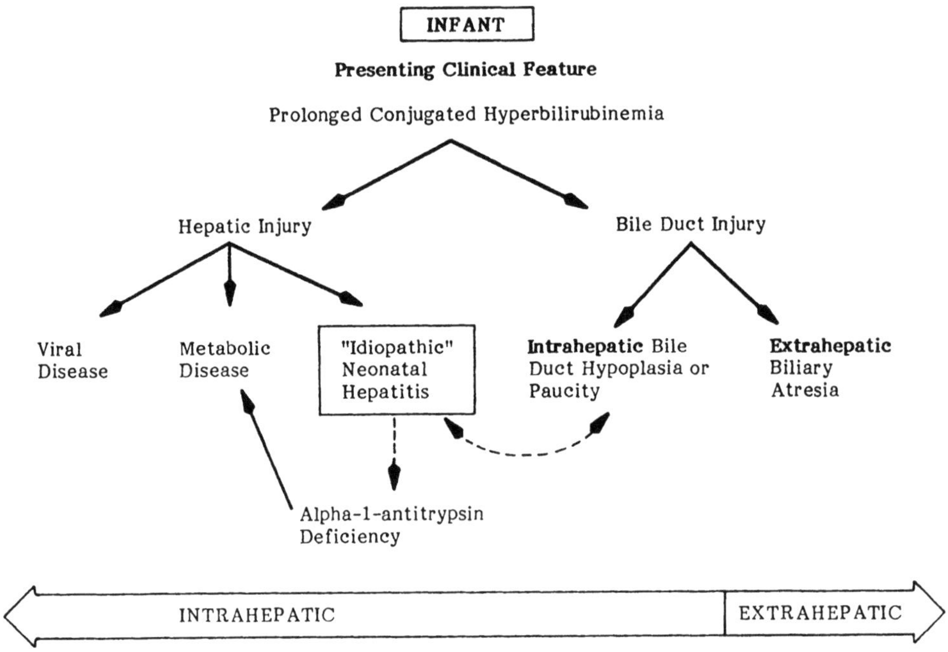

Figure 1. Neonatal cholestasis, a conceptual approach.

Table I. Neonatal Cholestasis: Recognized Disease Entities[a]

- Extrahepatic disorders
  - Biliary atresia
  - Biliary hypoplasia
  - Bile duct stenosis/sclerosing cholangitis
  - Anomalies of choledochal–pancreatico–ductal junction
  - Spontaneous perforation of bile duct
  - Mass (neoplasia, stone)
  - Bile/mucous plug
- Intrahepatic disorders
  - Idiopathic
    - Idiopathic neonatal hepatitis
    - Intrahepatic cholestasis, persistent
      - Arteriohepatic dysplasia (Alagille syndrome)
      - Byler disease (severe intrahepatic cholestasis with progressive hepatocellular disease)
      - Trihydroxycoprostanic acidemia (defective bile acid metabolism and cholestasis)
      - Zellweger syndrome (cerebrohepatorenal syndrome)
      - Nonsyndromic paucity of intrahepatic ducts (apparent absence of bile ductules)
    - Intrahepatic cholestasis, recurrent (syndromic?)
      - Familial benign recurrent cholestasis
      - Hereditary cholestasis with lymphedema (Aagenaes)

Table I. (Continued)

Anatomic
Congenital hepatic fibrosis/infantile polycystic disease
Caroli disease (cystic dilatation of intrahepatic ducts)
Metabolic disorders
Disorders of amino acid metabolism
Tyrosinemia
Disorders of lipid metabolism
Wolman disease
Niemann–Pick disease
Gaucher disease
Disorders of carbohydrate metabolism
Galactosemia
Fructosemia
Glycogenosis IV
Metabolic disease in which defect is uncharacterized
α_1-antitrypsin deficiency
Cystic fibrosis
Idiopathic hypopituitarism
Hypothyroidism
Neonatal iron storage disease
Infantile copper overload
Multiple acyl-CoA dehydrogenation deficiency (glutaric acid type II)
Familial erythrophagocytic lymphohistiocytosis
Hepatitis
Infectious
Cytomegalovirus
Hepatitis B virus (? non-A, non-B virus)
Rubella virus
Reovirus type 3
Herpes virus
Varicella virus
Coxsackie virus
Echovirus
Toxoplasmosis
Syphilis
Tuberculosis
Listeriosis
Toxic
Cholestasis associated with parenteral nutrition
Sepsis with possible endotoxemia (urinary tract infection, gastroenteritis)
Genetic/chromosomal
Trisomy E
Down syndrome
Donahue syndrome (leprechaunism)
Miscellaneous
Histiocytosis X
Shock/hypoperfusion
Intestinal obstruction
Polysplenia syndrome

[a]Modified from Balistreri.[1]

bilirubinemia involves a predominant elevation of unconjugated bilirubin and is rarely associated with a significant elevation of the conjugated fraction, even in the presence of confounding factors, such as hemolysis and breast feeding. However, the jaundiced child who manifests an elevation of the conjugated bilirubin fraction (i.e., >20% of the total) meets the commonly accepted criteria for neonatal cholestasis, which is never a benign phenomenon. The clinical presentation of infants with neonatal cholestasis is fairly stereotypic and provides very few clues regarding the underlying etiology. Affected infants have jaundice, dark urine, light or acholic stools, and hepatomegaly. The decreased bile flow can be due to either liver cell injury or bile duct obstruction (Fig. 1). There may also be variable degrees of hepatic synthetic dysfunction with hypoprothrombinemia manifested as a bleeding disorder.

2.2. Early Recognition of Specific Diseases

The next step in evaluation is prompt recognition of the specific and potentially treatable primary causes of cholestasis, which, if unrecognized, can eventuate in a progressive downhill course. These causes include (1) sepsis, (2) endocrinopathies (e.g., hypothyroidism and panhypopituitarism), (3) nutritional hepatotoxicity due to specific metabolic illnesses (e.g., galactosemia), and (4) other rare metabolic illnesses (e.g., tyrosinemia). Recognition of these entities may permit institution of appropriate therapy and the possible prevention of further morbidity or hepatobiliary injury. Neonatal liver injury is associated rarely with congenital infection due to specific viruses; however, these should be considered. Cystic fibrosis (sweat chloride analysis) and α_1-antitrypsin deficiency (see Section 2.4) can also be addressed quickly.

2.3. Biliary Atresia versus Neonatal Hepatitis

In the remaining cases, a specific diagnostic category cannot be assigned; therefore, the differential diagnosis revolves around separation of intrahepatic from extrahepatic forms of cholestasis. Clinical examination and historical features may be of some help in divination. Patients with extrahepatic cholestasis (i.e., biliary atresia) have a higher incidence and earlier onset of acholic stools than do infants with intrahepatic cholestasis. Infants with extrahepatic cholestasis are also of normal birthweight, while those with intrahepatic cholestasis (i.e., neonatal hepatitis) may be of lower birthweight, have splenomegaly, and manifest signs of generalized disease. Hepatomegaly is more frequent in patients with extrahepatic cholestasis; their liver is often firm or hard in consistency. In patients with intrahepatic cholestasis, hepatomegaly is less prominent and is less frequently associated with a palpable change in liver consistency.

No single biochemical test or imaging procedure has entirely satisfactory discriminatory value. The use of percutaneous transhepatic cholangiography (PTC) and endoscopic retrograde cholangiopancreatography (ERCP) has not been found to be of great help in the evaluation of the infant with cholestasis. Ultrasonography should be carried out early, however, since it may detect unsuspected causes of cholestasis associated with dilation of the biliary tract or the presence of a choledochal cyst. Radionucleotide hepatobiliary scintigraphy, using technetium-labeled iminodiacetic acid analogues, has been useful in evaluating hepatic clearance and the time for appearance of isotope in the intestinal tract. In biliary atresia, hepatic cell function is intact; therefore, uptake of the imaging agent is unimpaired, but excretion into the intestine is absent. The reverse is commonly seen in idiopathic neonatal hepatitis. Administration of phenobarbital (5 mg/kg for 5 days) prior to the study may enhance biliary excretion in patients with intrahepatic disease.

Liver biopsy provides the most reliable discriminatory evidence.[1] The histologic features noted in extrahepatic biliary atresia are bile ductular proliferation, the presence of bile plugs, and portal or periacinar edema and fibrosis. The basic hepatic acinar architecture remains intact. By contrast, infants with intrahepatic disease (i.e., idiopathic neonatal hepatitis) may have diffuse hepatocellular distortion accompanied by marked inflammation and focal hepatocellular necrosis. Paucity of intrahepatic bile ducts may be detected even during the first week of life; however, subsequent biopsies from these patients may be needed to demonstrate the characteristic pattern and evolution of bile ductal hypoplasia. The later histologic feature can be associated with syndromic features (Table II) or may be seen in a wide variety of viral, metabolic, and idiopathic diseases.[2] Liver biopsy may also provide clues to previously unrecognized entities, if storage material, viral inclusions, or specific patterns of injury are visualized.[3]

The schema outlined above will permit proper delination of patients into the classic categories. As an additional step, careful thought in search of a novel metabolic basis for those with idiopathic neonatal hepatitis may prove fruitful. It is this approach that has enabled clinicians to delineate α_1-antitrypsin deficiency as a specific cause of neonatal liver disease.

3. α_1-ANTITRYPSIN DEFICIENCY

Polymorphic α_1-antitrypsin, a glycoprotein synthesized by the liver, accounts for 80% of the serum α_1-globulin fraction.[4–6] α_1-Antitrypsin is the major inhibitor of destructive enzymes, such as leukocyte elastase, which is able to cleave the connective tissue components of the extracellular matrix of tissue. Therefore, α_1-antitrypsin normally protects the lung from destruction. In the presence of low serum protease activity (i.e., serum α_1-antitrypsin levels <40–50% of normal), elastases are unchecked and emphysema may ensue. The rise in serum α_1-antitrypsin levels in response to injury is assumed to preserve a balance between released cellular proteinases and proteinase inhibitors within vascular and extravascular fluids during injury. Deficiency of the major serum protease inhibitor, α-antitrypsin, is also associated with neonatal cholestasis, as well as cirrhosis in later childhood in a percentage of homozygous persons.[4,5]

4. BIOCHEMISTRY

α_1-Antitrypsin is encoded in the human genome by a single autosomal locus on the long arm of chromosome 14.[6,7] This locus is termed Pi (for protease inhibitor), and each of the multiple variant forms of α-antitrypsin is indicated by a single letter. The designation relates to their relative mobility on acid-starch gel. Isoelectric focusing (IEF) techniques and resolution of the polymorphic variants in the prealbumin zone suggest that the normal phenotype of the Pi system is M; the slowest migrating phenotype is PIZ.[5,7]

Determination of the phenotypic codominant alleles that control the electrophoretic mobility

Table II. Frequency of Major Abnormalities in Patients with Syndromic Paucity of Interlobular Bile Ducts[a]

Abnormality	Number present	Number of patients studied	Percent
Chronic cholestasis	73	80	91
Characteristic facies	76	80	95
Cardiac murmur	68	80	85
Vertebral abnormalities	70	80	87
Embryotoxon	55	62	88

[a]From Alagille et al.[2]

should be carried out in any patient with liver disease. Patients with liver disease are almost universally PiZZ; the genetic deficiency is inherited as an autosomal-recessive trait. α_1-Antitrypsin of the Z type is present in low concentration in serum—<0.2 mg/ml, approximately 10–20% of normal. Intermediate types (MZ, MS, and SZ) are associated with reduction in serum levels of α_1-antitrypsin; most are not definitively associated with the presence of liver disease, although neonatal hepatitis has been reported in a few heterozygous SZ children. The incidence of the PiZZ (homozygous-deficient) phenotype is estimated to be 1 in 2000 live births in Scandinavians and 1 in 7600 live births in North American whites.[8] A single amino acid substitution (lysine for glutamic acid at residue 342, related to a G-to-A transition at a corresponding location in the gene) is responsible for the production of a biochemically abnormal α_1-antitrypsin. The abnormal protein is poorly processed by the liver, aggregating and accumulating in the hepatocytes, with resultant low circulating antiprotease activity.

5. PATHOGENESIS

The cause of the liver disease in specific α_1-antitrypsin-deficient persons is uncertain. It appears that the abnormal α_1-antitrypsin is blocked in the secretory pathway prior to entrance into the Golgi apparatus.[6] Liver damage is presumably secondary either to retention of the α_1-antitrypsin in the liver or to a decreased availability of protease inhibitor to prevent tissues from injury. The fact that liver disease is not universal in homozygous-deficient persons suggests a complex pathogenesis. Udall et al.,[9] who had previously shown that transport of proteases occurs readily across the neonatal intestinal tract, allowing their entry into the systemic circulation, postulated that lumenal enzymes enter the systemic circulation of the neonate and, in the absence of protease inhibitors, initiate inflammation and fibrosis. Breast milk, with inherent antiproteases, seems to offer protection against the development of liver injury[10] (Fig. 2). Early feeding practices may therefore offer a confounding variable in the genesis of liver disease.

6. INCIDENCE

A perspective on α_1-antitrypsin deficiency and liver disease in childhood was initially provided by the prospective studies of Sveger[11] performed in Sweden between 1972 and 1974. Sveger screened via Pi-typing 200,000 newborn infants (representing 95% of all births in Sweden during that period); thus, he detected 122 infants with PiZZ and 48 with PiSZ. At-risk infants were monitored by periodic clinical evaluations and liver-function studies. Twelve percent of PiZZ

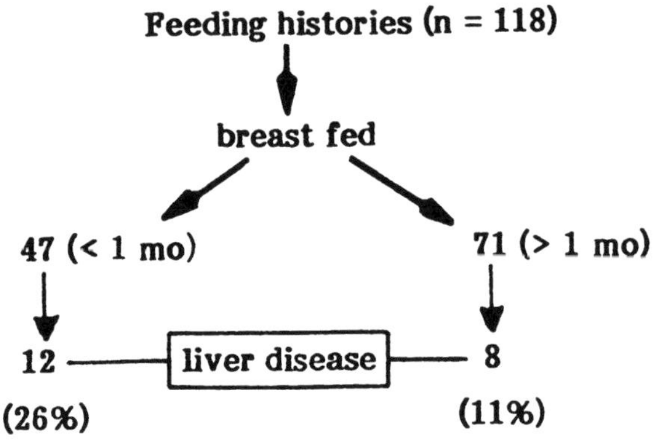

Figure 2. Analysis of feeding patterns of infants with α-1-antitrypsin deficiency. The incidence of liver disease was higher in those infants who had been breast fed for less than one month. (Adapted from Sveger.[29])

subjects had cholestasis, while an additional 7% had clinical evidence of liver disease in infancy. At 6 months of age, these infants appeared to be clinically recovered from their liver disease. The remaining PiZZ infants were clinically normal; however, 47% of these infants had elevated liver enzymes at 3 months of age. Therefore, only 34% of the PiZZ infants were found to have no clinical or laboratory evidence of liver injury. None of the PiSZ infants had clinical evidence of liver disease. In subsequent studies, it was noted that of the 120 PiZZ children followed prospectively for the first 4 years of life, 2.5% died.[12,13] Cholestasis had been found in 14 of PiZZ infants. At age 4, two had symptoms of cirrhosis; 45% of PiZZ children had increased serum transaminases suggesting persisting liver disease at 4 years.

When viewed from another perspective, approximately 5–10% of all infants presenting with undefined neonatal cholestasis (i.e., idiopathic neonatal hepatitis) may be subsequently shown to be homozygous α_1-antitrypsin deficient.[1,14] Sveger's initial suggestion that of all homozygous-deficient persons, less than 20% will develop neonatal cholestasis, has been confirmed by other series. These patients are clinically indistinguishable from other infants with idiopathic neonatal hepatitis. The only distinguishing features are the serum electrophoretic pattern and the histologic features.

7. CLINICAL MANIFESTATIONS

The presentation and clinical course of liver disease in patients with α_1-antitrypsin deficiency are highly variable. Jaundice, acoholic stools, and hepatomegaly are often present during the first week of life. Ghishan et al.[15] described a patient with α_1-antitrypsin deficiency (PiZZ) presenting with ascites and cirrhosis in the neonatal period, suggesting that liver insult may occur in utero and present as cryptogenic cirrhosis. The average birthweight of the homozygous-deficient infant may be below normal and unrelated to prematurity, suggesting once again the possibility of intrauterine hepatic damage.

The pattern of neonatal liver injury may also be highly variable. There is hepatocellular damage with giant cell transformation, minimal inflammation, and bile stasis, along with varying degrees of portal fibrosis with bile duct proliferation. These features are those of idiopathic neonatal hepatitis; further evaluation (i.e., special stains), however, will indicate the "hidden" diagnosis. There may be subsequent complete histologic resolution, persisting liver disease, or the development of cirrhosis. The jaundice usually clears during the second to fourth month, and the child may appear clinically well.

Similarly, chronic liver disease or undefined cryptogenic cirrhosis may present in an older child with portal hypertension or another manifestation, such as hematemesis. The risk of the development of liver disease in 115 adults with homozygous α_1-antitrypsin deficiency (PiZZ), evaluated by Cox and Smyth,[16] was relatively high for men between 51 and 60 years of age; the risk for women was lower. Cox and Smyth suggested that periodic assessment of liver function may be warranted for patients with α_1-antitrypsin deficiency who are over 40 years of age. The relative risk of cirrhosis could not be estimated, however, since no comparison group was included. Eriksson et al.[17] conducted a populated-based autopsy study in Malmö, Sweden, in order to assess the risk of cirrhosis as well as the risk of primary liver cancer in patients with homozygous α_1-antitrypsin deficiency (PiZZ). These workers found a strong relationship between α_1-antitrypsin and both entities; the point estimate of risk for cirrhosis and primary liver cancer were significant only for men. Similar to tyrosinemia and hemochromatosis, α_1-antitrypsin can therefore be viewed as a premalignant metabolic liver disease. The role of exogenous factors needs to be carefully examined.

Hodges et al.[18] suggested that heterozygous (MZ) α_1-antitrypsin deficiency in adults is associated with chronic active liver disease and cirrhosis. In 1055 patients biopsied over a 5-year period, there was an increased prevalence of MZ in patients with cryptogenic cirrhosis and with chronic active hepatitis (CAH) ($p < 0.001$). Inclusions in these cases appeared to be small in size. The study suggested that phenotyping of serum of every patient with undefined liver disease may provide important information.

8. DIAGNOSIS

The diagnosis of α_1-antitrypsin deficiency is first suggested by determination of α_1-antitrypsin phenotype and confirmed by liver biopsy. While the histologic features of chronic liver disease secondary to α_1-antitrypsin deficiency disease are well described,[4,5] i.e., mixed macro-/micronodular cirrhosis, and periodic acid-Schiff (PAS)-positive/diastase-resistant globules in periportal hepatocytes, the morphologic changes in utero and during the first few months of life may be nonspecific or easily confused with disease processes of other etiologies. The neonatal cholestasis clinically seen in 12% of PiZZ infants is associated with a variety of morphologic features.[11] The lobular architecture of the liver is usually retained with only mild disruption of hepatocyte cords. Portal areas are often expanded by an infiltrate of lymphocytes, plasma cells, and residual extramedullary hematopoiesis primarily of eosinophilic and neutrophilic precursors (Fig. 3). Bile ductules are increased in number (cholangiolar proliferation), contributing to the expanded portal areas. Fine strands of connective tissue may further expand the portal area and extend into the adjacent parenchyma. Bile pigment may be present in hepatocytes, Kupffer cells, portal area macrophages, and canaliculi (Fig. 4). This canalicular stasis may occasionally impart a pseudoglandular appearance to the surrounding hepatocytes. Finely granular hemosiderin pigment is also present in hepatocytes and Kupffer cells related to the extramedullary hematopoiesis. Giant cell transformation of hepatocytes with 3–10 hepatocytes coalescing to form a single cell with multiple nuclei is occasionally seen but with less frequency than in neonatal hepatitis from other causes (e.g., viral other metabolic defects). Hepatocellular necrosis is usually mild, but ballooning degeneration is rarely seen.

α_1-Antitrypsin globules are difficult to identify on hematoxylin and eosin (H&E)-stained

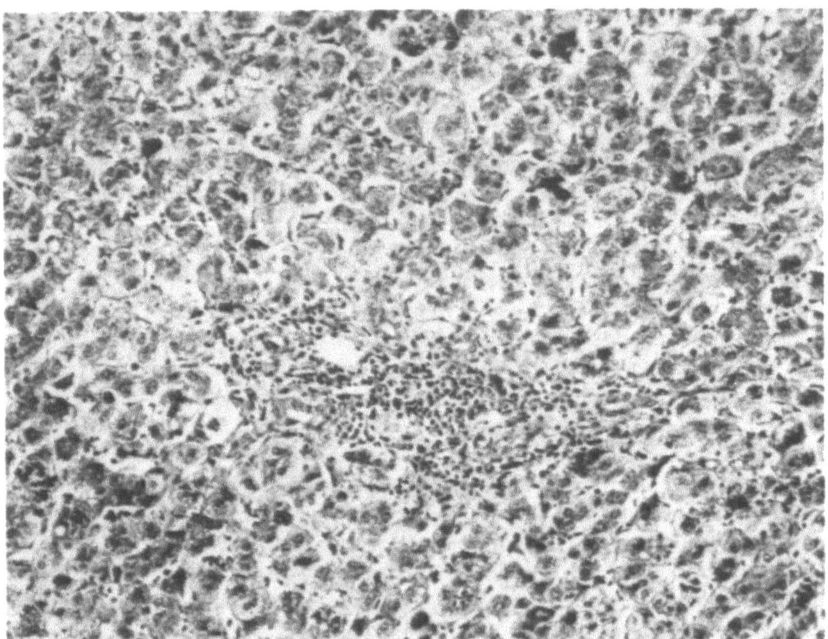

Figure 3. Neonatal hepatitis in a 3-week-old boy. The normal lobular architecture is disrupted by pseudoglandular transformation of hepatocytes, canalicular and hepatocellular cholestasis, and expansion of portal areas by lymphocytes and residual extramedullary hematopoiesis. (H&E, ×180)

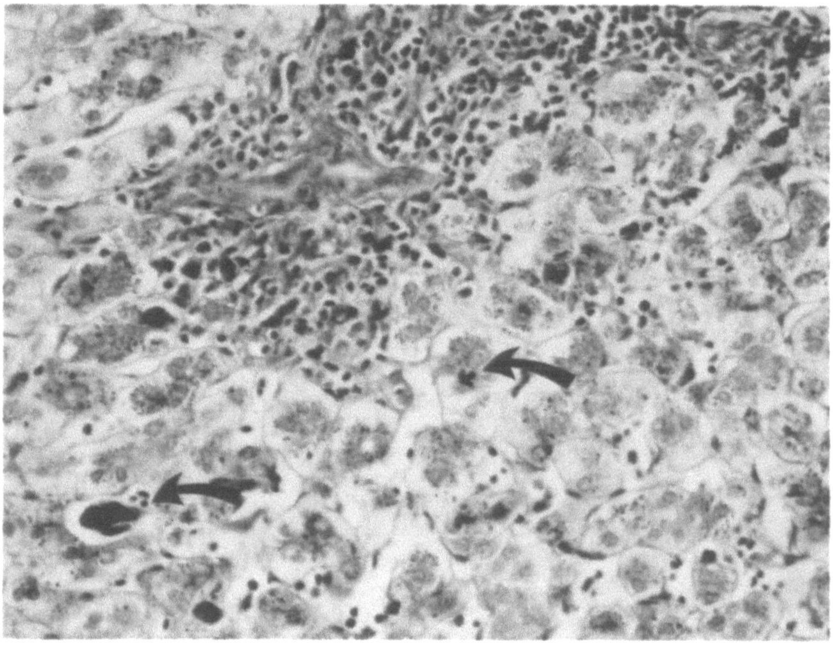

Figure 4. Neonatal hepatitis in a 3-week-old boy. Bile is present within the canaliculi (arrows) and in the cytoplasm of hepatocytes. The finely granular material in this periodic acid-Schiff (PAS) stain with diastase digestion represents both bile and small α_1-antitrypsin bodies (confirmed by immunoperoxidase stains). Note the portal infiltrate of lymphocytes and extramedullary hematopoiesis (top center).

sections in the first 4–6 months of life; PAS stain with diastase digestion (PAS/D) enhances their visibility only mildly, since they are usually quite small (1–3 μm) and may be confused with bile and hemosiderin pigment, which may also be PAS/D positive.[4,5] Globules, however, may be readily identified with immunofluorescent and immunoperoxidase techniques (Fig. 5).

Electron microscopy in these (and older) patients displays amorphous electron-dense material (α_1-antitrypsin) in dilated rough endoplasmic reticulum (RER) concentrated in the part of the cell lying toward the space of Disse but occasionally found throughout the whole cytoplasm[19,20] (Figs. 6 and 7). Dilated peroxisomes and lysosomes containing amorphous material may also be present. Evidence of cell injury and death may be seen in cells with stored α_1-antitrypsin in the dilated, RER while cells without this material will be unremarkable. Hepatocytes in patients with the genotype Pi^{--}, however, in which no serum concentration of α_1-antitrypsin can be detected, show no ultrastructural abnormality of the RER.[21]

In infants in whom neonatal cholestasis develops, a variety of morphologic changes may follow the initial injury. Resolution may occur in approximately 25% of cases, with only minimal fibrosis remaining. In another 25%, a more severe portal/periportal fibrosis develops; these children live into adulthood, when complications may include the development of cirrhosis and hepatocellular carcinoma.[17] In the remaining 50%, extensive liver disease develops, culminating in cirrhosis, portal hypertension, ascites, and liver failure in the first or second decade of life. Cirrhosis may develop rapidly (ascites and cirrhosis have been seen in a 2-week-old infant with α_1-antitrypsin deficiency[15]) or may progress slowly over months to years. The mixed macro-/micronodular cirrhosis is characterized by nodules of residual and regenerative hepatocytes, varying from a few millimeters to 1–2 cm in diameter, separated by thin to broad bands of connective tissue (Figs. 8 and 9). Hepatocytes near

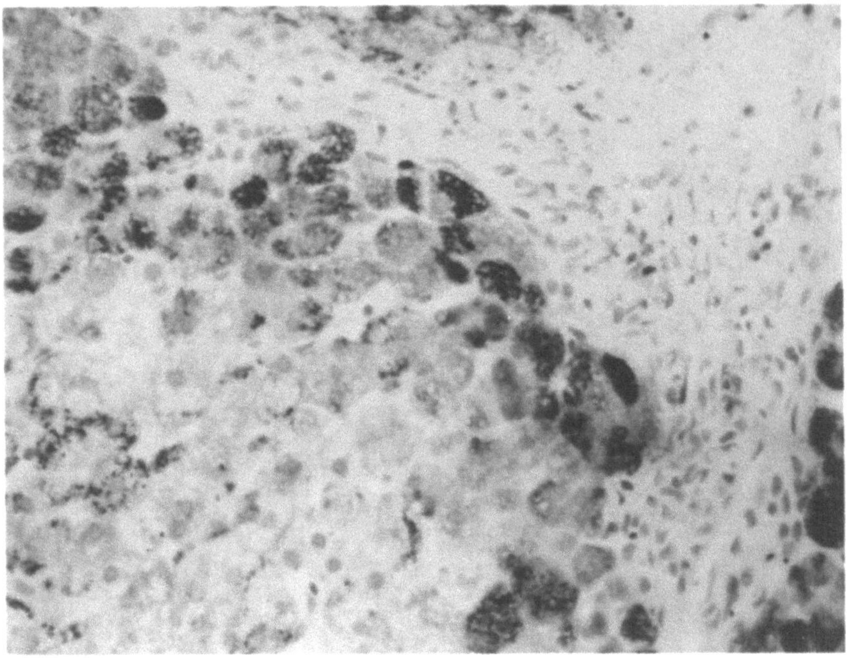

Figure 5. Macronodular cirrhosis in a 1-year-old girl. While not readily visible on H & E stain in this case, numerous α_1-antitrypsin bodies are noted with immunoperoxidase stain. (IP, ×400)

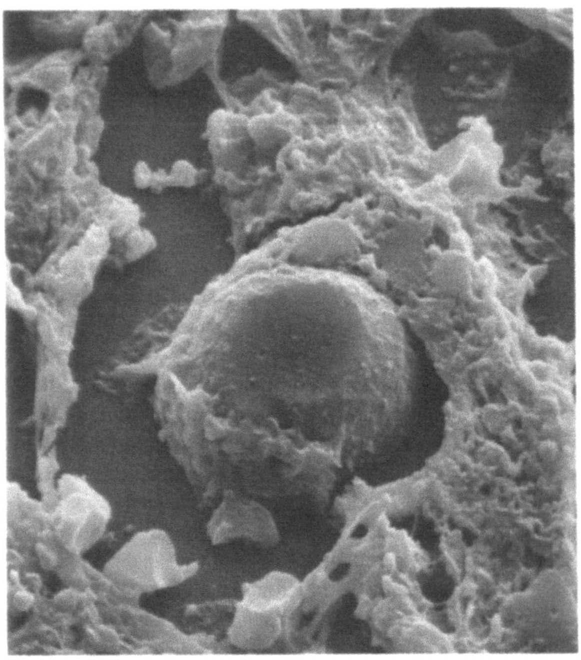

Figure 6. Macronodular cirrhosis in a 4-year-old boy. By scanning electron microscopy (SEM), a large inclusion (center) lies within a hepatocyte. Note the red blood cells (lighter material at lower left) along the wall of a sinusoid. (×2250) (Courtesy of K. G. Ishak, M.D., Ph.D., Washington, D.C.)

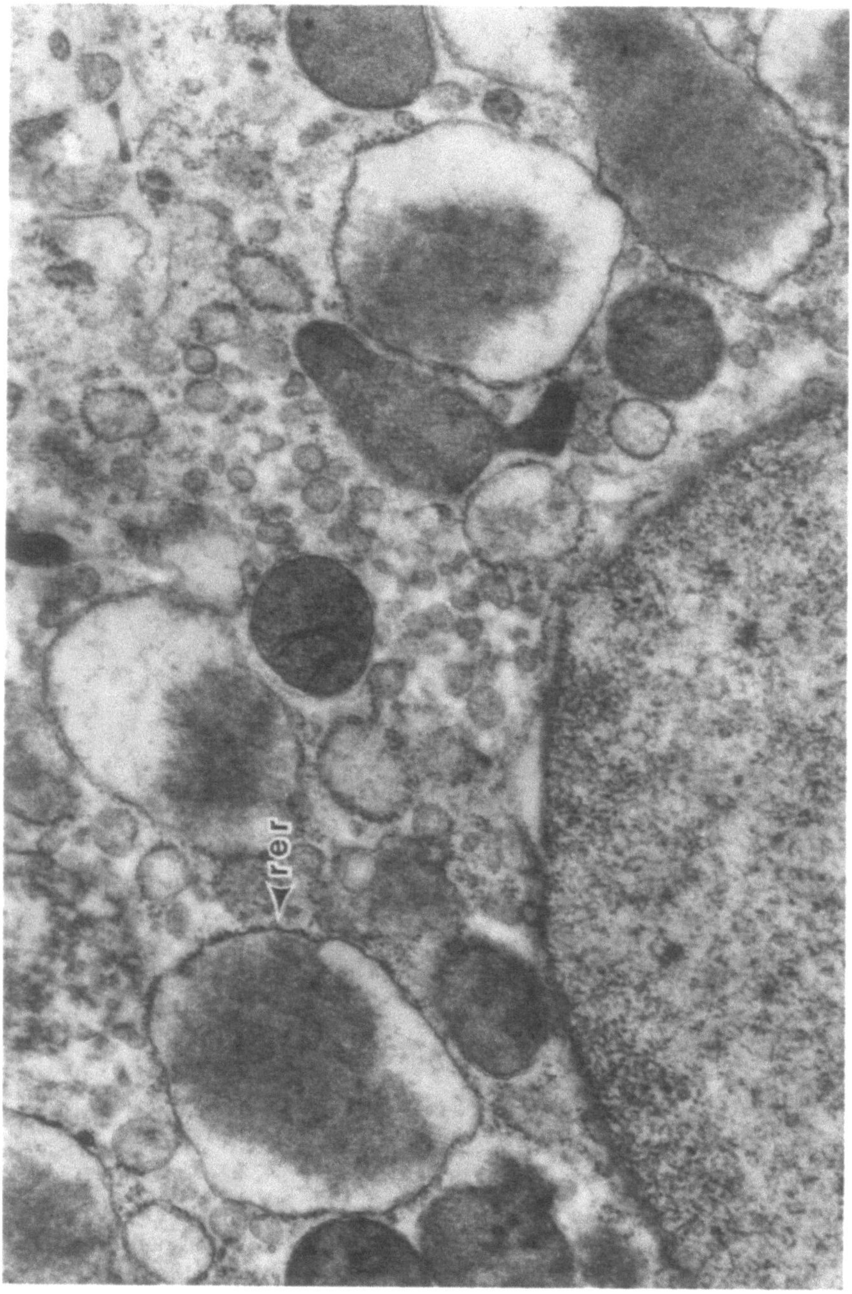

Figure 7. Cytoplasm of hepatocyte from a patient with α_1-antitrypsin deficiency. Note the dilated sacs of the rough endoplasmic reticulum (rer) partially filled with electron-dense homogeneous material; these correspond to the periodic acid-Schiff (PAS)-positive diastase-resistant globules seen on light microscopy. The material retained within the endoplasmic reticulum is the abnormal α_1-antitrypsin protein. (Transmission electron micrograph, lead citrate stain, ×31,350) (Courtesy of M. James Phillips, M.D., Toronto, Ontario.)

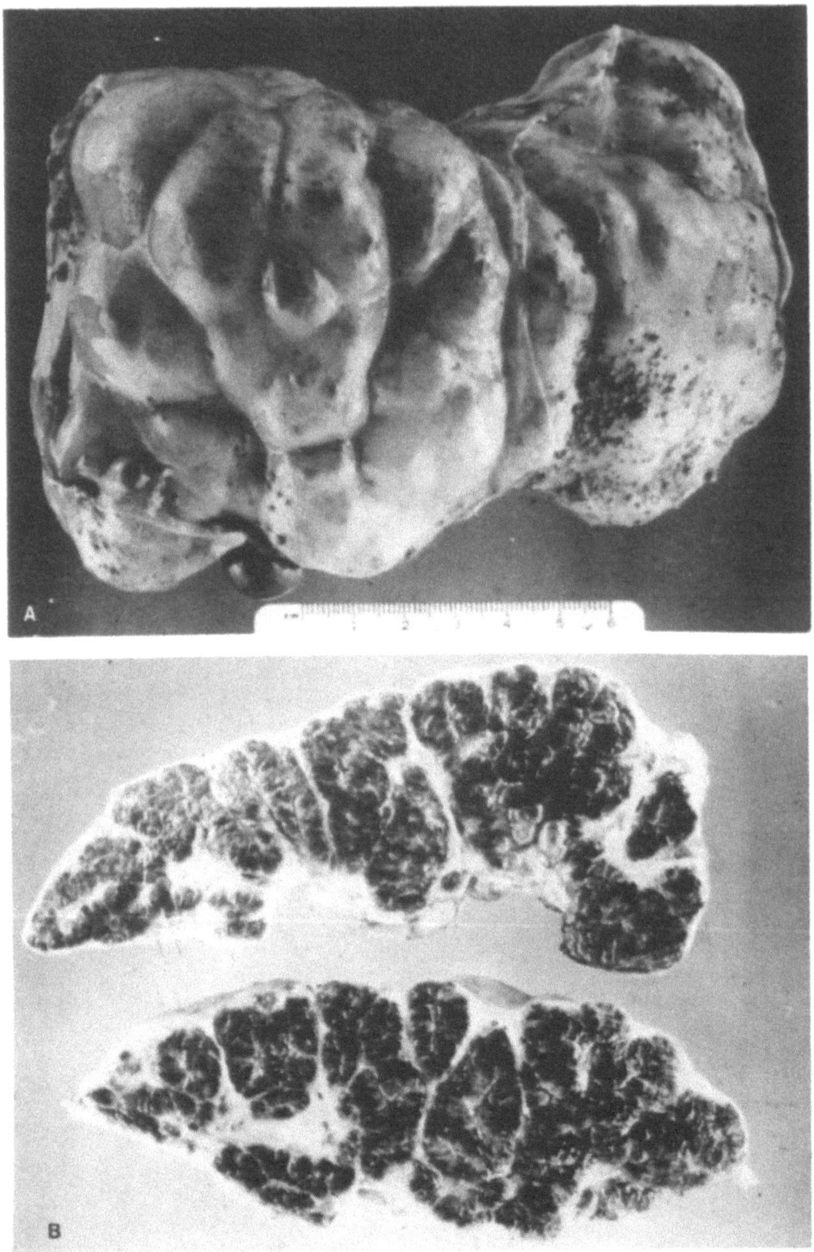

Figure 8. Macronodular cirrhosis in a 9-year-old boy. (A) The external surface of the liver is markedly distorted by large regenerative nodules separated by connective tissue. (B) On cut surface, the macronodules are separated and subdivided by irregular bands of dense connective tissue.

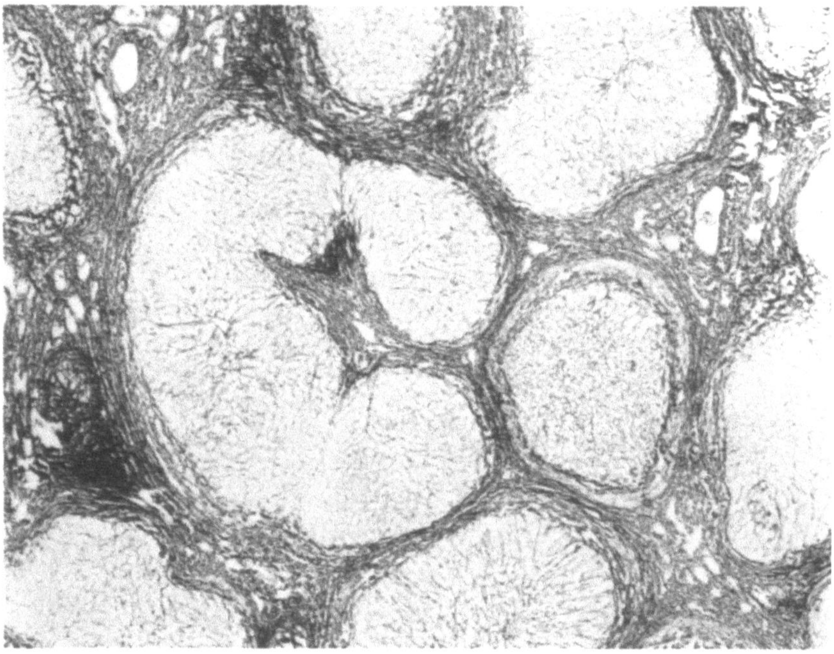

Figure 9. Macronodular cirrhosis in a 2-year-old boy. Broad septal bands of connective tissue containing vessels and bile ducts surrounding variable-sized nodules of hepatocytes. Note the absence of portal areas within the regenerative nodules. (Reticulin, ×15)

these septae contain the classic smooth, round, pink α_1-antitrypsin globules. A single large (10–25 μm in diameter) globule may occupy most of the cytoplasm of a cell, or a mixture of smaller globules may be present (Figs. 10 and 11). Cholangiolar and canalicular cholestasis may be seen along with focal bile duct proliferation, increased copper storage, Mallory bodies, and fatty metamorphosis. Hepatocellular necrosis and inflammation may be focally present at the junction of septa and hepatocyte nodule.

9. TREATMENT

Management of a child with liver disease associated with α_1-antitrypsin deficiency is non-specific, i.e., that of chronic cholestasis and/or cirrhosis with possible resultant end-stage liver disease; there is currently no specific therapy. Since liver disease is apparently associated with accumulation of aggregated α_1-antitrypsin (Z type), prevention or direct treatment is theoretically possible through (1) phenotypic conversion via liver transplantation, (2) induction of secretion of the abnormal protein, or (3) modulation of the regulatory gene. Orthotopic liver transplantation has been successfully performed in a large number of patients with advanced liver disease associated with α_1-antitrypsin deficiency. The remaining modalities, however, are the subject of much investigation.

Danazol, a 17α-substituted alkyl steroid is capable of increasing serum α_1-antitrypsin levels; however, there is no evidence that this is of clinical value. Replacement therapy looms as a possible treatment for lung disease. Rosenberg et al.[22] recently described the synthesis, in yeast, of a functional oxidation-resistant mutant of human α_1-antitrypsin. Gene-transfer experiments, i.e.,

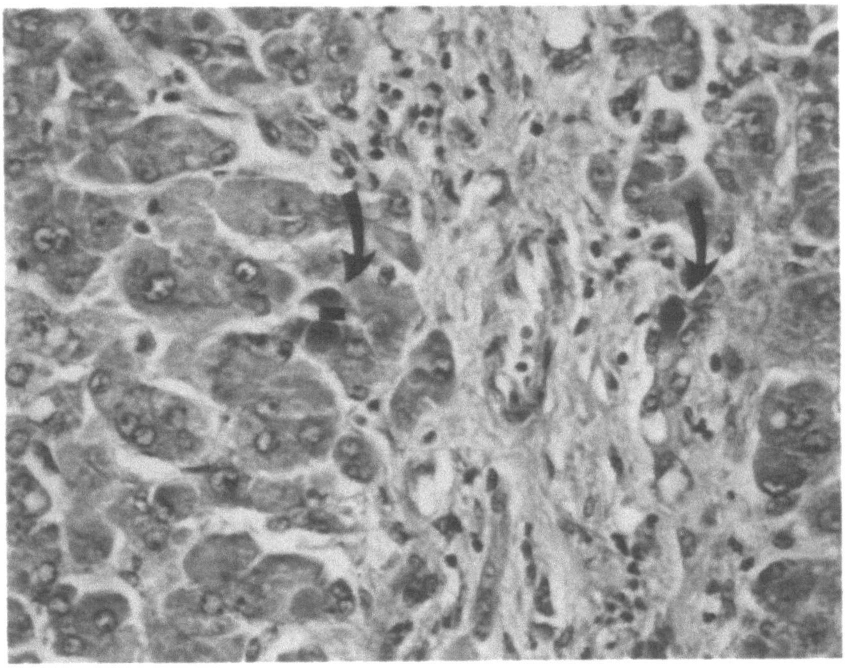

Figure 10. Macronodular cirrhosis in a 9-year-old boy. Hepatocytes adjacent to the fibrous septa contain variable-sized smooth round cytoplasmic bodies (arrows) representing collections of α_1-antitrypsin. (H&E, ×400)

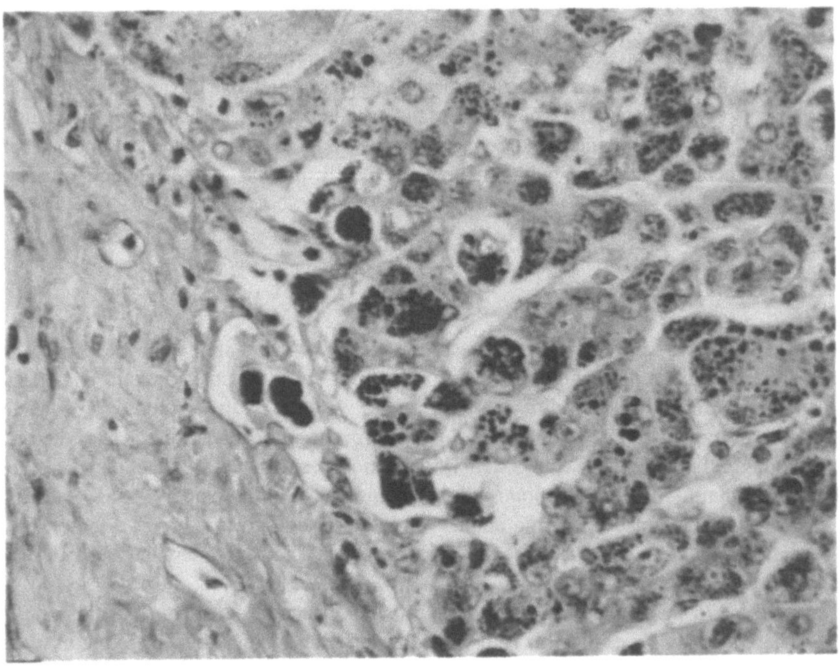

Figure 11. Macronodular cirrhosis in a 9-year-old boy. Using periodic acid-Schiff stain with diastase digestion, large numbers of α_1-antitrypsin bodies can be seen within hepatocytes. (PAS/D, ×300)

introduction of cloned normal human α_1-antitrypsin into cells lacking α_1-antitrypsin, is theoretically possible to ameliorate lung disease in the future.[23] Infusion of a plasma-derived concentrate of α_1-antitrypsin or synthetic protease have also been postulated as future therapeutic modalities.[24]

10. PROGNOSIS

The outcome of α_1-antitrypsin-deficient children with liver disease has been suggested by several studies since the initial observations of Sveger, and the results are remarkably uniform.[19,25] Approximately 25% of these children will persist in having abnormal liver-function tests and increasing evidence of cirrhosis may develop, such as portal hypertension and ascites; they will die of hepatic complications in the first 10 years of life unless orthotopic liver transplantation is successfully accomplished. Another 25% will have evidence of persistently abnormal liver function but will have a slow progression to cirrhosis. Another 25% will have minimal liver dysfunction and less severe fibrosis on liver biopsy and will live to adulthood. Another 25% will recover from the initial insult and return to normal liver function and normal liver and spleen size, except for minor evidence of residual fibrosis. Nebbia et al.[26] studied 45 children with a history of neonatal cholestasis associated with α_1-antitrypsin deficiency (PiZZ), 20 of whom apparently recovered. The 25 children in whom cirrhosis developed had been noted earlier on to have more fibrosis. The intrafamilial prognosis is also remarkably similar. Subtle differences suggest that genetic and environmental influences coexist.

11. PRENATAL DIAGNOSIS

The gene for α_1-antitrypsin has been cloned and sequenced, and the precise genetic differences have been defined; prenatal diagnosis of α_1-antitrypsin deficiency is therefore possible through molecular genetic techniques and analysis of tissue obtained by chorionic villus biopsy or amniocentesis. Direct analysis of the mutation site in the gene using oligonucleotide probes specific for the M, S, or Z alleles[27] and analysis of restriction fragment length polymorphisms (RFLP) are the currently employed modalities.[28] The possibility exists for direct first-trimester prenatal diagnosis of PiZZ α_1-antitrypsin deficiency via analyses of fetal DNA.[8] Prenatal diagnosis had previously been carried out via Pi typing of blood samples obtained by fetoscopy, which entailed significant risk. Despite the availability of detection of the PiZZ fetus, there is very little to justify intervention. No currently available methodology will predict which infant with PiZZ will have liver disease, but the fact that there is a high degree of intrafamilial correlation (i.e., the liver disease "breeds true") may provide some justification.

REFERENCES

1. Balistreri WF: Neonatal cholestasis. *J Pediatr* **106:**171–184, 1985.
2. Alagille D, Estrada A, Hadchouel M, et al: Syndromic paucity of interlobular bile ducts (Alagille syndrome or arteriohepatic dysplasia): Review of 80 cases. *J Pediatr* **110:**195–200, 1987.
3. Balistreri WF, Schubert WK: Liver disease in infancy and childhood, in Schiff L, Schiff E (eds): *Diseases of the Liver,* 6th ed. Lippincott, Philadelphia, 1986, pp. 1337–1426.
4. Sharp HL, Bridges R,A, Krivit W, et al: Cirrhosis associated with α-1-antritrypsin deficiency: A previously unrecognized inherited disorder. *J Lab Clin Med* **73:**934–939, 1969.
5. Sharp HL: Alpha-1-antitrypsin. An ignored protein in understanding liver disease. *Semin Liver Dis* **20:**314–328, 1982.
6. Bathurst IC, Travis J, George PM, et al: Structural and functional characterization of the abnormal Z α-1-antitypsin isolated from human liver. *FEBS* **177:**179–183, 1984.

7. Laurell CB, Eriksson S: The electrophoretic α-1-antiglobulin pattern of serum in α-1-antitrypsin deficiency. *Scand J Clin Lab Invest* **15:**132–140, 1965.
8. Cox DW, Mansfield T: Prenatal diagnosis of α-1-antitrypsin deficiency and estimates of fetal risk for disease. *J Med Genet* **24:**52–59, 1987.
9. Udall JN, Bloch KJ, Walker WA: Transport of proteases across neonatal intestine and development of liver disease in infants with α-1-antitrypsin deficiency. *Lancet* **1:**1441–1443, 1982.
10. Udall JN Jr, Dixon M, Newman AP, et al: Liver disease in α-1-antitrypsin deficiency: A retrospective analysis of the influence of early breast- vs. bottle-feeding. *JAMA* **253:**2679–2683, 1985.
11. Sveger T: Liver disease in α-1-antitrypsin detected by screening of 200,000 infants. *N Engl J Med* **294:**1316–1319, 1976.
12. Sveger T: Prospective study of children with α-1-antitrypsin deficiency: Eight-year-old follow-up. *J Pediatr* **104:**91–93, 1984.
13. Sveger T, Thelin T: Four-year-old children with α-1-antitrypsin deficiency: Clinical follow-up and parental attitudes towards neonatal screening. *Acta Paediatr Scand* **70:**171–177, 1981.
14. Danks DM, Campbell PE, Jack I, et al: Studies of the aetiology of neonatal hepatitis and biliary atresia. *Arch Dis Child* **52:**360–365, 1977.
15. Ghishan FK, Gray GF, Greene HL: Alpha-1-antitrypsin deficiency presenting with ascites and cirrhosis in the neonatal periods. *Gastroenterology* **85:**435–439, 1983.
16. Cox DW, Smyth S: Risk for liver disease in adults with α-1-antitrypsin deficiency. *Am J Med* **74:**221–227, 1983.
17. Eriksson S, Carlson J, Velez R: Risk of cirrhosis and primary liver cancer in α-1-antitrypsin deficiency. *N Engl J Med* **314:**736–739, 1986.
18. Hodges JR, Millward-Sadler GH, Barbatis C, et al: Heterozygous MZ α-1-antitrypsin deficiency in adults with chronic active hepatitis and cryptogenic cirrhosis. *N Engl J Med* **304:**557–560, 1981.
19. Nemeth A, Strandvik B, Glaumann H: Alpha-1-antitrypsin deficiency and juvenile liver disease: Ulstrastructural observations compared with light microscopy and routine liver tests. *Virchows Arch* **44:**15–33, 1983.
20. Hultcrantz R, Mengarelli S: Ultrastructural liver pathology in patients with minimal liver disease and α-1-antitrypsin deficiency: A comparison between heterozygous and homozygous patients. *Hepatology* **4:**937–945, 1984.
21. Feldman G, Martin J-P, Sesboue R, et al: The ultrastructure of hepatocytes in alpha-1-antitrypsin deficiency with the genotype Pi⁻⁻. *Gut* **16:**796–799, 1975.
22. Rosenberg S, Barr PJ, Najarian RC, et al: Synthesis in yeast of a functional oxidation-resistant mutant of human α-1-antitrypsin. *Nature (Lond)* **312:**77–80, 1984.
23. Ledley FD, Woo SLC: Molecular basis of α-1-antitrypsin deficiency and its potential therapy by gene transfer. *J Inher Metab Dis* **9:**85–91, 1986.
24. Cohen AB: Unraveling the mysteries of α-1-antitrypsin deficiency. *N Engl J Med* **314:**778–779, 1986.
25. Psacharopoulos HT, Mowat AP, Cook PJL, et al: Outcome of liver disease associated with α-1-antitrypsin deficiency (PiZ): Implications for genetic counselling and antenatal diagnosis. *Arch Dis Child* **58:**882–887, 1983.
26. Nebbia G, Hadchouel M, Odievre M, et al: Early assessment of evolution of liver disease associated with α-1-antitrypsin deficiency in childhood. *J Pediatr* **102:**661–664, 1983.
27. Kidd VJ, Golbus MS, Wallace RB, et al: Prenatal diagnosis of α-1-antitrypsin deficiency by direct analysis of the mutation site in the gene. *N Engl J Med* **310:**639–642, 1984.
28. Hejtmancik JF, Ward PA, Mansfield T, et al: Prenatal diagnosis of α-1-antirrypsin deficiency by restriction fragment length polymorphisms, and comparison with oligonucleotide probe analysis. *Lancet* **2:**767–770, 1986.
29. Sveger T: *JAMA* **254:**3036, 1985.

23

Hemochromatosis: Clinical Aspects and Response to Therapy

Norman D. Grace

1. INTRODUCTION

One hundred years ago, von Recklinghausen introduced the term hemochromatosis to describe the triad of diabetes mellitus, hyperpigmentation of the skin, and cirrhosis of the liver with iron overload. Since that time, a few milestones have greatly contributed to our understanding of the disorders of iron metabolism. In a classic monograph published in 1935, Sheldon[1] reviewed 311 published cases of hemochromatosis and proposed that the disease was the result of a genetic abnormality in iron metabolism. Seven years later, Balfour et al.[2] introduced venesection therapy as a method to deplete the excessive iron stores. During the early 1960s, MacDonald[3] published a series of papers questioning the genetic concept of the disease and raising a possible role for alcohol. He argued that cirrhosis and iron deposition may occur together but were not causally related. The difficulties in developing an animal model for the disease raised doubts about the hepatotoxicity of iron.[4] These concerns have been resolved by recent major advances. The toxicity of iron has been demonstrated at the cellular level, and histocompatability typing has verified the inheritance of hemochromatosis as an autosomal-recessive disorder in most, but not all, affected patients.[5]

The pathogenesis and pathologic features of hemochromatosis are discussed in Chapter 24. This chapter emphasizes the clinical features of the disease and their response to depletion of hepatic iron stores by venesection therapy.

2. DEFINITION AND CLASSIFICATION

Hemochromatosis may be defined as cirrhosis or fibrosis of the liver with increased iron stores, primarily in the hepatocyte with lesser amounts in Kupffer cells, associated with iron deposition in other organs, especially the pancreas, heart, and pituitary. These patients demonstrate increased iron absorption, inappropriate for the level of iron stores. All the entities listed in Table I would be included in this definition. Diagnosis of the familial form is based upon the appropriate history, HLA documentation of the inheritance pattern, and exclusion of the other potential causes of hepatic iron overload. The remainder of this chapter deals only with genetic hemochromatosis.

Norman D. Grace • Tufts University School of Medicine; Gastroenterology Service, The Faulkner Hospital, Boston, Massachusetts 02130.

Table I. Classification of Liver Disease Associated with Iron Overload

Genetic hemochromatosis
Liver disease associated with iron-loading anemias (ineffective erythropoiesis)
Thalassemia
Pyridoxine responsive anemias
Hereditary spherocytosis, glucose 6-phosphate dehydrogenase deficiency
Folic acid and vitamin B_{12} deficiency
Cirrhosis of the liver with secondary iron overload
Alcoholic cirrhosis
Postportasystemic shunt
Liver disease associated with excess iron ingestion
Dietary (i.e., Bantu)
Prolonged iron therapy

3. ABNORMALITIES IN HEMOCHROMATOSIS

Although the precise nature of the defect that allows patients with hemochromatosis to absorb iron inappropriate to their level of iron stores remains unclear, several potential abnormalities have been identified:

1. In vitro demonstration of increased iron uptake by duodenal mucosal cells[6–8]
2. Decreased avidity for iron by the reticuloendothelial system (RES), leading to continuous saturation of plasma transferrin[9–10]
3. Increased hemosiderin/ferritin ratio in hepatocytes (in patients with untreated hemochromatosis)[11]
4. Increased lysosomal fragility, leading to a release of iron into the cytoplasm, resulting in cellular damage and death[4,5]

4. MODE OF INHERITANCE

During the past decade, major advances have taken place in our understanding of the genetics in hemochromatosis. A strong association between HLA-A3 and, to a lesser extent, HLA-B7 and -B14 antigens, has been established.[5] The hemochromatosis locus is located on chromosome 6 in close proximity to the HLA-A locus.[12] Several large family studies have demonstrated an association between siblings with the same two haplotypes as the proband and the presence of genetic hemochromatosis.[13,14] This association was not as significant for offspring.[13] Using HLA typing to classify family members of probands with histologically proven hemochromatosis, elevation of serum ferritin, and transferrin saturation were found in almost all relatives who were homozygotes.[15] Family members who were heterozygous had minor increases in hepatic iron stores, whereas members who were nonidentical were similar to a control population.[16] Long-term follow-up studies in heterozygous patients failed to show clinical or histologic evidence of hepatic damage despite slight increases in hepatic iron stores.[17] By contrast, patients with alcoholic liver disease and increased iron stores have HLA haplotypes similar to a control population.[18] In summary, genetic hemochromatosis has been shown to be an autosomal-recessive disorder, with only homozygous patients developing the disease. The major clinical value of HLA typing lies in identifying those family members at risk of the development of hemochromatosis.

Hemochromatosis ranks among the most common hereditary disorders. Recent estimates of the prevalence of the homozygous state have been 1 : 200–1 : 300, as evidenced by elevations of serum ferritin and transferrin saturation in healthy male subjects.[19] This finding is in contrast to previous estimates, based on autopsy studies, of 1 : 450–500.[20,21]

5. DIAGNOSIS

Since hemochromatosis is a relatively common and treatable form of chronic liver disease, early diagnosis of the syndrome is critical (Table II). Although there is some controversy as to whether the serum ferritin or transferritin saturation is the best screening test, the combination yields a sensitivity of 83%, a specificity of 98%, and a predictive accuracy of 93%.[22] Isolated examples of false negatives using the serum ferritin as a screening test have been reported.[23] Therefore, if both the serum ferritin and transferrin saturation are within normal limits, the patient has a 99% probability that there is not an increase in iron stores.[12,14] Once a potential patient is identified by biochemical screening, a liver biopsy is strongly suggested, to determine the extent of fibrosis and the level of iron stores. Using chemical measurements of hepatic iron concentration (milligrams iron per gram dry weight of tissue) that has been adjusted for the age of the patient, genetic hemochromatosis can be distinguished from other types of liver disease with iron overload including alcoholic liver disease.[24] These studies also suggest a threshold level of hepatic iron above which there is a high risk of fibrosis. Radiologic evaluation using either an abdominal computed tomography (CT) scan (double energy source) or magnetic resonance imaging (MRI) has been advocated by some investigators.[25,26] However, these techniques may lack the sensitivity to detect early cases. Also, they do not give an accurate estimate of hepatic fibrosis. The desferroxamine excretion test can be used for problem cases (i.e., where a liver biopsy might be precluded because of coagulation disturbances) but, in general, is a research test.[5]

6. CLINICAL FEATURES AND THERAPY

Is there evidence that depletion of iron stores by venesection therapy enhances survival or results in improvement of the clinical features of hemochromatosis? For years, the assumption has

Table II. Diagnostic Tests in Patients with Genetic Hemochromatosis

Patient
Laboratory
Serum ferritin
Transferrin Saturation
Desferrioxamine excretion test (optional)
Radiologic
CT scan (double energy source)
MRI (experimental)
Pathology
Liver biopsy (histology, iron content)
Family members
Laboratory
Serum ferritin and transferrin saturation
HLA typing for siblings of affected person
Pathology
Liver biopsy (histology, iron content)

been that if excess iron stores cause tissue damage, removal of these stores should benefit the patient. Ever since the introduction of phlebotomy therapy by Balfour et al.[2] in 1942, this has been the standard therapy for patients with genetic hemochromatosis. Support for this approach to therapy has been based on a number of case reports citing improvement in clinical features associated with depletion of iron stores. More recently, three retrospective studies using either untreated patients or age- and sex-matched controls have supported the use of venesection therapy.[27–30] No controlled, prospective studies have been attempted and it is unlikely, given the evidence to be presented, that one ever will be done. The following sections summarize the clinical features of the disease and, based on data from these retrospective studies, response to therapy is reviewed.

7. CLINICAL FEATURES

Genetic hemochromatosis is a disease of middle age, insidious in onset, often presenting with arthritis or complaints of abdominal pain. Nonspecific complaints including weakness, lethargy, loss of libido, impotence, and weight loss are common.[31] It is five times more common in males than in females, the lower incidence in females being attriuted to a combination of menstrual loss and a lower dietary intake of iron.[27,32] Cardiac symptoms tend to be more common in younger patients[33] and, in the prephlebotomy era, heart disease was the third most common cause of death.[32]

Niederau et al.[30] found that in the 75 patients presenting with weakness and lethargy, 51% improved with depletion of iron stores, 40% remained unchanged, and 9% actually worsened (Table III). In addition, 11% of previously asymptomatic patients developed weakness and lethargy during the course of treatment. Abdominal pain was present initially in 64 patients, 64% improved with venesection therapy, 33% remained unchanged, and 3% were worse.

8. LIVER DISEASE

Hepatomegaly is common, occurring in 75–90% of patients, but jaundice is present in only 10% at the time of presentation. Manifestations of portal hypertension are infrequent and occur late in the disease. The reported incidence of hepatoma varies, depending on the length of follow-up, but averages about 14%.[5] Histologic features progress from increased iron stores with minimal tissue damage to hepatic fibrosis and, finally, a macronodular cirrhosis.

Niederau et al.[30] noted that hepatomegaly decreased in 70% of patients with depletion of iron stores, while Williams et al.[29] found that 21 of 26 patients who had a palpable liver prior to treatment returned to normal upon completion of venesection therapy. Abnormal liver-function tests

Table III. Presenting Symptoms in Patients with Genetic Hemochromatosis: Response to Venesection Therapy[a]

Feature	Improved		Unchanged		Worsened	
	N	Percent	*N*	Percent	*N*	Percent
Weakness/lethargy	38	51	30	40	7	9
Present (75)	—		31	89	4	11
Absent (35)						
Abdominal pain						
Present (64)	41	64	21	33	2	3
Absent (46)	—		45	98	1	2

[a]From Niederan et al.[30]

improved in 50–70% of patients.[28,30] Bomford and Williams[28] noted improvement in histologic features in only three of 75 patients evaluated by serial liver biopsies, while 68 patients remained unchanged and two had progressive damage despite removal of iron stores. Niederau et al.[30] noted that improvement in the degree of fibrosis was frequently observed, but reversal of cirrhosis was not achieved in any patients. Despite successful depletion of iron stores, 29–30% of patients ultimately died of a hepatoma.[28,30] However, all these patients had cirrhosis at the time of presentation. Hepatoma has not been reported as a complication of the disease in patients who were in the precirrhotic stage at the time of presentation. This observation emphasizes the need for early diagnosis and treatment.

9. CARDIAC DISEASE

Two types of cardiac abnormality occur as complications of hemochromatosis. Patients develop iron deposition in the myocardium, which leads to a biventricular failure.[34] Cardiac arrhythmias occur, especially in younger patients, and autopsy studies have shown iron deposition confined to the atrioventricular node with sparing of the sinus nodes.[35,36] Echocardiography can detect changes before they are evident by electrocardiography (ECG) or chest roentgenography.[37] Since sudden cardiac death is an occasional consequence of myocardial iron deposition, early detection by echocardiography may be life-saving.

Niederau et al.[30] found ECG abnormalities in 35% of patients at presentation. Of these, 37% improved with therapy, 58% were unchanged, and 5% worsened. Bomford and Williams[28] noted that two patients with congestive heart failure (CHF) improved but two patients with arteriosclerotic heart disease remained unchanged. Echocardiographic studies in 22 patients, pre- and postvenesection therapy, showed that impaired left ventricular variables clearly improved during the course of therapy.[38]

10. DIABETES MELLITUS

As part of the original triad, the presence of diabetes mellitus in association with chronic liver disease has alerted the clinician to the diagnosis of hemochromatosis. In fact, only 60–70% of patients with hemochromatosis demonstrate abnormal glucose tolerance, while impairment of glucose tolerance is also quite common in other forms of chronic liver disease.[39,40] The pathogenesis of the diabetes is multifactorial, with iron deposition in the pancreatic acinar cells and the islets of Langerhans, hepatic cirrhosis, and genetic factors all contributing.[39–42] The diabetic complications in hemochromatosis are similar to those in the genetic form of the disease and include coronary artery and peripheral vascular disease, nephropathy, retinopathy, peripheral neuropathy, and fat atrophy. A potential distinguishing feature is the plasma insulin response to a glucose load, which is deficient and delayed in diabetes mellitus, excessive and delayed in cirrhosis, and relatively deficient but prompt in hemochromatosis.[39] Patients with hemochromatosis and a normal tolerance to carbohydrates show a normal insulin response to glucose. In contrast to the impairment of pancreatic endocrine function, patients with hemochromatosis have no clinical evidence of exocrine pancreatic insufficiency and have a normal response to secretin stimulation.[43]

Less then one half of patients completing venesection therapy to deplete hepatic and pancreatic iron stores demonstrate improvement in diabetes mellitus[28,30] (Table IV). Niederau et al.[30] show improvement in 45–50% of patients, while 5% demonstrate deterioration. Bomford and Williams[28] found improvement in only 28%, with a 13% worsening. Niederau et al.[44] suggested that the improvement in diabetes may in part be due to the improvement in liver disease, especially in the non-insulin-dependent patient whose abnormal glucose metabolism may be due to impaired hepatic function rather than irreversible destruction of pancreatic beta cells by excess iron.

Table IV. Diabetes Mellitus: Response to Venesection Therapy

Investigators/features	Improved		Unchanged		Worsened	
	N	Percent	*N*	Percent	*N*	Percent
Niederau et al.[30]						
Insulin-dependent diabetes mellitus (40)	18	45	20	50	2	5
Non-insulin dependent diabetes mellitus (24)	12	50	11	46	1	4
Impaired glucose tolerance (11)	5	45	5	45	1	10
Normal glucose tolerance (35)	—		34	97	1	3
Bomford and Williams[28] (56)	16	28	33	59	7	13

11. OTHER ENDOCRINE DEFICIENCIES

Pituitary insufficiency occurs in up to 65% of patients with hemochromatosis, usually presenting as loss of libido and testicular atrophy due to a decrease in gonadotropins.[45,46] Hypothyroidism associated with a deficiency of thyroid-stimulating hormone (TSH) is rare.[45] Iron deposition occurs in adrenal, thyroid, and parathyroid glands but is not associated with functional impairment.

In response to venesection therapy, 22% of patients with initial impairment of pituitary function demonstrated improvement, 69% were unchanged, and 10% deteriorated[30]; 16% of patients in whom pituitary function was normal at the time of diagnosis demonstrated impairment upon completion of venesection therapy. Williams et al.[29] noted that hypogonadism was unaffected by venesection therapy, with a number of patients becoming completely impotent. Most of these patients required testosterone therapy. Kelly et al.[47] evaluated gonadal function in 64 patients who were homozygous for the HLA-linked hemochromatosis allele. Ten of the 41 males showed reduced libido or impotence and six had testicular atrophy. All 23 women had a normal libido and did not develop premature menopause. Four males were evaluated pre- and postvenesection therapy, with two showing a return of normal testosterone levels and sexual function. Lufkin et al.[48] also failed to demonstrate improvement in hypothalamic–pituitary function by venesection therapy.

12. SKIN PIGMENTATION

Abnormal skin pigmentation is part of the classic triad of hemochromatosis and most commonly occurs in exposed areas and in surgical scars. The pigmentation is of two types—the more commonly found bronze pigmentation due to melanin deposition, and a slate gray pigmentation due to iron located in the basal cell of the epidermis and sweat glands.[1,31,41] Pigmentation may also be found in the gums, buccal mucosa, and in the conjunctiva, corneal epithelium, and ciliary body of the eye.[49]

Niederau et al.[30] found that 77% of patients with pigmentation present at the time of diagnosis improved with venesection therapy. Williams et al.[29] noted a "decrease in skin color as venesection proceeded" but that "slight pigmentation . . . particularly around scars, often remained."

13. ARTHROPATHY

Although not recognized as a complication of hemochromatosis until the initial description in 1964, recent series have found this fairly specific arthropathy to be present in up to 50% of the patients, often as the presenting complaint.[31,50–52] The arthropathy is a chondrocalcinosis or pseudogout and is diagnosed by the finding of calcium pyrophosphate crystals in the joint fluid. Deposits of iron can be found in the synovial intimal cells and phagocytic cells of the stroma.[53] Initially, the small joints of the hands, especially the second and third metacarpophalangeal joints, are involved. Other joints involved include the wrists and larger weight-bearing joints, such as the hips. Radiologic features include sclerosis in the subchondral bone, loss of articular cartilage, subchondral cyst formation, and chondrocalcinosis of articular cartilage.

Although Walker et al.[53] found that "synovial iron was unusual in patients who had completed venesection therapy," Williams et al.[29] noted a lack of improvement with treatment and commented on "the development in some patients of clinical symptoms of arthritis after excess iron had been removed." Niederau et al.[30] concurred with these observations, finding improvement in 20% of patients and no change in 80% as a result of venesection therapy. These observations have raised some questions about the role of iron in the development of this arthropathy.

14. SURVIVAL

Although most investigators would agree that excess iron stores result in tissue damage and the development of hemochromatosis, does removal of these excess stores, once the disease is present, lead to improvement in survival? There are no prospective randomized controlled trials to establish the value of venesection therapy. Therefore, we must rely on retrospective reports,[27–31] with the potential bias associated with this form of analysis.

The most convincing of these studies is the report by Niederau et al.,[30] in which 163 patients with hemochromatosis (112 with cirrhosis, 51 in the precirrhotic stage) who underwent venesection therapy were compared with age- and sex-matched controls. Depletion of iron stores was documented by liver biopsy in 110 of the 163 patients. 28 patients died before iron depletion could be achieved and 25 were continuing therapy at the time of the publication. The mean follow-up period was 10.5 years with no patient lost to follow-up. Several important conclusions can be derived from the data: (1) comparing the total population of patients with hemochromatosis with an age- and sex-matched normal population, there was a significant reduction in survival; (2) survival was significantly reduced in the cirrhotic patients as compared with the noncirrhotic patients ($p<0.05$); (3) survival was significantly worse in patients who had diabetes at the time of diagnosis than in those who did not ($p<0.002$); (4) patients in whom the iron stores could be depleted within 18 months fared better than those who took longer ($p<0.001$); and (5) most importantly, patients in whom the diagnosis was made prior to the development of cirrhosis, and in whom venesection therapy was successfully performed, had a normal life expectancy.

Bomford and Williams[28] compared 85 patients treated with venesection therapy with 26 untreated patients and found a mean survival of 63.4 months for the treated group compared with 17.8 months for those not receiving phlebotomy therapy. These data must be interpreted with some caution, as there were major differences between the two groups. For example, most untreated patients had been seen prior to 1960, whereas, starting in 1952, most patients were treated with venesection therapy. In those untreated patients seen after 1952, it is unclear why this form of therapy was not used, i.e., were they too sick to tolerate venesection? Also, diabetes mellitus with its complications was more common in the untreated group. Powell[27] compared 19 venesected patients with seven untreated patients and found a significant improvement in survival for the venesected group. However, no explanation is given as to why the seven untreated patients did not receive venesection therapy. Finally, Milder et al.[31] reported a median survival of 12.5 years from the date of diagnosis for 49 patients with genetic hemochromatosis with a mean follow-up of 3.5 years. No comparisons were made, either with untreated patients or with a control population. They did find that nonalcoholic patients with hemochromatosis did significantly better than those with a history of increased alcohol intake (2-year survival, 84% versus 53%). The survival data from these studies can be seen in Table V. The improved survival reported by Niederau et al.[30] may be a

Table V. Survival Data for Treated Patents with Genetic Hemochromatosis

Investigators	Number of patients	Hepatic fibrosis or cirrhosis (%)	Survival (%) 5 yr	10 yr	15 yr
Bomford and Williams (1976)[28]	85	91	66	32	10
Powell et al. (1970)[7]	51	100	70	—	—
Milder et al. (1980)[31]	34	94	71	—	—
Niederau et al. (1985)[30a]	163	69	92	76	59
Cirrhotic	112	—	90	72	55
Noncirrhotic	51	—	98	82	68

[a]Patients without cirrhosis and diabetes mellitus had a normal life expectancy.

consequence of the use of screening methods to detect patients at an earlier stage than might occur when the patients are diagnosed by the presence of symptoms or signs of the disease.

Comparison of the causes of death in the studies by Niederau et al.[30] and Bomford and Williams[28] exhibits a remarkable similarity (Table VI). Both studies report a striking incidence of hepatoma as the cause of death despite successful completion of venesection therapy. It should be noted that in both studies only patients with cirrhosis at the time of diagnosis developed hepatoma. Bomford reports a relatively high incidence of extrahepatic malignancies, whereas Niederau found the frequency of extrahepatic malignancies to be similar to the general population. Ammann et al.[54] and Viteri et al.[55] also reported a higher than expected incidence of extrahepatic carcinomas associated with hemochromatosis. A recent carefully controlled study by Bradbear et al.[56] supports Niederau's finding that the incidence of extrahepatic malignancies is not increased.

Conclusions about the value of venesection therapy to deplete excess iron stores in patients with genetic hemochromatosis must be qualified by the lack of prospective randomized trials.

Table VI. Causes of Death in Patients Treated with Venesection Therapy

Causes of death	Bomford and Williams[28] *N*	Percent	Niederau et al.[30] *N*	Percent
Neoplasms	23	51	23	43
Hepatoma	13	29	16	30[a]
Extrahepatic	10	22	7	13
Diabetes mellitus	1	2	3	6[a]
Cardiovascular	8	18	10	19[a]
Cirrhosis	7	15	10	19[a]
Other	6	14	7	13
Total deaths	45		53	

[a]Significantly greater than age- and sex-matched normal population.

However, based on the studies reviewed in this chapter, the following statements seem justified:

1. In the precirrhotic, prediabetic patient, treatment by depletion of iron stores is associated with a normal life expectancy.
2. Depletion of iron stores does not prevent the development of hepatoma unless treatment is initiated in the precirrhotic stage.
3. In those patients who are able to complete venesection therapy successfully, especially if it can be accomplished in under 1½ years, survival is improved.
4. Venesection therapy has a beneficial effect on liver-function tests, hepatomegaly, abdominal pain, cardiac abnormalities, and skin pigmentation. The results for diabetes mellius and lethargy are equivocal. No improvement occurs in hepatic histology, esophageal varices, hypogonadism, or arthropathy.

These conclusions strongly support the use of biochemical screening (serum ferritin, saturation of iron-binding capacity) and HLA typing of family members of patients with genetic hemochromatosis. Whether large-scale biochemical screening of the general population is warranted (i.e., cost effective) is yet to be determined.

REFERENCES

1. Sheldon JH: Hemochromatosis. Oxford University Press, London, 1935.
2. Balfour, WM, Hahn PF, Bale WF, et al: Radioactive iron absorption in clinical conditions: Normal, pregnancy, anemia and hemochromatosis. *J Exp Med* **76:**15–30, 1942.
3. MacDonald RG: *Hemochromatosis and Hemosiderosis*. Charles C. Thomas, Springfield, Illinois, 1964.
4. Grace ND: Evidence for hepatic toxicity of iron, in Powell LW (ed): *Metals and the Liver*. Dekker, New York, 1978, pp. 131–144.
5. Grace ND: Iron metabolism and hemochromatosis, in Zakim D, Boyer TD (eds): *Hepatology: A Textbook of Liver Disease*. W. B Saunders Co., Philadelphia, 1982, pp. 1159–1176.
6. Cox TM, Peters TJ: Uptake of iron by duodenal biopsy specimens from patients with iron deficiency anemia and primary haemochromatosis. *Lancet* **1:**123–124, 1978.
7. Powell LW, Campbell CB, Wilson E: Intestinal mucosal uptake of iron and iron retention in idiopathic haemochromatosis as evidence for a mucosal abnormality. *Gut* **11:**727–731, 1970.
8. Cox TM, Peters TJ: *In vitro* studies of duodenal iron uptake in patients with primary and secondary iron storage disease. *Q J Med* **49:**249–257, 1980.
9. Blitzer BL, Weiss GB, Osbaldiston GW, et al: Early idiopathic hemochromatosis with absent stainable bone marrow iron stores. *Gastroenterology* **75:**886–888, 1978.
10. Valberg LS: Tissue iron distribution in idiopathic hemochromatosis. *Gastroenterology* **75:**915–916, 1978.
11. Beaumont C, Simon M, Smith PM, et al: Hepatic and serum ferritin concentrations in patients with idiopathic hemochromatosis. *Gastroenterology* **79:**877–883, 1980.
12. Bassett ML, Halliday W, Powell LW: Genetic hemochromatosis. *Semin Liver Dis* **4:**217–227, 1984.
13. Simon M, Bourel M, Genetet B., et al: Idiopathic hemochromatosis demonstration of recessive transmission and early detection by family HLA typing. *N Engl J Med* **297:**1017–1021, 1977.
14. Bassett ML, Halliday JW, Powell LW, et al: Early detection of idiopathic hemochromatosis: Relative value of serum ferritin and HLA typing. *Lancet* **2:**4–7, 1979.
15. Beaumont C, Simon M, Fauchet R, et al: Serum ferritin as a possible marker of the hemochromatosis allele. *N Engl J Med* **301:**169–174, 1979.
16. Cartwright GE, Edwards CQ, Kravitz K, et al: Hereditary hemochromatosis: Phenotypic expression of the disease. *N Engl J Med* **301:**175–179, 1979.
17. Bassett ML, Halliday W, Powell LW: HLA typing in idiopathic hemochromatosis: Distinction between homozygotes and heterozygotes with biochemical expression. *Hepatology* **1:**120–126, 1981.
18. Simon M, Bourel M, Genetet B, et al: Idiopathic hemochromatosis and iron overload in alcoholic liver disease: Differentiation by HLA phenotype. *Gastroenterology* **73:**655–658, 1977.

19. Olsson KS, Ritter B, Rosen U, et al: Prevalence of iron overload in central Sweden. *Acta Med Scand* **213:**145–150, 1983.
20. MacSween RNM, Jackson JM: Haemochromatosis: A clinical-pathological review of 37 cases. *Scott J Med* **11:**395–400, 1966.
21. MacDonald RA, Mallory GK: Hemochromatosis and hemosiderosis: Study of 211 autopsied cases. *Arch Intern Med* **105:**686–701, 1960.
22. Powell LW, Halliday JW, Bryant S: Screening for Hemochromatosis *Ann NY Acad Sci* (in press), 1988.
23. Wands JR, Rowe JA, Mezey SE, et al: Normal serum ferritin concentrations in pre-cirrhotic hemochromatosis. *N Engl J Med* **294:**302–305, 1976.
24. Bassett ML, Halliday JW, Powell LW: Value of hepatic iron measurement in early hemochromatosis and determination of the critical iron level associated with fibrosis. *Hepatology* **6:**24–29, 1986.
25. Howard J, Ghent C, Carey L, et al: Diagnostic efficacy of hepatic computed tomography in the detection of body iron stores. *Gastroenterology* **84:**209–215, 1983.
26. Brittenham GM, Farrell DE, Harris JW, et al: Magnetic susceptibility measurement of human iron stores. *N Engl J Med* **307:**1671–1675, 1982.
27. Powell LW: Changing concepts in haemochromatosis. *Postgrad Med J* **46:**200–209, 1970.
28. Bomford A, Williams R: Long-term results of venesection therapy in idiopathic haemochromatosis. *Q J Med* **45:**611–623, 1976.
29. Williams R, Smith PM, Spicer EJF, et al: Venesection therapy in idiopathic haemochromatosis. *Q J Med* **38:**1–16, 1969.
30. Niederau C, Fischer R, Sonnenberg A, et al: Survival and causes of death in cirrhotic and in non-cirrhotic patients with primary hemochromatosis. *N Engl J Med* **313:**1256–1262, 1985.
31. Milder MS, Cook JD, Stray S, et al: Idiopathic hemochromatosis, an interim report. *Medicine (Baltimore)* **59:**34–49, 1980.
32. Finch SC, Finch CA: Idiopathic hemochromatosis: An iron storage disease. *Medicine (Baltimore)* **34:**381–430, 1955.
33. Charlton RW, Abrahams, C, Bothwell TH: Idiopathic hemochromatosis in young subjects. Clinical, pathological and chemical findings in four patients. *Arch Pathol Lab Med* **83:**132–140, 1967.
34. Buja LM, Roberts WC: Iron in the heart. Etiology and clinical significance. *Am J Med* **51:**209–221, 1971.
35. James TN: Pathology of the cardiac conduction system in hemochromatosis. *N Engl J Med* **271:**92–94, 1964.
36. Aranow WS, Meister L, Kent JR: Atrioventricular block in familial hemochromatosis treated by permanent synchronous pacemaker. *Arch Intern Med* **123:**433–435, 1969.
37. Henry WL, Neinhaus AW, Wiener M, et al: Echocardiographic abnormalities in patients with transfusion dependent anemia and secondary myocardial iron deposition. *Am J Med* **64:**547–555, 1978.
38. Candell-Riera J, Lu L, Seres L, et al: Cardiac hemochromatosis. Beneficial effects of iron removal therapy, an echocardiographic study. *Am J Cardiol* **52:**824–829, 1983.
39. Stocks AE, Powell LW: Carbohydrate intolerance in idiopathic haemochromatosis and cirrhosis of the liver. *Q J Med* **42:**733–749, 1973.
40. Dymock IW, Cassar J, Pyke DA, et al: Observations on the pathogenesis, complications and treatment of diabetes in 115 cases of haemochromatosis. *Am J Med* **52:**203–210, 1972.
41. Bell ET: The relation of portal cirrhosis to hemochromatosis and to diabetes mellitus. *Diabetes* **4:**435–446, 1955.
42. Balcerzak SP, Mintz DH, Westerman MP: Diabetes mellitus and idiopathic hemochromatosis. *Am J Med Sci* **255:**53–62, 1968.
43. Perman G, Bonera E: The secretin test in patients with hemochromatosis. *Acta Med Scand* **175:**787–790, 1964.
44. Niederau C, Berger M, Stremmel W, et al: Hyperinsulinaemia in non-cirrhotic haemochromatosis: Impaired hepatic insulin degradation? *Diabetologia* **26:**441–444, 1984.
45. Stocks AE, Martin FIR: Pituitary function in haemochromatosis. *Am J Med* **45:**839–845, 1968.
46. Stocks AE, Powell LW: Pituitary function in idiopathic hemochromatosis and cirrhosis of the liver. *Lancet* **2:**298–300, 1972.
47. Kelly TM, Edwards CQ, Meikle AW, et al: Hypogonadism in hemochromatosis: Reversal with iron depletion. *Ann Intern Med* **101:**629–632, 1984.
48. Lufkin EG, Baldus WP, Bergstralh EJ, et al: Influence of phlebotomy treatment in abnormal hypothalamic–Pituitary function in genetic hemochromatosis. *Mayo Clinic Proc* **62:**473–479, 1987.

49. Davies G, Dymock I, Harry J, et al: Deposition of iron and melanin in ocular structures in haemochromatosis. *Br J Ophthalmol* **56**:338–342, 1972.
50. Schumaker HR: Hemochromatosis and arthritis. *Arthritis Rheum* **7**:41–50, 1964.
51. Dymock IW, Hamilton EBD, Laws JW, et al: Arthropathy of Haemochromatosis: Clinical and radiological analysis of 63 patients with iron overload. *Ann Rheum Dis* **29**:469–476, 1970.
52. deSeze S, Ryckewaert A, Hubault A, et al: Les chondrocalcinoses articulaires. *Semin Hop (Paris)* **42**:2461–2482, 1966.
53. Walker RJ, Dymock IW, Ansell ID, et al. Synovial biopsy in haemochromatosis arthropathy: Histological findings and iron deposition in relation to total body iron overload. *Ann Rheum Dis* **31**:98–102, 1972.
54. Ammann RW, Muller E, Bansky J, et al: High incidence of extrahepatic carcinomas in idiopathic hemochromatosis. *Scand J Gastroenterol* **15**:733–736, 1980.
55. Viteri A, Vernace SJ, Schaffner F: Extrahepatic malignancy in chronic liver disease: Report of six cases. *Gastroenterology* **71**:1075–1078, 1976.
56. Bradbear R, Bain C, Siskind V, et al: Cohort study of internal malignancy in genetic hemochromatosis and other chronic or alcoholic liver diseases. *J Natl Cancer Inst* **75**:81–84, 1985.

24

Hemochromatosis: Pathology

Peter J. Scheuer

1. DEFINITIONS

Iron overload in tissues, including the liver, can be designated as siderosis. This may be transient as in temporary post-transfusion overload, static as in a site of old hemorrhage, or progressive as in hemochromatosis. The amount of iron in hepatocytes can be roughly graded by visual assessment into grades 0–4. The relationship between histologic grade and iron content is not linear, grades 1 and 2 representing relatively small amounts, and grades 3 and 4 substantial increase.[1] Image analysis offers the possibility of more precise evaluation.[2]

The term hemochromatosis is reserved for a disease state characterized by progressive iron deposition in liver and other tissues, accompanied by fibrosis and ultimately, in some patients, by cirrhosis. It should be noted, however, that in the early stages of genetic hemochromatosis there is iron overload, principally affecting hepatocytes, without fibrosis. Recognition of this phase by the combined efforts of clinician and laboratory is vital if cirrhosis and its complications and sequelae are to be prevented.

2. SITES AND FORMS OF IRON DEPOSITION IN THE LIVER

Iron is deposited in the form of hemosiderin and ferritin in hepatocytes, bile duct epithelium, macrophages, endothelial cells, and connective tissue. Much of the iron apparently lying free in connective tissue by light microscopy is probably within macrophages. Hemosiderin may be a breakdown product of ferritin.[3]

3. GENETIC HEMOCHROMATOSIS

Genetic hemochromatosis, inherited in an autosomal-recessive pattern, is characterized by excess absorption of iron from the intestine and by progressive deposition of iron in tissues. The reason for the increased absorption is not clear. About three fourths of patients with genetic hemochromatosis have histocompatibility antigen HLA-A3; -B7 and -B14 are also commonly

Peter J. Scheuer • Royal Free Hospital and School of Medicine, London NW3 2QG, England.

found. While this does not permit definitive diagnosis in the individual patient, it is helpful in determining the likelihood that a sibling is homozygous for the disease.[4]

In the early stages of genetic hemochromatosis, there is excess stainable iron in hepatocytes, predominantly around the portal tracts, in acinar zones 1. The iron is in the form of hemosiderin granules, giving the Prussian blue reaction, mainly concentrated at the biliary poles of the hepatocytes. A small amount of diffuse cytoplasmic staining may also be seen. At this stage, macrophage iron is usually scanty or unstainable, and portal tracts and their contents are negative. The relatively small amounts of excess hepatocellular iron (1 or 2 in a 0–4 grading system) reflect only slight increase in chemical iron content of the liver. Histologically, they cannot be confidently distinguished from iron overload resulting from other factors, or even of undetermined cause. Mild siderosis is a common unexplained finding in liver biopsy material from patients who are not known to have genetic or secondary hemochromatosis. In a consecutive series of 200 liver biopsies, 92 (46%) showed stainable iron (L. Petrovic and P. J. Scheuer, unpublished data); 13 patients had known iron storage disease. When these were excluded, 47 of the remaining 187 biopsies (25%) showed iron in hepatocytes, 51 (27%) had iron in Kupffer cells, and 45 (24%) iron in endothelial cells. Overall positivity was 79 of 187 (42%).

As iron continues to accumulate, the density of staining increases, and the siderosis extends from acinar zones 1 into zones 2 and 3. The hemosiderin, by accentuating the pericanalicular regions of hepatocytes, often outlines the bile canalicular network (Fig. 1). The likelihood that the siderosis is due to genetic hemochromatosis now increases sharply, even in alcoholic subjects from populations in whom genetic hemochromatosis is relatively common.[5] Some macrophage iron may now be present, and the epithelium of some bile ducts becomes positive.

At this stage, with substantial iron deposits in liver cells both histochemically (grades 3 and 4) and as assessed by chemical liver iron measurement,[2] fibrosis begins to develop in the portal tracts, expanding them and forming septa without markedly altering the overall acinar–lobular architecture. The pattern of fibrosis is sometimes described as resembling holly leaves, with sharp spikes

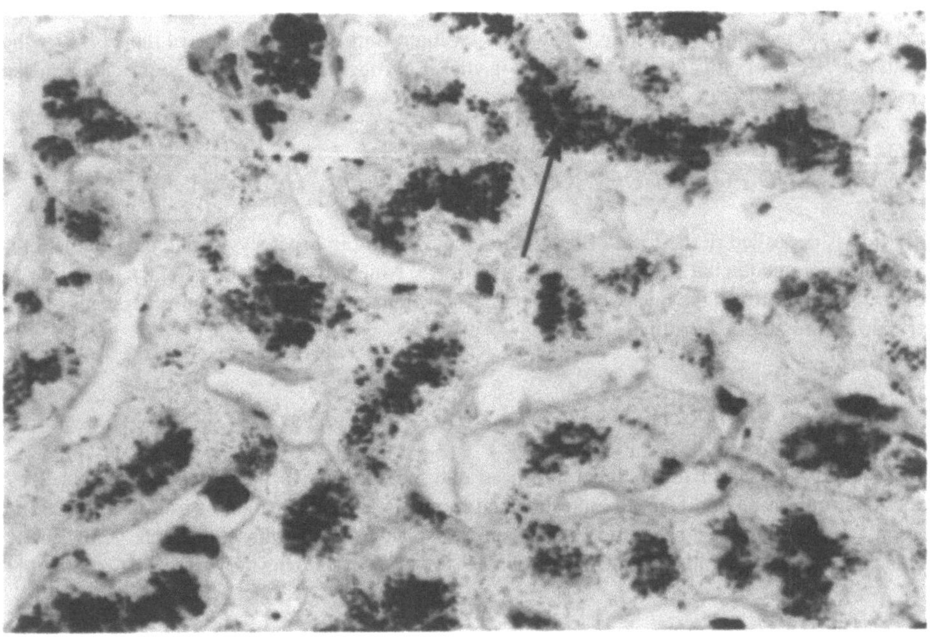

Figure 1. Heavy iron overload in hepatocytes. Deeply stained hemosiderin granules are mainly located at the biliary poles of hepatocytes, in places outlining the bile canaliculi (arrow). (Perls' stain, ×495)

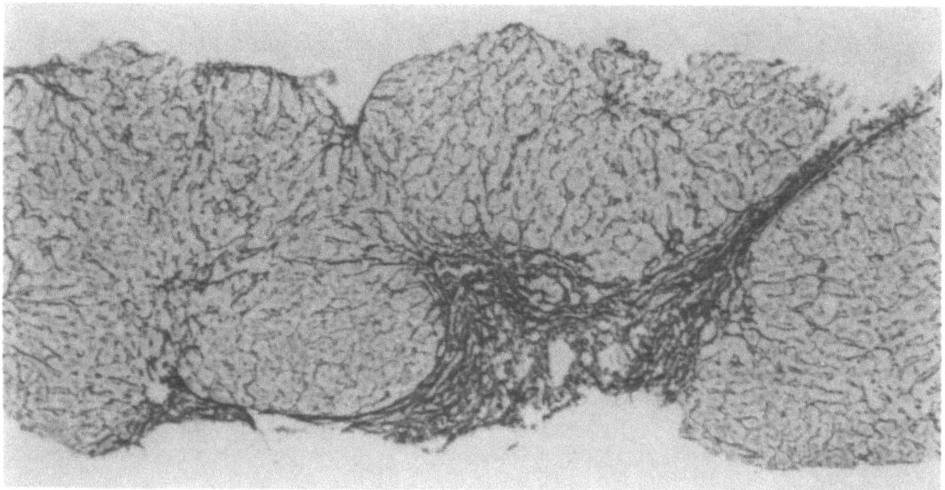

Figure 2. Genetic hemochromatosis. Fibrous septa extend from an expanded portal tract. (Reticulin, ×72)

extending from the thickened tracts (Fig. 2). Terminal hepatic venules (centrilobular veins) remain in their normal relationship to the portal zones, and hepatocytes show little change apart from the accumulation of iron. Inflammation is usually absent or very mild, and there is neither cholestasis nor hepatocellular necrosis.

The method of progression of the histologic lesion has been stressed because it has important bearing on the clinical picture and on patient management. Liver function, as measured by standard laboratory tests, is almost always good. The lack of necrosis, of regeneration and of interference with the hepatic microarchitecture indicates that the lesion is not at this time one of cirrhosis, and it may thus be potentially reversed or arrested if the iron overload can be eliminated, although the more severe examples of fibrosis are unlikely to be reversed completely. Study of the pathogenesis of the portal fibrosis seems more relevant to the earlier phases of hemochromatosis than mechanisms of hepatocellular damage, since the latter is conspicuously absent or mild. However, hepatocellular damage may occur at some stage as a result of destabilization of lysosomes by hemosiderin[6] or by increased lipid peroxidation resulting from the presence of free iron in the cytoplasm.[7] It is likely that there is a toxic threshold above which tissue damage occurs.[5,8]

Eventually, fibrous septa come to link portal tracts and, as seen in two dimensions, form serpiginous bands around irregularly shaped islands of liver parenchyma. The overall pattern is reminiscent of that seen in chronic biliary disease. True cirrhosis, with regenerative hyperplasia of the parenchyma, develops very late, usually after many years.

Effective treatment of hemochromatosis by venesection leads to the gradual removal of stainable iron from the liver. Iron encrusted onto collagen fibers in portal tracts often remains and resembles a form of iron seen in the spleen in the Gamna–Gandy body of severe chronic venous congestion. After removal of iron from hepatocytes, macrophages or connective tissue, abundant iron-negative pigment of lipofuscin type usually remains (Fig. 3). This is the residual organic matrix of the hemosiderin granules.

Monitoring of the effects of venesection may be achieved by simple visual grading of hepatocellular iron, but chemical estimation is usually carried out as well. If necessary, paraffin-embedded tissue can be rehydrated and analysed, in which case the type of tissue in which iron has been chemically assayed can be histologically controlled. Assessment of structural changes is sometimes more difficult, because in patients in whom cirrhosis has developed before venesection is started, increasing nodule size may give a false impression of improvement.

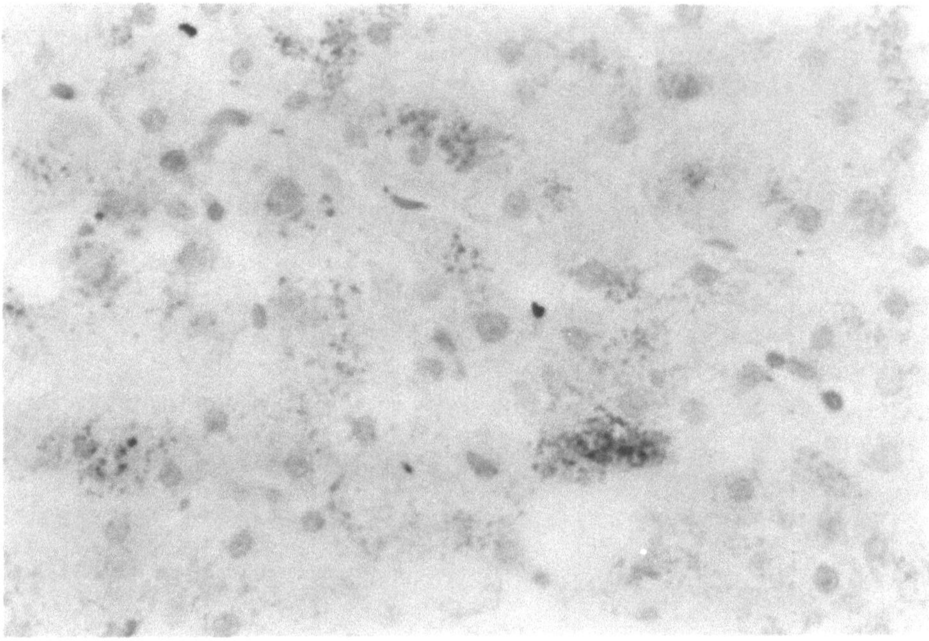

Figure 3. Treated hemochromatosis. Hepatocytes contain abundant iron-negative brown pigment. From the same patient, whose liver biopsy is illustrated in Fig. 1. (Perls' stain, ×523)

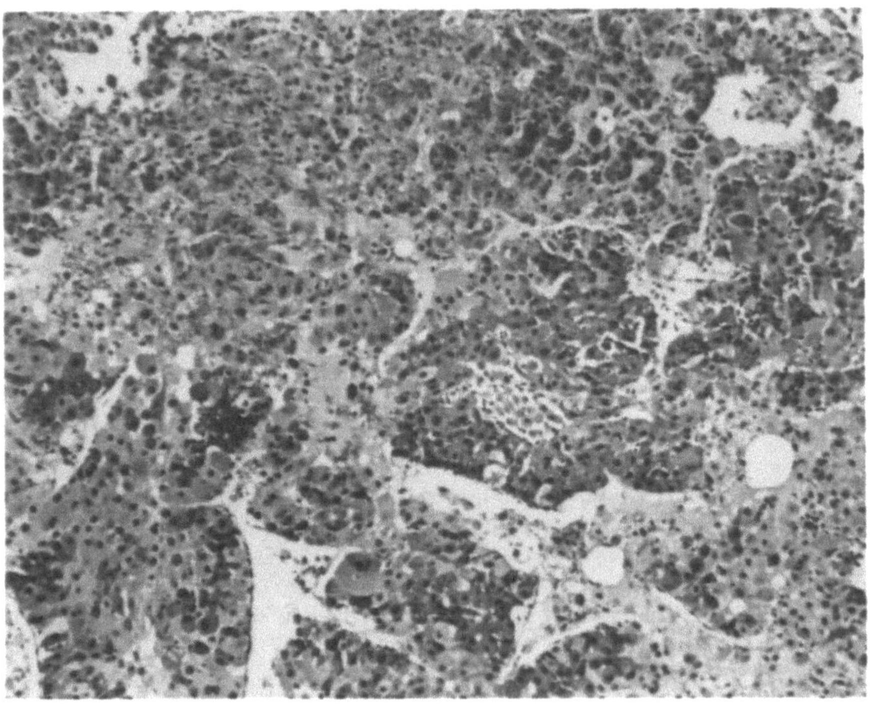

Figure 4. Hepatocellular carcinoma in a patient with hemochromatosis, whose earlier liver biopsies are illustrated in Figs. 1 and 3. (H&E, ×210)

Cirrhosis resulting from genetic hemochromatosis may be complicated by hepatocellular carcinoma (Fig. 4). This tumor does not appear to develop in the absence of cirrhosis, and in a recent series of 163 patients[9] effective treatment of patients in the precirrhotic stage of the disease was associated with a normal life expectancy.

The distinction of genetic hemochromatosis from nongenetic forms of iron overload usually presents little difficulty, because of the characteristic pattern of fibrosis in the genetic form and, in the early stages, the abundant tissue iron in the absence of substantial fibrosis. Occasionally, large amounts of stainable iron are found in patients with alcoholic cirrhosis. Attention should then be paid to the presence of specific features of alcoholic hepatitis, and previous biopsies should be examined if available, in order to clarify the pathogenesis of the patient's liver disease. Chemical measurement in the alcoholic usually shows lower levels of iron than in genetic hemochromatosis.[5] The finding of high liver iron levels chemically or histochemically suggests that the patient has genetic hemochromatosis in addition to any element of alcoholic liver disease.[5,10] In some populations, hepatic siderosis in alcohol abusers is uncommon.[11]

4. SECONDARY HEMOCHROMATOSIS

Hemochromatosis may complicate a number of hematological diseases, notably thalassemia. In this condition, iron overload associated with the disease itself is exacerbated by regular blood transfusions. Histologically, more iron is seen in macrophages within acini and portal tracts than in the genetic form, although iron also accumulates in hepatocytes. In patients with anemia, hematopoietic cells may be seen in the sinusoids. A striking difference from genetic hemochromatosis is the presence of inflammatory cells, mainly lymphocytes, in portal tracts and sinusoids[12,13] (Fig. 5).

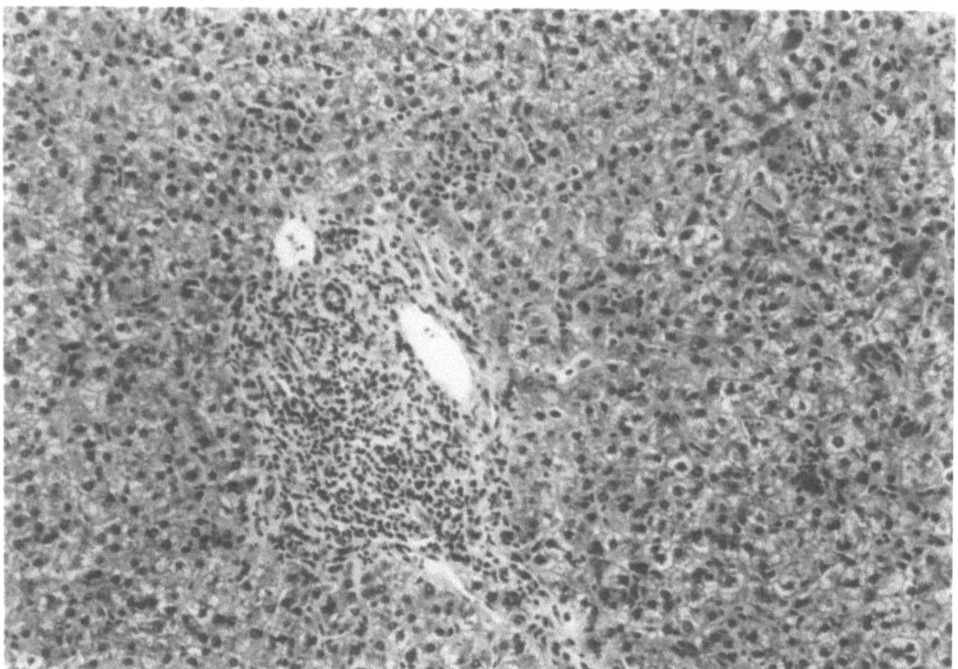

Figure 5. Thalassemia. The lymphocytic infiltration of portal tract and sinusoids is the result of transfusion-related non-A, non-B hepatitis. (H&E, ×162)

This is due to transfusion-related hepatitis, which plays an important role in progression to cirrhosis.[14,15] A recent study of thalassemic patients in whom iron overload was successfully controlled with desferrioxamine showed that parenterally transmitted non-A, non-B hepatitis was the main reason for progression of liver damage.[16] The pattern of fibrosis in patients with thalassemia is, as might be expected, a variable mixture of that seen in genetic hemochromatosis and that found in patients with chronic viral hepatitis.

5. NEONATAL HEMOCHROMATOSIS

Some degree of iron deposition in liver is common during the neonatal period because of the normal breakdown of large numbers of erythrocytes. Tissue siderosis is also characteristic of some inherited metabolic disorders, notably tyrosinemia and Zellweger syndrome.

Rarely, massive overload develops in the liver and leads to death within days or weeks of birth.[17] This neonatal form of hemochromatosis is usually not diagnosed in life. Histologically iron is found in hepatocytes as well as biliary epithelium and macrophages. Other organs are also affected. The iron presumably accumulates in utero but the reasons for this are obscure.

6. OTHER FORMS OF IRON OVERLOAD

6.1. Acute Hepatitis

Iron is sometimes seen in clumped hepatic macrophages in acute hepatitis, whether viral or drug related (Fig. 6). This may be due to release of iron from damaged hepatocytes.[18] Iron is also found in the form of dense granules in endothelial cells (Fig. 7). By electron microscopy, this is seen to be associated with the formation of basement membrane material by the cells and might play a role in the development of chronic liver disease[19]; however, this requires further study.

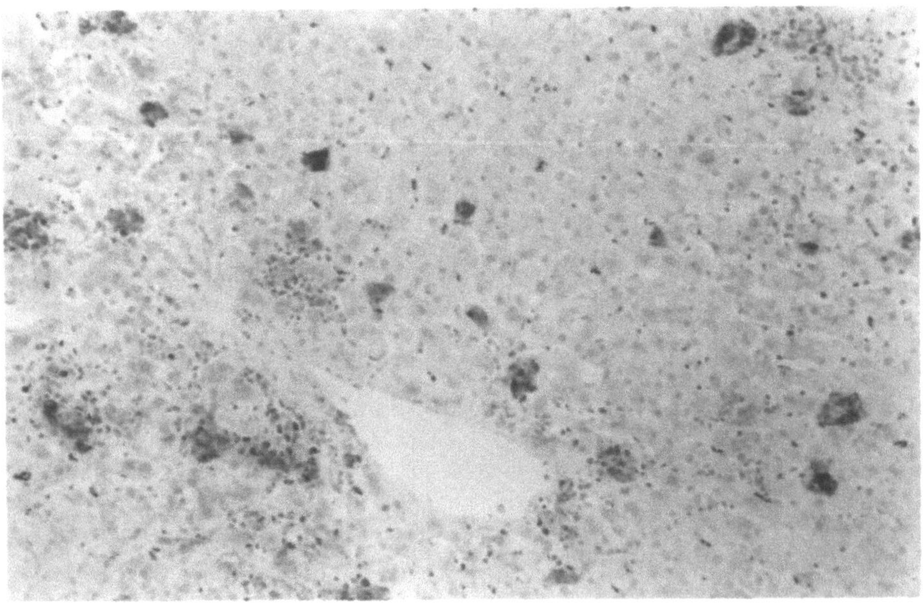

Figure 6. Acute viral hepatitis. Much iron is seen in clumped macrophages, especially around the terminal hepatic venule (below center). (Perls' stain, ×145)

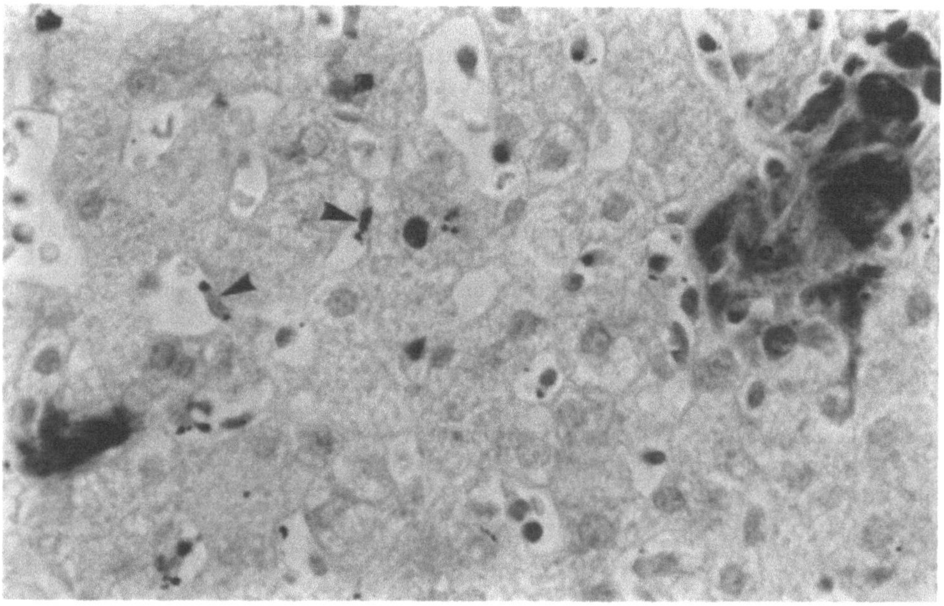

Figure 7. Acute viral hepatitis. In addition to iron in macrophages, well seen above right, there are dense Prussian blue-positive granules in endothelial cells (arrowheads). (Perls' stain, ×578)

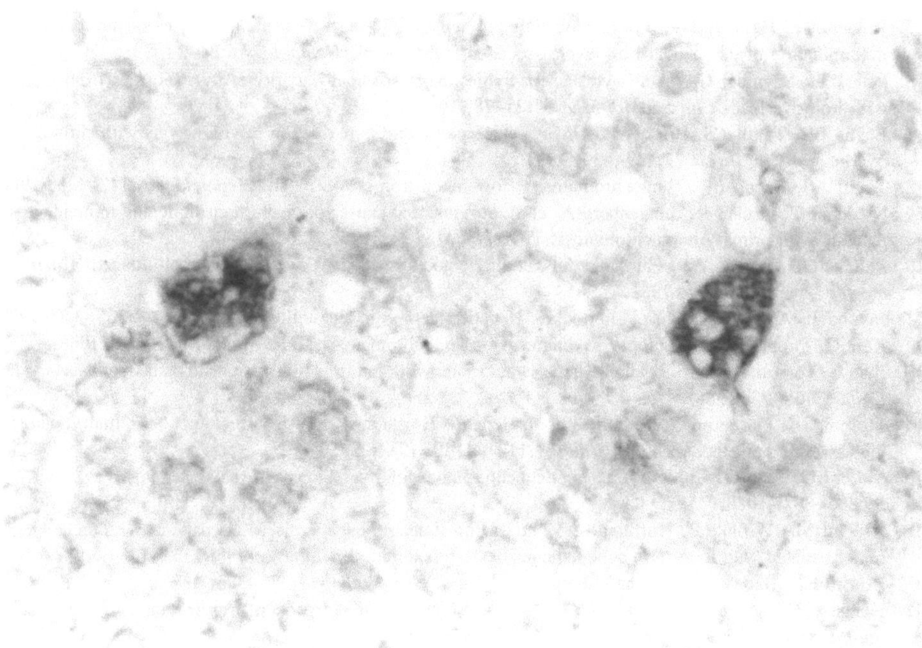

Figure 8. Porphyria cutanea tarda. Positive staining for iron is seen in macrophages. (Perls' stain, ×680)

6.2. Porphyria Cutanea Tarda

Most patients with porphyria cutanea tarda have stainable iron on liver biopsy.[20,21] This is most characteristically seen in macrophages, the cytoplasm of which contains hemosiderin granules and also shows diffuse staining for iron (Fig. 8).

6.3. Renal Transplantation

Histologic evidence of iron overload is common in patients receiving renal allografts.[22–24] This may progress to serious liver disease, making removal of iron desirable. The iron overload does not appear to be related to transfusion or hemolysis, although these may be contributory factors.

6.4. Hemolysis

In hemolytic anemia, iron is mainly seen in macrophages, but hepatocytes may be involved as well. Breakdown of erythrocytes following blood transfusion also leads to accumulation of iron in the liver.

REFERENCES

1. Barry M: Liver iron concentration, stainable iron, and total body storage iron. *Gut* **15**:411–415, 1974.
2. Deugnier Y, Margules S, Brissot P, et al: Comparative study between biochemical and histological methods and image analysis in liver iron overload. *J Clin Pathol* **35**:45–51, 1982.
3. Weir MP, Sharp GA, Peters TJ: Electron microscopic studies of human haemosiderin and ferritin. *J Clin Pathol* **38**:915–918, 1985.
4. Gollan JL: Diagnosis of hemochromatosis. *Gastroenterology* **84**:418–431, 1983.
5. Bassett ML, Halliday JW, Powell LW: Value of hepatic iron measurements in early hemochromatosis and determination of the critical iron level associated with fibrosis. *Hepatology* **6**:24–29, 1986.
6. Peters TJ, Seymour CA: Acid hydrolase activities and lysosomal integrity in liver biopsies from patients with iron overload. *Clin Sci Mol Med* **50**:75–78, 1976.
7. Bacon BR, Tavill AS, Brittenham GM, et al: Hepatic lipid peroxidation in vivo in rats with chronic iron overload. *J Clin Invest* **71**:429–439, 1983.
8. Tavill AS, Bacon BR. Hemochromatosis: How much iron is too much? *Hepatology* **6**:142–145, 1986.
9. Niederau C, Fischer R, Sonnenberg A, et al: Survival and causes of death in cirrhotic and in noncirrhotic patients with primary hemochromatosis. *N Engl J Med* **313**:1256–1262, 1985.
10. LeSage GD, Baldus WP, Fairbanks VF, et al: Hemochromatosis: Genetic or alcohol-induced? *Gastroenterology* **84**:1471–1477, 1983.
11. Jakobovits AW, Morgan MY, Sherlock S: Hepatic siderosis in alcoholics. *Dig Dis Sci* **24**:305–310, 1979.
12. Kent G, Popper H: Liver biopsy in diagnosis of hemochromatosis. *Am J Med* **44**:837–841, 1968.
13. Jean G, Terzoli S, Mauri R, et al: Cirrhosis associated with multiple transfusions in thalassaemia. *Arch Dis Child* **59**:67–70, 1984.
14. Moroni GA, Piacentini G, Terzoli S, et al: Hepatitis B or non-A, non-B virus infection in multitransfused thalassaemic patients. *Arch Dis Child* **59**:1127–1130, 1984.
15. Masera G, Jean G. Conter V, et al: Sequential study of liver biopsy in thalassaemia. *Arch Dis Child* **55**:800–802, 1980.
16. Aldouri MA, Wonke B, Hoffbrand AV, et al: Iron state and hepatic disease in patients with thalassaemia major, treated with long term subcutaneous desferrioxamine. *J. Clin Pathol* **40**:1353–1359, 1987.
17. Blisard KS, Bartow SA: Neonatal hemochromatosis. *Hum Pathol* **17**:376–383, 1986.
18. Hengeveld P, Zuyderhoudt FMJ, Jöbsis AC, van Gool J: Some aspects of iron metabolism during acute viral hepatitis. *Hepatogastroenterology* **29**:138–141, 1982.
19. Bardadin KA, Scheuer PJ: Endothelial cell changes in acute hepatitis. A light and electron microscopic study. *J Pathol* **144**:213–220, 1984.

20. Cortés JM, Oliva H, Paradinas FJ, Hernadez-Guío C: The pathology of the liver in porphyria cutanea tarda. *Histopathology* **4**:471–485, 1980.
21. Lefkowitch JH, Grossman ME: Hepatic pathology in porphyria cutanea tarda. *Liver* **3**:19–29, 1983.
22. Rao KV, Anderson WR: Hemosiderosis: An unrecognized complication in renal allograft recipients. *Transplantation* **33**:115–117, 1982.
23. Rao KV, Anderson WR: Hemosiderosis and hemochomatosis in renal transplant recipients. *Am J Nephrol* **5**:419–430, 1985.
24. Anderson WR, Rao KV: Hepatic iron overload in renal transplant recipients: Ultrastructural observations. *Ultrastruct Pathol* **10**:227–234, 1986.

25

Granulomatous Liver Disease: Clinical Aspects

Willis C. Maddrey

1. INTRODUCTION

The finding of hepatic granulomas may tantalize, challenge, frustrate, or guide the clinician to the correct diagnosis of a systemic illness. Hepatic granulomas are frequent, having been reported in 2–10% of large series of liver biopsies.[1–14] Granulomas represent a specialized (albeit nonspecific) type of inflammatory response of the mononuclear phagocytic (reticuloendothelial) system. The liver is a common site for granuloma formation most likely because of its rich blood supply and the large number of reticuloendothelial (Kupffer) cells. Granulomas may be circumscribed, nodular, well-delineated, and distinct from the surrounding parenchyma or found in areas of diffuse inflammation.[11] The inciting agents that lead to granuloma formation may enter the liver via the hepatic artery, portal vein, or lymphatics.[15] Most infectious agents that cause granulomas probably reach the liver through the blood. Granulomas are likely to occur whenever there is uptake by phagocytic cells of bacteria, fungi, parasites, or other pathogens that persist within the macrophages, thereby eliciting an inflammatory response that may be either an immunologic or nonimmunologic reaction.[6,11,15]

Conditions in which hepatic granulomas have been reported cover a remarkable spectrum of disorders of infectious and noninfectious etiologies. Often the underlying disease has predominantly extrahepatic manifestations, and the liver is only incidentally involved in a multisystemic process. A number of the disorders in which hepatic granulomas are found are rare, and often the relationship between the disorder and the finding of granulomas is suspect.[16] In many patients (10–40%), no etiology is found that adequately explains the granulomas.[1–14]

A variety of types of acute and chronic inflammatory cells are found within granulomas, including monocytes and macrophages as well as fibroblasts, and in some eosinophils and polymorphonuclear cells. The large pale-staining epithelioid cells are specialized macrophages. Multinucleated giant cells, present in many granulomas, presumably result from fusion of macrophages. Occasionally, granulomas have central suppurative or caseous necrosis. Well-established granulomas may have a fibrous capsule or may be totally or partly replaced by scar. Granulomas in histoplasmosis, coccidioidomycosis, and a variety of other disorders may calcify. Occasionally foreign material such as talc or silica is found in granulomas.

Willis C. Maddrey • Department of Medicine, Jefferson Medical College, Philadelphia, Pennsylvania 19107.

Hepatic granulomas are most frequently found in or near the portal tract but may occur anywhere within the hepatic lobule. Well-delineated granulomas are characteristic in patients with sarcoidosis, tuberculosis, schistosomiasis, and histoplasmosis, whereas granulomatous inflammation (less well-formed granulomas) are found in many infectious diseases, including tularemia, Q fever and many drug reactions.[5,7,13,14,16]

In most patients, granulomas in the liver are associated with few if any signs or symptoms of liver disease. The nature and extent of evidence of liver or systemic disease often depend on the characteristics and extent of underlying disease. Often hepatic granulomas are found during an evaluation of fever, night sweats, abdominal pain, weight loss, hepatomegaly, splenomegaly, erythema nodosum, or lymphadenopathy or when a liver biopsy is performed as part of an evaluation for an apparent multisystem disorder associated with abnormalities of one or more biochemical tests of the liver.[1–14,17,18] An elevated serum alkaline phosphatase or γ-glutamyltranspeptidase level is frequently found in patient with hepatic granulomas in whom there are no other abnormal laboratory findings. Hepatic granulomas may be found in patients in whom there are no biochemical abnormalities suggestive of liver damage.[18] Peripheral (and intragranuloma) eosinophilia may be found in patients with drug-induced granulomas, parasites, or Hodgkin disease.

It is unusual for an etiologic diagnosis to be made from histologic examination of hepatic granulomas. Granulomas from a wide variety of conditions look alike, emphasizing that granuloma formation is a type of inflammatory response that may be quite nonspecific. Special stains of the granulomas are occasionally helpful in diagnosing such diverse disorders as tuberculosis, leprosy, atypical mycobacterial infection, schistosomiasis, syphilis, visceral larval migrans, histoplasmosis, coccidioidomycosis and talc.[5–7,11,13,14] In most instances, the finding of hepatic granulomas is of most value in indicating the need for, and the direction of, other diagnostic studies to establish a cause.

The identification of hepatic granulomas may lead to an extensive review, or re-review, of the patient's residence, travel, occupation, therapeutic (or illicit) drug usage, pets, or avocational history. The evaluations necessary to establish a diagnosis may include imaging studies, skin tests, serologic analyses, and biopsies of other tissues.

There are major geographic considerations in constructing a differential diagnostic list to guide an evaluation for the cause of hepatic granulomas. Leprosy, schistosomiasis, coccidioidomycosis, histoplasmosis, and exposure to parasites are all disorders that must be considered in patients who reside in, or who have visited, endemic areas. Furthermore, known industrial or occupational exposures such as to beryllium (miners or workers in atomic energy plants) or brucellosis (abattoir workers or veterinarians) may direct the evaluation to the correct diagnosis in a patient found to have hepatic granulomas. Evaluation of a patient following recognition of one or more granulomas on liver biopsy may be extensive, and in many patients a satisfactory well-supported diagnosis is not obtained. In such situations, it is preferable to designate the patient as having hepatic granulomas of unknown etiology rather than to label all such persons as having sarcoidosis. Often with long-term follow-up, a cause for the granulomas such as tuberculosis, histoplasmosis, Hodgkin disease, or inflammatory bowel disease will become apparent. To a clinician liberal with the use of the diagnosis of sarcoidosis, there are few if any granulomas considered to be of unknown etiology.

From the many possible causes of granulomas in the liver listed in comprehensive reviews,[1,4–9,11,13,14] we can identify a shorter list of diagnostic possibilities that account for most hepatic granulomas encountered in patients in the United States (Table I).

2. CHARACTERISTICS OF SEVERAL FREQUENTLY ENCOUNTERED CONDITIONS ASSOCIATED WITH HEPATIC GRANULOMAS

2.1. Sarcoidosis

Sarcoidosis is defined as a systemic granulomatous disorder of unknown etiology that may affect almost any organ with frequent clinical manifestations relating to involvement of the lungs,

Table I. Causes of Hepatic Granulomas Encountered in the United States[a]

- Sarcoidosis
- Infectious diseases
  - Bacterial infections
    - Tuberculosis
    - Atypical mycobacterial infection (especially in AIDS)
    - Brucellosis
    - Tularemia
    - BCG infection
  - Viral infections
    - Cytomegalovirus
    - Epstein–Barr virus
  - Fungal infections
    - Histoplasmosis
    - Coccidioidomycosis
  - Parasitic infections
    - Schistosomiasis (in patients from Puerto Rico or other endemic areas)
  - Rickettsial diseases
    - Q fever
  - Spirochetal
    - Syphilis (secondary)
- Primary liver disease
  - Primary biliary cirrhosis
- Malignancies
  - Hodgkin disease
  - Non-Hodgkin lymphoma
  - Renal cell carcinoma
- Drug reactions (see Table III)
- Miscellaneous disorders
  - Lipogranulomas (often related to mineral oil)
  - Berylliosis
  - Talc
  - Inflammatory bowel disease
  - Postjejunoileal bypass
  - Lymphomatoid granulomatosis
  - Wegener's granulomatosis
  - Chronic granulomatous disease
- Idiopathic hepatic granulomas

[a]More extensive lists are found in references 1, 9, 11, 13, and 14.

lymph nodes, and skin.[19,20] Most patients with sarcoidosis have granulomas on percutaneous needle biopsy, and sarcoidosis is the most frequent diagnosis made in large series of patients with hepatic granulomas in the United States. The incidence of granulomas in series of patients with sarcoidosis ranges from approximately 60% in some reports to 94% of the 231 patients reported by Klatskin.[7,11,13]

The diagnosis of sarcoidosis is based on the finding of granulomas in two or more organs in a patient with a compatible clinical setting. At many centers (including ours), a diagnosis of sarcoidosis is suspect if a liver biopsy is performed and there is no evidence of hepatic granulomas.

Klatskin[7] estimated there may be a remarkable number of granulomas (up to 75 million) in the liver of patients with sarcoidosis and emphasized the value of serial sectioning of a generous liver biopsy. The most consistent biochemical abnormality in patients with sarcoidosis involving the liver is an elevation in serum alkaline phosphatase. Many patients with sarcoidosis have increased gammaglobulin levels that may be increased to remarkable levels. The serum angiotensin-converting enzyme level (ACE) is increased in 50–80% of patients. Finding an elevated ACE level is not specific for sarcoidosis, however, as elevations have been found in patients with primary biliary cirrhosis and other granulomatous disorders.[21,22] Gallium-67 scanning may be helpful in diagnosing sarcoidosis, with the isotope often taken up by the granulomas.[21] The Kveim test, frequently positive in patients with sarcoidosis, is not well standardized and is no longer widely used.[13,23]

The hepatic granulomas found in patients with sarcoidosis are usually not associated with any evidence of liver disease and are found during elevation to confirm the diagnosis in a patient with diffuse pulmonary infiltrates, paratracheal lymphadenopathy, a papular rash, uveitis, fever of unknown etiology, or an elevated serum alkaline phosphatase. Hepatic granulomas from sarcoidosis may be found in patients with normal alkaline phosphatase levels. The granulomas are most often found in or around the portal tract and do not caseate. Schaumann bodies, inclusions that are often found in granulomas in lymph nodes in patients with sarcoidosis, are less frequently found in hepatic granulomas. As granulomas from sarcoidosis age and involute, collagen deposition develops around the periphery, and the granuloma is replaced by scar tissue.

Some patients with sarcoidosis develop symptomatic liver disease[19,24–26] (Table II). Some have hepatomegaly, splenomegaly, and biochemical abnormalities suggestive of chronic hepatitis.[19,26] Approximately 20% of patients with sarcoidosis have hepatomegaly.[19] Occasionally, a patient with sarcoidosis will present with evidence of considerable inflammation throughout the liver and marked perigranulomatous inflammation. These patients may have clinical, biochemical, and histologic evidence of a chronic active hepatitis (CAH) that may progress to cirrhosis with portal hypertension, hemorrhage from gastroesophageal varices, and ascites.[19,24–26] Sarcoidosis is therefore a rare cause of CAH and cirrhosis. In patients with evidence of severe liver disease from sarcoidosis, the granulomas are usually found throughout the hepatic lobule, and generally many areas of inflammation are apparently not associated with granulomas. In patients with advanced disease, there may be considerable fibrosis and cirrhosis with portal hypertension. Portal hypertension may be present in the absence of cirrhosis.[19] The pathogenesis of the portal hypertension in patients with hepatic sarcoidosis is unknown but may reflect the destruction of portal veins within the portal triads or the development of arteriovenous fistulas in the portal triad caused by the granulomatous inflammation or may result from the hepatic inflammation and resultant fibrosis.[13,19,26]

In addition, a syndrome of prolonged cholestatic liver injury that may mimic primary biliary cirrhosis has been reported in patients with sarcoidosis.[19,27–32] In such patients, there is apparent destruction of the interlobular bile ducts by the granulomas. In one series, five young males with apparent sarcoidosis had manifestations of severe prolonged cholestasis with progressive jaundice and pruritus.[32] In three of these five patients, biliary cirrhosis developed, and in the other two,

Table II. Spectrum of Hepatic Sarcoidosis

Incidental granulomas
Focal inflammation with granulomas
Chronic active hepatitis
Primary biliary cirrhosis-like disorder
Cirrhosis

hepatic fibrosis developed. All these patients had negative tests for antimitochondrial antibody (AMA). Other patients have been reported in whom an illness compatible with either sarcoidosis or primary biliary cirrhosis, or both, has been found.[27–30] A few such patients have been AMA positive.[27,30] Both sarcoidosis and primary biliary cirrhosis are disorders that may lead to a diminishing (vanishing) bile duct syndrome in adults.[33] Whether there is etiologic overlap between primary biliary cirrhosis and sarcoidosis will remain an area of speculation until the etiology of one or both disorders is found.[31]

Several instances of Budd–Chiari syndrome have been reported in patients with sarcoidosis.[34–36] It is uncertain how the granulomatous process of sarcoidosis might promote hepatic vein thrombosis.

Treatment of patients with symptomatic hepatic sarcoidosis with corticosteroids may be effective in improving biochemical abnormalities and in reducing hepatic size and tenderness. However, there is no conclusive proof that corticosteroid therapy retards the fibrotic process, thereby delaying the development or progression to cirrhosis and portal hypertension.[19] We use corticosteroid therapy in patients with sarcoidosis in whom there is evidence of CAH with bridging necrosis and in whom we would use corticosteroid therapy were the granulomas not present. At most Western centers, sarcoidosis is therefore the most common diagnosis applied in patients with hepatic granulomas. However, it must be recalled that there is no definitive diagnostic test for sarcoidosis, and the diagnosis remains one of exclusion.

2.2. *Infectious Etiologies*

The remarkable variety of infectious causes of granulomas is evident from a review of Table I. Bacterial organisms, especially those that tend to invade and persist in macrophages (e.g., tuberculosis, fungi, and migrating parasites) have been implicated.[1–16]

2.2.1. Bacterial Infections

2.2.1a. Tuberculosis. The diagnosis of tuberculosis is considered in almost every patient in whom hepatic granulomas are found.[1–14,37,38] In a series of 164 patients with tuberculosis who had a liver biopsy, Klatskin[7] reported hepatic granulomas in 94% of patients with disseminated (miliary) tuberculosis, in 71% of 14 patients with involvement of the lung and other tissues, and in 25% of 93 patients with tuberculosis apparently confined to the lungs. Tuberculosis was second only to sarcoidosis as a cause of hepatic granulomas in Klatskin's series of 565 patients with hepatic granulomas. In another series, the liver was often involved in extrapulmonary tuberculosis, with granulomas found on liver biopsy in 80% of patients.[37] Patients with miliary tuberculosis are often quite ill, and the hepatic granulomas may be poorly developed or may show caseating necrosis. The finding of hepatic granulomas in patients in whom tuberculosis is thought to be confined to the lungs indicates that there has, at some time, been hematogenous spread of the disease.

The finding of granulomas on liver biopsy may be an important clue that leads to the diagnosis of tuberculosis in a patient who presents with nonspecific symptoms, anorexia, fever, anemia, or weight loss and in whom there are no obvious signs of pulmonary involvement.[38,39] Tuberculosis is an important consideration in any patient with fever of unknown origin, and liver biopsy is a most valuable diagnostic tests.[6,13,17,18]

Even when the liver contains many granulomas from tuberculosis, there are usually few signs of symptoms of liver disease. The liver may be of normal size or enlarged and tender. The granulomas are most often found in or near portal tracts. Caseation may occur in hepatic granulomas caused by tuberculosis but is less frequent than in granulomas found in lymph nodes. Slight jaundice may be present. The increased incidence of disseminated tuberculosis in patients who are alcoholic is well established, and liver biopsy may reveal a mixture of alcohol-induced liver injury and granulomas from tuberculosis.[13] Rarely, there is involvement of the bile ducts with tuberculosis; instances of tuberculous cholangitis and biliary tract obstruction presumably secondary to tuberculous adenitis have been reported.[40]

Special stains to identify acid-fast bacilli in hepatic granulomas are occasionally useful in establishing the diagnosis of tuberculosis.[7,9,41] Fluorescent stains have a higher yield in identifying acid-fast bacilli than the classic Ziehl–Nielsen stains.[41] In the usual absence of finding acid-fast bacilli in hepatic granulomas, the diagnosis of tuberculosis must be established from other evidence. Culture of a portion of the liver biopsy for acid-fast bacilli may be useful.[13,42–44] In some patients with prolonged fevers and granulomas on liver biopsy, a therapeutic trial of antituberculous therapy is performed. In this setting, patients with tuberculosis usually demonstrate a clinical response within several weeks with reduction of fever. A patient with sarcoidosis will not have a response to antituberculous therapy.

2.2.1b. Brucellosis. Hepatic granulomas are found in patients with several types of brucellosis, especially in the more chronic forms of the illness.[45–53] The major brucellar organisms associated with granulomatous reactions are *Brucella abortus* (cows), *B. suis* (pigs), and less frequently *B. melitensis* (goats). Rarely, human infection from *B. canis* (dogs) has been reported.[48] Brucellosis is often an occupational disorder that may be acquired by farmers, abattoir workers, veterinarians who come in contact with infected animals, or persons who ingest unpasteurized dairy products. Patients with brucellosis may present with fever of unknown origin, often associated with prolonged weakness, depression, and fatigue associated with musculoskeletal pains. Brucellosis has been called undulant fever in the past because of the tendency for remissions and relapses.

The liver is often slightly enlarged in patients with brucellosis, and lymphadenopathy is a frequent finding. Minimal increases in serum alkaline phosphatase and aminotransferase levels are usually found.[16] Examination of the liver biopsy often reveals granulomas intermingled with nonspecific hepatitis. There are no characteristic features of the granulomas in brucellosis. Occasionally, *Brucella* organisms may be cultured from a liver biopsy.

Granulomatous reactions are most commonly found in patients with chronic *B. abortus*, in which the granulomas are typically found throughout the hepatic lobule rather than localized in the portal tract. The granulomas in *B. abortus* infection are often quite circumscribed. Patients with *B. suis* infection may have an invasive suppurative liver disease associated with calcification in the liver and spleen. Patients with *B. suis* infection may present with hepatic abscesses after years of apparent dormancy.[52] *B. melitensis* is often an acute disease that may lead to a diffuse hepatocellular injury without granulomas.[53] Brucellosis, even in the chronic form, rarely (if ever) leads to cirrhosis.[16] It is difficult to culture *Brucella* organisms, and the diagnosis of brucellosis is usually established by identification of increasing appropriate serum agglutinin titers.

2.2.1c. Tularemia. Tularemia, which may be acquired from contact with infected wild animals, is a cause of hepatic granulomatous inflammation that may caseate.[16] Patients with tularemia are often extremely ill, and the usual pathologic findings include diffuse areas of intense necrosis in which there may be granulomatous changes. Well-formed discrete granulomas are not found in patients with tularemia.

2.2.1d. Leprosy. Hepatic granulomas are found in approximately 60–90% of patients with lepromatous leprosy and in 20% of patients with tuberculoid leprosy.[54,55] Clinical manifestations of liver disease are usually absent or mild. The acid-fast *Lepra* bacilli may be found by the use of special stains, such as the auramine stain or Fite stain. Only minor abnormalities in biochemical functions of the liver are found in patients with leprosy, even when many granulomas are present.

2.2.2. Fungal Infections

2.2.2a. Histoplasmosis. Occasionally, patients with disseminated histoplasmosis will have hepatomegaly with granulomatous changes. Histoplasmosis is most often encountered in the central or eastern United States, and in highly endemic areas, histoplasmosis is a frequent cause of hepatic granulomas.[4,56–59] Hepatomegaly may be present. The granulomas may caseate and, with healing, may calcify. The diagnosis of histoplasmosis is made from identification and culture of the fungus from blood, bone marrow, or sputum. In rare instances, *Histoplasma capsulatum* has been cultured from liver biopsy specimens.[56–59] *Histoplasma* skin tests are of limited diagnostic value.

2.2.2b. Coccidioidomycosis. Coccidioidomycosis is a fungal disease that is an established cause of hepatic granulomas.[60,61] Coccidioidomycosis is found in the southwest United States, including parts of California (especially the San Joaquin Valley), Arizona, Texas, and neighboring areas, and is spread by inhalation of spores. The liver may be involved with granulomas that may be found near microabscesses. Hepatomegaly may be noted. Healing granulomas may hyalinize and later calcify. The diagnosis of coccidioidomycosis is established by demonstration of a rising titer of the approximate complement-fixing immunoglobulin G (IgG) antibodies and, in some patients, by identification of the organisms in the granulomas.

2.2.3. Viral Infections

2.2.3a. Cytomegalovirus Infection. Patients with acute hepatitis from infection with cytomegalovirus (CMV) have been found to have nonspecific acute hepatic granulomas in association with hepatic inflammation.[62–64] The diagnosis of CMV infection is established by finding characteristic increases in antibody tests. CMV infection has been shown to be a cause of hepatic granulomas in patients with acquired immune deficiency syndrome (AIDS).[65,66]

2.2.3b. Epstein–Barr Virus. Hepatic granulomas and diffuse hepatitis have been found in liver biopsies from patients with infectious mononucleosis caused by the Epstein–Barr virus (EBV).[16] The diagnosis of infectious mononucleosis (EBV infection) is established by demonstrating a characteristic rise in titer of antibodies directed against various EBV antigens.

2.2.3c. Hepatic Granulomas in AIDS. Hepatic granulomas are frequently found in patients with AIDS and may result from a variety of infections or drug reactions.[65–68] There is no evidence that the HIV virus itself causes granulomas. In one series, 48% of 21 patients with AIDS had granulomas on liver biopsy, the most frequent cause of which was *Mycobacterium avium-intracellulare*.[65] Other causes of hepatic granulomas in patients with AIDS include tuberculosis, CMV infection, histoplasmosis, or a drug reaction. In patients with AIDS in whom there is an elevated serum alkaline phosphatase level, the liver biopsy may be helpful in identifying an infection that may be amenable to treatment.

2.2.4. Rickettsial Diseases

2.2.4a. Q Fever. Granulomas are frequently found in liver biopsies from patients with the rickettsial disease Q fever (*Coxiella burnetti*).[69–73] Patients with Q fever often have clinical manifestations of prolonged fever, hepatosplenomegaly, and evidence of hepatic inflammation. Q fever occurs worldwide, except in Scandinavia, and *Coxiella burnetti* infection is common in goat and sheep herds. A history of contact with livestock may be the initial clue to the diagnosis. Q fever is usually acquired by inhalation of the rickettsia from animal products. Hepatomegaly and hepatic tenderness may be present along with slight increases in serum alkaline phosphatase and aminotransferases. Occasionally, jaundice is found. The hepatic granulomas are usually small and may be characterized by a fibrinoid ring formation with a central empty space.[72] The diagnosis of Q fever is established by the finding of rising titers of appropriate complement-fixing antibodies.

2.2.5. Parasitic Diseases

2.2.5a. Schistosomiasis. Schistosomiasis is likely the most common worldwide cause of hepatic granulomas.[13,15,74] The hepatic granulomas frequently found in patients with schistosomiasis (*Schistosoma mansoni* and *S. japonicum*) result from a reaction to schistosomal eggs released by adult female worms into the mesenteric veins and subsequently lodge in the small portal venules, inciting a granulomatous reaction.[15,74] The granulomas that develop are an immunologic response to egg components and lead to portal and periportal fibrosis and portal hypertension. Often part of the schistosomal egg is found in the granulomas, and the value of serial sectioning of the liver biopsy searching for the characteristic egg fragments is established. Schistosomiasis is not endemic in the United States, but the disorder should be considered in patients with granulomatous liver disease who come from endemic areas or in whom a travel history suggests possible exposure. Most patients with schistosomiasis from the Western hemisphere come from Puerto Rico. *S. mansoni* is the only type of schistosomiasis found in the Western hemisphere. The diagnosis of schistosomiasis is made by finding eggs within the granulomas, in the feces, or in biopsies of the rectal mucosal.

2.2.6. Other Infections

A remarkable spectrum of infections in which hepatic granulomas have been reported are listed in Table I and in comprehensive review articles.[1–14] The relative contribution of these infections to series of patients with hepatic granulomas will vary, depending on local disease prevalences and the abilities of the clinician. The geographic considerations are often extremely helpful in establishing a diagnosis. For example, granulomas resulting from the gram-negative infection melioidosis were found in American military personnel returning from Southeast Asia.[75,76] Coccidioidomycosis is an important consideration in evaluating hepatic granulomas found in a patient from the southwest United States but is rare in patients from the eastern United States.[13,60] Histoplasmosis is especially prevalent in the central and eastern United States. Even further afield, infection by nymphs of the pentastome *Linguatula serrata* is a problem in Malaysian aborigines who become infected by ingesting embryonated eggs from infected snakes and may develop hepatic granulomas.[77] Rarely patients in the United States have had hepatic granulomas from infection with the nymphs of *Lingualata serrata.*[78] Disseminated granulomatous infection with bacille Calmette-Guérin (BCG) used either in a vaccination program or for immunotherapy, especially for malignant melanoma, has been reported.[79,80] It is therefore most important to obtain a careful social, occupational, and travel history in patients with hepatic granulomas in order to consider and identify rare, often exotic, disorders.

Rare instances of hepatic granulomas related to infections have been reported in Whipple disease,[81] giardiasis,[82] and listeriosis.[83] Hepatic granulomas may be found in patients with secondary syphilis.[84]

2.3. Malignancies

2.3.1. Hodgkin Disease

The finding of hepatic granulomas may be the initial clue to the diagnosis of Hodgkin disease. Extensive studies of patients with Hodgkin disease have revealed granulomas in as many as 12% of patients.[85–87] These granulomas are most often located in the portal tracts.[85–90] The granulomas may occur in areas of the liver in which there is no evidence of Hodgkin disease and in persons in whom there has been no prior lymphangiography. Granulomas may be found in the liver months to years before Hodgkin disease is diagnosed.[91,92] Thus, follow-up evaluation for the development of Hodgkin disease is indicated in patients with hepatic granulomas of unknown etiology.[85] The presence of granulomas is not considered important in the staging of Hodgkin disease. However, it has been suggested that the presence of epithelioid granulomas may be a favorable prognostic sign.[92,93] In follow-up studies, patients with Hodgkin disease who had hepatic granulomas had fewer relapses and longer survival than did patients without granulomas.

Granulomas have also been found in the spleen, bone marrow, and abdominal lymph nodes in patients with Hodgkin disease, but granulomas are less frequently found in these sites than in the liver.[87] Rarely, granulomas have been found in patients with non-Hodgkin lymphomas.[87,88]

The cause of the granulomas in Hodgkin and in non-Hodgkin lymphomas is unknown. It has been suggested that the granulomas are a manifestation of a host response to the neoplasm. Hepatic granulomas have been noted in patients with a variety of other tumors, including hairy cell leukemia and renal cell carcinoma.[94,95]

2.4. Drug-Induced Hepatic Granulomas

Hepatic granulomas are found as part of the hepatic injury caused by many drugs, and a careful history of exposure to therapeutic drugs is an important part of the evaluation.[96–99] Several therapeutic drugs in which there is conclusive or highly suggestive evidence of drug-induced hepatic granulomas are listed in Table III.[96–124] It is often difficult, or impossible, to separate the contribution of the drug to the causation of the hepatic granulomas from that of the condition for which the drug is being given. Drug-induced injury should be considered as the cause for hepatic granulomas whenever there is a suitable temporal relationship between the institution of the drug and the appearance of liver injury. Whenever possible, all potential inciting drugs should be discontinued. The proof of a drug-related injury afforded by a rechallenge is rarely available. Blood eosinophilia and eosinophils in or around the granulomas are frequent in patients with drug-induced gran-

Table III. Drugs Reported to Cause Hepatic Granulomas

Drug	References
Allopurinol	100–103
Carbamazepine	104,105
Chlorpropamide	106
Diltiazem	107
Gold	108
Halothane	109
Hydralazine	110
Methyldopa	111,112
Nitrofurantoin	96,97
Phenylbutazone	96,113–116
Phenytoin	117
Procainamide	118
Quinine	119
Quinidine	120,121
Sulfonamides	122,123
Tocainide	124

ulomatous liver disease, but the finding of eosinophils is quite nonspecific and may be found in granulomas caused by many other conditions such as Hodgkin disease.

In a series of 23 patients with liver injury from phenylbutazone, nine had evidence of hepatic granulomas.[116] Hepatic granulomas in phenylbutazone-induced injury were usually found in patients with evidence of a hypersensitivity-type reaction (fever and rash) and only mild hepatocellular injury. The granulomas were usually found in or near the portal tract, and eosinophils were detected in the granulomas in eight of the nine patients. In two patients, no granulomas were found in follow-up liver biopsies 6 months after withdrawal of phenylbutazone. Patients with more severe hepatic injury from phenylbutazone did not have evidence of granulomas. Therefore, it appears that there are at least two types of phenylbutazone-induced liver injury and that those patients who have a granulomatous response have a milder injury. In one patient, a deliberate rechallenge with phenylbutazone was followed by reappearance of hepatic injury, thereby supporting the relationship of the drug to the injury.[114]

Patients with allopurinol-induced hepatic injury may have signs and symptoms suggestive of a hypersensitivity reaction with fever, rash, and eosinophilia in addition to abnormal liver tests.[100–103] One patient with allopurinol-induced liver injury had fibrin-ring granulomas previously observed in patients with Q fever and Hodgkin disease.[72]

2.5. Primary Liver Disease

2.5.1. Primary Biliary Cirrhosis

Granulomas are found in approximately 40–50% of liver biopsies from patients with primary biliary cirrhosis.[125] The cause of the granulomas, and indeed the cause of primary biliary cirrhosis, remains unknown. The hepatic granulomas in primary biliary cirrhosis are not associated with fever. The granulomas are most often found around bile ducts and in the periportal region. In a series of 295 liver biopsy specimens from 100 patients with primary biliary cirrhosis, granulomas were found in 54 patients and were less frequently found as the histologic stage of the disease increased.[125] These observations suggest the findings of granulomas is a favorable prognostic sign indicating a milder or earlier form of primary biliary cirrhosis. There were no differences in age or serum bilirubin levels between patients with and those without granulomas, and therefore the presence of granulomas was considered an independent favorable prognostic indicator. When patients with late primary biliary cirrhosis were separately analyzed, 23 of 57 had granulomas, but granulomas were present in only one of 14 patients who died. In another study of patients with primary biliary cirrhosis, the presence of granulomas on liver biopsy was not of prognostic value.[126]

When serial sections of wedge liver biopsies from 39 patients with primary biliary cirrhosis from Japan were examined, granulomas were found in 76.9% of patients.[127] There was an apparent decrease in the number of granulomas in patients as hepatic fibrosis developed and bile duct loss occurred.

2.6. Idiopathic Hepatic Granulomas

Despite extensive evaluation and follow-up, the cause of many hepatic granulomas remains unknown.[1–14] Simon and Wolff[128] reported a series of 13 patients with hepatic granulomas associated with a chronic febrile illness that often lasted for years, was frequently associated with abdominal pain and weight loss, and was designated granulomatous hepatitis. Other series of patients with granulomas of unknown etiology have emphasized the presentation of the syndrome as chronic abdominal pain.[129] Whether this disorder is a variant of sarcoidosis or deserves to stand as a separate diagnosis of unknown etiology remains to be determined.[130]

Patients with unexplained granulomas should be carefully followed. In some patients, a diagnosis, such as primary biliary cirrhosis, tuberculosis, sarcoidosis, underlying malignancy, or inflammatory bowel disease, will subsequently be established. If extensive investigations do not lead to a specific diagnosis in a symptomatic patient with hepatic granulomas, a trial of corticosteroid therapy may be considered. A course of antituberculous therapy is often instituted before the patient is given corticosteroid therapy to protect against the emergence of undiagnosed tuberculosis.[128]

Rarely, patients have been described with an acute, short-term, febrile illness resembling infectious mononucleosis with lymphocytosis characterized by hepatic granulomas.[131,132] The etiology (or etiologies) of the disorder is unknown and may represent a viral infection.

2.7. Miscellaneous Disorders

2.7.1. Jejunoileal Bypass Surgery

During the era of popularity of jejunoileal bypass surgery, hepatic granulomas were frequently found.[133,134] The etiology of the granulomas was uncertain. There was little evidence to incriminate a specific causative agent in most patients, although a few instances of tuberculosis were encountered.[135]

2.7.2. Lipogranulomas

Lipid-containing granulomas are found in liver biopsies from patients with a variety of conditions, including alcoholic liver disease and obesity, and in some with no apparent underlying disease.[136–140] These lipogranulomas are often small and are more likely to be around the terminal hepatic venule (central vein) than are epithelioid granulomas. It appears the lipogranulomas develop in response to the ingestion of lipids by macrophages. Some lipogranulomas occur as a reaction to mineral oil, which is ingested in a large number of food and medicinal products.[136,140]

2.7.3. Berylliosis

If beryllium is inhaled, a chronic multisystem granulomatous disease develops affecting the liver, lung, and other organs.[141,142] Beryllium exposure is more likely to occur in beryllium miners or in workers in atomic energy facilities. The clinical and histologic manifestations of berylliosis may resemble sarcoidosis or tuberculosis and is diagnosed by the demonstration of increased tissue levels of beryllium.[142]

2.7.4. Extrahepatic Bile Duct Obstruction

In one series from Scotland of 77 patients with hepatic granulomas, seven patients were reported in whom the granulomas were thought related to extrahepatic bile duct obstruction.[10] The Scottish experience differed from series from the United States in that extrahepatic biliary obstruction, neoplasm, and bacterial infection were found to be more common causes of granulomas as compared with the predominance of sarcoidosis and tuberculosis in compilations from the United States.

2.7.5. Talc

Granulomas containing talc may be found in the liver of patients who are intravenous drug abusers.[143,144] The talc is recognized as birefringent foreign-body material, which is used as filler material for the injected drugs.

2.7.6. Lymphomatoid Granulomatosis

Lymphomatoid granulomatosis is a rare disorder in which hepatic granulomas are found.[145–147] Lymphomatoid granulomatosis is characterized by infiltration of many organs with a polymorphic infiltrate, including lymphocytoid and plasmacytoid cells and granulomatous inflammation. The major organs affected are the lungs, skin, kidneys, and central nervous system (CNS). The liver is involved in approximately one third of patients.[147] Hepatomegaly and jaundice may be present. The disease may progress to lymphoma.[145–147]

2.7.7. Chronic Granulomatous Disease

Chronic granulomatous disease (CGD) is a disorder found in children and occasionally in adults, characterized by an inability of granulocytes to destroy phagocytized microorganisms.[148–150] CGD is more frequent in males and is apparently an inherited disorder.[148–150] The continuing presence of microorganisms within the granulocytes leads to chronic granulomatous inflammation related to the inability of neutrophils from these patients to destroy the microorganism. The inability to reduce the dye nitroblue tetrazolium (NBT) because of defective production of oxygen metabolites is a useful diagnostic test.

2.8. Other Disorders

Granulomas in the liver have also been reported in patients with a variety of other disorders, including Crohn disease,[151] rheumatoid arthritis,[152] polymyalgia rheumatica,[153] allergic granulomatosis,[154] and Wegener's granulomatosis.[155]

3. COMMENTS

The finding of one or more granulomas on a liver biopsy is often a challenge to the diagnostic skills of the clinician. If an etiologic agent is identified in the granuloma, an infrequent finding, the task is simple. More often, however, other extensive investigations may be required. The list of diagnostic possibilities may be remarkably long, covering a variety of infectious and noninfectious conditions. Only a few of the causes of hepatic granulomas have been reviewed in this chapter. In many patients, no firm diagnosis is ever established. Just because an hepatic granuloma is found in a patient with an established disorder does not prove that the granuloma is caused by the condition. The rewards when evaluation of a patient with hepatic granulomas leads to the identification of a systemic disorder amenable to treatment are considerable. Treatment, such as is available, is directed toward the underlying condition, and not toward the granulomas.

We have much more to learn regarding granulomatous inflammation. A few of the interesting clinical observations that need to be explored further include whether (and if so why) the finding of hepatic granulomas in patients with primary biliary cirrhosis and with Hodgkin disease signifies a favorable prognosis; whether primary biliary cirrhosis and sarcoidosis are related disorders; and the nature of the inciting agent for the granulomas in patients with Hodgkin disease.

Establishing the exact etiology for hepatic granulomas may require patience and repeat evaluations. A patient with a diagnosis of granuloma of unknown etiology should be followed carefully, with special attention to the appearance of signs or symptoms indicating an underlying malignancy (e.g., Hodgkin disease), inflammatory bowel disease, arteritis, tuberculosis, or fungal disease.

REFERENCES

1. Guckian JC, Perry JE: Granulomatous hepatitis. An analysis of 63 cases and review of the literature. *Ann Intern Med* **65**:1081–1100, 1966.
2. Guckian JC, Perry JE: Granulomatous hepatitis of unknown etiology. An etiologic and functional evaluation. *Am J Med* **44**:207–215, 1968.

3. Iversen K, Christoffersen P, Poulsen H: Epithelioid cell granulomas in liver biopsies. *Scand J Gastroenterol* **7**(suppl):61–67, 1970.
4. Mir-Madjlessi SH, Farmer RG, Hawk WA: Granulomatous hepatitis: A review of 50 cases. *Am J Gastroenterol* **60**:122–134, 1973.
5. Klatskin G: Hepatic granulomata: Problems in interpretation. *Ann NY Acad Sci* **278**:427–432, 1976.
6. Fauci AS, Wolff SM: Granulomatous hepatitis, in Popper H, Schaffner F (eds): *Progress in Liver Diseases,* Vol. 5. Grune & Stratton, Orlando, Florida, 1976, pp. 609–621.
7. Klatskin G: Hepatic granulomata; problems in interpretation. *Mt Sinai J Med* **44**:798–812, 1977.
8. Irani SK, Dobbins WO III: Hepatic granulomas: A review of 73 patients from one hospital and survey of the literature. *J Clin Gastroenterol* **1**:131–143, 1979.
9. Harrington PT, Gutierrez JJ, Ramirez-Ronda CH, et al: Granulomatous hepatitis. *Rev Infect Dis* **4**:638–655, 1982.
10. Cunningham D, Mills PR, Quigley EMM, et al: Hepatic granulomas: Experience over a 10-year period in the west of Scotland. *Q J Med* **202**:162–170, 1982.
11. Ishak KG: Granulomas of the liver, in Ioachim HL (ed): *Pathology of Granulomas.* Raven, New York, 1983, pp. 307–369.
12. Mills PR, Russell RI: Diagnosis of hepatic granulomas: A review. *J Roy Soc Med* **76**:393–397, 1983.
13. Reynolds TB, Campra JL, Peters RL: Hepatic granulomas, in Zakim D, Boyer TD (eds): *Hepatology. A Textbook on Liver Diseases.* WB Saunders, Philadelphia, 1982, pp. 995–1009.
14. Berk JE, Cohen M: Hepatic granulomas, in Berk JE (ed): *Bockus Gastroenterology,* 4th ed. WB Saunders, Philadelphia, 1985, pp. 3189–3202.
15. Warren KS: A Functional classification of granulomatous inflammation. *Ann NY Acad Sci* **278**:7–18, 1976.
16. Klatskin G: Hepatitis associated with systemic infection, in Schiff L (ed): *Diseases of the Liver,* 2nd ed. JB Lippincott, Philadelphia, 1963, pp. 539–572.
17. Petersdorf RG, Beeson PB: Fever of unexplained origin: Report on 100 cases. *Medicine (Baltimore)* **40**:1–30, 1961.
18. Dinarello CA, Wolff SM: Approach to the patient with fever of unknown origin, in Mandell GL, Douglas RG Jr, Bennett JE (eds): *Principles and Practice of Infectious Diseases.* Wiley, New York, 1984, pp. 347–350.
19. Maddrey WC, Johns CJ, Boitnott JK, et al: Sarcoidosis and chronic hepatic disease: A clinical and pathological study of 20 patients. *Medicine (Baltimore)* **49**:375–395, 1970.
20. Israel HL, Margolis ML, Rose LJ: Hepatic granulomatosis and sarcoidosis. Further observations. *Dig Dis Sci* **29**:353–356, 1984.
21. Nosal A, Schleissner LA, Mishkin FS, et al: Angiotensin-1-converting enzyme and gallium scan in noninvasive evaluation of sarcoidosis. *Ann Intern Med* **90**:328–331, 1979.
22. Rohatgi PK, Singh R, Vieras F: Extrapulmonary localization of gallium in sarcoidosis. *Clin Nucl Med* **12**: 9–16, 1987.
23. Israel HL, Goldstein RA: Relation of Kveim-antigen reaction to lymphadenopathy. *N Engl J Med* **284**: 345–349, 1971.
24. Porter GH: Hepatic sarcoidosis. A cause of portal hypertension and liver failure. A review. *Arch Intern Med* **108**:483–495, 1961.
25. Tekeste H, Latour F, Levitt RE: Portal hypertension complicating sarcoid liver disease: Case report and review of the literature. *Am J Gastroenterol* **79**:389–396, 1984.
26. Valla D, Pessegueiro-Miranda H, Degott C, et al: Hepatic sarcoidosis with portal hypertension. A report of seven cases with a review of the literature. *Q J Med* **242**:531–544, 1987.
27. Karlish AJ, Thompson RPH, Williams R: A case of sarcoidosis and primary biliary cirrhosis. *Lancet* **2**: 599, 1969.
28. Stanley NN, Fox RA, Whimster WF, et al: Primary biliary cirrhosis or sarcoidosis—or both. *N Engl J Med* **287**:1282–1284, 1972.
29. Bass NM, Burroughs AK, Scheuer PJ, et al: Chronic intraheptic cholestasis due to sarcoidosis. *Gut* **23**: 417–421, 1982.
30. Fagan EA, Moore-Gillon JC, Turner-Warwick M: Multiorgan granulomas and mitochondrial antibodies. *N Engl J Med* **308**:572–575, 1983.
31. Maddrey WC: Sarcoidosis and primary biliary cirrhosis: Associated disorders? *N Engl J Med* **308**:588–590, 1983.

32. Rudzki C, Ishak KG, Zimmerman HJ: Chronic intrahepatic cholestasis of sarcoidosis. *Am J Med* **59**:373–387, 1975.
33. Sherlock S: The syndrome of disappearing intrahepatic bile ducts. *Lancet* **2**:493–496, 1987.
34. Natalino MR, Goyette RE, Owensby LC, et al: The Budd–Chiari syndrome in sarcoidosis. *JAMA* **239**:2657–2658, 1978.
35. Mitchell MC, Boitnott JK, Kaufman S, et al: Budd–Chiari syndrome: Etiology, diagnosis and management. *Medicine (Baltimore)* **61**:199–218, 1982.
36. Russi EW, Bansky, G, Pfaltz M, et al: Budd–Chiari syndrome in sarcoidosis. *Am J Gastroenterol* **81**:71–75, 1986.
37. Korn RJ, Kellow WF, Heller P, et al: Hepatic involvement in extrapulmonary tuberculosis—Histologic and functional characteristics. *Am J Med* **27**:60–71, 1969.
38. Bowry S, Chan CH, Weiss H, et al: Hepatic involvement in pulmonary tuberculosis. Histologic and functional characteristics. *Am Rev Respir Dis* **101**:941–948, 1970.
39. Frank BB, Raffensperger EC: Hepatic granulomata. Report of a case with jaundice improving on antituberculous therapy and review of the literature. *Arch Intern Med* **115**:223–234, 1965.
40. Murphy TF, Gray GF: Biliary tract obstruction due to tuberculous adenitis. *Am J Med* **68**:452–454, 1980.
41. Yamaguchi BT Jr, Braunstein H: Fluorescent stain for tubercle bacilli in histologic sections. *Am J Clin Pathol* **43**:184–187, 1965.
42. Rumball JM, Baum GL: Liver biopsy culture in the diagnosis of miliary tuberculosis. *Gastroenterology* **22**:124–127, 1952.
43. Healey RJ, Leff AA, Rosenak BD: Needle biopsy in tuberculosis of the liver, with culture of acid-fast bacilli. A case report. *Am J Dig Dis* **4**:638–641, 1959.
44. Cucin RL, Coleman, M, Eckhardt JJ, et al: The diagnosis of miliary tuberculosis: Utility of peripheral blood abnormalities, bone marrow, and liver needle biopsy. *J Chron Dis* **26**:355–361, 1973.
45. Spink WW, Hoffbauer FW, Walker WW, et al: Histopathology of the liver in human brucellosis. *J Lab Clin Med* **36**:40–58, 1949.
46. Joske RA, Finckh ES: Hepatic changes in human brucellosis. *Med J Aust* **1**:266–269, 1955.
47. Hunt AC, Bothwell PW: Histological findings in human brucellosis. *J Clin Pathol* **20**:267–272, 1967.
48. Fox MD, Kaufman AF: Brucellosis in the United States 1965–1974. *J Infect Dis* **136**:312–316, 1977.
49. Bruguera M, Cervantes F: Hepatic granulomas in brucellosis. *Ann Intern Med* **92**:571–572, 1980.
50. Masana L, Bernardo L, Bacardi R, et al: Granulomas in *Brucella melitensis* infect. *Ann Intern Med* **92**:264–265, 1980.
51. Fernandez-Guirrero ML, Diaz M, Cortes JM, et al: Hepatic granulomas in brucellosis. *Ann Intern Med* **92**:572, 1980.
52. Williams RK, Crossley K: Acute and chronic hepatic involvement of brucellosis. *Gastroenterology* **83**:455–458, 1982.
53. Jordans HGM, De Bruin KD: Granulomas in *Brucella melitensis* infection. *Ann Intern Med* **92**:264–265, 1980.
54. Karat AB, Job CK, Rao PSS: Liver in leprosy: Histological and biochemical findings. *Br Med J* **1**:307–310, 1971.
55. Chen TSN, Drutz DJ, Whelan GE: Hepatic granulomas in leprosy. Their relation to bacteremia. *Arch Pathol Lab Med* **100**:182–185, 1976.
56. Israel HL, DeLamater E, Sones M: Chronic disseminated histoplasmosis—An investigation of its relationship to sarcoidosis. *Am J Med* **12**:252–260, 1952.
57. Lanza FL, Nelson RS, Somayaji BN: Acute granulomatous hepatitis due to histoplasmosis. *Gastroenterology* **58**:392–396, 1970.
58. Reddy P, Gorelick DF, Brasher CA et al: Progressive disseminated histoplasmosis as seen in adults. *Am J Med* **48**:629–636, 1970.
59. Smith JW, Utz, JR: Progressive disseminated histoplasmosis. A prospective study of 26 patients. *Ann Intern Med* **76**:557–565, 1972.
60. Forbus WD, Bestebreurtje AM: Coccidioidomycosis: A study of 95 cases of the disseminated type with special reference to the pathogenesis of the disease. *Milit Surg* **99**:653–719, 1946.
61. Ward JR, Hunter RC Jr: Disseminated coccidioidomycosis demonstrated by needle biopsy of the liver. *Ann Intern Med* **48**:157–163, 1958.
62. Reller LB: Granulomatous hepatitis associated with acute cytomegalovirus infection. *Lancet* **1**:20–22, 1973.

63. Bonkowsky HL, Lee RV, Klatskin G: Acute granulomatous hepatitis. Occurrence in cytomegalovirus mononucleosis. *JAMA* **233:**1284–1288, 1975.
64. Clarke J, Craig RM, Saffro R, et al: Cytomegalovirus granulomatous hepatitis. *Am J Med* **66:**264–269, 1979.
65. Kahn SA, Saltzman BR, Klein RS, et al: Hepatic disorders in the acquired immune deficiency syndrome: A clinical and pathological study. *Am J Gastroenterol* **81:**1145–1148, 1986.
66. Lebovics E, Thung SN, Schaffner F, et al: The liver in the acquired immunodeficiency syndrome: A clinical and histological study. *Hepatology* **5:**293–298, 1985.
67. Orenstein MS, Tavitian A, Yonk B, et al: Granulomatous involvement of the liver in patient with AIDS. *Gut* **26:**1220–1225, 1985.
68. Glasgow BJ, Anders K, Layfield LJ, et al: Clinical and pathological findings of the liver in the acquired immune deficiency syndrome (AIDS). *Am J Clin Pathol* **83:**582–588, 1985.
69. Bernstein M, Edmondson HA, Barbour BJ: The liver lesion in Q fever. Clinical and pathological features. *Arch Intern Med* **116:**491–498, 1965.
70. Dupont HL, Hornick RB, Levin HS, et al: Q fever hepatitis. *Ann Intern Med* **74:**198–206, 1971.
71. Pellegrin M, Delsol G, Auvergnat JC, et al: Granulomatous hepatitis in Q fever. *Human Pathol* **11:**51–57, 1980.
72. Qizilbash AH: The pathology of Q fever as seen on liver biopsy. *Arch Pathol Lab Med* **107:**364–367, 1983.
73. Thung SN, Gerber MA, Lebovics E, et al: Granulomatous hepatitis in Q fever. *Mt Sinai J Med* **53:**283–285, 1986.
74. Dunn MA, Kamel R: Hepatic schistosomiasis. *Hepatology* **1:**653–661, 1981.
75. Greenawald KA, Nash G, Foley FD: Acute systemic melioidosis. Autopsy findings in four patients. *Am J Clin Pathol* **52:**188–198, 1969.
76. Piggott JA, Hochholzer L: Human melioidosis. A histopathologic study of acute and chronic melioidosis. *Arch Pathol Lab Med* **90:**101–111, 1970.
77. Prathap K, Lau KS, Bolton JM: Pentastomiasis: A common finding at autopsy among Malaysian aborigines. *Am J Trop Med Hyg* **18:**20–27, 1969.
78. Gardiner CH, Dyke JW, Shirley SF: Hepatic granuloma due to a nymph of linguatula serrata in a woman from Michigan: A case report and review of the literature. *Am Soc Trop Med Hyg* **33:**187–189, 1984.
79. Hunt JS, Silverstein MJ, Sparks FC, et al: Granulomatous hepatitis: A complication of B.C.G. immunotherapy. *Lancet* **2:**820–821, 1973.
80. Aungst CW, Sokal JE, Jager BV: Complications of BCG vaccination in neoplastic disease. *Ann Intern Med* **82:**666–669, 1975.
81. Girardin MFSM, Zafrani ES, Chaumette MT, et al: Hepatic granulomas in Whipple's disease. *Gastroenterology* **86:**753–856, 1984.
82. Roberts-Thomson IC, Anders RF, Bhathal PS: Granulomatous hepatitis and cholangitis associated with giardiasis. *Gastroenterology* **83:**480–483, 1982.
83. Buchner LH, Schneierson SS: Clinical and laboratory aspects of *Listeria monocytogenes* infections. A report of ten cases. *Am J Med* **45:**904–921, 1968.
84. Lee RV, Thornton GF, Conn HO: Liver disease associated with secondary syphilis. *N Engl J Med* **284:** 1423–1425, 1971.
85. Kadin ME, Donaldson SS, Dorfman RF: Isolated granulomas in Hodgkin's disease. *N Engl J Med* **283:** 859–861, 1970.
86. Bagley CM Jr, Roth JA, Thomas LB, et al: Liver biopsy in Hodgkin's disease. Clinicopathological correlations in 127 patients. *Ann Intern Med* **76:**219–225, 1972.
87. Kim H, Dorfman RF, Rosenberg SA: Pathology of malignant lymphomas in the liver: Application in staging, in Popper H, Schaffner F (eds): *Progress in Liver Diseases,* Vol. 5, Grune & Stratton, Orlando, Florida, 1976, pp. 683–698.
88. Braylan RC, Long JC, Jaffe ES, et al: Malignant lymphoma obscured by concomitant extensive epithelioid granulomas: Report of three cases with similar clinicopathologic features. *Cancer* **39:**1146–1155, 1977.
89. Abt AB, Kirschner RH, Belliveau RE, et al: Hepatic pathology associated with Hodgkin's disease. *Cancer* **33:**1564–1571, 1974.
90. Pak HY, Friedman NB: Pseudosarcoid granulomas in Hodgkin's disease. *Hum Pathol* **12:**832–837, 1981.
91. Aderka D, Kraus M, Avidor I, et al: Hodgkin's and non-Hodgkin's lymphomas masquerading as "idiopathic" liver granulomas. *Am J Gasteroenterol* **79:**642–644, 1984.

92. O'Connell MJ, Schimpff SC, Kirschner RH, et al: Epithelioid granulomas in Hodgkin's disease. A favorable prognostic sign? *JAMA* **233**:886–889, 1975.
93. Sacks EL, Donaldson SS, Gordon J, et al: Epithelioid granulomas associated with Hodgkin's disease. Clinical correlations in 55 previously untreated patients. *Cancer* **41**:562–567, 1978.
94. Bendix-Hansen K, Kristensen IB: Granulomas of spleen and liver in hairy cell leukaemia. *Acta Path Microbiol Immunol Scand* **92**:157–160, 1984.
95. Chagnac A, Gal R, Kimche D, et al: Liver granulomas: A possible paraneoplastic manifestation of hypernephroma. *Am J Gastroenterol* **80**:989–992, 1985.
96. Zimmerman HJ: *Hepatotoxicity. The Adverse Effects of Drugs and Other Chemicals on the Liver.* Appleton & Lange, East Norwalk, Connecticut, 1978.
97. McMaster KR III, Hennigar GR: Drug-induced granulomatous hepatitis. *Lab Invest* **44**:61–73, 1981.
98. Maddrey WC: Drug and chemical-induced hepatic injury, in Berk JE (ed): *Bockus, Gastroenterology,* 4th ed. WB Saunders, Philadelphia, 1985, pp. 2922–2956.
99. Zimmerman H, Maddrey WC: Toxic and drug-induced hepatitis, in Schiff L (ed): *Diseases of the Liver,* 6th ed. JB Lippincott, Philadelphia, 1987, pp. 591–667.
100. Medline A, Cohen LB, Tobe BA, et al: Liver granulomas and allopurinol. *Br Med J* **1**:1320–1231, 1978.
101. Swank LA, Chejfe G, Nemchausky BA: Allopurinol-induced granulomatous hepatitis with cholangitis and a sarcoid-like reaction. *Arch Intern Med* **138**:997–998, 1978.
102. Al-Kawas FH, Seeff LB, Berendson RA, et al: Allopurinol hepatotoxicity. Report of two cases and review of the literature. *Ann Intern Med* **95**:588–590, 1981.
103. Vanderstigel M, Zafrani ES, Lejonc JL, et al: Allopurinol hypersensitivity syndrome as a cause of hepatic fibrin-ring granulomas. *Gastroenterology* **90**:188–190, 1986.
104. Mitchell MC, Boitnott JK, Arregui A, et al: Granulomatous hepatitis associated with carbamazepine therapy. *Am J Med* **71**:733–735, 1981.
105. Levy M, Goodman MW, Van Dyne BJ, et al: Granulomatous hepatitis secondary to carbamazepine. *Ann Intern Med* **95**:64–64, 1981.
106. Rigberg LA, Robinson MJ, Espiritu CR: Chlorpropamide-induced granulomas. A probable hypersensitivity reaction in liver and bone marrow. *JAMA* **235**:409–410, 1976.
107. Sarachek NS, London RL, Matulewicz TJ: Diltiazem and granulomatous hepatitis. *Gastroenterology* **88**: 1260–1262, 1985.
108. Harats N, Ehrenfeld M, Shalit M, et al: Gold-induced granulomatous hepatitis. *Isr J Med Sci* **21**:753–756, 1985.
109. Dordal E, Glagov S, Orlando RA, et al: Fatal halothane hepatitis with transient granulomas. *N Engl J Med* **283**:357–359, 1970.
110. Jori GP, Peschle C: Hydralazine disease associated with transient granulomas in the liver. A case report. *Gastroenterology* **64**:1163–1167, 1973.
111. Bezahaler GH: Case report: Fatal methyldopa-associated granulomatous hepatitis and myocarditis. *Am J Med Sci* **283**:41–45, 1982.
112. Miller AC, Reid WM: Methyldopa-induced granulomatous hepatitis. *JAMA* **235**:2001–2002, 1976.
113. Goldstein G: Sarcoid reaction associated with phenylbutazone hypersensitivity. *Ann Intern Med* **59**:97–100, 1963.
114. Ishak KG, Kirchner JP, Dhar JK: Granulomas and cholestatic-hepatocellular injury associated with phenylbutazone. Report of two cases. *Dig Dis* **22**:611–617, 1977.
115. Lebacq EG, Desmet V: Sarcoid granulomas associated with phenylbutazone treatment. *Mt Sinai J Med NY* **44**:778–781, 1977.
116. Benjamin SB, Ishak KG, Zimmerman HJ, et al; Phenylbutazone liver injury: A clinical–pathological survey of 23 cases and review of the literature. *Hepatology* **1**:255–263, 1981.
117. Lee TJ, Carney CN, Lapis JL, et al: Diphenylhydantoin-induced hepatic necrosis. A case study. *Gastroenterology* **70**:422–424, 1976.
118. Rotmensch HH, Yust I, Siegman-Igra Y, et al: Granulomatous hepatitis: A hypersensitivity response to procainamide. *Ann Intern Med* **89**:646–647, 1978.
119. Katz B, Weetch M, Chopra S: Quininc-induced granulomatous hepatitis. *Br Med J* **286**:264–265, 1983.
120. Chajek T, Lehrer B, Geltner D, et al: Quinidine-induced granulomatous hepatitis. *Ann Intern Med* **81**: 774–776, 1974.
121. Geltner D, Chajek T, Rubinger D, et al: Quinidine hypersensitivity and liver involvement. *Gastroenterology* **70**:650–652, 1976.

122. Espiritu CR, Kim TS, Levine RA: Granulomatous hepatitis associated with sulfadimethoxine hypersensitivity. *JAMA* **202**:161–164, 1976.
123. Callen JP, Soderstrom RM: Granulomatous hepatitis associated with salicylazosulfapyridine therapy. *South Med J* **71**:1159–1160, 1978.
124. Tucker LE: Tocainide-induced granulomatous hepatitis. *JAMA* **255**:3362, 1986.
125. Lee RG, Epstein O, Jauregui H, et al: Granulomas in primary biliary cirrhosis: A prognostic feature. *Gastroenterology* **81**:983–986, 1981.
126. Portmann B, Popper H, Neuberger J, et al: Sequential and diagnostic features in primary biliary cirrhosis based on serial histologic study in 209 patients. *Gastroenterology* **88**:1777–1790, 1985.
127. Nakanuma Y, Ohta G: Quantitation of hepatic granulomas and epithelioid cells in primary biliary cirrhosis. *Hepatology* **3**:423–427, 1983.
128. Simon HB, Wolff SM: Granulomatous hepatitis and prolonged fever of unknown origin: A study of 13 patients. *Medicine (Baltimore)* **52**:1–21, 1973.
129. Shee CD, Creamer B: Idiopathic granulomatous hepatitis and abdominal pain. *Postgrad Med J* **56**:342–343, 1980.
130. Israel HL, Goldstein RA: Hepatic granulomatous and sarcoidosis. *Ann Intern Med* **79**:669–678, 1973.
131. Eliakim J, Eisenberg S, Lebij IS, et al: Granulomatous hepatitis accompanying a self-limited febrile disease. *Lancet* **1**:1348–1352, 1968.
132. Gelb AM, Brazenas N, Sussman H, et al: Acute granulomatous disease of the liver. *Am J Dig Dis* **15**:842–847, 1970.
133. Peters RL, Gay T, and Reynolds TB: Post-jejunoileal-bypass hepatic disease. Its similarity to alcoholic hepatic disease. *Am J Clin Pathol* **63**:318–331, 1975.
134. Banner BF, Banner AS: Hepatic granulomas following ileal bypass for obesity. *Arch Pathol Lab Med* **102**:655–657, 1978.
135. Pickleman JR, Evans LS, Kane JM, et al: Tuberculosis after jejunoileal bypass for obesity. *JAMA* **234**:744, 1975.
136. Boitnott JK, Margolis S: Mineral oil in human tissues. II. Oil droplets in lymph nodes of the porta hepatis. *Bull Johns Hopkins Hosp* **118**:414–422, 1966.
137. Christoffersen P, Braendstrup O, Juhl E, et al: Lipogranulomas in human liver biopsies with fatty change. A morphological, biochemical and clinical investigation. *Acta Pathol Microbiol Scand* **79**:150–158, 1971.
138. Keen ME, Engstrand DA, Hafez G-R: Hepatic lipogranulomatosis simulating veno-occlusive disease of the liver. *Arch Pathol Lab Med* **109**:70–72, 1975.
139. Dincsoy HP, Weesner RE, MacGee J: Lipogranulomas in non-fatty human livers: A mineral oil induced environmental disease. *Am J Clin Pathol* **78**:35–41, 1982.
140. Wanless IR, Geddie WR: Mineral oil lipogranulomata in liver and spleen: A study of 465 autopsies. *Arch Pathol Lab Med* **109**:283–286, 1985.
141. Stoeckle JD, Hardy HL, Weber AL: Chronic beryllium disease. Long-term follow-up of sixty cases and selective review of the literature. *Am J Med* **46**:545–561, 1969.
142. Sprince NL, Kazemi H, Hardy HL: Current (1975) problem of differentiating between beryllium disease and sarcoidosis. *Ann NY Acad Sci* **278**:654–664, 1976.
143. Min K-W, Gyorkey F, Cain GD: Talc granulomata in liver disease in narcotic addicts. *Arch Pathol Lab Med* **98**:331–335, 1974.
144. Molos MA, Litton N, Schubert TT: Talc liver. *J Clin Gastroenterol* **9**:198–203, 1987.
145. Liebow AA, Carrington CRB, Friedman PJ: Lymphomatoid granulomatosis. *Hum Pathol* **3**:457–558, 1972.
146. Katzenstein A-LA, Carrington CB, Liebow AA: Lymphomatoid granulomatosis: A clinico-pathologic study of 152 cases. *Cancer* **43**:360–373, 1979.
147. Fauci AS, Haynes BF, Costa J, et al: Lymphomatoid granulomatosis. Prospective clinical and therapeutic experience over 10 years. *N Engl J Med* **306**:68–74, 1982.
148. Azimi PH, Bodenbender JG, Hintz RL, et al: Chronic granulomatous disease in three siblings. *JAMA* **206**:2865–2870, 1968.
149. Balfour HH Jr, Shehan JJ, Speicher CE, et al: Chronic granulomatous disease of childhood in a 23-year-old man. *JAMA* **217**:960–961, 1971.
150. Burns DA, Sarkany I: Chronic granulomatous disease in an adult. *J Roy Soc Med* **72**:139–142, 1979.
151. Maurer LH, Hughes RW Jr, Folley JH, et al: Granulomatous hepatitis associated with regional enteritis. *Gastroenterology* **53**:301–305, 1967.

152. Roberts WN, Coblyn JS: Rheumatoid arthritis and granulomatous hepatitis: A new association. *J Rheumatol* **10**:969–972, 1983.
153. Burke M, Sasson E, Baratz M, et al: Hepatic granuloma in polymyalgia rheumatica. *J Am Geriatr Soc* **32**: 472–473, 1984.
154. Churg J: Allergic granulomatosis and granulomatous-vascular syndromes. *Ann Allergy* **21**:619–628, 1963.
155. Fauci AS, Wolff SM: Wegener's granulomatosis: Studies in eighteen patients and a review of the literature. *Medicine (Baltimore)* **52**:535–561, 1973.

26

Granulomatous Liver Disease: Pathology

Jay H. Lefkowitch

1. INTRODUCTION

Granulomas are found in up to 10% of liver biopsies[1,2] and thereby represent a significant diagnostic challenge for the histopathologist. These focal collections of mature apposed macrophages participate in an immunologic reaction to foreign material or other antigenic stimuli. Participating macrophages may attain epithelium-like features (epithelioid macrophages) or may fuse (giant cells). Interleukins 1 and 2 (IL-1 and IL-2), T-helper (T4) and T-suppressor (T8) lymphocytes, and variable numbers of eosinophils and plasma cells contribute to the formation of these localized lesions.[3] The pathologic features of hepatic granulomas have been comprehensively reviewed by Ishak[1] and others.[3–9]

2. GENERAL FEATURES

Liver granulomas may be located either within portal tracts or in the lobular parenchyma, or both. The noncaseating variety far exceeds caseating granulomas in frequency, the latter seen most often in tuberculosis. In most cases, little architectural damage is produced by granulomas, and healing results in either complete restitution of tissue or focal hyalinization. Conspicuous exceptions, however, include the damage and destruction of bile ducts associated with granulomas in primary biliary cirrhosis[10] or occasional cases of sarcoidosis,[11] the "pipestem" fibrosis surrounding portal vein radicles containing *Schistosome* eggs[12] and the rare instances of cirrhosis following hyalinization of sarcoid granulomas.[13] Focal Kupffer cell hyperplasia in liver parenchyma adjacent to granulomas may be present.

The size of a granuloma usually exceeds 50 μm in diameter[9]; Klatskin[6] estimated that in granulomatous diseases such as sarcoidosis the liver may contain 15–75 million granulomas. When granulomatous liver disease is suspected, multiple sections through the needle biopsy or larger specimen should therefore be studied. Serial sections should be reserved for evaluating the specific contents of an individual granuloma. Once a granuloma is identified, the routine pathologic examination should include polarization and special staining procedures, including acid-fast, fungal, and bacterial stains.

Jay H. Lefkowitch • Department of Pathology, College of Physicians and Surgeons, Columbia University, New York, New York 10032.

3. SYSTEMATIC PATHOLOGIC APPROACH TO HEPATIC GRANULOMAS

Because of the diverse causes of hepatic granulomas (Table I), the pathologist must adopt a pragmatic approach to diagnosis. According to several large series,[3,5–7,14] the major causes of hepatic granulomas (in decreasing order of frequency) are sarcoidosis, primary liver disease (i.e., primary biliary cirrhosis), tuberculosis, drugs, and schistosomiasis (Table II). The cause may not be identified in up to 36% of cases.[4] Upon identification of a granuloma, the following stepwise evaluation by pathologists will help elucidate the cause of most hepatic granulomas.

3.1. Workup of Liver Granulomas

1. Consider statistical likelihood of cause (Table II).
2. Examine granuloma for the causative agent (e.g., *Schistosome* egg, talc, silicone particles, mycobacteria, bacilli, fungi, damaged bile duct).
3. Consider pathologic features and clinical setting (e.g., hyalinizing portal granulomas in sarcoid; damaged bile duct in a woman with positive antimitochondrial antibodies and primary biliary cirrhosis; known systemic granulomatous disease, such as chronic granulomatous disease of childhood).
4. Consider drugs (Table III).
5. Consider systemic granulomatous disease or neoplasm (e.g., chronic granulomatous disease of childhood, regional enteritis, Hodgkin lymphoma).
6. Consider granulomatous hepatitis of Simon and Wolff.[15]
7. Determine that the cause is unknown.

3.2. Histologic Features of Hepatic Granulomas

3.2.1. Sarcoidosis

Sarcoid granulomas may be scattered randomly throughout the parenchyma but are most often portal and periportal and frequently confluent (Fig. 1). Hyalinization is common and may infrequently result in frank cirrhosis.[13] These granulomas are noncaseating. A syndrome of chronic intrahepatic cholestasis in sarcoidosis, with destruction of bile ducts, hepatic copper retention, and progressive micronodular biliary cirrhosis has been described in young black males.[11]

3.2.2. Primary Biliary Cirrhosis

Damage and destruction of intrahepatic bile ducts in primary biliary cirrhosis (PBC) is a process mediated by lymphocytes and plasma cells, resulting in four histologic stages, including stage 1 (florid bile duct lesion), stage 2 (bile ductular proliferation), stage 3 (scarring), and stage 4 (cirrhosis). Granulomas and (more commonly) poorly formed granulomatous lesions may be found within or adjacent to portal tracts in proximity to damage bile ducts in as many as 50% of patients.[10] Occasionally, granulomas are located within the lobule or near central veins. When in these latter sites, the diagnosis may be confused with sarcoidosis or other conditions, but clinical features, serologic data, and histologic changes in portal tracts usually clarify the diagnosis. Granulomas in PBC predominate in stage 1 disease and diminish in subsequent stages.[10,16] Several recent studies have suggested that granulomas in PBC indicate a favorable prognosis,[10,17] particularly for long-term survival in asymptomatic patients,[17] although this has not been uniformly observed.[18,19] It may be necessary to examine multiple (or serial) sections in order to identify the diagnostic damaged bile duct within portal granulomas.

Table I. Causes of Hepatic Granulomas—Selected Examples

Infectious	
	Bacterial (tuberculosis, atypical Mycobacteria, leprosy, brucellosis, tularemia, neonatal listeriosis)
	Fungal (histoplasmosis, coccidioidomycosis, blastomycosis, cryptococcosis, candidiasis, aspergillosis)
	Parasitic (schistosomiasis, visceral larva migrans, i.e., *Toxocara*)
	Viral (cytomegalovirus, infectious mononucleosis)
	Rickettsial (Q fever, i.e., *Coxiella burnetii*)
	Spirochetal (syphilis, i.e., secondary and tertiary)
Sarcoidosis	
Primary biliary cirrhosis	
Drugs	
Vascular diseases	
	Polyarteritis nodosa
	Temporal arteritis
	Wegener's granulomatosis
Sytemic diseases	
	Chronic granulomatous disease of childhood
	Inflammatory bowel disease
	Whipple disease
	Granulomatous hepatitis of Simon and Wolff
Neoplasms	
	Hodgkin and non-Hodgkin lymphoma
	Primary and metastatic carcinoma
Foreign bodies	
	Talc (heroin abusers)
	Silicone (hemodialysis)
	Suture

Table II. Causes of Hepatic Granulomas: Approximate Anticipated Frequencies[a]

Etiology	Percent of cases
Sarcoidosis	40–60
Primary liver disease (primary biliary cirrhosis)	20–30
Tuberculosis	15–30
Drugs	20
Schistosomiasis	<5
Other	5–10

[a]These approximate percentages, based on several series,[3,5–7,14] are provided only as general diagnositic guidelines in the pathologic workup of granulomas. Geographic and institutional differences may account for fairly large variations from the proposed scheme.

Table III. Drugs Responsible for Hepatic Granulomas[a]

Allopurinol	Mineral oil
α-Methyldopa	Nitrofurantoin
Aspirin	Oral contraceptives
Carbamazepine	Oxyphenbutazone
Cephalexin	Penicillin
Diazepam	Phenylbutazone
Diphenylhydantoin	Procainamide
Halothane	Procarbazine
Hydralazine	Pronestyl
Isoniazid	Quinidine
Metahydrin	Sulfonamides
Metolazone	Sulfonylurea derivaties

[a]Adapted from Ishak.[1]

3.2.3. Tuberculosis

Hepatic granulomas are very common in patients with widely disseminated miliary tuberculosis (nearly 100%) and chronic pulmonary tuberculosis (79–99%), according to Klatskin.[20] They are less common (20% of cases) in primary pulmonary tuberculosis. In so-called primary miliary tuberculosis of the liver, granulomatous liver disease is the presenting clinical problem, and the initial (usually pulmonary) focus of tuberculosis is rarely demonstrated; virtually 100% of these cases show granulomas. Hepatic tuberculomas (Fig. 2) and granulomatous involvement of bile ducts (tuberculous cholangitis) are other rare forms of tuberculosis.

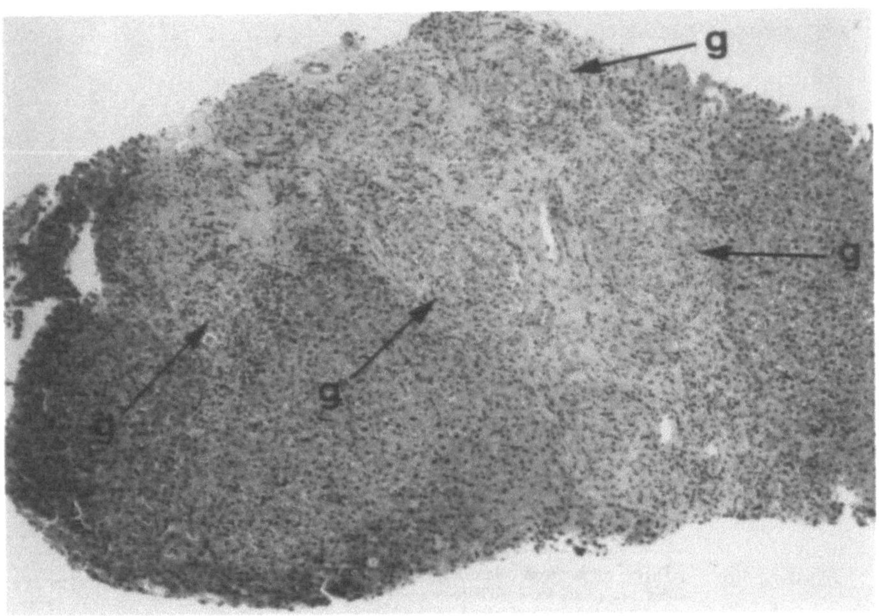

Figure 1. Sarcoidosis. Noncaseating granulomas (g) cluster in portal and periportal regions with production of pale hyalinized fibrous tissue. (H&E, ×100)

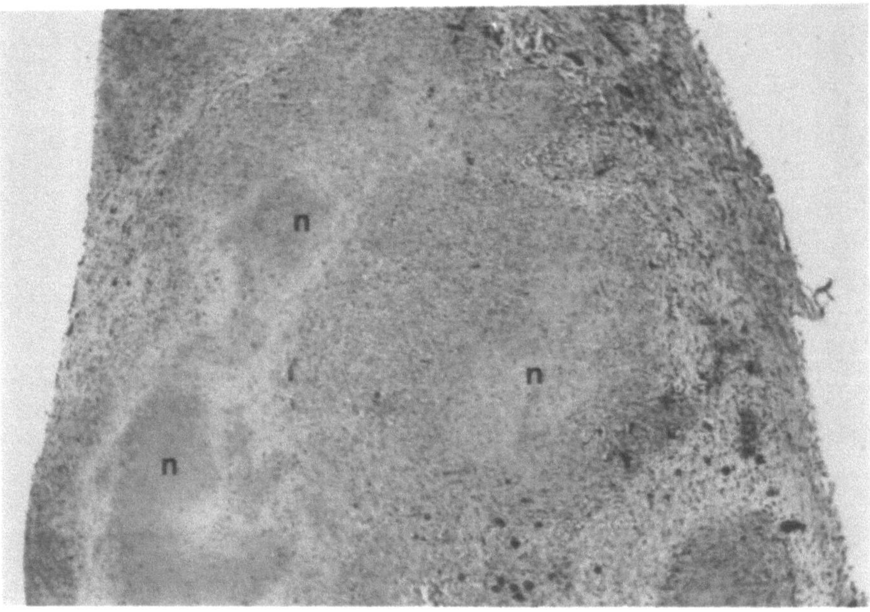

Figure 2. Tuberculoma of liver. Subcapsular mass of confluent granulomas with caseation necrosis at their centers (n). (H&E, ×40)

Tuberculous granulomas in the liver (Fig. 3) show caseation infrequently, more often in autopsy specimens than in biopsy tissue. Other diseases may result in necrosis of liver granulomas (e.g., melioidosis, typhoid fever, tularemia, botryomycosis).[1] Acid-fast stains are positive in approximately 13% of biopsy specimens and in 31% of autopsy specimens.[8]

3.2.4. Drugs

The major feature distinguishing drug-related granulomas from other causes is the presence of eosinophils[14] (Fig. 4). Drugs may account for as many as 29% of cases in large series of patients with hepatic granulomas,[14] and numerous agents have been implicated (see Table III).

3.2.5. Schistosomiasis

Clinically significant granulomatous liver disease and presinusoidal portal hypertension results from infections by *Schistosoma mansoni* and *japonicum*. Lodging of schistosomal eggs in portal vein branches results in a local cell-mediated immune response in the form of a granuloma (Fig. 5), as well as the Splendore–Hoeppli phenomenon (radiating acidophilic filaments and eosinophils around the periphery of the egg). Progressive development of "pipestem" fibrosis is a function of both collagen synthesis and collagenolysis.[12] Fine dark brown birefringent schistosome pigment (a hemoglobin derivative from parasitic ingestion of host erythrocytes) is a useful marker in portal tracts. The cuticle of schistosome eggs is positive on acid-fast stains. Excessive portal inflammation superimposed on portal fibrosis should be investigated for possible concomitant chronic hepatitis B virus (HBV) infection, as there is a significant HBV carrier rate in areas in which schistosomiasis is endemic.

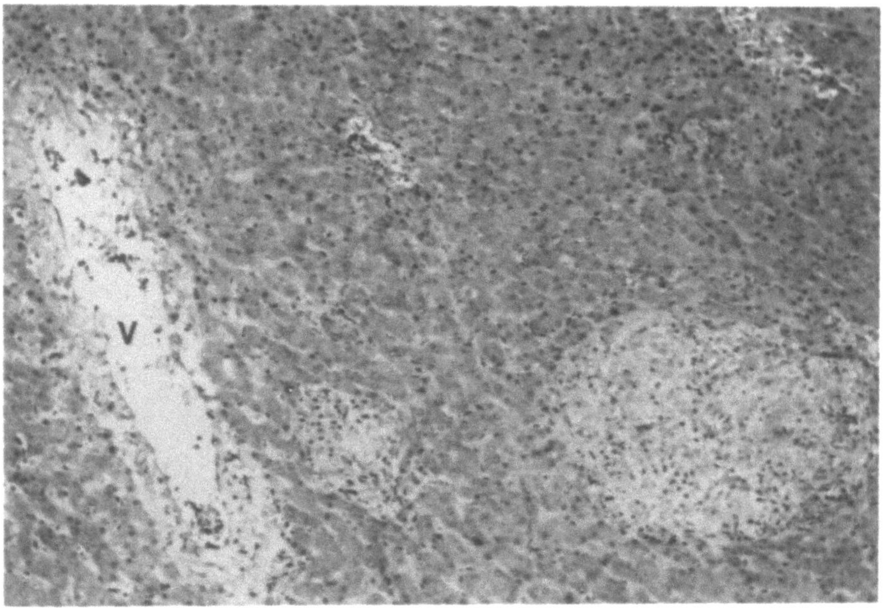

Figure 3. Noncaseating tuberculous granulomas. Lobular granulomas of several sizes. V, central vein. (H&E, ×100)

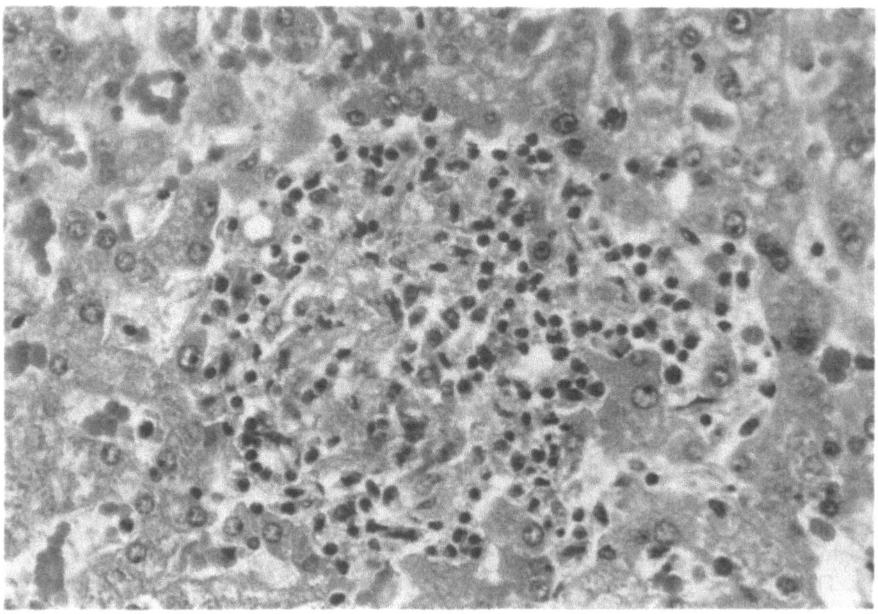

Figure 4. Drug-induced hepatic granuloma. Numerous eosinophils are present in this granuloma, caused by a sulfonamide antibiotic. (H&E, ×325)

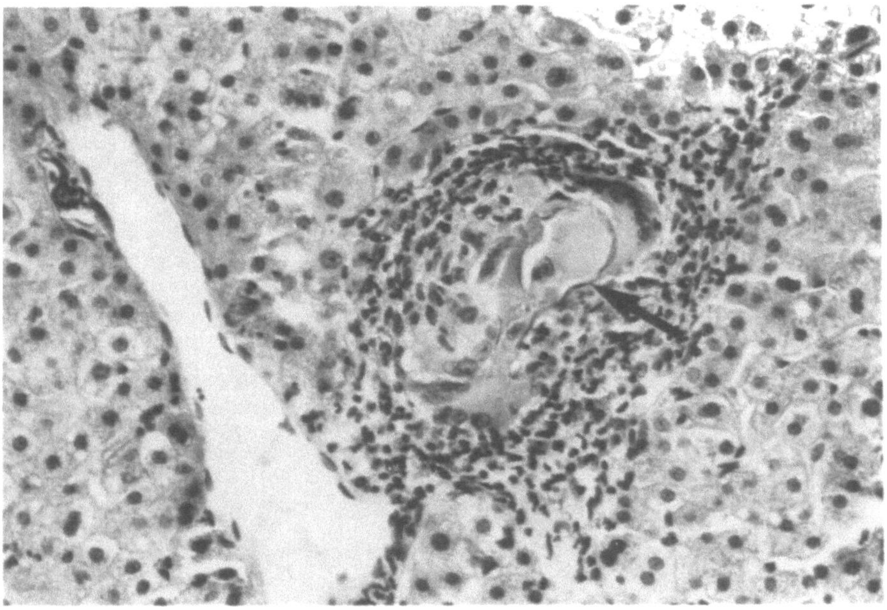

Figure 5. Hepatic schistosomiasis. *Schistoma mansoni* egg (arrow) surrounded by epithelioid macrophages and a multinucleate giant cell within a portal granuloma. Note the refractile outer cuticle of the egg (at arrow tip). (H&E, ×250)

3.2.6. Acquired Immune Deficiency Syndrome

Hepatic involvement in acquired immune deficiency syndrome (AIDS)[21] may be indicated by elevated serum alkaline phosphatase levels reflecting the presence of multiple granulomas in biopsy and autopsy liver tissue.[22] Granulomatous liver disease may represent one fourth or more of significant hepatic pathology in AIDS. Other lesions include fatty change, hemosiderosis, HBV carrier state, mild chronic hepatitis, cytomegalovirus (CMV) hepatitis, and Kaposi sarcoma.[21–24]

Liver granulomas in AIDS are most often due to *Mycobacterium avium-intracellulare* (MAI) infection. These mycobacteria are usually found in abundant clusters, packing individual macrophages within each granuloma (Fig. 6). The routine hematoxyline and eosin (H&E) appearance of these MAI granulomas consists of plump occasionally foamy or vacuolated macrophages associated with a few lymphocytes; they are located anywhere within the liver parenchyma or portal tracts. Atypical mycobacteria are positive on acid-fast and methenamine silver stains. However, antituberculous drug therapy prior to liver biopsy may eliminate any stainable mycobacteria on acid-fast stain.[21–24] Other agents responsible for granulomas in AIDS patients include fungi (*Histoplasma, Cryptococcus*), viruses (CMV), and drugs (e.g., trimethoprim-sulfamethoxasole for pneumocystis pneumonia).[21–24]

3.2.7. Other Infections

While numerous other infective agents may produce liver granulomas, many are seen infrequently, and the histopathologic features are not specific.[1] Brief mention should be made of the Q-fever granuloma caused by *Coxiella burnetti*.[25] These granulomas contain a central empty space surrounded by an acidophilic ring of fibrinoid material, mononuclear cells, and macrophages. The "empty space" is believed to be an entrapped lipid vacuole.

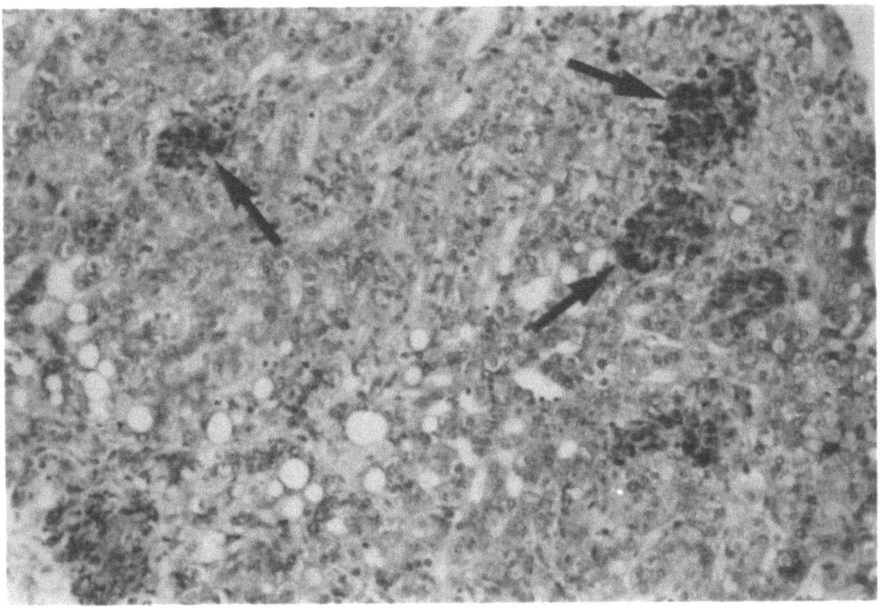

Figure 6. Liver of AIDS patient with atypical mycobacterial granulomas. Multiple noncaseating granulomas throughout the parenchyma contain packed acid-fast bacilli (arrows). (Ziehl-Neelsen stain, ×160)

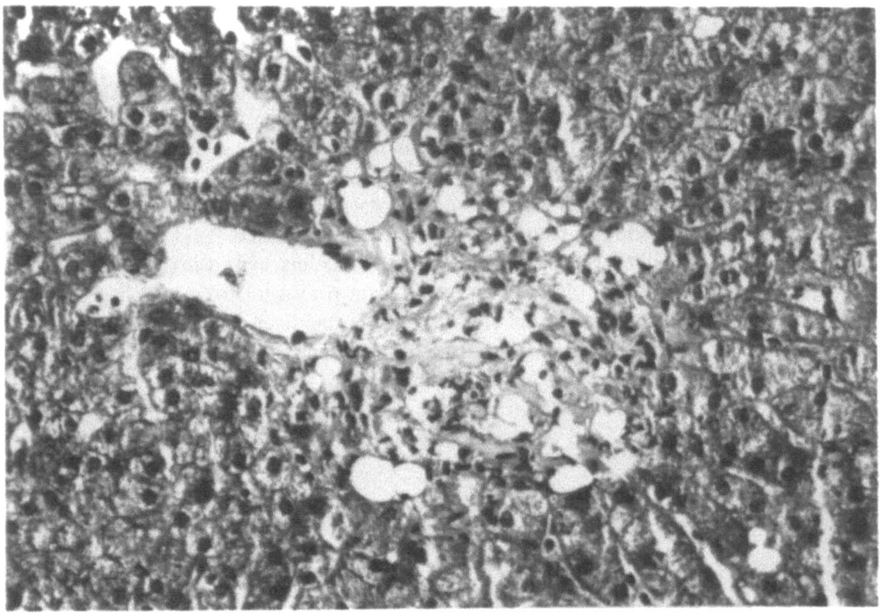

Figure 7. Lipogranuloma. Collection of lipid vacuoles, lymphocytes, and macrophages adjacent to the wall of a central vein. These may also be located within the lobule or portal tracts. (H&E, ×250)

3.2.8. Lipogranulomas and Foreign Bodies

In a recent autopsy series,[26] hepatic lipogranulomas were found in nearly one half of cases. Lipogranulomas are focal collections of lipid vacuoles surrounded by lymphocytes and macrophages (Fig. 7). They are commonly adjacent to central vein walls, in the lobule, or in portal tracts. Although they may be related to the presence of fatty liver (with rupture of intracellular lipid as the stimulus for granuloma formation), current suggestions favor mineral oil (in laxatives or food products) as the inciting agent. These lesions produce no significant clinical sequelae. On histologic examination, they may be associated with focal fibrosis within the lipogranuloma and around its periphery. Extraneous foreign materials within the liver, including talc (in heroin users)[27] or silicone (in renal dialysis patients, from blood-pump tubing)[28] may be visible within portal tract granulomas on routine and polarizing microscopy.

3.2.9. Granulomatous Hepatitis of Simon and Wolff

When the potential causes of hepatic granulomas in patients with fever of unknown origin have been examined, and no source is apparent, the granulomatous hepatitis described by Simon and Wolff[15] should be considered. The histopathology of these noncaseating granulomas is nonspecific, and the clinical features and steroid responsiveness of the condition serve to establish the diagnosis.

REFERENCES

1. Ishak KG: Granulomas of the liver, in Ioachim HL (ed): *Pathology of Granulomas*. Raven, New York, 1983, pp. 307–369.
2. Petersdorf RG, Beeson PB: Fever of unexplained origin—Report on 100 cases. *Medicine (Baltimore)* **40:**1–30, 1961.
3. James DG: Hepatic granulomas, in Brunner H, Thaler H (eds): *Hepatology. A Festschrift for Hans Popper*. Raven, New York, 1985, pp. 269–280.
4. Fauci AS, Wolff SM: Granulomatous hepatitis, in Popper H, Schaffner F (eds): *Progress in Liver Diseases*, Vol. V. Grune & Stratton, Orlando, Florida, 1976, pp. 609–621.
5. Cunningham D, Mills PR, Quigley EMM, et al: Hepatic granulomas—Experience over a 10-year period in the West of Scotland. *Q J Med* **51:**162–170, 1982.
6. Klatskin G: Hepatic granulomata: Problems in interpretation. *Mt Sinai J Med* **44:**798–812, 1977.
7. Neville E, Piyasena KHG, James DG: Granulomas of the liver. *Postgrad Med J* **51:**361–365, 1975.
8. Guckian JC, Perry JE: Granulomatous hepatitis: An analysis of 63 cases and review of the literature. *Ann Intern Med* **65:**1081–1100, 1966.
9. Christoffersen P, Poulsen H: Granulomatous inflammatory diseases, in Peters RL, Craig JR (eds): *Liver Pathology*. Churchill Livingstone, New York, 1986, pp. 147–160.
10. Lee RG, Epstein O, Jauregui H, et al: Granulomas in primary biliary cirrhosis: A prognostic feature. *Gastroenterology* **81:**983–986, 1981.
11. Rudzki C, Ishak KG, Zimmerman HJ: Chronic intrahepatic cholestasis of sarcoidosis. *Am J Med* **59:**373–387, 1975.
12. Warren KS: The kinetics of hepatosplenic schistosomiasis. *Semin Liver Dis* **4:**293–300, 1984.
13. Maddrey WC, Johns CJ, Boitnott JK, et al: Sarcoidosis and chronic hepatic disease: A clinical and pathological study of 20 patients. *Medicine (Baltimore)* **49:**375–395, 1970.
14. McMaster KR, Hennigar GR: Drug-induced granulomatous hepatitis. *Lab Invest* **44:**61–73, 1981.
15. Simon HB, Wolff SM: Granulomatous hepatitis and prolonged fever of unknown origin: A study of 13 patients. *Medicine (Baltimore)* **52:**1–21, 1973.
16. Nakanuma Y, Ohta G: Quantitation of hepatic granulomas and epithelioid cells in primary biliary cirrhosis. *Hepatology* **3:**423–427, 1983.
17. Beswick DR, Klatskin G, Boyer JL: Asymptomatic primary primary biliary cirrhosis. A progress report on long-term follow-up and natural history. *Gastroenterology* **89:**267–271, 1985.

18. Portmann B, Popper H, Neuberger J, Williams R: Sequential and diagnostic features in primary biliary cirrhosis based on serial histologic study in 29 patients. *Gastroenterology* **88:**1777–1790, 1985.
19. Kaplan MM: Primary biliary cirrhosis. *N Engl J Med* **316:**521–528, 1987.
20. Klatskin G: Hepatitis associated with systemic infections, in Schiff L (ed): *Diseases of the Liver*, 4th ed. JB Lippincott, Philadelphia, 1975, pp. 711–754.
21. Lebovics E, Thung SN, Schaffner F, Radensky PW: The liver in acquired immune deficiency syndrome. *Hepatology* **5:**293–298, 1985.
22. Orenstein MS, Tavitian A, Yonk B, et al: Granulomatous involvement of the liver in patients with AIDS. *Gut* **26:**1220–1225, 1985.
23. Nakanuma Y, Liew CT, Peters RL, Govindarajan S: Pathologic features of the liver in acquired immune deficiency syndrome. *Liver* **6:**158–166, 1986.
24. Dworkin BM, Stahl RE, Giardina MA, et al: The liver in acquired immune deficiency syndrome: Emphasis on patients with intravenous drug abuse. *Am J Gastroenterol* **82:**231–236, 1987.
25. Pellegrin M, Delsol G, Auvergnat JC, et al: Granulomatous hepatitis in Q fever. *Hum Pathol* **11:**51–57, 1980.
26. Wanless IR, Geddie WR: Mineral oil lipogranulomata in liver and spleen. *Arch Pathol Lab Med* **109:**283–286, 1985.
27. Edland JF: Liver disease in heroin addicts. *Hum Pathol* **3:**75–84, 1972.
28. Leong A S-Y, Disney APS, Gore DW: Spallation and migration of silicone from blood-pump tubing in patients in hemodialysis. *N Engl J Med* **306:**135–140, 1982.

27

Jaundice of Systemic Infection

Charles O. Abernathy, J. Thomas Stocker, Riccardo Utili, and Leonard B. Seeff

1. INTRODUCTION

A variety of infectious diseases may produce jaundice or other biochemical abnormalities, even though the liver is not the primary site of infection.[1–3] Despite the often serious nature of the infection or underlying disease process, the hepatic aspects are generally not life-threatening. However, the assorted liver aspects can mimic extrahepatic obstructive jaundice, making it important to identify the source of the hepatic dysfunction using such imaging techniques as ultrasonography or computed tomography (CT) or performing the appropriate cholangiographic procedures.[4]

This chapter reviews selected bacterial, rickettsial, and viral diseases that may alter hepatic function. Obviously excluded from this discussion are the hepatitis viruses, types A, B, and non-A, non-B (NANB), since they are direct hepatotrophic agents.

2. BACTERIAL INFECTION

The occurrence of jaundice in neonates with extrahepatic bacterial infections, especially gram-negative, is well documented,[2,5–15] with an incidence reported to range from 6 to 60%.[5,7,14] This syndrome may also occur in adults[2,16–21] but much less commonly. For example, in one retrospective study, the frequency of jaundice in adult bacteremic patients was less than 1%.[20] Subclinical hepatic dysfunction, however, is not rare. In a recent prospective study of 82 patients with bacteremia, more than 50% had hyperbilirubinemia, most without overt jaundice.[22]

Infections by many organisms, including *Escherichia coli, Salmonella* species, *Klebsiella pneumonia, Pseudomonas aeruginosa, Hemophilus influenza,* various *Bacteroides* and *Proteus*

The opinions expressed in this review are those of the authors and do not necessarily reflect the policies of the U.S. Environmental Protection Agency or of the Department of the Army or the Department of Defense.

Charles O. Abernathy • Health Effects Branch (WH-550D), Office of Drinking Water, U.S. Environmental Protection Agency, Washington, D.C. 20460. *J. Thomas Stocker* • Armed Forces Institute of Pathology, Washington, D.C. 20306-6000. *Riccardo Utili* • Clinic of Tropical and Subtropical Diseases, First Medical School, University of Naples, I-800135 Naples, Italy. *Leonard B. Seeff* • Georgetown University; Gastroenterology/Hepatology/Nutrition, Veterans Administration Medical Center, Washington, D.C. 20007.

species, aerobic and anaerobic *Streptococcus* species, and *Staphylococcus aureus*, have been reported to cause septic jaundice.[5–22] Generally, the jaundice is cholestatic in nature with little or no parenchymal damage.[2,5,7,13,14,21]

The pattern of biochemical abnormalities is consistent with a cholestatic type of disease. Bilirubin values may occasionally exceed 30 mg% but are usually less than 10 mg%; the conjugated form accounts for approximately 75% of the increase in serum bilirubin. Although serum alkaline phosphatase (SAP) levels are increased in more than one half of cases, they are seldom elevated more than threefold. In addition, the transaminases are usually normal or slightly elevated, except in severe sepsis.[2,18,19,21]

The diagnosis of septic jaundice should be entertained in a patient who has a sudden onset of icterus with pyrexia, conjugated hyperbilirubinemia, and normal or slightly elevated SAP and transaminase values. The primary diagnostic problem is to separate this entity from those cases of jaundice resulting from extrahepatic obstruction or those arising from a direct bacterial colonization of the liver with consequent abscess formation. Data obtained from the patient's history, physical examination, biochemical and microbiologic tests, and imaging procedures permit distinction of this syndrome from other possible causes of jaundice.

2.1. Gram-Negative Cocci

2.1.1. Gonococcal Infection

In patients with disseminated dermal lesions or bacteremia resulting from *Neisseria gonorrhoeae*, hepatic dysfunction has been reported to occur in approximately one half of cases.[23] Before the advent of penicillin, the jaundice in many cases may have resulted, in part, from the use of acriflavine, an antibiotic with hepatotoxic potential.[24] Hepatic abscess has also been reported in a few cases, and a direct invasion of the liver may account for some of the abnormalities. In others, a severe anemia occurs and hemolysis may also play a role.[1] Biopsies from patients with elevated transaminases have demonstrated a pattern of parenchymal and portal-tract infiltration suggestive of subacute or chronic viral hepatitis.[3]

Acute perihepatitis (Fitz-Hugh–Curtis syndrome) is the most common hepatic complication, occurring in 9–15% of patients with cervical gonorrhea.[3,25] This syndrome has also been reported to occasionally occur in males[26] and in adolescent females.[27]

2.2. Gram-Negative Bacilli

2.2.1. Conditions Caused by *Escherichia coli* and Related Species

The syndrome of cholestatic jaundice during gram-negative bacterial infection has frequently been described in neonates[5–15] and is a significant cause of jaundice in newborns.[2] For example, in one study of icteric neonates that excluded cases of hemolytic jaundice from fetomaternal blood incompatibility, jaundice of sepsis accounted for 25 of 76 cases.[7] Affected patients are usually male, under 3 months of age; the most common cause is urinary tract infection (UTI) with *E. coli* (Fig. 1). It is characterized by conjugated hyperbilirubinemia and slight to moderate increases in SAP and transaminase levels. Indeed, jaundice may be the only clinical sign of infection, as fever may not be present.[5,6,11] Rapid identification of the infective agent and appropriate antibiotic therapy usually leads to a complete recovery.

In older children or adults, this condition is occasionally observed but is generally mild,[16,19] unless associated with pregnancy[28] or severe sepsis.[17–22] In cases of severe sepsis, the prognosis may be poor due to the underlying infection.[2] The incidence of jaundice during severe infection is not known, but when shock occurs, it is relatively high. Banks et al.[29] reported that 36 of 57 septic shock patients were icteric (*E. coli* was the most commonly isolated organism). They also reported

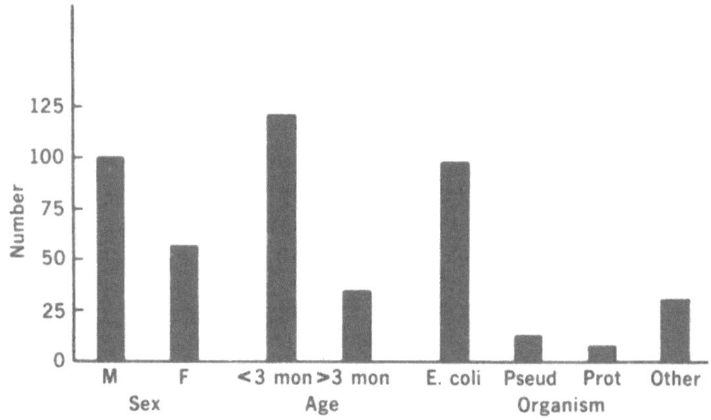

Figure 1. Sex and age distribution of patients and infective organisms in jaundice caused by gram-negative bacterial infections. Data compiled from references 5–13 and 17–21.

that 85% of patients had abnormalities in liver-function tests within 2 days of the episode of shock and that the presence of a persistent hyperbilirubinemia augured a poor prognosis.

Morphologic changes in the liver may be minimal with only focal hepatocellular necrosis, Kupffer cell hyperplasia, mild hepatocellular and canalicular cholestasis, and bile duct proliferation. In some cases of chronic cholestasis and obstructive symptoms, however, extensive inspissated bile plugs may be present in proliferated cholangioles and periportal canaliculi occasionally coalescing as small "bile lakes" (Figs. 2 and 3). Interlobular bile ducts, surprisingly, are rarely involved, although adjacent cholangioles may display prominent intra- and periductular infiltration by neutrophils (Fig. 4A,B) along with the luminal cholestasis.[2,5,18,30] Portal and periportal fibrosis may be present subdividing lobules. Ultrastructural studies have described marked canalicular dilation with blunting or loss of microvilli in both children[13] and adults.[17]

Clinical and experimental reports suggest that endotoxin may be involved in the pathogenesis of this syndrome. For example, it may occur in the absence of bacteremia; its manifestations are similar during infections with different gram-negative bacteria.[2,5,7,18,21] In addition, endotoxins from *E. coli*[31–34] and *Salmonella enteritidis*[35] have been reported to inhibit bile flow and sulfobromophthalein excretion in both in vitro and in vivo models. The lower bile acid pool sizes and synthetic rates in neonates[36] and in premature infants[37] may also play a role in their greater susceptibility to the clinical manifestations of this syndrome.

2.2.2. Typhoid Fever

Bacteremia has been reported to occur in most patients with *Salmonella typhi* infections.[38] Jaundice may occur in 4–16% of cases and elevated alanine transaminase (ALT) in an additional 25% of cases. In addition, bilirubin, SAP, and aspartate transaminase (AST) values were reported to be elevated in about one fourth of patients.[39]

Histologically, *S. typhi* may produce a nonspecific reactive hepatitis characterized by focal hepatocellular necrosis, mild cholestasis, Kupffer cell hyperplasia, and infiltration of portal areas by lymphocytes (Fig. 5). This mononuclear cell infiltrate may aggregate in periportal sinusoids along with hyperplastic Kupffer cells, producing a typhoid nodule (Fig. 6). Granulomas composed of necrotic debris, histiocytes, and lymphocytes may rarely be observed. In more severe cases, hepatocytes display anisocytosis, anisonucleosis, fatty metamorphosis, and increased mitotic activity.[40,41]

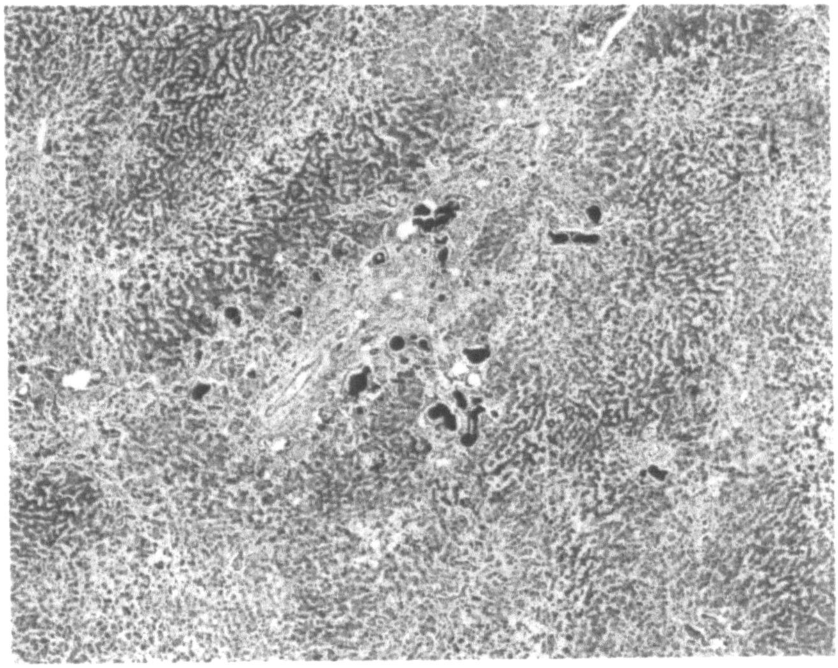

Figure 2. Escherichia coli sepsis with chronic cholestasis. Inspissated bile plugs present in cholangioles and canaliculi surrounding a portal area (center). Hepatocytes surrounding central veins display anoxic coagulative necrosis. (H&E, ×30; AFIP Neg. 87-5865)

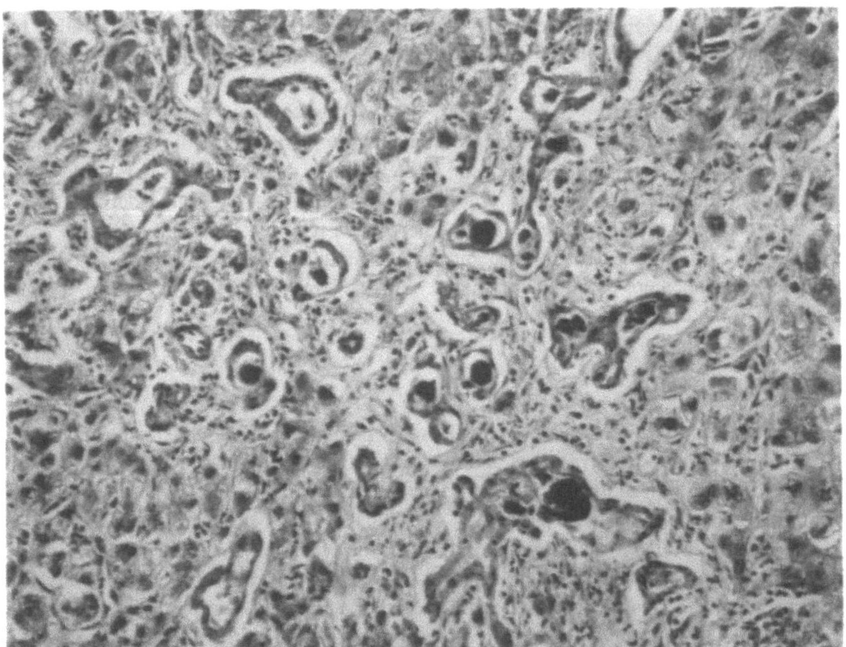

Figure 3. Escherichia coli sepsis with chronic cholestasis. Proliferated cholangioles containing dark smooth bile plugs, surrounded by increased fibrous connective tissue infiltrated by neutrophils. (H&E, ×150; AFIP Neg. 87-5863)

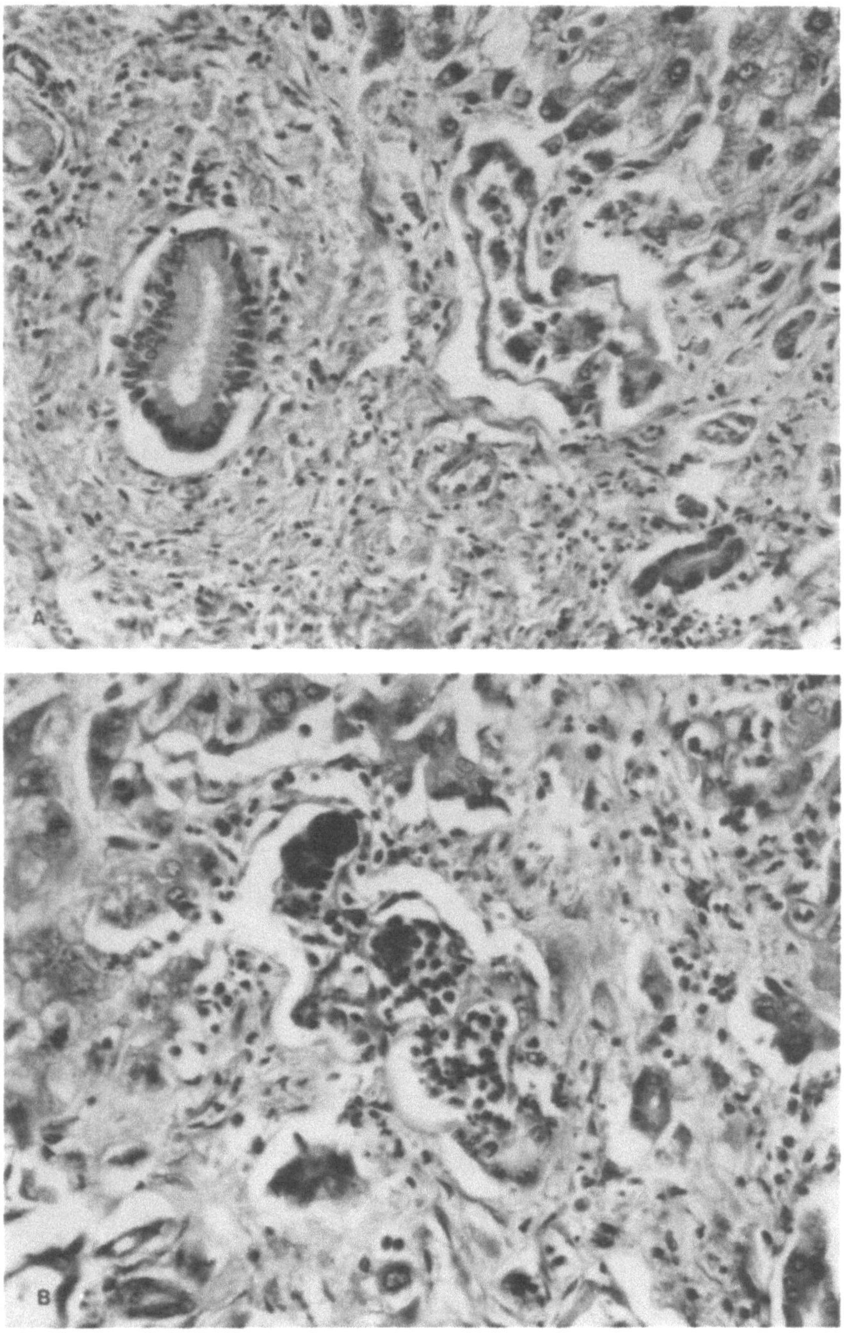

Figure 4. Escherichia coli sepsis with chronic cholestasis. (A) Unremarkable interlobular bile duct (left) lies adjacent to a cholangiole filled with amorphous debris and bile. (H&E, ×240; AFIP Neg. 87-5861) (B) Another cholangiole filled with a mixture of bile and neutrophils. Note neutrophils within the lining epithelium and in connective tissue surrounding the cholangiole. (H&E, ×300; AFIP Neg. 87-5862)

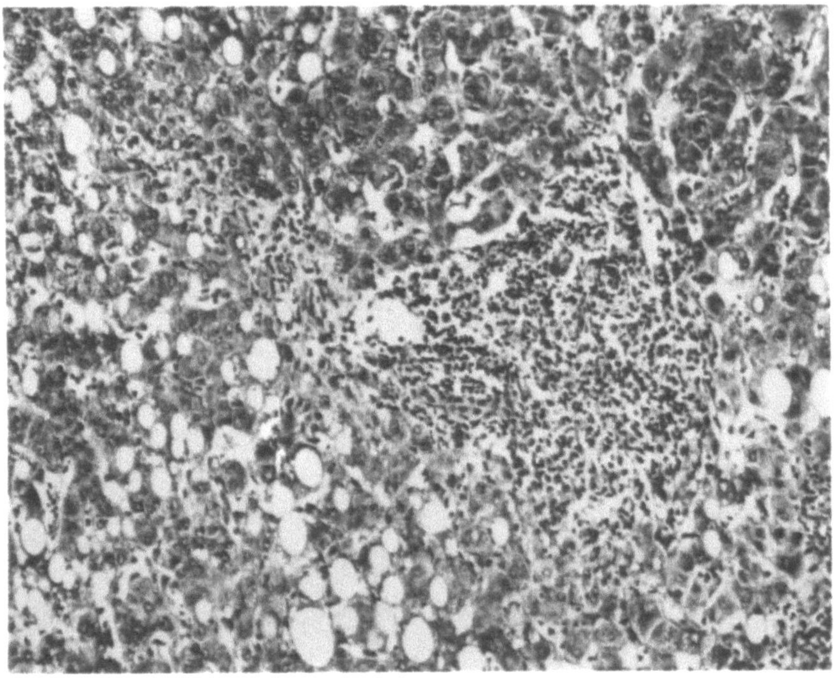

Figure 5. Salmonella typhi sepsis. Portal area (right) infiltrated by lymphocytes surrounded by hepatocytes displays focal necrosis and large droplet fatty metamorphosis. (H&E, ×150; AFIP Neg. 87-5873)

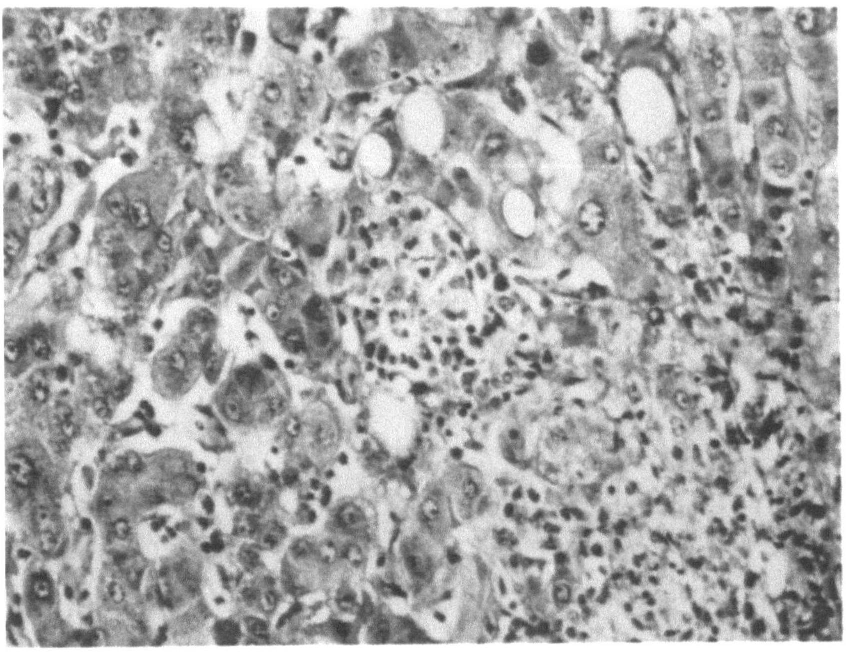

Figure 6. Salmonella typhi sepsis. Typhoid nodule (center) composed of lymphocytes and hyperplastic Kupffer cells distends a sinusoid. The edge of a portal area is at lower right. (H&E, ×300; AFIP Neg. 87-5870)

Although typhoid fever patients exhibit symptoms, such as fever, leukopenia, Kupffer cell hyperplasia, cholestasis, shock, and disseminated intravascular coagulation (DIC), attributed to endotoxemia,[2,31,42–44] the role of endotoxin in the pathogenesis of typhoid fever is controversial. For example, Butler et al.[45] did not find endotoxin in the blood of 21 Vietnamese typhoid fever patients. However, a recent report[46] found a close association between endotoxemia and various indices of hepatic dysfunction, especially the 2-hr postprandial serum bile acid (SBA) levels (Table I). In addition, the highest elevations in SBA and AST values occurred in those patients having the highest endotoxin blood titers.[46] Another possible cause for the liver involvement is direct parenchymal invasion by the bacteria, since *Salmonella* have been found in liver tissue by fluorescent microscopy.[47] Resolution of the role of endotoxin and other factors in the pathogenesis of typhoid fever awaits further investigation.

2.2.3. Paratyphoid Fever

During infection with *Salmonella paratyphi*, jaundice occurs less frequently than with typhoid fever.[39,48] There may be moderate elevations in bilirubin (less than fivefold) and SAP (two- to threefold), and occasionally the transaminases may be markedly elevated. The liver histology has not been fully characterized but appears to be similar to that of typhoid fever[3] (Fig. 7).

2.2.4. Legionnaires' Disease

The epidemic of pneumonia, due to *Legionella pneumophila*, at the American Legion convention in 1976 was first described clinically by Fraser et al.[49] In a subsequent study, jaundice was reported to develop in 12% (3 of 24 cases) of patients, while the transaminase and SAP levels were increased in less than 20%.[50] Histologically, the liver changes were slight, and only microvesicular steatosis and focal areas of necrosis were noted. The underlying mechanism is unknown, but the organism has been found in the liver.[51]

2.3. Gram-Positive Cocci

2.3.1. Pneumonia

The occurrence of jaundice during *Streptococcus pneumoniae* infection is well known.[1,52] In various studies, the incidence of jaundice has been reported to range from 5 to almost 70%.[3] More

Table I. Endotoxemia and Hepatic Function Tests in 21 Typhoid Fever Patients[a]

Test	Normal values	Patients with abnormal test values on admission: N	Percent
Endotoxin in blood	0	21	100
Fasting serum bile acids	<6 μmoles/liter	13	62
2-hr postprandial serum bile acids	<8 μmoles/liter	19	90
Asparatate transaminase	<40 U/liter	12	60
Alkaline phosphatase	<170 U/liter	4	20
Total bilirubin	<1 mg%	4	20

[a]Data from Adinolfi et al.[46]

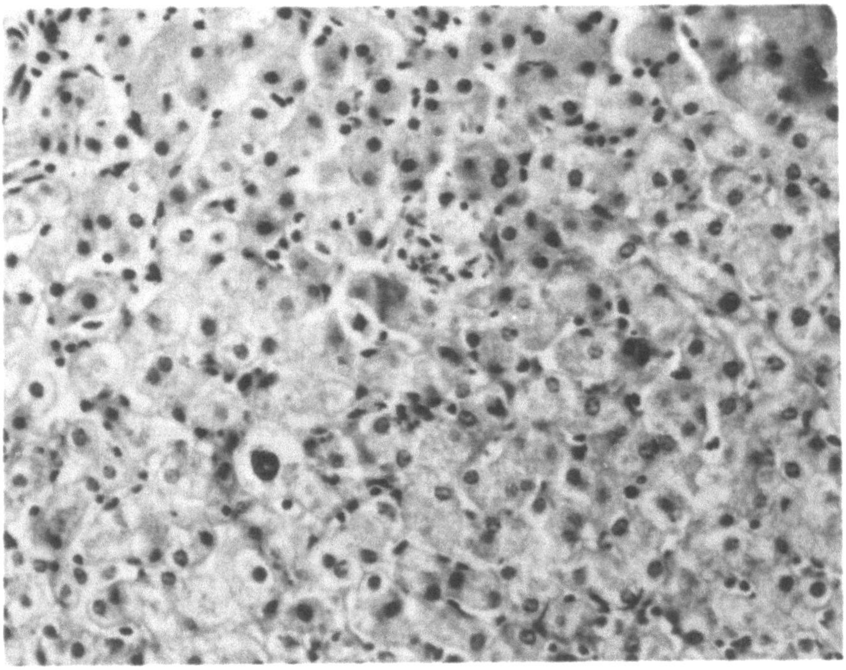

Figure 7. Salmonella paratyphi sepsis. Nonspecific reactive changes include focal hepatocellular necrosis, sinusoidal infiltration by lymphocytes, and scattered large regenerative hepatocytes. (H&E, ×300; AFIP Neg. 87-5874)

recently, it has been reported to occur primarily in black males,[53–55] but the reasons for this predilection are unclear.

Although several theories have been proposed, the mechanism underlying the liver injury is not known. For example, hemolysis, due to glucose 6-phosphate dehydrogenase (G6PD) deficiency, has been proposed to be a factor,[54] but another study did not find a correlation.[55] Other factors, such as fever, anoxia, or bacterial serotype, also do not correlate with the severity of the hepatic involvement.[2] Klatskin[1] has suggested that the liver dysfunction is related to the adverse toxic effects of the underlying infection. The degree of liver involvement, however, does not play a role in the outcome of the infection.[52,54,56]

Biochemically, the disease is characterized by elevations in conjugated bilirubin and by increased urinary excretion of bilirubin and urobilinogen.[52,56] The pathology is one of nonspecific liver injury, including hepatocyte swelling, focal necrosis, and cholestasis.[2,3,57]

2.3.2. Staphylococcal Infection

Except for those patients with toxic shock syndrome (TSS), jaundice associated with staphylococcal infections is rare.[3,58] During TSS, however, the frequency of hepatic dysfunction is high. In one study,[59] ALT, AST, and bilirubin values were elevated in 40–50% of cases, while in another,[60] every patient had abnormal values for at least one hepatic function test, including 16 of 16 who had SBA determinations. In fact, Gourley et al.[60] consider cholestasis a universal finding in TSS. Although predominantly seen in women during menses,[59,60] it was first described in adolescents of either sex[61] and has been observed in males and nonmenstruating females.[62] In addition, TSS has recently been recognized as a complication of influenza.[63,64]

Histologic examination of the liver of TSS patients has demonstrated an acute cholangitis[65] (Fig. 8). It was suggested that the cholangitis could be responsible for the cases of hyperbilirubinemia and jaundice reported during TSS.[65] The pathogenesis of TSS is uncertain, but the lack of a bacteremic stage[59] suggests that an exotoxin liberated by *S. aureus* may play a direct role[59–61,65] or an indirect role by sensitizing the patient to the adverse effects of endotoxin.[60] Other bacterial infections that may lead to abnormal liver function and jaundice are listed in Table II.

3. RICKETTSIAL INFECTION

The rickettsiae are small coccoids that are obligate intracellular parasites. They evoke strong immunologic reactions and confer lengthy immunity against reinfection. Except for *Coxiella burnetii*, all are transmitted by insect vectors and usually present with a characteristic rash.[89,90]

3.1. Q Fever

Q fever, caused by *C. burnetii*, is acquired by contact with infected animals, usually by inhalation of the organism.[91] Hepatomegaly (65%) and abnormal liver-function tests (85%) are often seen, but jaundice occurs in only about 5% of cases.[92] Although transaminases may be elevated, and occasionally markedly, the most commonly observed enzyme abnormality is an increase in SAP.[92,93] However, there may be histologic evidence of liver injury when serum enzymes are normal or minimally elevated[93]; conversely, the liver may not be affected,[94] even in fatal cases.

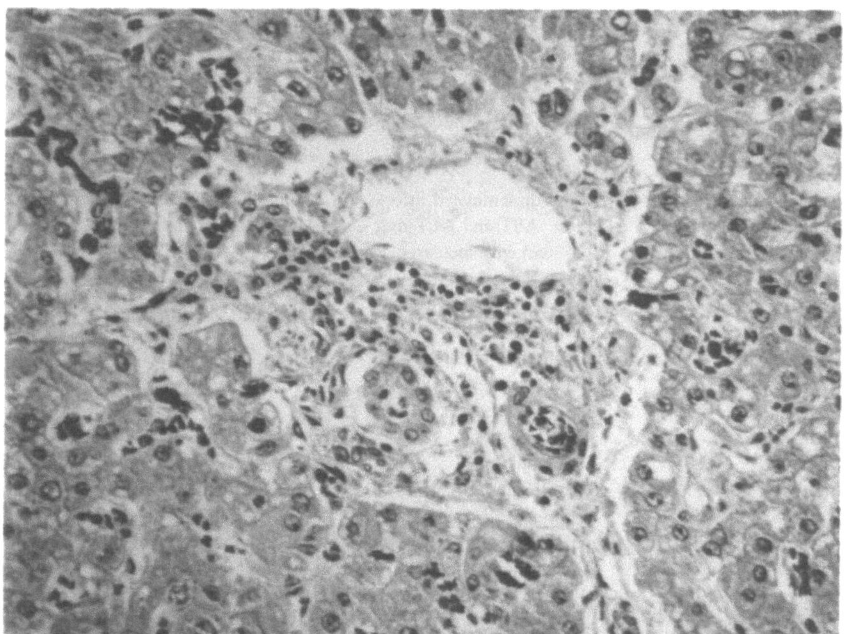

Figure 8. Toxic shock syndrome in a 17-year-old girl. Neutrophils are present within the surrounding and interlobular bile duct in the center lower portion of this portal area. Mild hepatocellular unrest and regenerative activity are noted in the lobules adjacent to the portal area. (H&E, ×250; AFIP Neg. 87-6892)

Table II. Hepatic Involvement during Bacterial Infection[a]

Infection (etiologic agents)	Liver involvement	Notes	Reference
Gram-positive			
Coccal			
Streptococcus (β-hemolytic)	Vascular injury, mononuclear cell infiltrate, vacuolation and congestion	Jandice rare; early reports may have included cases of viral hepatitis	3, 66
Bacilli			
Clostridial *Clostridium perfringens* (*C. welchii*)	Severe anemia and jaundice; gas pockets in liver	Organism may be cultured from liver; exotoxin probably plays role in the anemia	67–70
Actinomycosis *Actinomycetes israelii*	Liver involved in disseminated form; multiple abscesses of liver with sulfur granules	Liver probably not primary site of infection; direct invasion of liver; focal hepatic gallium accumulation	71–73
Gram-negative			
Bacilli			
Shigellosis *Shigella sonnei* *S. flexneri* *S. dysenteriae*	AST, ALT, and SAP may be increased; periportal inflammatory infiltrate, cholestasis, fatty changes	Possibility of direct effect on liver	74, 75
Meliodidosis *Pseudomonas pseudomallei*	Abscesses with inflammatory infiltrate, focal necrosis; may be fatty change; jaundice rare	In chronic infection, liver may be only organ affected	3, 76–78
Tularemia			
Francisella (*Pasteurella*) tularensis	During disseminated infection, AST and ALT may be markedly increased; large foci of necrosis, and rare epitheloid granulomas	Acquired by contact with ticks, biting flies, or rabbits	3, 79, 80
Campylobacter enteritis *Campylobacter fetus* spp. *jejuni*	No jaundice, but transaminases elevated in 25%; nonspecific focal necrosis and lipogranulomas	Possible invasion of liver	81–83
Brucellosis *Brucella abortus* *B. melitensis* *B. suis*	SAP, BR, transaminases often abnormal; jaundice rare; periportal fibrosis and inflammation, Kupffer cell hypertrophy	Organism found in liver biopsy specimens; disease may be acute, subacute, chronic, or relapsing; *B. melitensis* is more invasive and causes a more acute form of illness	3, 84–88

[a]AST, aspartate transaminase; ALT, alanine transaminase; BR, bilirubin; SAP, serum alkaline phosphatase.

Microscopically, Kupffer cell proliferation, granulomas, focal necrosis, and portal tract infiltration can be seen. Granulomas juxtaposed with fatty change and eosinophilic necrosis of the sinusoidal wall have been considered pathognomonic,[95,96] but these changes have not been reported in all cases.[93] Since the organism has been located in hepatic parenchyma under experimental conditions,[97] a direct effect on the liver is possible. In this connection, it is of interest to note that infection of guinea pigs with *C. burnetii* has been reported to cause changes in their liver plasma membranes.[98]

3.2. Rocky Mountain Spotted Fever

The patient's history, specifically in relationship to tick exposure, and a characteristic rash are important in separating this disease, caused by *Rickettsia rickettsii*, from leptospirosis.[3] It should be mentioned, however, that the typical rash is not always present[99,100] and that it occurs more frequently in the eastern United States than in the Rocky Mountain area.[100]

Jaundice as a complication of this infection is rare, but two cases were recently described.[101] In the adolescent boy, there were elevations in ALT, AST, and conjugated bilirubin but a minimal increase in SAP (less than twofold). The liver biopsy from the other patient, a 55-year-old man, showed a nonspecific acute hepatitis with cholestasis. In both cases, Ramphal et al.[101] suggested that hemolysis and renal insufficiency may have played a role in the development of the jaundice.

The pathogenesis of this disease is unknown, but studies using chick embryo cells have shown that the rickettsiae are located primarily in the cytosol and that they cause a severe dilation of the rough endoplasmic reticulum (RER).[102] Walker and Cain[102] postulated that the organism may exert a direct cytotoxic effect.

4. VIRAL INFECTION

Viral infections, including the "flu," probably constitute the most common group of human diseases. They may be transmitted by inhalation, human contact, insect and animal bites, contaminated biologic specimens and instruments, and during birth.[89,90] While such known factors as stress, alteration of immune status, menstruation, and pregnancy can precipitate a recurrence of the disease, other factors undoubtedly play a role. The relative contribution of various factors in the recrudescence of viral diseases is currently the subject of intense investigation.

4.1. Herpetoviridae

There are many viruses that can cause disease with hepatic involvement.[1,90] The present discussion, however, is limited to some members of the Herpetoviridae family. These double-stranded DNA viruses are among the most common viral infections of humans.[103] Hepatic complications are rare and are dependent on viral dissemination.

4.1.1. Epstein–Barr Virus

Infectious mononucleosis is a lymphoproliferative disease characterized by a sore throat, fever, lymphadenopathy, and atypical lymphocytes in the blood. It occurs primarily in adolescents and young adults and is known to be transmitted by kissing.[89]

In almost all cases of infectious mononucleosis, serum transaminases are elevated,[104,105] but jaundice occurs in only 5–15% of cases.[104,106,107] In addition, the degree of hepatic dysfunction is not directly related to the severity of the clinical disease.[104] It may resemble infectious hepatitis but can usually be differentiated by means of serologic markers.[108] Histologically, there is a marked inflammation of the portal and sinusoidal areas after producing a characteristic "Indian filing" of lymphocytes within the sinusoids. Generally, there is only slight liver damage, but marked regenerative activity with numerous mitotic figures may be present.[109] However, cases of fatal hepatic necrosis have been reported.[110]

4.1.2. Herpes Simplex Virus

Herpes simplex virus (HSV) is composed of two strains—HSV-1 and HSV-2—and is a common human infection. Viral antibodies to HSV-1 and HSV-2 can be found in 30–50% and 80–100% of adults from higher and lower socioeconomic groups, respectively. HSV-1 is transmitted by oral secretions and dermal contact and primarily affects nongenital areas, while HSV-2 is contracted during birth or by sexual contact.[111,112] HSV infection occurs most frequently in neonates,[113,114] in immunosuppressed adults,[115] and in pregnant women.[116]

Hepatitis arising from HSV infection is very rare, occurring mainly in neonates infected with HSV-2 during birth,[117–119] but has been reported to occur in supposedly immunocompetent adults.[120]

On gross examination of the liver in fatal cases of herpes infection, numerous small (0.1- to 0.3-cm) soft tan-white nodules are noted randomly scattered throughout the parenchyma. On microscopic examination, these foci consist of areas of coagulative hepatocellular necrosis involving irregular portions of hepatic lobules, including central veins and portal areas (Fig. 9A). Rarely, these foci of necrosis may become confluent producing massive areas of necrotic liver.

Herpes virus infects individual cells and is first visible as a fine nuclear granularity. As the virus multiplies, the nuclear chromatin is pushed against the nuclear membrane by a smooth eosinophilic Cowdry type A inclusion body (Fig. 9B). The nucleus itself is not enlarged, in contradistinction to cytomegalovirus (CMV) infection, and the cytoplasm is unremarkable until the cell undergoes a coagulative necrosis with dissolution of the nuclear and cell membranes. Infected cells with the typical intranuclear inclusions can usually be identified only near the margin of the necrotic foci. Reactive and regenerative changes may be seen in surviving hepatocytes and bile duct epithelium.[113,115,120] In some cases, macrovesicular fat and mild to moderate portal inflammation may be observed.[120]

4.1.3. Cytomegalovirus Infection

Cytomegalovirus infection is found throughout the world, and more than 50% of tested adults had antibodies against the virus.[121] Although infection is common, it seldom results in clinically evident symptoms. Neonates and immunosuppressed patients, however, are at risk and may develop serious illness from disseminated CMV. It may present as a febrile systemic illness, hepatitis, atypical mononucleosis or as the Guillain-Barre syndrome.[122]

Cytomegalovirus involvement of the liver is limited primarily to the bile duct epithelial cells with marked enlargement of the cells (i.e., cytomegalo-) by both intranuclear and cytoplasmic inclusion bodies. The intranuclear inclusion, when fully developed, consists of a large smooth eosinophilic body separated from the marginated chromatin by a clear halo (Fig. 10). Periodic acid-Schiff-positive granules may greatly distend the cytoplasm of the bile duct cells. Portal areas may display marked infiltration by lymphocytes, occasionally producing lymphoid aggregates or germinal centers.[123–125] Less frequently, focal (and rarely) massive necrosis and bile stasis may be present. Several other viral diseases that can also affect hepatic function are listed in Table III.

The brief nature of this review precludes a complete listing of infectious agents that may alter hepatic function. For additional information, the reader is referred to several reviews.[1–3,90,121,122,128,156,157]

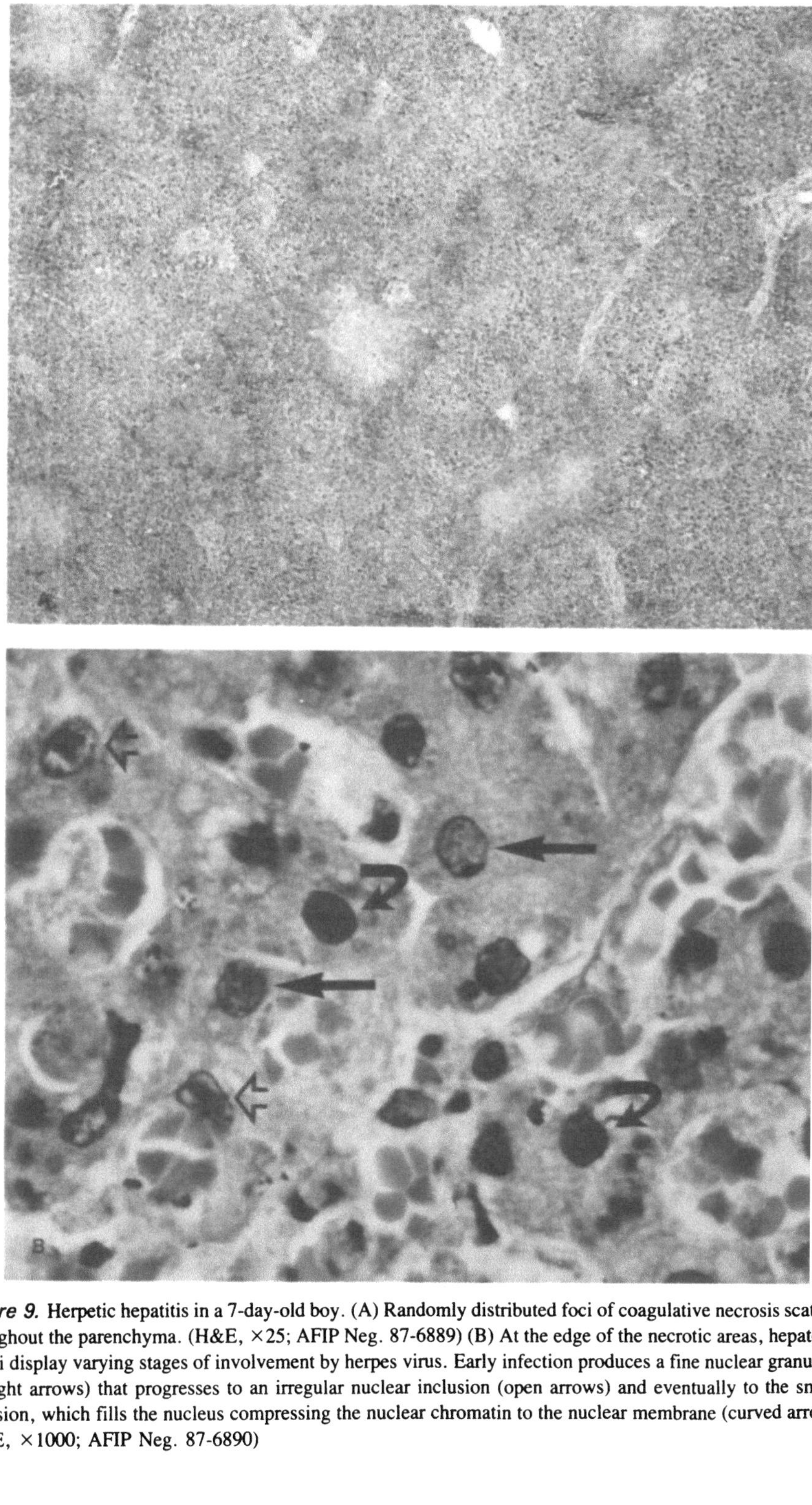

Figure 9. Herpetic hepatitis in a 7-day-old boy. (A) Randomly distributed foci of coagulative necrosis scattered throughout the parenchyma. (H&E, ×25; AFIP Neg. 87-6889) (B) At the edge of the necrotic areas, hepatocyte nuclei display varying stages of involvement by herpes virus. Early infection produces a fine nuclear granularity (straight arrows) that progresses to an irregular nuclear inclusion (open arrows) and eventually to the smooth inclusion, which fills the nucleus compressing the nuclear chromatin to the nuclear membrane (curved arrows). (H&E, ×1000; AFIP Neg. 87-6890)

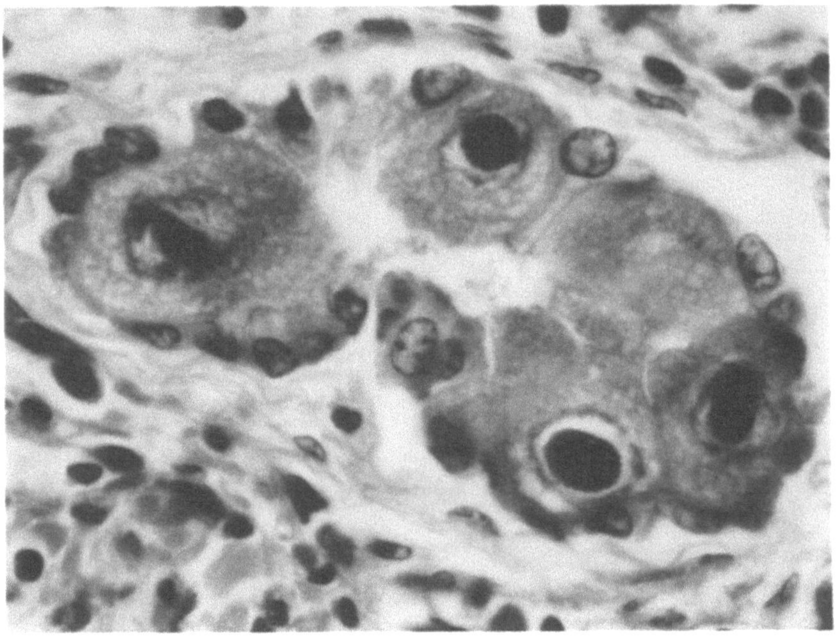

Figure 10. Cytomegalovirus infection in a newborn boy. Four massively enlarged bile duct epithelial cells contain large smooth intranuclear inclusion bodies separated from the nuclear membrane by a clear halo area. Note the normal-size epithelial cells adjacent to these cells. (H&E, ×1000; AFIP Neg. 87-6891)

Table III. Hepatic Dysfunction Caused by Some Viruses[a]

Virus	Hapatic dysfunction	Notes	Reference
Yellow fever	Midzonal necrosis; acidophilic fatty change; inflammatory reactions rare	Experimental data duggests Kupffer cells as first site of necrosis; virus may replicate in Kupffer cells	126–130
Coxsackie B	Approx. 10% may be jaundiced; moderate rises in SAP, BR, and transaminases; central hemorrhagic necrosis; nonspecific portal tract infiltration; ^{99m}Tc sulfur uptake inhibited	Infants at high risk; other complications as meningitis or myocarditis often present; virus-like particles found in liver; jaundice more frequent in fatal cases	131–135
Lassa fever	Nonzonal necrosis; level of inflammation does not correspond to degree of necrosis; acidophilic bodies and Kupffer cell hyperplasia	Hemorrhagic fevers caused by Junin and Machupo viruses similar; viruses found in liver and may exert cytolytic action	128, 129, 136–140
Marburg	Mild jaundice occasionally present; focal acidophilic necrosis of liver and Kupffer cells; AST may be markedly elevated with respect to ALT;	Ebola virus similar, but more virulent; virus can develop in liver; may persist in body fluids for 2–3 months	128, 129, 141–147

Table III. (Continued)

Virus	Hapatic dysfunction	Notes	Reference
	BR, SAP, and BSP retention may be normal		
Rift Valley fever	Hepatomegaly and jaundice; LDH elevated in 2 of 4 cases in one study; necrosis may be diffuse or localized in periportal midzonal areas	Hemorrhage and jaundice indicate poor prognosis; virus found in liver; transmitted by mosquitoes or contact with live or dead animals	128, 129, 148–151
Mumps	Jaundice, hepatomegaly, BR elevation, and abnormal BSP retention in one case	Very rare complication of mumps	152
Rubella	Hepatosplenomegaly common; occasional jaundice; pathology varies from severe giant cell hepatitis and marked Kupffer cell reaction to cholestasis with periportal inflammation; ALT, AST, and SAP may be markedly increased	Primarily in neonates; virus can be isolated from liver	153–155

[a]ALT, alanine transaminase; AST, aspartate transaminase; BR, bilirubin; BSP, sulfobromophthalein; LDH, lactic dehydrogenase; SAP, serum alkaline phosphatase; Tc, technetium.

ACKNOWLEDGMENT. The authors would like to thank the U.S. Environmental Protection Agency Headquarters Library staff for their assistance in the literature search and article acquisition and Dr. James J. Murphy for a critical reading of the manuscript. Dr. Abernathy also holds an appointment as a Research Toxicologist at the Veterans Administration Medical Center, Washington, D.C.

REFERENCES

1. Klatskin G: Hepatitis associated with systemic infection, in Schiff L (ed): *Diseases of the Liver*, 4th ed. JB Lippincott, Philadelphia, 1975, pp. 711–754.
2. Zimmerman HJ, Fang M, Utili R, et al: Jaundice due to bacterial infection. *Gastroenterology* **77**:362–374, 1979.
3. Lewis JH, Zimmerman HJ: Bacterial infection as a cause of jaundice. *Intern Med Spec Gastroenterol* **5**:94–113, 1984.
4. Scharschmidt, BF, Goldberg, HI, Schmid R: Approach to the patient with cholestatic jaundice. *N Engl J Med* **308**:1515–1519, 1983.
5. Bernstein J, Brown AK: Sepsis and jaundice in early infancy. *Pediatrics* **29**:873–882, 1962.
6. Hamilton JR, Sass-Kortsak S: Jaundice associated with severe bacterial infection in young infants. *J Pediatr* **63**:121–132, 1963.
7. Danks DM, Campbell PE, Connelly JF: An aetiological study of neonatal jaundice in a children's hospital. *Aust Paediatr J* **1**:193–201, 1965.
8. Kenny JF, Medearis DN, Kleyn S, et al: An outbreak of urinary tract infections and septicemia due to *Escherichia coli* in male infants. *J Pediatr* **68**:530–541, 1966.
9. Arthur AB, Wilson BDR: Urinary infection presenting with jaundice. *Br Med J* **1**:539–540, 1967.
10. Seeler RA, Hahn K: Jaundice in urinary tract infection in infancy. *Am J Dis Child* **118**:553–558, 1969.
11. Rooney JC, Hill DJ, Danks DM: Jaundice associated with bacterial infection in the newborn. *Am J Dis Child* **122**:39–41, 1971.

12. Ng SH, Rawstron JR: Urinary tract infections presenting with jaundice. *Arch Dis Child* **46:**173–176, 1971.
13. Borges MAG, DeBrito T, Borges JMG: Hepatic manifestations in bacterial infections of infants and children. Clinical features, biochemical data and morphologic hepatic changes (histological and ultrastructural). *Acta Hepatogastroenterol* **19:**328–344, 1972.
14. Escobedo MB, Barton LL, Marshall RE, et al: The frequency of jaundice in neonatal bacterial infections. *Clin Pediatr* **13:**656–657, 1974.
15. Kunzer W Jr, Niederhoff H, Sutor AH, et al: Cholestatic icterus and "shock liver" resulting from disseminated intravascular coagulation in newborn and babies. *Klin Paediatr* **192:**254–263, 1980.
16. Naveh Y, Friedman A: Urinary tract infection presenting with jaundice. *Pediatrics* **62:**524–525, 1978.
17. Fahrlander H, Huber F, Gloor F: Intrahepatic retention of bile in severe bacterial infections. *Gastroenterology* **47:**590–599, 1964.
18. Eley A, Hargreaves T, Lambert HP: Jaundice in severe infections. *Br Med J* **2:**75–77, 1965.
19. Miller DF, Irvine RW: Jaundice in acute appendicitis. *Lancet* **1:**321–323, 1969.
20. Vermillon SE, Gregg JA, Baggenstoss AH, et al: Jaundice associated with bacteremia. *Arch Intern Med* **124:**611–618, 1969.
21. Miller DJ, Keeton GR, Webber BL, et al: Jaundice in severe bacterial infection. *Gastroenterology* **71:**94–97, 1976.
22. Franson TR, Hierholzer WJ, LaBrecque DR: Frequency and characteristics of hyperbilirubinemia associated with bacteremia. *Rev Infect Dis* **7:**1–9, 1985.
23. Holmes KK, Counts GW, Beaty HN: Disseminated gonococcal infection. *Ann Intern Med* **74:**979–993, 1971.
24. Zimmerman HJ: *Hepatotoxicity: The Adverse Effects of Drugs and Other Chemicals on the Liver.* Appleton & Lange, East Norwalk, Connecticut, 1978.
25. Trimble C: Gonococcal perihepatitis simulating acute cholecystitis. *Surg Gynecol Obstet* **130:**54–56, 1970.
26. Kimball MW, Knee S: Gonococcal perihepatitis in a male. The Fitz-Hugh–Curtis syndrome. *N Engl J Med* **282:**1082–1084, 1970.
27. McLain LG, Decker M, Nye D, et al: Gonococcal perihepatitis in a female adolescent. Fitz-Hugh–Curtis syndrome. *JAMA* **239:**339–340, 1978.
28. Monges A, Tronconi JC, Legre M, et al: L'Ictere satellite des infections urinaires gravidiques. *Med Chir Dig* **2:**345–350, 1973.
29. Banks JG, Foulis AK, Ledingham IMcA, et al: Liver function in septic shock. *J Clin Pathol* **35:**1249–1252, 1982.
30. Lefkowitch JH: Bile ductular cholestasis: An ominous histopathologic sign related to sepsis and "cholangitis lenta." *Hum Pathol* **13:**19–24, 1982.
31. Utili R, Abernathy CO, Zimmerman HJ: Cholestatic effects of *Escherichia coli* endotoxin on the isolated perfused rat liver. *Gastroenterology* **70:**248–253, 1976.
32. Utili R, Abernathy CO, Zimmerman HJ: Studies on the effects of *E. coli* endotoxin on canalicular bile formation in the isolated perfused rat liver. *J Lab Clin Med* **89:**471–482, 1977.
33. Utili R, Abernathy CO, Aron SA, et al: *In vivo* effects of *Escherichia coli* endotoxin on sulfobromophthalein clearance in the guinea pig. *Experientia* **33:**1631–1632, 1977.
34. Boelsterli U, Abernathy CO, Balazs T, et al: Effects of endotoxin tolerance on hepatic excretory function: *In vivo* study. *Toxicol Lett* **11:**207–212, 1982.
35. Utili R, Abernathy CO, Zimmerman HJ: Effects of *Salmonella enteritidis* endotoxin on the excretory function of the isolated perfused rat liver. *Proc Soc Exp Biol Med* **155:**184–188, 1977.
36. Watkins JB, Ingall D, Szczepanik P, et al: Bile-salt metabolism in the newborn. Measurement of pool size and synthesis by stable isotope technic. *N Engl J Med* **288:**431–434, 1973.
37. Watkins JB, Szczepanik P, Gould JB, et al: Bile-salt metabolism in the human premature infant. Preliminary observations of pool size and synthesis rate following prenatal administration of dexamethasone and phenobarbital. *Gastroenterology* **69:**706–713, 1975.
38. Stuart BM, Pullen RL: Typhoid: Clinical analysis of 360 cases. *Arch Intern Med* **78:**629–661, 1946.
39. Ramachandran S, Godfrey JJ, Perera MVF: Typhoid hepatitis. *JAMA* **230:**236–240, 1974.
40. DeBrito T, Trench-Vieira W, Diagostino-Dias M: Jaundice in typhoid hepatitis. A light and electron microscopy study based on liver biopsies. *Acta Hepatogastroenterol* **24:**426–433, 1977.
41. Mallory FB: A histological study of typhoid fever. *J Exp Med* **3:**139–151, 1975.
42. Nolan JP: Bacteria and the liver. *N Engl J Med* **299:**1069–1071, 1978.

43. Wolff SM: Biological effects of bacterial endotoxins in man, in Kass EH, Wolff SM (eds): *Bacterial Lipopolysaccharides*. University of Chicago Press, Chicago, 1973, pp. 251–256.
44. Gunnar RM, Loeb HS, Winslow EJ, et al: Hemodynamic measurements in bacteremia and septic shock in man, in Kass EH, Wolff SM (eds): *Bacterial Lipopolysaccharides*. University of Chicago Press, Chicago, 1973, pp. 287–290.
45. Butler T, Bell WR, Levin J, et al: Typhoid fever: Studies of blood coagulation, bacteremia, and endotoxemia. *Arch Intern Med* **138**:407–410, 1978.
46. Adinolfi LE, Utili R, Gaeta GB, et al: Presence of endotoxemia and its relationship to liver dysfunction in patients with typhoid fever. *Infection* **15**:359–362, 1987.
47. Calva JJ, Ruiz-Palacios GM: Salmonella hepatitis: Detection of *Salmonella* antigens in the liver of patients with typhoid fever. *J Infect Dis* **154**:373–374, 1986.
48. Meals RA: Paratyphoid fever: A report of 62 cases with several unusual findings and a review of the literature. *Arch Intern Med* **136**:1422–1428, 1976.
49. Fraser DW, Tsai TR, Orenstein W, et al: Legionnaires' disease: Description of an epidemic of pneumonia. *N Engl J Med* **297**:1189–1197, 1977.
50. Kirby BD, Snyder KM, Meyer RD, et al: Legionnaires' disease: Clinical features of 24 cases. *Ann Intern Med* **89**:297–309, 1978.
51. Watts JC, Hicklin MD, Thomason BM, et al: Fatal pneumonia caused by *Legionella pneumophila*, serogroup 3: Demonstration of the bacilli in extrathoracic organs. *Ann Intern Med* **92**:186–188, 1980.
52. Zimmerman HJ, Thomas LJ: The liver in pneumonoccal pneumonia: Observations in 94 cases on liver function and jaundice in pneumonia. *J Lab Clin Med* **35**:556–567, 1950.
53. Mekel RCPM, Theron JJ, Simson IW: Pneumonia with jaundice in the Bantu. *Proc Third World Cong Gastroenterol* **3**:283, 1967.
54. Tugswell P, Williams O: Jaundice associated with lobar pneumonia. *Q J Med* **66**:97–118, 1977.
55. Parent MA: G-6 PD deficiency in jaundice associated with lobar pneumonia. *Lancet* **2**:155, 1973.
56. Radford AJ, Rhodes FA, Matz LR: The association of jaundice with lobar pneumonia in the territory of Papua and New Guinea. *Med J Aust* **2**:678–681, 1967.
57. Theron JJ, Pepler WJ, Mekel RCPM: Ultrastructure of the liver in Bantu patients with pneumonia and jaundice. *J Pathol* **106**:113–117, 1972.
58. Tuazon CU, Cardella TA, Sheagren JN: Staphylococcal endocarditis in drug users. Clinical and microbiologic aspects. *Arch Intern Med* **135**:1555–1561, 1975.
59. Shands KN, Schmid GP, Dan BB, et al: Toxic-shock syndrome in menstruating women. Association with tampon use and *Staphylococcus aureus* and clinical features in 52 cases. *N Engl J Med* **303**:1436–1442, 1980.
60. Gourley GR, Chesney PJ, Davis JP, et al: Acute cholestasis in patients with toxic-shock syndrome. *Gastroenterology* **81**:928–931, 1981.
61. Todd J, Fishaut M, Kapral F, et al: Toxic-shock syndrome associated with phage-group-1 staphylococci. *Lancet* **2**:1116–1118, 1978.
62. Davis JP, Chesney PJ, Wand PJ, et al: Toxic-shock syndrome. Epidemiologic features, recurrence, risk factors, and prevention. *N Engl J Med* **303**:1429–1435, 1980.
63. MacDonald KL, Osterholm MT, Hedberg CW, et al: Toxic shock syndrome. A newly recognized complication of influenza and influenzalike illness. *JAMA* **257**:1053–1058, 1987.
64. Sperber SJ, Francis JB: Toxic shock syndrome during an influenza outbreak. *JAMA* **257**:1086–1087, 1987.
65. Ishak KG, Rogers WA: Cryptogenic acute cholangitis—Association with toxic shock syndrome. *Am J Clin Pathol* **76**:619–626, 1981.
66. Fishbein WN: Jaundice as an early manifestation of scarlet fever. Report of three cases in adults and review of the literature. *Ann Intern Med* **57**:60–72, 1962.
67. Pyrtek LJ, Bartus SH: *Clostridium welchii* septicaemia following cholecystectomy. *N Engl J Med* **266**:689–693, 1962.
68. Bennett JM, Healey PJM: Spherocytic hemolytic anemia and acute cholecystitis caused by *Clostridium welchii*. *N Engl J Med* **268**:1070–1072, 1963.
69. Clancy MT, O'Briain S: Fatal *Clostridium welchii* septicaemia following acute cholecystitis. *Br J Surg* **62**:518–519, 1975.
70. de Gier J, de Haas GH, van Deenen LLM: Action of phospholipases from *Clostridium welchii* and *Bacillus coreus* on red-cell membranes. *Biochem J* **81**:33P–34P, 1961.
71. Brown JR: Human actinomycosis. A study of 181 subjects. *Hum Pathol* **4**:319–330, 1973.

72. Golematis B, Hatzitheofilou C, Melissas J: Liver actinomycosis. *Am J Gastroenterol* **67**:148–150, 1977.
73. Chandarlapaty SKC, Dusol M, Edwards R, et al: ^{67}Gallium accumulation in hepatic actinomycosis. *Gastroenterology* **69**:752–755, 1975.
74. Hornsey JT, Schwartzmann SW, Galambos JT: *Shigella* hepatitis. *Am J Gastroenterol* **66**:146–149, 1976.
75. Stern MS, Gitnick GL: *Shigella* hepatitis. *JAMA* **235**:2628, 1976.
76. Brundiage WG, Thuss CJ, Walden DC: Four fatal cases of melioidosis in U.S. soldiers in Vietnam. Bacteriologic and pathologic characteristics. *Am J Trop Med Hyg* **17**:183–191, 1968.
77. Greenwald KA, Nash G, Foley FD: Acute systemic melioidosis. Autopsy findings in four patients. *Am J Clin Pathol* **52**:188–198, 1969.
78. Piggott JA, Hochholzer L: Human melioidosis. A histopathologic study of acute and chronic melioidosis. *Arch Pathol Lab Med* **90**:101–111, 1970.
79. Forshay L: Tularemia. A summary of certain aspects of the disease including methods for early diagnosis and the results of serum treatment in 600 patients. *Medicine (Baltimore)* **19**:1–83, 1940.
80. Pullen RL, Stuart BM: Tularemia. Analysis of 225 cases. *JAMA* **129**:495–500, 1945.
81. Drake AA, Gilchrist MJR, Washington JA, et al: Diarrhea due to *Campylobacter fetus* subspecies *jejuni*. A clinical review of 63 cases. *Mayo Clin Proc* **56**:414–423, 1981.
82. Pitkanen T, Ponka A, Pettersson T, et al: *Campylobacter* enteritis in 188 hospitalized patients. *Arch Intern Med* **143**:215–219, 1983.
83. Reddy KR, Farnum JB, Thomas E: Acute hepatitis associated *Campylobacter* colitis. *J Clin Gastroenterol* **5**:259–262, 1983.
84. Nushan H, Bailey AA: Acute hepatitis due to brucellosis. *Ann Intern Med* **39**:915–919, 1953.
85. Spink WW: Suppuration and calcification of the liver and spleen due to long-standing infection with *Brucella suis*. *N Engl J Med* **257**:209–210, 1957.
86. Cohen FB, Robins B, Lipsten W: Isolation of *Brucella abortus* by percutaneous liver biopsy. *N Engl J Med* **257**:228–230, 1957.
87. Fogel R, Lewis S: Diagnosis of *Brucella melitensis* infection by percutaneous needle biopsy of the liver. *Ann Intern Med* **53**:204–215, 1960.
88. Young EJ: *Brucella melitensis* hepatitis: The absence of granulomas. *Ann Intern Med* **91**:414–415, 1979.
89. Robbins SL, Cotran RS: *Pathologic Basis of Disease*. WB Saunders, Philadelphia, 1979.
90. World Health Organization: Bacterial and viral zoonoses. WHO Tech Rep Ser **682**:1–146, 1982.
91. Spelman DW: Q fever. A study of 111 consecutive cases. *Med J Aust* **1**:547–553, 1982.
92. Powell OW: Liver involvement in "Q" fever. *Aust Ann Med* **10**:52–58, 1961.
93. DuPont HL, Hornick RB, Levin HS, et al: Q fever hepatitis. *Ann Intern Med* **74**:198–206, 1971.
94. Urso FP: The pathologic findings in rickettsial pneumonia. *Am J Clin Pathol* **64**:335–342, 1975.
95. Bernstein M, Edmondson HA, Barbour BH: The liver lesion in Q fever. Clinical and pathologic features. *Arch Intern Med* **116**:491–498, 1965.
96. Hofmann CE, Heaton JW Jr: Q fever hepatitis. Clinical manifestations and pathological findings. *Gastroenterology* **83**:474–479, 1982.
97. Mitchell R, Grist NR, Bazaz G, et al: Pathological, rickettsiological and immunofluorescence studies of a case of Q fever endocarditis. *J Pathol* **91**:317–323, 1966.
98. Marecki N, Becker F, Baca OG, et al: Changes in liver and L-cell plasma membranes during infection with *Coxiella burnetii*. *Infect Immun* **19**:272–280, 1978.
99. Westerman EL: Rocky Mountain spotless fever. A dilemma for the clinician. *Arch Intern Med* **142**:1106–1107, 1982.
100. Ramsey PG, Press OW: Successful treatment of Rocky Mountain "spotless" fever. *West J Med* **140**:94–96, 1984.
101. Ramphal R, Kluge R, Cohen V, et al: Rocky Mountain spotted fever and jaundice. Two consecutive cases acquired in Florida and a review of the literature on this complication. *Arch Intern Med* **138**:260–263, 1978.
102. Walker DH, Cain BG: The rickettsial plaque. Evidence for direct cytopathic effect of *Rickettsia rickettsii*. *Lab Invest* **43**:388–396, 1980.
103. Kaplan AS (ed): *The Herpesviruses*. Academic, New York, 1973.
104. Dunnet WN: Infectious mononucleosis. *Br Med J* **1**:1187–1191, 1963.
105. Gelb D, West M, Zimmerman HJ: Serum enzymes in disease. IX. Analysis of factors responsible for elevated values in infectious mononucleosis. *Am J Med* **33**:249–261, 1962.
106. Abrams HL: Infectious mononucleosis with intense jaundice of long duration. *N Engl J Med* **238**:295–297, 1948.

107. Jordan WS, Albright RW: Liver function tests in infectious mononucleosis. *J Lab Clin Med* **35**:688–698, 1950.
108. Hoagland RJ: *Infectious Mononucleosis*. Grune & Stratton, Orlando, Florida, 1967.
109. Gowing NFC: Infectious mononucleosis: Histophathologic aspects, in Sommers SC (ed): *Haematologic and Lymphoid Pathology. Decennial 1966–1975*. Appleton & Lange, East Norwalk, Connecticut, 1975, pp. 261–280.
110. Allen UR, Bass BH: Fatal hepatic necrosis in glandular fever. *J Clin Pathol* **16**:337–341, 1963.
111. Nahmias AJ, Roizman B: Infection with herpes-simplex viruses 1 and 2. *N Engl J Med* **289**:667–674, 719–725, 781–789, 1973.
112. Amstey MS: Management of pregnancy complicated by genital herpes virus infection. *Obstet Gynecol* **37**:515–520, 1971.
113. White JG: Fulminating infection with herpes-simplex virus in premature and newborn infants. *N Engl J Med* **269**:455–460, 1963.
114. Miller DR, Hanshaw JB, O'Leary DS, et al: Fatal disseminated herpes simplex virus infection and hemorrhage in the neonate. Coagulation studies in a case and a review. *J Pediatr* **76**:409–415, 1970.
115. Lee JC, Fortuny IE: Adult herpes simplex hepatitis. *Hum Pathol* **3**:277–281, 1972.
116. Taina E, Hanninen P, Gronroos M: Viral infections in pregnancy. *Acta Obstet Gynecol Scand* **64**:167–173, 1985.
117. Nahmias AJ, Alford CA, Korones SB: Infection of the newborn with herpes virus hominus. *Adv Pediatr* **17**:185–226, 1970.
118. Overall JC Jr, Glasgow LA: Virus infections of the fetus and newborn infant. *J Pediatr* **77**:315–333, 1970.
119. Hanshaw JB: Herpes virus hominis infection in the fetus and newborn. *Am J Dis Child* **126**:546–555, 1973.
120. Goodman ZD, Ishak KG, Sesterhenn IA: Herpes simplex hepatitis in apparently immunocompetent adults. *Am J Clin Pathol* **85**:694–699, 1986.
121. Schiff GM: Viral diseases of the liver other than infectious and serum hepatitis, in Schiff L (ed): *Diseases of the Liver*, 4th ed. JB Lippincott, Philadelphia, 1975, pp. 594–603.
122. Wright R, Millward-Sadler GH, Bull FG: Acute viral hepatitis, in Wright R, Millward-Sadler GH, Alberti KGMM, Karran S (eds): *Liver and Biliary Disease*, 2nd ed. WB Saunders, London, 1985, pp. 677–767.
123. Chiba S, Hori S, Kawamura N, et al: Primary cytomegalovirus infection and liver involvement in early infancy. *Tohoku J Exp Med* **117**:143–151, 1975.
124. Fisher ER, Davis E: Cytomegalic-inclusion disease in the adult. *N Engl J Med* **258**:1036–1040, 1958.
125. Shusterman NH, Frauenhoffer C, Kinsey MD: Fatal massive hepatic necrosis in cytomegalovirus mononucleosis. *Ann Intern Med* **88**:810–812, 1978.
126. Francis TI, Moore, DL, Edington GM, et al: A clinicopathological study of human yellow fever. *Bull WHO* **46**:659–667, 1972.
127. Kerr JA: Liver pathology in yellow fever. *Trans R Soc Trop Med Hyg* **67**:882, 1973.
128. World Health Organization: Viral haemorrhagic fevers. *WHO Tech Rep Ser* **721**:1–126, 1985.
129. Howard CR, Ellis DS, Simpson DIH: Exotic viruses and the liver. *Semin Liver Dis* **4**:361–374, 1984.
130. Mims CA: Aspects of the pathogenesis of virus diseases. *Bacteriol Rev* **28**:30–71, 1964.
131. O'Shaughnessey WJ, Buechner HA: Hepatitis associated with a coxsackie B5 virus infection during late pregnancy. *JAMA* **179**:71–72, 1962.
132. Sun NC, Smith VM: Hepatitis associated with myocarditis. Unusual manifestation of infection with coxsackie virus group B, type 3. *N Engl J Med* **274**:190–193, 1966.
133. Gregor GR, Geller SA, Walker GF, et al: Coxsackie hepatitis in an adult with ultrastructural demonstration of the virus. *Mt Sinai J Med* **12**:575–580, 1975.
134 Hinkle GH, Leonard JC, Krous HF, et al: Absence of hepatic uptake of Tc-99mm sulfur colloid in an infant with coxsackie B_2 viral infection. *Clin Nucl Med* **8**:246–248, 1983.
135. Kaplan MH, Klein SW, McPhee J, et al: Group B coxsackievirus infections in infants younger than three months of age: A serious childhood illness. *Rev Infect Dis* **5**:1019–1032, 1983.
136. Edington GM, White HA: The pathology of Lassa fever. *Trans R Soc Trop Med Hyg* **66**:381–389, 1972.
137. Winn WC Jr, Walker DH: The pathology of human Lassa fever. *Bull WHO* **52**:535–545, 1975.
138. Child PL, McKenzie RB, Valverde LR, et al: Bolivian haemorrhagic fever: A pathogenic description. *Arch Pathol Lab Med* **83**:434–435, 1967.
139. Elsner B, Schwarz E, Mando OG, et al: Pathology of 12 fatal cases of Argentine hemorrhagic fever. *Am J Trop Med Hyg* **22**:229–236, 1973.
140. Howard CR, Simpson DIH: The biology of arenaviruses. *J Gen Virol* **51**:1–14, 1980.

141. Smith CE, Simpson DI, Simpson ET, et al: Fatal human disease from vervet monkeys. *Lancet* **2:**1119–1121, 1967.
142. Bechtelsheimer H, Korb G, Gedigk P: The morphology and pathogenesis of "Marburg virus" hepatitis. *Hum Pathol* **3:**255–264, 1972.
143. Gear JSS, Cassel GA, Gear AJ, et al: Outbreak of Marburg virus disease in Johannesburg. *Br Med J* **4:**489–493, 1975.
144. Murphy FA, Simpson DIH, Whitfield SG, et al: Marburg virus infection in monkeys: Ultrastructural studies. *Lab Invest* **24:**279–291, 1971.
145. Editorial: World Health Organization. *Wkly Epidemiol Rec* **52:**177, 1976.
146. Bowen ETW, Platt GS, Lloyd G, et al: Viral hemorrhagic fever in southern Sudan and Northern Zaire. *Lancet* **1:**571–573, 1977.
147. Ellis DS, Simpson DIH, Francis DP, et al: Ultrastructure of Ebola virus particles in human liver. *J Clin Pathol* **31:**201–208, 1978.
148. Van Velden DJJ, Meyer JD, Olivier J, et al: Rift Valley fever affecting humans in South Africa. A clinicopathological study. *S Afr Med J* **51:**867–871, 1977.
149. El Shinnawi BM, Sobhy F, El Zawahry A: Laboratory findings in some cases of Rift Valley fever: Histopathological, haematological, and biochemical. *J Egypt Public Health Assoc* **53:**187–189, 1978.
150. Laughlin LW, Meegan JM, Strausbaugh LJ, et al: Epidemic Rift Valley fever in Egypt: Observations of the spectrum of human illness. *Trans R Soc Trop Med Hyg* **73:**630–633, 1979.
151. World Health Organization: Rift Valley fever: An emerging human and animal problem. *WHO Pub* **63:**1–69, 1982.
152. Warren WR: Hepatitis complicating mumps. *Arch Intern Med* **98:**525–528, 1956.
153. Korones SB, Ainger LE, Monif GRG, et al: Congenital rubella syndrome: New clinical aspects with recovery of virus from affected infants. *J Pediatr* **67:**166–181, 1965.
154. Esterly JR, Slusser RJ, Ruebner BH: Hepatic lesions in the congenital rubella syndrome. *J Pediatr* **71:**676–685, 1967.
155. Ali Z, Hull B, Lewis M: Neonatal manifestation of congenital rubella following an outbreak in Trinidad. *J Trop Pediatr* **32:**79–82, 1986.
156. Evans AS (ed): *Viral Infections of Humans*. Plenum, New York, 1976.
157. Holdstock G, Balasegaram M, Millward-Sadler GH, et al: The liver in infection, in Wright R, Millward-Sadler GH, Alberti KGMM, Karran S (eds): *Liver and Biliary Disease*, 2nd ed. WB Saunders, London, 1985, pp. 1077–1119.

V

Miscellaneous Liver Diseases

28

Hepatic Vein Thrombosis, Veno-Occlusive Disease, and Ischemic Hepatitis

Eugene R. Schiff

1. INTRODUCTION

Hepatic vein thrombosis, veno-occlusive disease, and ischemic hepatitis (shock liver) all produce pathologic changes in zone 3 of the hepatic lobules. Obstruction of the major outflow tracts of the liver will readily lead to congestion of the central veins and, if severe enough, hemorrhagic necrosis will ensue. Endothelial injury to the smaller hepatic venules will result in a similar centrilobular injury. Finally, any compromise of the delivery of oxygen to the liver as occurs in ischemic hepatitis can be anticipated to preferentially injure those hepatocytes that are the last to receive oxygen; zone 3 of the lobule. It is altogether fitting that this trio of centrilobular vascular disorders be included in this volume honoring Hyman Zimmerman. Indeed Dr. Zimmerman and his colleagues have provided the largest review on the management of oral contraceptive induced hepatic vein thrombosis.[1]

2. HEPATIC VEIN THROMBOSIS

Budd–Chiari syndrome or hepatic vein thrombosis is a relatively uncommon entity, but it is important to recognize because of newer treatment modalities that may alter an otherwise fatal course. The most common causes (Table I) are myeloproliferative disorders, paroxysmal nocturnal hemoglobinuria, oral contraceptives, malignancies (particularly hepatocellular carcinoma), liver abscesses, and membranous webs in the inferior vena cava. At least 30 percent of patients with this syndrome have no established cause. However, an increasing number of reports have demonstrated a thrombotic predisposition among patients with hepatic vein thrombosis of unknown etiology.

Valla et al.[2] cultured the bone marrow or peripheral blood mononuclear cells in 20 patients with Budd–Chiari syndrome. Erythroid colony formation was seen in 16 patients, yet the conventional criteria for the diagnosis of a primary myeloproliferative disorder were met in only two cases. These results suggest that a primary myeloproliferative disorder is a more common cause of the Budd–Chiari syndrome than was previously established. Thirteen of the patients were female, but only four had used oral contraceptives up to the onset of the hepatic vein thrombosis. Whether the

Eugene R. Schiff • Division of Hepatology, University of Miami School of Medicine; Hepatology Section, Veterans Administration Medical Center, Miami, Florida 33125.

Table I. Etiologic Factors in Patients with Hepatic Vein Thrombosis[a]

Idiopathic
Hematologic disorders
Polycythemia rubra vera
Paroxysmal nocturnal hemoglobinuria
Other myeloproliferative disorders
Lupus anticoagulant, antithrombin III deficiency
Oral contraceptives
Pregnancy and postpartum
Tumors
Hepatocellular carcinoma
Renal cell carcinoma
Adrenal carcinoma
Leiomyosarcoma of the inferior vena cava
Angiosarcoma of the right atrium
Epithelioid hemangioendothelioma
Infections
Amebic abscess
Pyogenic liver abscesses
Aspergillosis
Hydatid cyst
Syphilis
Vasculitis
Behçet disease
Conditions of uncertain relevance
Ulcerative colitis
Nephrotic syndrome
Caroli disease
Sarcoidosis
Miscellaneous
Membranous webs in inferior vena cava
Congenital narrowing of inferior vena cava
Trauma

[a]Modified from Maddrey.[41]

oral contraceptives have further stimulated an underlying thrombogenic potential is not clear. Lupus anticoagulant and antiphospholipid antibodies have also been found among patients with hepatic vein thrombosis.[3,4] It can be anticipated that future studies will uncover cases with protein C and protein S deficiencies, known thrombogenic disorders.

The mechanism of polycythemia associated with Budd–Chiari syndrome is unknown. Levy et al.[5] determined serum erythropoietin levels and cultured bone marrow specimens for erythroid progenitors in ten patients with Budd–Chiari syndrome. Their results suggest that in some cases of Budd–Chiari syndrome the polycythemia seen acutely resolves and may be secondary to the liver disease rather than the cause of the hepatic vein thrombosis. The lupus anticoagulant interferes with the phospholipid fraction of the prothrombin activator complex. The presence of antiphospholipid antibodies is strongly associated with the lupus anticoagulant. Fibrous webs across the inferior vena cava at or just above the entrance of the hepatic veins can lead to hepatic vein thrombosis.[6,7] This lesion is more commonly found in South Africa and the Orient, but has been described in the United States. It has been proposed that the membranous web results from a defect in the closure of the ductus venosus.

2.1. Clinical Picture

Typically the patient will present with either an acute or insidious onset of ascites associated with abdominal pain and hepatomegaly. The pain is related both to stretching of the liver capsule and abdominal distension from ascites. Marked leg edema and prominent venous patterns over the abdomen and back are suspicious of inferior vena cava obstruction along with the hepatic vein thrombosis. Jaundice is uncommon except when there has been severe centrilobular necrosis which may lead to a clinical picture of fulminant hepatic failure. In some cases, the hepatorenal syndrome ensues. Splenomegaly may be difficult to detect on physical examination because of massive ascites but, if present, is a reflection of portal hypertension and/or an underlying myeloproliferative disease. The liver chemical profile is not very helpful and certainly is not characteristic. The alkaline phosphatase is invariably elevated and serum aminotransferases are slightly increased, generally less than twice normal.[6] Paracentesis, although occasionally bloody, is not characteristic. The protein concentration is quite variable but averages approximately 2g/dl.[7]

2.2. Diagnostic Methods

There are three important diagnostic steps: imaging of the liver, liver biopsy, and hepatic angiography. The sulfur-colloid scan may be characteristic in about 40% of patients when there is a markedly increased uptake in an enlarged caudate lobe, in contrast to a relatively decreased uptake in the rest of the liver.[8–10] This hot spot is thought to result from an engorgement of the caudate lobe, which drains into the inferior vena cava through venous branches independent of the main hepatic veins. Intrahepatic venous abnormalities may be visualized by ultrasound, computed tomography (CT), and magnetic resonance imaging (MRI).[8,11] Hepatic venous abnormalities without nodularity of the hepatic parenchyma and the presence of comma-shaped intrahepatic varices are characteristic of the Budd–Chiari syndrome.[12] Thrombosis of the inferior vena cava and/or portal vein may further complicate Budd–Chiari syndrome and should be looked for at the time of scanning. Doppler sonography may also be a useful screening method to determine the patency of vessels and the direction of blood flow.

Liver biopsy will be characteristic and, because of the associated ascites, is best performed by laparoscopy. The gross appearance of the liver is swollen, blunt edged, and reddish purple. Microscopically, there is severe centrilobular congestion and extravasation of red cells into the space of Disse. Cell atrophy and necrosis secondary to local ischemia are often present.

Hepatic angiography is critical in establishing the diagnosis and the presence of additional vascular involvement and in planning therapy. Arteriography demonstrates an enlarged liver with stretching and bowing of the hepatic arteries. Corkscrewing of the branches of the hepatic artery is indicative of underlying cirrhosis and may be helpful in the differential diagnosis as well as assessing the progression of the disease. Retrograde flow into portal veins occurs as a result of the hepatic venous block. Wedged hepatic venography, if possible, will demonstrate a classic and characteristic spider web pattern; however, there may be an inability to fill or catheterize the hepatic veins. At venography, the inferior vena cava will be visualized, and it is imperative to search for the presence of a membranous web, thrombosis, or extrinsic compression. Pressure gradients should be determined particularly if there is partial occlusion of the inferior vena cava to access the feasibility of decompressive shunting procedures.

2.3. Prognosis

Until recently, the course of Budd–Chiari syndrome was almost universally characterized by progressive deterioration, with most patients dying within 3 years of the onset of the illness. Gupta et al.[13] (Fig. 1) studied 18 patients over a 20-year period. Although eight patients died within the first 3 years, nearly 50% were alive after 5 years. The presence of bleeding esophageal varices was

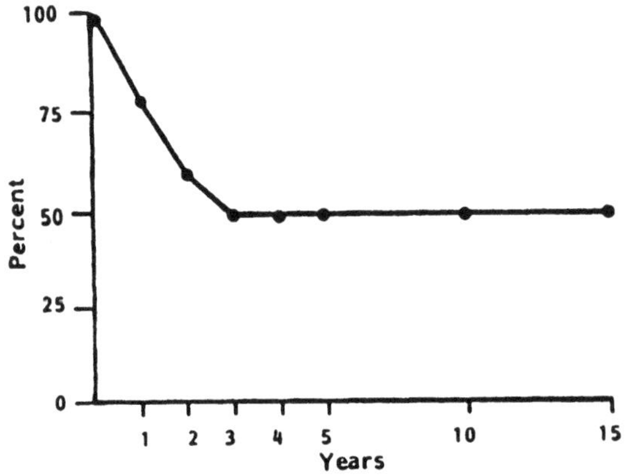

Figure 1. Budd–Chiari syndrome. Actuarial survival based on life-table analysis showing the pattern of mortality. (From Gupta et al.[13])

indicative of a poor prognosis. Patients with functioning intrahepatic collaterals demonstrated angiographically had the best prognosis.

2.4. Medical Therapy

Medical management initially includes measures directed at amelioration of the ascites. Diuretics and therapeutic paracentesis will control the ascites but, unless there is definitive therapy to relieve the hepatic venous outflow block, or spontaneous resolution of the illness evolves, the ascites may become refractory and peritoneovenous shunting may be necessary. Anticoagulants are unlikely to bring about lysis of the thrombi but may prevent further propagation of the clots. Thrombolytic therapy is fraught with complications of hemorrhage, however, would seem to be indicated in patients with acute hepatic vein thrombosis. Streptokinase and urokinase have been used successfully in some patients.[14] Percutaneous transluminal angioplasty has been successfully employed in the treatment of membranous obstruction of the inferior vena cava and hepatic veins.[15] In 14 cases in which this technique was successfully carried out, no serious complications were reported; however, reocclusion occurred in six patients, necessitating repeat angioplasty. Successful angioplasty has been followed by resolution of clinical symptoms. Fururi et al.[16] had successfully treated three cases of hepatic inferior vena cava obstruction associated with Budd–Chiari syndrome with percutaneous transluminal angioplasty, using a laser. The occluded areas were canalized with the laser and were further widened by simultaneous inflation of balloon catheters.

2.5. Surgical Therapy

In an attempt to decompress the congested liver, several types of shunting procedures have been tried.[17–19] Side-to-side portacaval and mesocaval shunts are among the more popular procedures employed in hepatic vein thrombosis.[20] For these types of central shunts to succeed, the inferior vena cava must be patent above the caval anastomosis, and there must be a favorable pressure gradient within the vena cava. Extrinsic compression of the cava by an enlarged caudate lobe will impede decompression by the shunt by raising the venous pressure proximal to the occlusion. In such cases, a mesoatrial shunt is preferred; however, there is limited experience with mesoatrial shunts, and thrombosis of the prosthetic grafts is likely to occur.[21] Nevertheless, initially a mesoatrial shunt may successfully decompress the liver and provide an opportunity to replace this shunt with a portacaval shunt that is less likely to occlude.

Bansky et al.[22] described and successfully used a dorsocranial liver resection and direct hepatoatrial anastomosis in seven patients. After establishing a partial cardiopulmonary bypass the lower part of the right atrium and the vena cava are opened by longitudinal incision continued into the intrahepatic portion of the vena cava. Thrombotic material is removed, and a wedge resection of the dorsocranial aspect of the liver including the confluence of the occluded hepatic veins is carried out. The vena cava and the right atrium are then sutured around the resected area to the liver capsule. One intraoperative death occurred, but in five patients the liver size returned to normal and ascites disappeared. A patent anastomosis has been demonstrated in the six surviving patients. In contrast to portacaval shunts, the hepatoatrial anastomosis can be performed regardless of the patency of the inferior vena cava.

In patients with membranous webs of the inferior vena cava, such approaches as surgical resection of the membrane under cardiopulmonary bypass, the use of bypass grafts, and transcardiac membranotomy have all been successful.[23] Finally, orthotopic liver transplantation has been successful in the treatment of hepatic vein thrombosis. Lerut et al.[29] reviewed their experience in 13 consecutive recipients of orthotopic liver grafts. Six of these patients were women with Budd–Chiari syndrome. Five achieved a prolonged survival with liver transplantation and only one had recurrence of the disease. Three were reported to be alive 2–6 years after the transplant was performed. The decision for liver transplantation is a difficult one, since some patients will spontaneously resolve. Extensive thrombosis of the hepatic veins resulting in a clinical picture of fulminant hepatic failure will most likely require liver transplantation to achieve survival, but this may be impossible to accomplish in a timely manner.

Whether medical or surgical therapy is used in Budd–Chiari syndrome, an attempt must be made to control or decrease the thrombogenic phenomenon that led to the hepatic vein thrombosis. In conclusion, Budd–Chiari syndrome can be more readily recognized by newer imaging techniques, and both medical and surgical therapy has provided a better prognosis for what was previously considered a universally terminal disease.

3. VENO-OCCLUSIVE DISEASE

Bush tea disease was described in Jamaica among people who took pyrrolizidine alkaloids derived from species of *Senecio* and *Crotolaria* used for medicinal or beverage purposes. This disorder has been observed in other parts of the world and was more recently described in four Chinese women who took an herbal tea for treatment of psoriasis.[25] Liver biopsy in all four cases confirmed hepatic veno-occlusive disease. The herbal medicine contained pyrrolizidine alkaloids of the *Senecio* species.

The primary pathologic changes are seen in the central and sublobular hepatic veins. Partial or complete occlusion of the terminal hepatic veins results from intimal thickening. Initially, there is fluid accumulation in the intima as well as extravasation of erythrocytes. Later collagen deposition in the intima takes place. In the United States, the most common cause of veno-occlusive disease is bone marrow transplantation.[26] This may be a result of radiation therapy and/or chemotherapy. Drugs that have been associated with the development of veno-occlusive disease are azathioprine, urethane, thioguanine, dacarbazine, busulfan, and dimethylbusulfan.[27,28] The incidence of hepatic veno-occlusive disease after bone marrow transplantation is as high as 20% with a mortality rate of up to 50%. Dulley et al.[29] suggested that the use of methotrexate and/or cylosporin contributes to the development of veno-occlusive disease after chemoradiation therapy. It has been proposed that the pathogenesis of veno-occlusive disease involves an initial injury to the endothelium of the central veins and/or sinusoids, triggering a coagulation cascade in the periadventitial zone of the central venules. Read et al.[30] described four renal transplant patients in whom hepatic veno-occlusive disease developed after immunosuppressive therapy with azathioprine. Veno-occlusive disease has been responsible for deaths among captive cheetahs.[31] Analysis of the commercial feline diet demonstrated large amounts of two vital estrogens identified as daidezein and genistein. These compounds were derived from a soybean product that was included in the cheetah diet and were thought to be responsible for the development of the veno-occlusive disease.

The clinical picture of veno-occlusive disease is similar to that of Budd–Chiari syndrome.[32] Patients develop ascites, abdominal pain, and hepatomegaly; however, jaundice is more likely to be present. The veno-occlusion may be progressive and lead to massive hepatocelluar necrosis. Therapy is primarily supportive in bone marrow transplant patients; however, side to side portacaval shunts have been successfully performed.[33] Epitheloid haemangioendothelioma, a rare malignancy, may mimic the clinical picture of veno-occlusive disease.[36]

4. ISCHEMIC HEPATITIS

Shock liver or ischemic hepatitis occurs as a result of decreased hepatic perfusion, leading to cellular anoxia and necrosis. The clinical syndrome is characterized by an abrupt elevation of the aminotransferases followed by resolution within 7–10 days.[35,36] The often striking elevation of the serum transaminases may mimic viral hepatitis. The syndrome is most often described in patients predisposed to sudden hypotension. This group includes those with myocardial infarcts, cardiac failure, arrhythmias, sepsis, cerebrovascular accidents (CVA), renal failure, and chronic obstructive pulmonary disease (COPD). There may be a transient rise in serum bilirubin and alkaline phosphatase levels as well as prolongation of the prothrombin time following the initial peak in serum aminotransferases. Systemic hypotension may not always be documented. Profound cardiogenic shock as occurs in cardiac arrest may result in severe centrilobular necrosis and a clinical presentation of fulminant hepatic failure. Gibson and Dudley[37] described 19 episodes of ischemic hepatitis, all of which occurred in high-risk patients, but only five episodes were associated with documented hypotension. Liver biopsy findings of centrilobular necrosis, and often passive congestion, are readily distinguishable from a viral etiology. The elevation of the serum aminotransferases correlates best with the presence of centrilobular necrosis. When there is congestion alone, there may be normal or minimal elevation in the aminotransferases. Lefkowitch and Mendez[38] examined 140 postmortem liver biopsies from patients with cardiac disease or preterminal hypotensive shock. Congestion with necrosis was present in 77% of specimens.

Reactive oxygen intermediates are thought to play an important pathogenic role in ischemic liver injury.[39] It has been hypothesized that oxygen supplied during ischemia is insufficient to maintain ATP production and, as a consequence, there is an inability to maintain normal cellular ionic gradients.[40] Intracellular calcium concentration rises and promotes the generation of xanthine oxidase. On reperfusion of the ischemic tissue xanthine oxidase gives rise to a series of metabolic steps. This leads to the formation of large quantities of superoxide, overwhelming the cellular protective mechanisms and promoting cell injury. Nevertheless, the association between hepatocellular injury and oxygen-derived free radicals is largely circumstantial.

Most cases of ischemic hepatitis are self-limited and not associated with liver failure. They should readily be distinguished from viral or drug-induced hepatitis, and no specific therapy should be given. The prognosis is primarily related to the underlying cardiopulmonary disorder. Liver biopsy may be necessary, particularly in patients who are candidates for liver transplantation or who are receiving potentially hepatotoxic drugs, such as amiodarone.

5. CONCLUSION

Although the three entities described—hepatic vein thrombosis, veno-occlusive disease, and ischemic hepatitis—are all pathologic processes involving the terminal hepatic venules and centrilobular regions of the liver, they are distinct entities that have different etiologies. Severe forms may all result in fulminant hepatic failure. Medical therapy is largely supportive in hepatic vein thrombosis and veno-occlusive disease but may be all that is necessary if spontaneous resolution occurs, particularly in hepatic vein thrombosis. Surgical therapy, including decompressive shunts and liver transplantation, are used primarily in hepatic vein thrombosis, although a side-to-side portacaval shunt may be helpful in selected cases with veno-occlusive disease. Patients with veno-occlusive disease who do not have an underlying malignancy and who are suitable candidates, e.g., those with bush tea disease, may respond favorably to liver transplantation. Finally, an awareness of the entity of ischemic hepatitis should avoid confusion with drug-induced and viral hepatitis.

REFERENCES

1. Lewis JH, Tice HL, Zimmerman HJ: Budd–Chiari syndrome associated with oral contraceptive steroids. A review of treatment of 47 cases. *Dig Dis Sci* **28:**673–682, 1983.
2. Valla D, Casadevall N, Lacombe C, et al: Primary myeloproliferative disorder and hepatic vein thrombosis. *Ann Intern Med* **103:**329–334, 1985.
3. Steenbergen WV, Beyls J, Vermylen J, et al: "Lupus" anticoagulant and thrombosis of the hepatic veins (Budd–Chiari syndrome). *J Hepatol* **3:**87–94, 1986.
4. Mackworth-Young CG, Melia WM, Harris EN, et al: The Budd–Chiari syndrome. Possible pathogenetic role of anti-phospholipid antibodies. *J Hepatol* **3:**83–86, 1986.
5. Levy VG, Ruskone A, Baillou C, et al: Polycythemia and the Budd–Chiari syndrome study of serum erythropoietin and bone marrow erythroid progenitors. *Hepatology* **5:**858–861, 1985.
6. Mitchell MC, Boitnott, JK, Kaufman S, et al: Budd–Chiari syndrome: Etiology, diagnosis and management. *Medicine (Baltimore)* **61:**199–218, 1982.
7. Reynolds TB: Budd–Chiari syndrome, in Schiff L, Schiff E (eds): *Diseases of the Liver,* 6th ed. JB Lippincott, Philadelphia, 1987, pp. 1466–1477.
8. Friedman AC, Ramchandani P, Black M, et al: Magnetic resonance imaging diagnosis of Budd–Chiari syndrome. *Gastroenterology* **91:**1289–1295, 1986.
9. Gupta S, Barter S, Phillips GW, et al: Comparison of ultrasonography, computed tomography and 99mTc liver scan in diagnosis of Budd–Chiari syndrome. *Gut* **28:**242–247, 1987.
10. Picard M, Carrier L, Chartrand R, et al: Budd–Chiari syndrome: Typical and atypical scintigraphic aspects. *J Nucl Med* **28:**803–809, 1987.
11. Mathieu D, Vasile N, Menu Y, et al: Budd–Chiari syndrome: Dynamic CT. *Radiology* **165:**409–413, 1987.
12. Stark DD, Hahn PF, Trey C, et al: MRI of the Budd–Chiari syndrome. *AJR* **146:**1141–1148, 1986.
13. Gupta S, Blumgart LH, Hodgson JHF: Budd–Chiari syndrome: Long-term survival and factors affecting mortality. *Q J Med* **232:**781–791, 1986.
14. Sholar PW, Bell WR: Thrombolytic therapy for inferior vena cava thrombosis in paroxysmal nocturnal hemoglobinuria. *Ann Intern Med* **103:**539–541, 1985.
15. Sparano J, Chang J, Trasi S, et al: Treatment of the Budd–Chiari syndrome with percutaneous transluminal angioplasty. *Am J Med* **82:**8821–8828, 1987.
16. Fururi S, Yamauchi T, Ohtomo K, et al: Hepatic inferior vena cava obstructions: Clinical results of treatment with percutaneous transluminal laser-assisted angioplasty. *Radiology* **166:**673–677, 1988.
17. Ahn SS, Yellin A, Sheng FC, et al: Selective surgical therapy of the Budd–Chiari syndrome provides superior survivor rates than conservative medical management. *J Vasc Surg* **5:**28–37, 1987.
18. McCarthy PM, va Heerden JA, Adson MA, et al: The Budd–Chiari syndrome. Medical and surgical management of 30 patients. *Arch Surg* **120:**657–662, 1985.
19. Vons C, Bourstyn E, Bonnet P, et al: Results of Portal systemic shunts in Budd–Chiari syndrome. *Ann Surg* **203:**366–370, 1986.
20. Sarr MG, Herlong HF, Cameron JL: Long-term patency of the mesocaval C shunt. *Am J Surg* **151:**98–103, 1986.
21. Chezmar JL, Bernardino ME: Mesoatrial shunt for the treatment of Budd–Chiari syndrome: Radiologic evaluation in eight patients. *AJR* **149:**707–710, 1987.
22. Bansky G, Ernest C, Jenni R, et al: Treatment of Budd–Chiari syndrome by dorsocranial liver resection and direct hepatoatrial anastomosis. *J Hepatol* **2:**101–112, 1986.
23. Rector WG, Xu Y, Goldstein L, et al. Membranous obstruction of the inferior vena cava in the United States. *Medicine (Baltimore)* **2:**134–143, 1985.
24. Lerut J, Tzakis AG, Bron K, et al: Complications of venous reconstruction in human orthotopic liver transplantation. *Ann Surg* **205:**404–414, 1987.

25. Kumana CR, Ng M, Hsiang JL, et al: Hepatic veno-occlusive disease due to toxic alkaloid in herbal tea. *Lancet* **2**:1360–1361, 1983.
26. Shulman HM, Gown AM, Nugent DJ: Hepatic veno-occlusive disease after bone marrow transplantation. Immunohistochemical identification of the material within occluded central venules. *Am J Pathol* **127**:549–558, 1987.
27. Zimmerman HJ, Maddrey WC: Toxic and drug-induced hepatitis, in Schiff L, Schiff E (eds): *Diseases of the Liver*. JB Lippincott, Philadelphia, 1987, pp. 591–667.
28. Doll DC, Ringenberg QS, Yarbro JW: Vascular toxicity associated with antineoplastic agents. *J Clin Oncol* **4**:1405–1417, 1986.
29. Dulley FL, Kanfer EJ, Appelbaum FR, et al: Venocclusive disease of the liver after chemoradiotherapy and autologous bone marrow transplantation. *Transplantation* **43**:870–873, 1987.
30. Read AE, Wiesner RH, LaBrecque DR, et al: Hepatic veno-occlusive disease associated with renal transplantation and azathioprine therapy. *Ann Intern Med* **104**:651–655, 1986.
31. Setchell KD, Gosselin SJ, Welsh MB, et al: Dietary estrogens—A probable cause of infertility and liver disease in captive cheetahs. *Gastroenterology* **93**:225–233, 1987.
32. Rollins BJ: Hepatic veno-occlusive disease. *Am J Med* **81**:297–306, 1986.
33. Murray JA, LaBrecque DR, Gingrich RD, et al: Successful treatment of hepatic veno-occlusive disease in a bone marrow transplant patient with side-to-side portacaval shunt. *Gastroenterology* **92**:1073–1077, 1987.
34. Clements D, Hubscher S, West R, et al: Epitheloid heamangioendothelioma. *J Hepatol* **2**:441–449, 1986.
35. Rawson JS, Achord JL: Shock liver. *South Med J* **78**:1421–1425, 1985.
36. Bynum TE, Boitnott JK, Maddrey WC: Ischemic hepatitis. *Dig Dis Sci* **24**:129–135, 1979.
37. Gibson PR, Dudley FJ: Ischemic hepatitis: Clinical features, diagnosis and prognosis. *Aust NZ J Med* **14**:822–825, 1984.
38. Lefkowitch JH, Mendez L: Morphologic features of hepatic injury in cardiac disease and shock. *J Hepatol* **2**:313–327, 1986.
39. Adkison D, Hollwarth ME, Benoit JN, et al: Role of free radicals in ischemia-reperfusion injury to the liver. *Acta Physiol Scand* **548**(suppl):101–107, 1986.
40. Arthur MJP: Reactive oxygen intermediates and liver injury. *J Hepatol* **6**:125–131, 1988.
41. Maddrey WC: Hepatic vein thrombosis (Budd–Chiari syndrome): Possible association with the use of oral contraceptives. *Semin Liver Dis* **7**:32–39, 1987.

29

Budd–Chiari Syndrome: Pathology

Kamal G. Ishak

1. ETIOLOGY AND PATHOGENESIS

Budd–Chiari syndrome (BCS) is a rare condition resulting from obstruction to the outflow of blood from the liver. It is characterized clinically by hepatomegaly, splenomegaly, right upper quadrant (RUQ) abdominal pain, and ascites.[1–16] Most patients have an acute onset, but occasionally the disorder appears insidiously. BCS is caused by many different conditions and diseases, including membranous webs, veno-occlusive disease (VOD), and hepatic vein thrombosis. Almost one third of cases of hepatic vein thrombosis are idiopathic.[1,5] Well-recognized underlying conditions associated with hepatic vein thrombosis include hematologic disorders, such as polycythemia rubra vera, paroxysmal nocturnal hemoglobinuria, lupus anticoagulant,[6] antithrombosis 3 deficiency,[7] and myeloproliferative disorders, as well as the use of oral contraceptives.[8] Worldwide, the most common cause of hepatic outflow obstruction is membranous obstruction of the inferior vena cava.[9] Cases related to oral contraceptives are discussed by Lewis et al.[10] and Maddrey.[11] In a case-control study from France, the relative risk of hepatic vein thrombosis among recent oral contraceptive users was 2.37, compared with nonusers.[12] The duration of oral contraception prior to development of the syndrome is variable, with a mean of approximately 30 months.[10] The etiopathogenesis of hepatic vein thrombosis in women on oral contraceptives remains undetermined. It has been suggested that oral contraceptives may increase the risk of thrombosis associated with primary myeloproliferative disorders, which was found to be a major cause of hepatic vein thrombosis in young women in one study.[13]

The relationship between polycythemia and BCS is controversial. Some investigators consider BCS a complication of polycythemia rubra vera,[1] while others believe that the polycythemia is secondary to the hepatic vein occlusion.[14] A recent study of serum erythropoietin and bone marrow erythroid progenitors in 10 patients with BCS indicates that, in some cases, the polycythemia (resolved after the acute phase) may be secondary to liver disease.[15]

There is generally little overlap between etiologic factors of hepatic vein thrombosis and VOD. Worldwide, the most common cause of VOD is the consumption of pyrrolizidine alkaloids.[16] Other causes of this lesion have come to include radiation together with consumption of pyrrolizidine alkaloids,[23] aflatoxicosis,[24,25] hypervitaminosis A,[26] urethane,[27,28] 6-thioguanine,[29–33] vincristine

Kamal G. Ishak • Department of Hepatic Pathology, Armed Forces Institute of Pathology, Washington, D.C. 20306-6000. The opinions or assertions contained herein are the private views of the author and are not to be construed as official or as reflecting the views of the Department of the Army or the Department of Defense.

and cytosine arabinoside,[34] 6-mercaptopurine,[35] dacarbazine,[36–38] indicine *N*-oxide,[39] chemoradiation therapy before bone marrow transplantation,[40–48] azathioprine for immunosuppression,[49–52] nitrosamines in experimental animals,[53,54] dietary estrogens in captive cheetahs,[55] and a familial immunodeficiency syndrome.[56] Alcoholic liver disease may be accompanied by VOD, whether due to injury produced by alcohol or contaminants, or as a consequence of the evolving alcoholic hepatopathy.[57–59]

The diagnosis of BCS is suggested by the constellation of clinical findings and radiographic studies. Liver biopsy can be diagnostic but may not be feasible because of coagulation abnormalities and ascites. Scintigraphy, hepatic venography, sonography, computed tomography (CT), and magnetic resonance imaging (MRI) have all been used in the diagnosis.[2–6,60–64]

Medical and surgical therapy for BCS is discussed by numerous groups of investigators.[2–5,8–10,65–68] The prognosis is poor, with most patients dying within several months to 3 years of diagnosis.[8] In the series of 30 patients reported by McCarthy et al.,[67] the overall mortality was 57%; hepatic failure was the most common cause of death. Medical treatment was associated with a worse mortality (86%) than was surgical treatment (31%). In a more recent study by Gupta et al.,[68] the prognosis of 18 patients with BCS studied over a 20-year period was found to be better than in previous studies. Thus, the initial high mortality diminished after the first 3 years, and actuarial analysis of survival showed that nearly 50% of patients were alive after 5 years.[68]

2. HISTOPATHOLOGY

Budd–Chiari syndrome is caused mainly by hepatic vein thrombosis or veno-occlusive disease. Morphologically, the venous lesions are quite different, but the secondary acute and late sequelae are fundamentally quite similar. Excellent pathologic descriptions of hepatic vein thrombosis and VOD were recently reported by Simson[69] and Bras and Brandt.[16]

2.1. Hepatic Vein Thrombosis

Gross inspection of the abdominal cavity in hepatic vein thrombosis shows ascites, hepatomegaly, splenomegaly, and thrombotic occlusion of hepatic veins at their junction with the inferior vena cava. Vena caval and intrahepatic extension is frequent. Sections of the liver reveal the nutmeg pattern of passive congestion, and red or white thrombi are often visible to the naked eye. Microscopically, the cases with a rapidly fatal course show recent thrombi of differing ages, with some having undergone organization and recanalization (Figs. 1–4). Other changes include severe dilation of sinusoids, most pronounced in acinar zone 1, and coagulative ischemic necrosis (Figs. 5–7). In subacute or chronic cases, there may be perisinusoidal fibrosis, central–central fibrous linkage, and even the reversed lobular pattern of congestive cirrhosis. Hemorrhagic infarcts (Fig. 9), calcification, and regeneration may be present. Regeneration begins in residual liver cells in zone 1, with the formation of thick liver plates and nodule formation (Figs. 10 and 11). The nodules gradually enlarge and may coalesce to form adenomatoid configurations (Figs. 12 and 13). One third to one half of all cases of membranous obstruction of the vena cava from Japan[70] and South Africa[71] may be complicated by the development of hepatocellular carcinoma.

2.2. Veno-Occlusive Disease

In VOD, thrombosis is not seen grossly or microscopically, but a nutmeg pattern is evident grossly in the acute stage. The changes, microscopically, are restricted to intrahepatic terminal hepatic venules. Initially, the lumens of the small veins are partially or completely occluded by intimal edema, with intramural extravasation of erythrocytes (Fig. 14). The acute congestion and the coagulative degeneration and necrosis are very similar to those caused by hepatic vein thrombosis. Survival is followed by proliferation of myofibroblasts and collagenization of the thickened

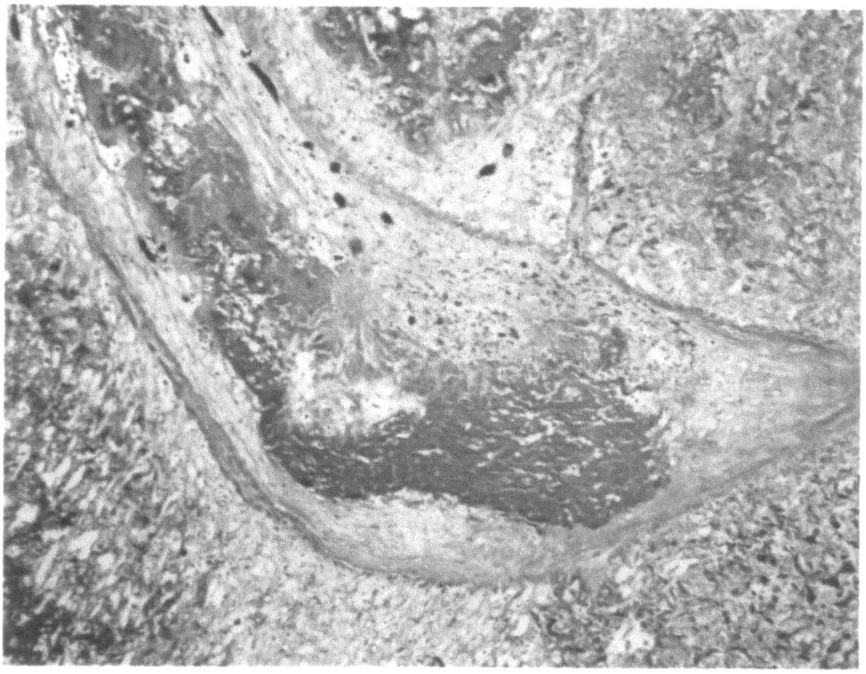

Figure 1. Case of hepatic vein thrombosis associated with lupus anticoagulant. Large intercalated vein is completely occluded by a recent thrombus. (H&E, ×60)

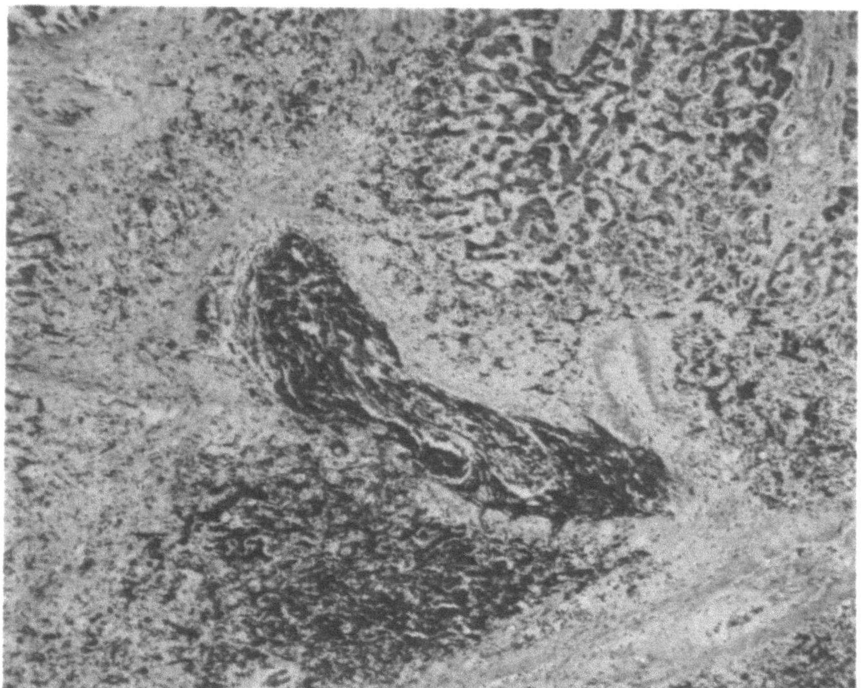

Figure 2. Case of hepatic vein thrombosis associated with long-term use of oral contraceptives. Sausage-shaped vein occupied by a darkly stained recent thrombus. This vessel is a tributary of a larger vein (bottom, right) completely occluded by an old thrombus. (Masson, ×60)

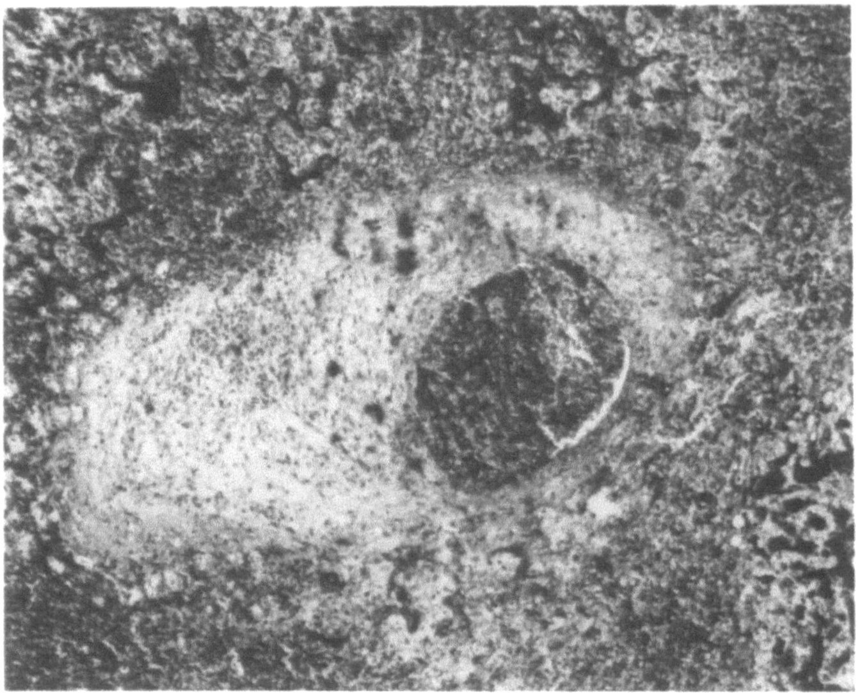

Figure 3. Same case illustrated in Fig. 2, showing terminal hepatic venule obliterated by fibrous tissue. The remaining lumen (right) is occluded by a recent thrombus. (Masson, ×100)

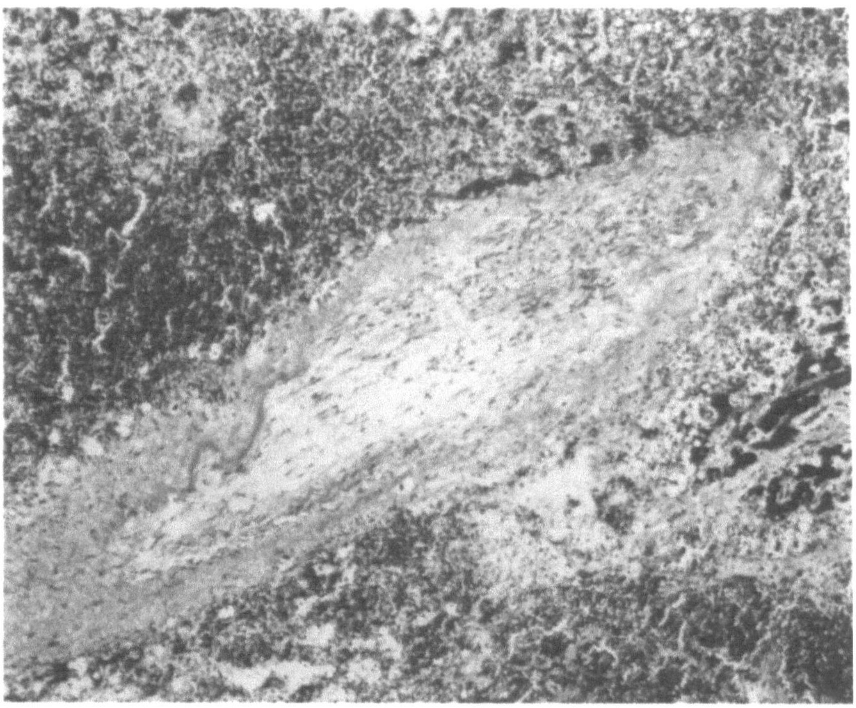

Figure 4. Same case illustrated in Figs. 2 and 3. Terminal hepatic venule completely obliterated by dense fibrous tissue. (Masson, ×100)

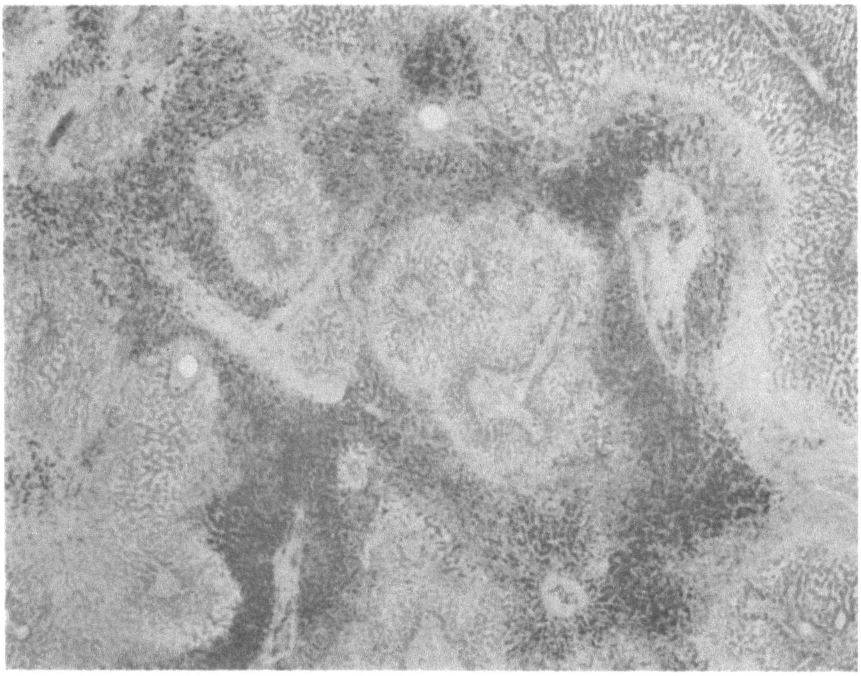

Figure 5. Acute hepatic vein thrombosis resulting in alternating light and dark areas. Darkly stained areas (zones 3 and 2) represent necrosis and intense congestion, while lightly stained areas are the spared zones 1. (H&E, ×25)

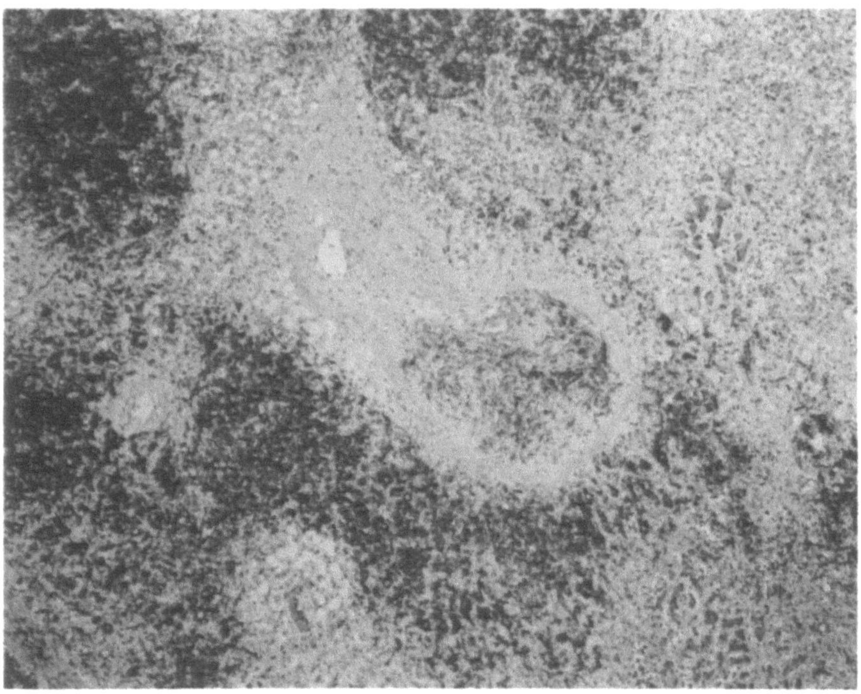

Figure 6. Terminal hepatic venule, completely occluded by a thrombus, surrounded by hemorrhagic necrosis with intense sinusoidal congestion. (H&E, ×60)

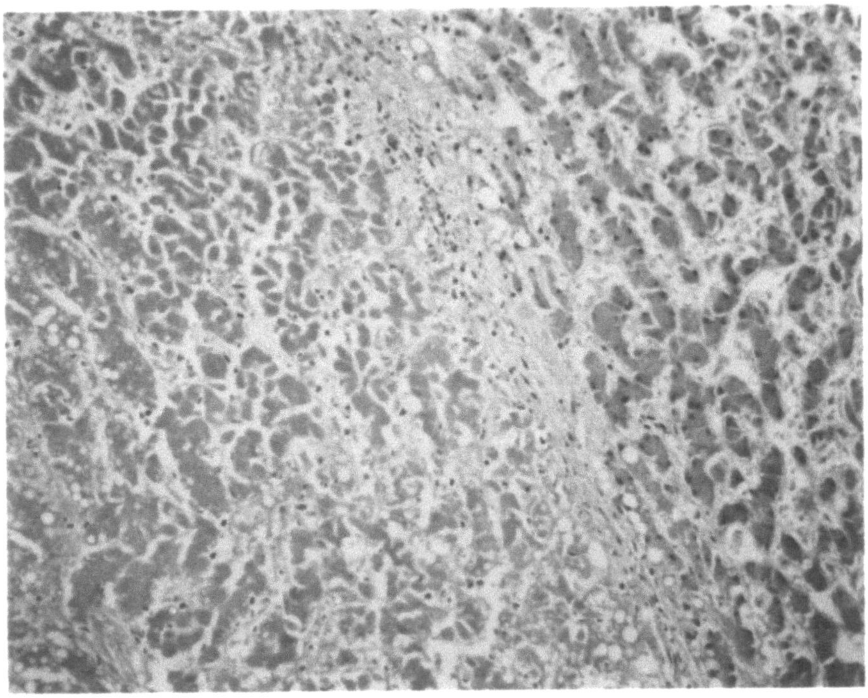

Figure 7. Hepatocytes affected by coagulative necrosis (left two thirds of field) contain no nuclei and have a blurred outline; there is also disruption of the plates. (H&E, ×160)

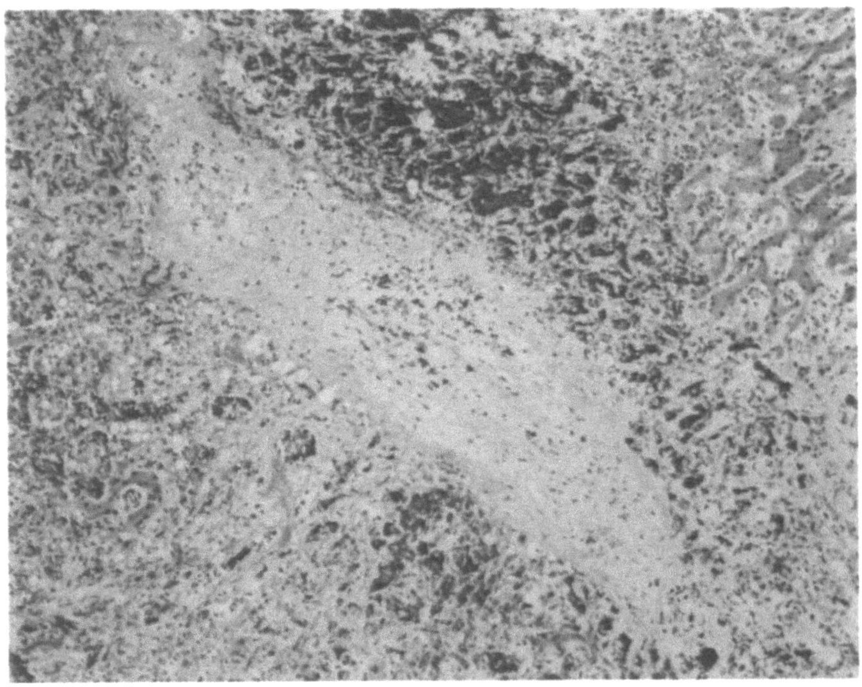

Figure 8. Subacute hepatic vein thrombosis. Fibrotically occluded THV surrounded by sinusoidal dilation, atrophy of liver cell plates and fibrosis. (×100)

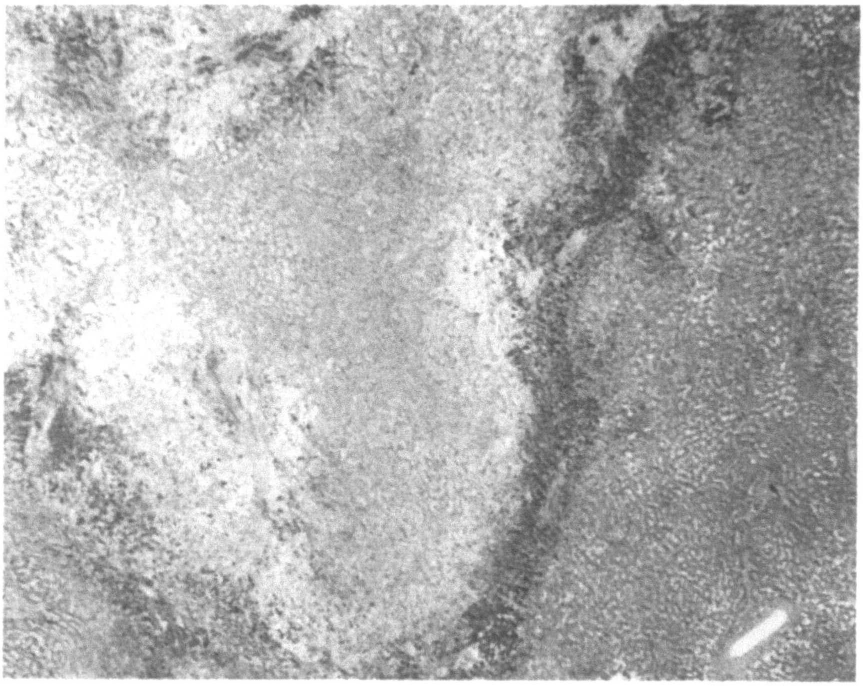

Figure 9. Infarct resulting from hepatic vein occlusion involves multiple contiguous acini. (H&E, ×25)

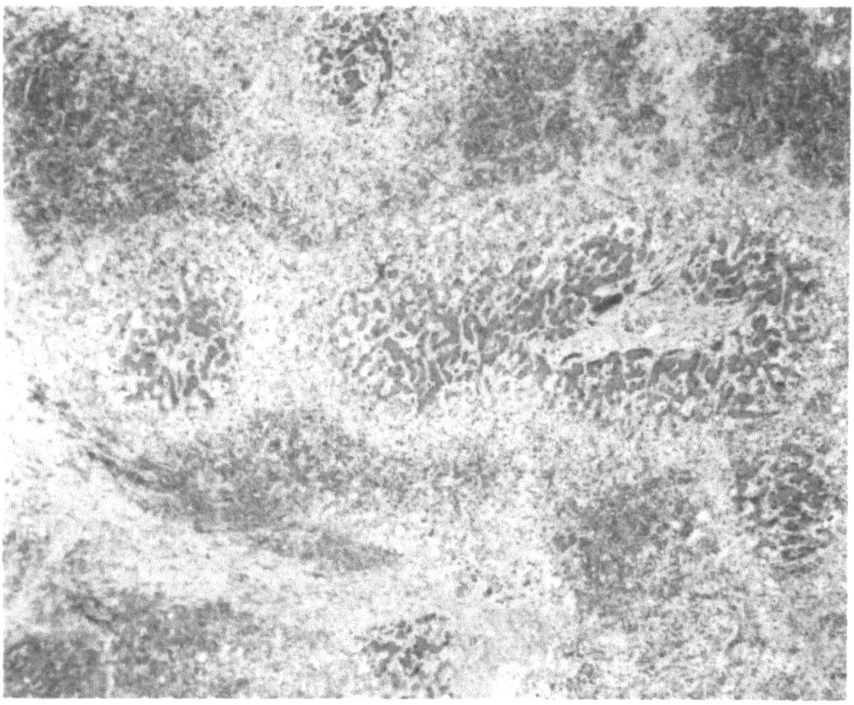

Figure 10. Residual hepatocytes in zone 1 show early regeneration. (H&E, ×60)

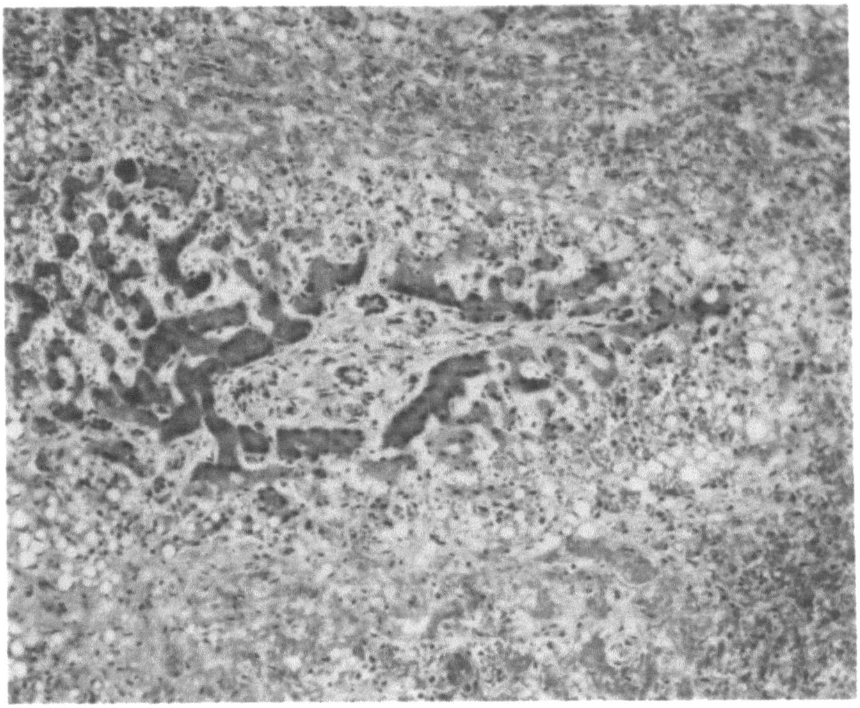

Figure 11. Higher magnification of case illustrated in Fig. 10. Periportal liver plates two cells thick. Note hepatocellular necrosis with dropout in the surrounding parenchyma. (H&E, ×160)

intima (Fig. 15). Small vessels grow into the fibrosed intima, leading to revascularization resembling that of the recanalization of vessels occluded by thrombi. Subacute and chronic cases are associated with fibrosis in spaces of Disse (most prominent in zone 3), sinusoidal dilation, and atrophy of liver cell plates. Thick liver plates are observed in zone 1, but nodular regeneration is infrequently observed.

An etiologic diagnosis of either hepatic vein thrombosis or VOD is not possible on a morphologic basis, with a few exceptions. Cases of hepatic vein thrombosis secondary to infections (e.g., hydatid cyst, amebic abscess) are clearly recognizable if the infectious lesions are aspirated or biopsied. VOD secondary to alcoholic hepatitis[57] is accompanied by perivenular "chicken-wire" fibrosis, Mallory bodies, megamitochondria, and variable degrees of steatosis. VOD lesions are also present in the cirrhotic stage of alcoholic liver disease (Figs. 16 and 17). The diagnosis of hepatic vein thrombosis related to primary or secondary malignancies is also feasible if tumor tissue is biopsied. An example of neoplastic VOD-like lesions characteristic of epithelioid hemangioendothelioma[72] is illustrated in Figs. 18 and 19. Other primary tumors, such as leiomyosarcoma,[73] angiosarcoma,[74] or hepatocellular carcinoma,[75] and secondary tumors, such as renal cell carcinoma, are also recognizable by their characteristic morphology. Both epithelioid hemangioendothelioma and angiosarcoma typically also involve portal vein branches. The neoplastic cells of the former tumor also synthesize factor VIII-related antigen that can be demonstrated in tissue sections by immunohistochemical staining.

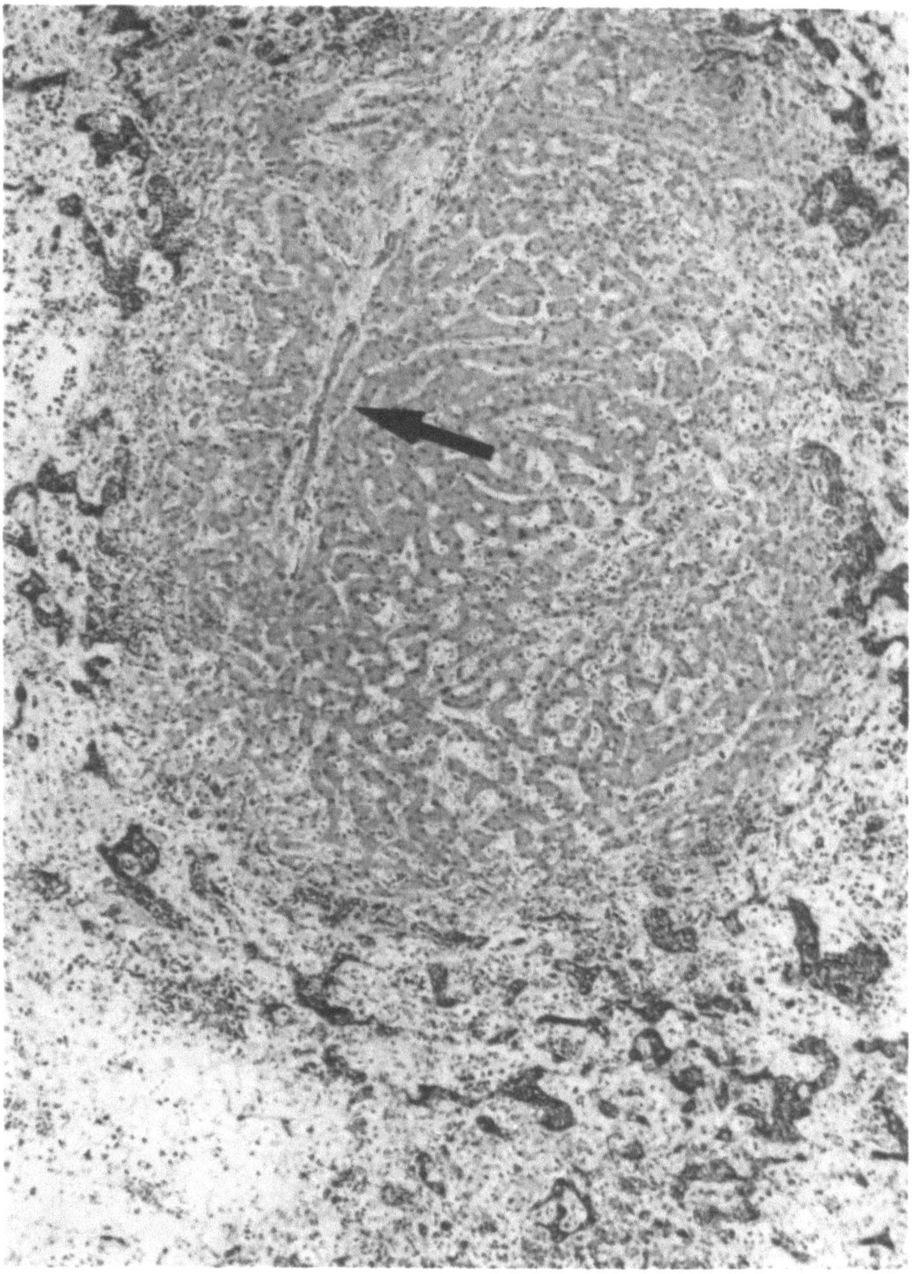

Figure 12. Small regenerative nodule surrounds a portal area (arrow). Surrounding area shows complete loss of liver cells and marked sinusoidal dilation and congestion. (H&E, ×60)

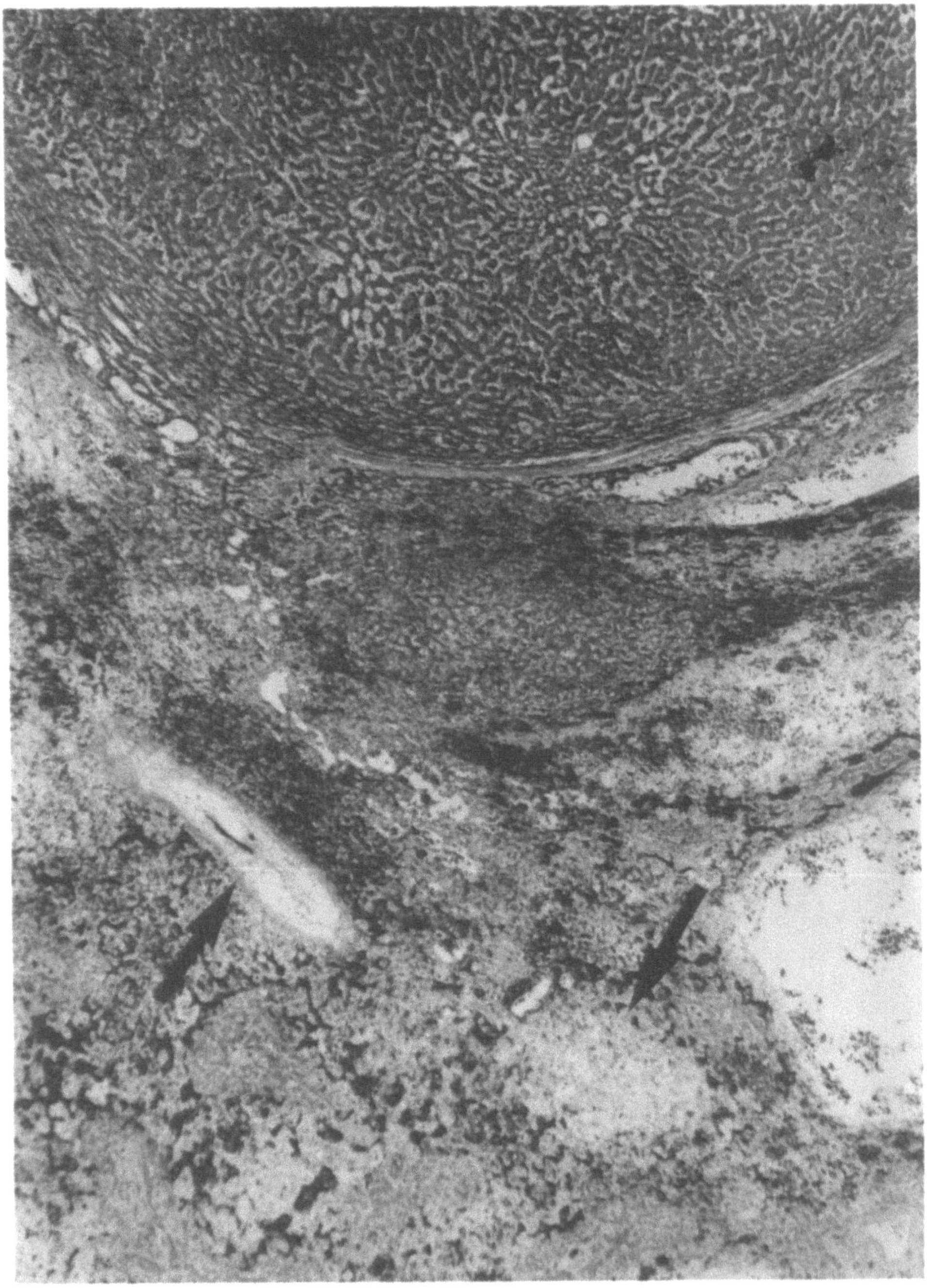

Figure 13. Segment of large adenoma-like regenerative nodule (top). Two occluded veins (arrows) surrounded by collapsed and fibrotic parenchyma, with marked sinusoidal dilation and congestion. (H&E, ×60)

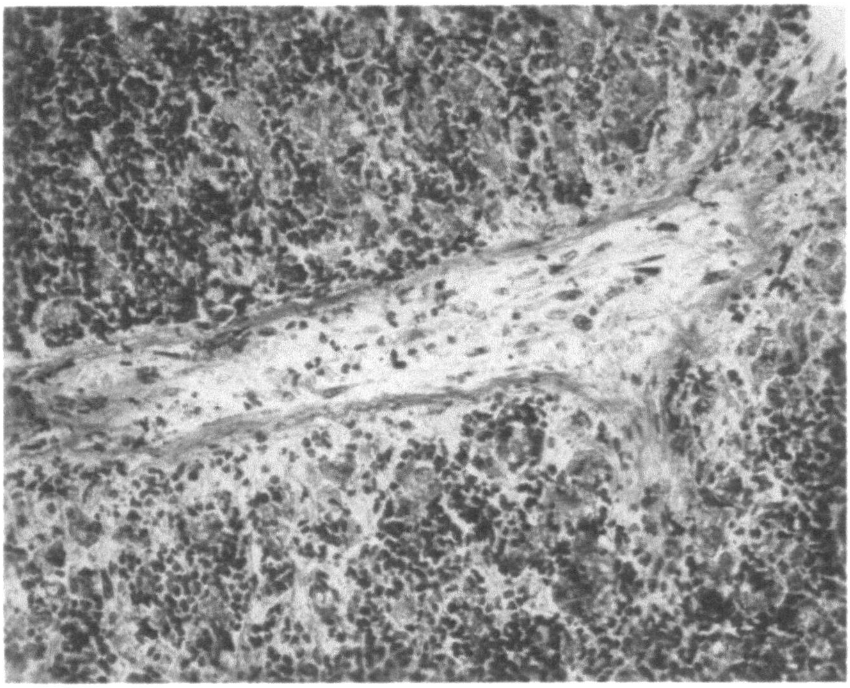

Figure 14. Acute veno-occlusive disease due to *Senecio* toxicity. Terminal hepatic venule completely occluded by an edematous intima in which extravasated erythrocytes are entrapped. Surrounding parenchyma is necrotic. (Masson, ×400)

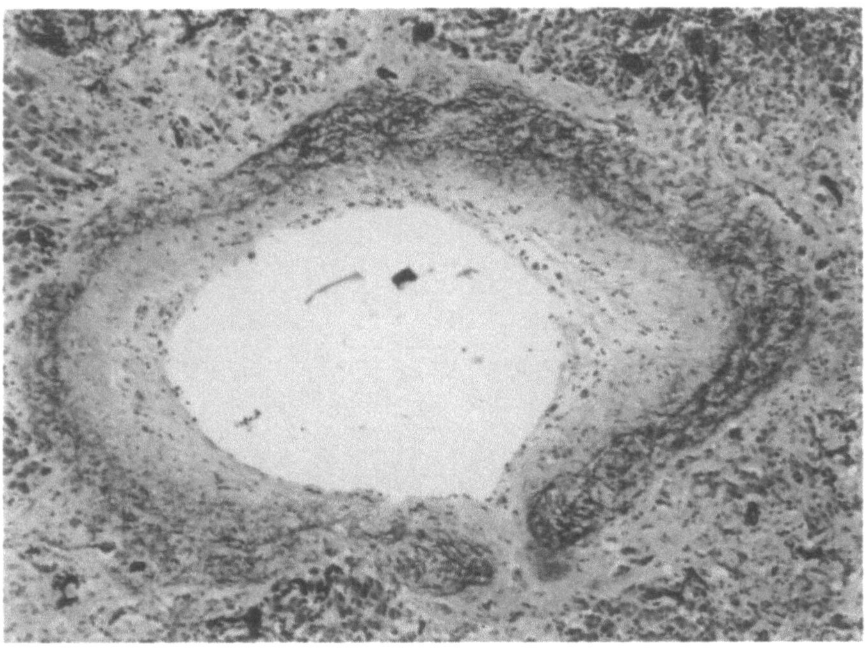

Figure 15. Chronic veno-occlusive disease due to radiation injury. Terminal hepatic venule has a narrowed lumen due to a fibrotically thickened intima. There is also a marked increase in the number of darkly stained elastic fibers. (Movat pentachrome stain, ×100)

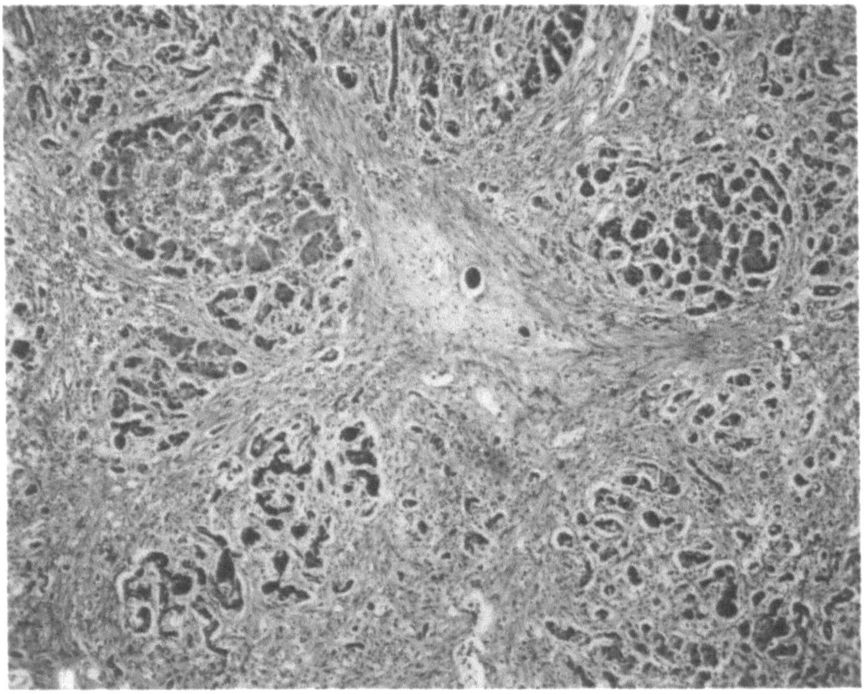

Figure 16. Occluded terminal hepatic venule surrounded by micronodules of alcoholic cirrhosis. (H&E, ×60)

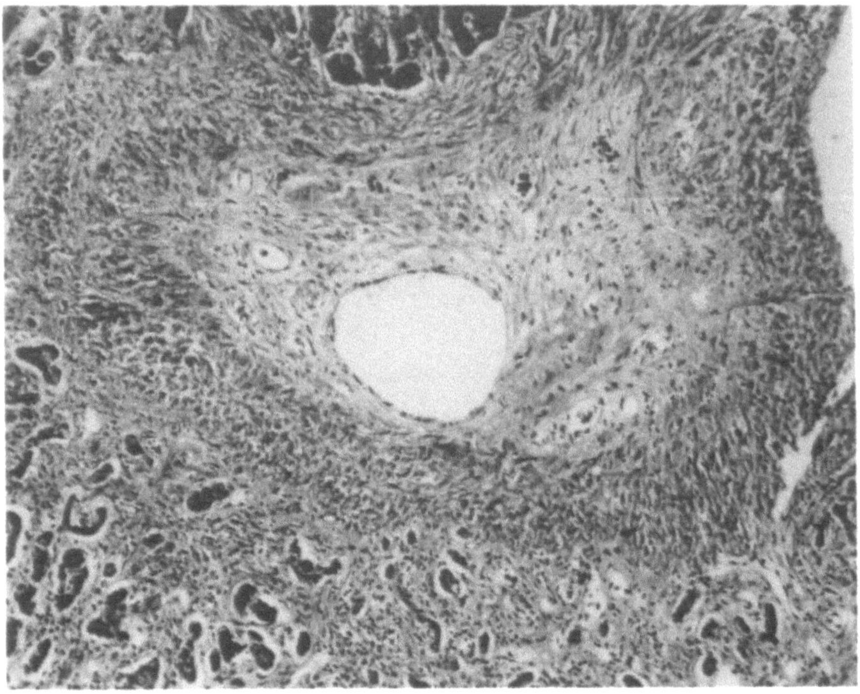

Figure 17. Same case illustrated in Fig. 16. Terminal hepatic venule occluded by fibrous tissue with re canalization. (Masson, ×160)

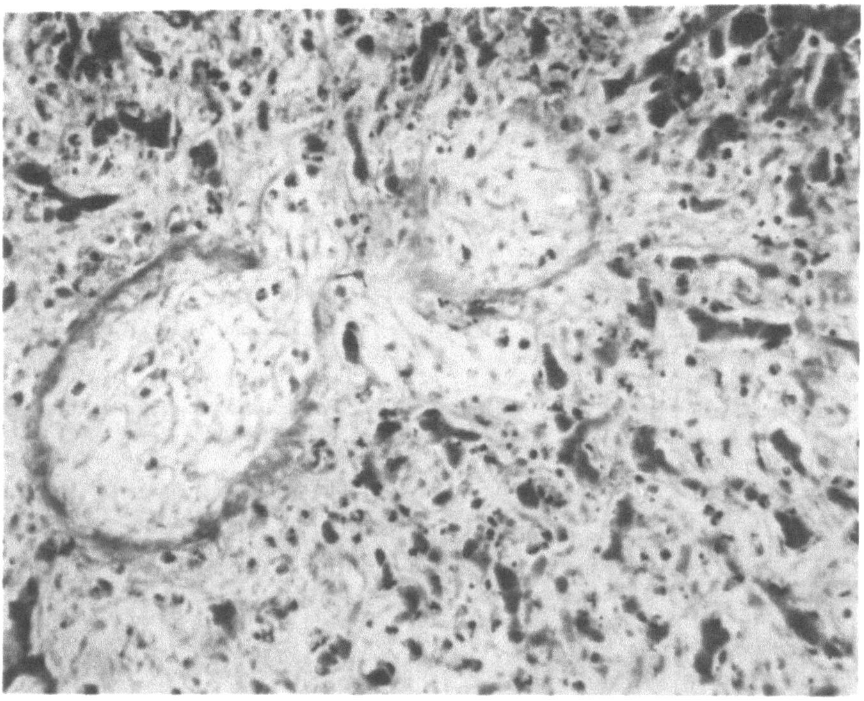

Figure 18. Epithelioid hemangioendothelioma. Terminal venules filled with neoplastic cells. (Masson, ×250)

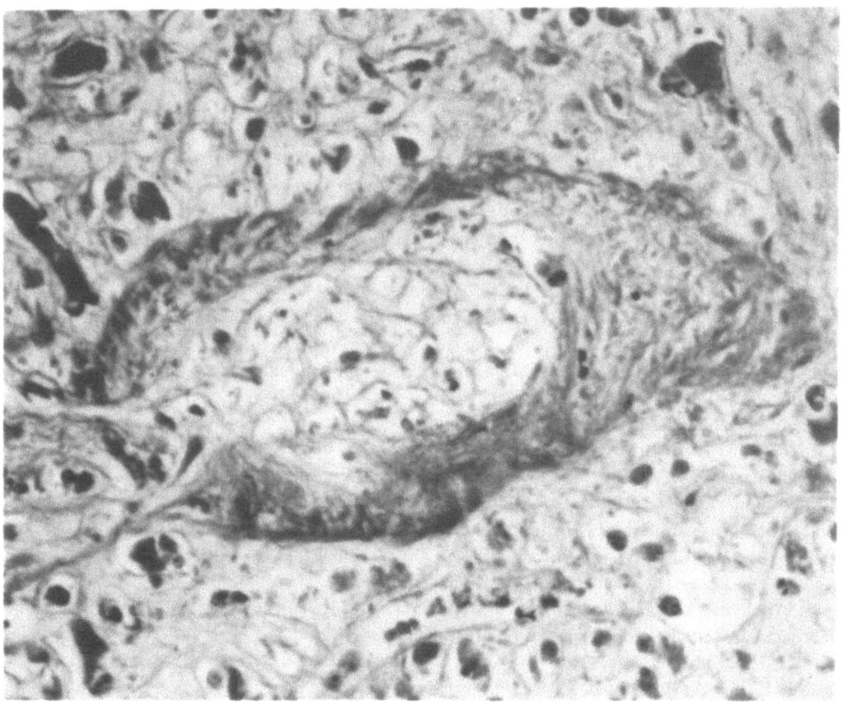

Figure 19. Same case illustrated in Fig. 18. Terminal hepatic venule completely occluded by neoplastic cells. (Masson, ×400)

REFERENCES

1. Parker RGF: Occlusion of the hepatic veins in man. *Medicine (Baltimore)* **38**:369–401, 1959.
2. Clain D, Freston J, Kreel L, et al: Clinical diagnosis of the Budd–Chiari syndrome. *Am J Med* **43**:544–554, 1967.
3. Tavill AS, Wood EJ, Kreel L, et al: The Budd–Chiari syndrome: Correlation between hepatic scintigraphy and the clinical, radiological, and pathological findings in nineteen cases of hepatic venous outflow obstruction. *Gastroenterology* **68**:509–518, 1975.
4. Powell-Jackson PR, Melia W, Canalese J, et al: Budd–Chiari syndrome: Clinical pattern and therapy. *Q J Med* **51**:79–88, 1982.
5. Mitchell MC, Boitnott JK, Kaufman S, et al: Budd–Chiari syndrome: Etiology, diagnosis and management. *Medicine (Baltimore)* **61**:199–218, 1982.
6. Van Steenbergen W, Beyls J, Vermylen J, et al: "Lupus" anticoagulant and thrombosis of the hepatic veins (Budd–Chiari syndrome). Report of three patients and review of the literature. *J Hepatol* **3**:87–94, 1986.
7. Das M, Carroll SF: Antithrombin III deficiency: An etiology of Budd–Chiari syndrome. *Surgery* **97**:242–245, 1985.
8. Maddrey WC: Hepatic vein thrombosis (Budd–Chiari syndrome). *Hepatology* **4**:44S–46S, 1984.
9. Rector WG, Yu Y, Goldstein L, et al: Membranous obstruction of the inferior vena cava in the United States. *Medicine (Baltimore)* **64**:134–143, 1985.
10. Lewis JH, Tice HL, Zimmerman HJ: Budd–Chiari syndrome associated with oral contraceptive steroids: Review and treatment of 47 cases. *Dig Dis Sci* **28**:673–683, 1985.
11. Maddrey WC: Hepatic vein thrombosis (Budd–Chiari syndrome): Possible association with the use of oral contraceptives. *Semin Liver Dis* **7**:32–39, 1987.
12. Valla D, Monique GL, Poynard T, et al: Risk of hepatic vein thrombosis in relation to recent use of oral contraceptives. A case-control study. *Gastroenterology* **90**:807–811, 1986.
13. Valla D, Casadevall N, Lacombe C, et al: Primary myeloproliferative disorder and hepatic vein thrombosis. *Ann Intern Med* **103**:329–334, 1985.
14. Thomas M, Caroli J: Polycythemie et syndrome de Budd–Chiari: A propos de 17 observations. *Ann Intern Med* **122**:1175–1186, 1971.
15. Levy VG, Ruskone A, Baillou C, et al: Polycythemia and the Budd–Chiari syndrome: Study of the serum erythropoietin and bone marrow erythroid progenitors. *Hepatology* **5**:858–861, 1985.
16. Bras G, Brandt KH: Vascular disorders, in MacSween RNM, Anthony PP, Scheuer PJ (eds): *Pathology of the Liver.* Churchill-Livingstone, Edinburgh, 1970, pp. 407–502.
17. Ingold JA, Reed GB, Kaplan HS, et al: Radiation hepatitis. *AJR* **93**:200–208, 1965.
18. Reed GB, Cox AJ: The human liver after radiation injury: A form of veno-occlusive disease. *Am J Pathol* **48**:597–612, 1966.
19. Fajardo LF, Berthrong M: Radiation injury in surgical pathology. *Am J Surg Pathol* **2**:159–199, 1978.
20. Fajardo LF, Colby TV: Pathogenesis of veno-occlusive disease after radiation. *Arch Pathol Lab Med* **104**:584–588, 1980.
21. Rowland R, Pieterse AS, Kimber RJ, et al: Radiation veno-occlusive disease. *Aust NZ J Med* **11**:534–538, 1981.
22. Dejaard A, Krogsgaard K, Jacobsen M: Veno-occlusive disease and peliosis of the liver after Thorotrast administration. *Virchows Arch Pathol Anat* **403**:87–94, 1984.
23. Feigen M: Fatal veno-occlusive disease of the liver associated with herbal tea consumption and radiation. *Aust NZ J Med* **14**:61–62, 1984.
24. Krishnamachari KAVR, Bhat RV, Nagarajan V, et al: Hepatitis due to aflatoxicosis: An outbreak in Western India. *Lancet* **1**:1061–1063, 1975.
25. Tandon BN, Krishnamurthy L, Koshy A, et al: Study of an epidemic of jaundice, presumably due to toxic hepatitis, in Northwest India. *Gastroenterology* **72**:488–494, 1977.
26. Russell RM, Boyer JL, Bagheri SA, et al: Hepatic injury from chronic hypervitaminosis A resulting in portal hypertension and ascites. *N Engl J Med* **291**:435–440, 1974.
27. Meacham GL, Tillotson FW, Heinle RW: Liver damage after prolonged urethane therapy. *Am J Clin Pathol* **22**:22–27, 1952.
28. Brodsky I, Johnson H, Killman SA, et al: Fibrosis of central and hepatic veins, and perisinusoidal spaces of the liver following prolonged administration of urethane. *Am J Med* **29**:976–980, 1961.
29. Satti MB, Weinbren K, Gordon-Smith EC: 6-Thioguanine as a cause of toxic veno-occlusive disease of the liver. *J Clin Pathol* **35**:1086–1091, 1982.

30. D'Cruz CA, Wimmer, RS, Harcke HT, et al: Veno-occlusive disease of the liver in children following chemotherapy for acute myelocytic leukemia. *Cancer* **52:**1803–1807, 1983.
31. Wasser JS, Coleman M: Leukemia chemotherapy and centrilobular hepatic necrosis. *Ann Intern Med* **86:**508–509, 1977.
32. Griner PF, Elbadawi A, Packman CH: Veno-occlusive disease of the liver after chemotherapy of acute leukemia: Report of two cases. *Ann Intern Med* **85:**578–582, 1976.
33. Gill RA, Onstad GR, Cardamone JM, et al: Hepatic veno-occlusive disease caused by 6-thioguanine. *Ann Intern Med* **96:**58–60, 1982.
34. Burkhardt A, Kloppel G: Unusual obliterative disease of the hepatic veins in an infant. *Virchows Arch Pathol Anat* **375:**225–232, 1977.
35. Clark PA, Hsia Ye, Huntsman RG: Toxic complications of treatment with 6-mercaptopurine: Two cases with hepatic necrosis and intestinal ulceration. *Br Med J* **1:**393–395, 1960.
36. Houghton AN, Shafi N, Rickles FR: Acute hepatic vein thrombosis occurring during therapy for Hodgkin's disease: A case report. *Cancer* **44:**2324–2329, 1979.
37. Asbury RF, Rosenthal SN, Decalzi ME, et al: Hepatic veno-occlusive disease due to DTIC. *Cancer* **45:**2670–2674, 1980.
38. Greenstone MA, Dowd PM, Mikhailidis DP, et al: Hepatic vascular lesions associated with dacarbazine treatment. *Br Med J* **282:**1744–1745, 1981.
39. Letendre L, Kovach JS, Ludwig J, et al: Hepatic veno-occlusive disease in patients with acute leukemia treated with indocine N-oxide. *Proc Am Soc Clin Oncol Annu Mtg* **22:**488, 1981 (abst).
40. Jacobs P, Miller JL, Uys CJ, et al: Fatal veno-occlusive disease of the liver after chemotherapy, whole-body irradiation and bone marrow transplantation for refractory acute leukemia. *S Afr Med J* **55:**5–10, 1979.
41. Schulman HM, McDonald GB, Mathews D, et al: An analysis of hepatic veno-occlusive disease and centrilobular hepatic degeneration following bone marrow transplantation. *Gastroenterology* **79:**1178–1191, 1980.
42. Woods WG, Dehner LP, Nesbit ME, et al: Fatal veno-occlusive disease of the liver following high dose chemotherapy, irradiation and bone marrow transplantation. *Am J Med* **68:**285–290, 1980.
43. Beschorner WE, Pino J, Boitnott JK, et al: Pathology of the liver with bone marrow transplantation: Effects of busulfan, carmustine, acute graft-versus-host disease, and cytomegalovirus infection. *Am J Pathol* **99:**369–386, 1980.
44. Lazarus HM, Gottfried MR, Herzig RH, et al: Veno-occlusive disease of the liver after high doses mitomycin C therapy and autologous bone marrow transplantation. *Cancer* **49:**1789–1795, 1982.
45. Gottfried MR, Sudilovsky O: Hepatic veno-occlusive disease after high-dose mitomycin C and autologous bone marrow transplantation therapy. *Hum Pathol* **13:**646–650, 1982.
46. Farthing MJG, Clark ML, Sloane JP, et al: Liver disease after bone marrow transplantation. *Gut* **23:**465–474, 1982.
47. McDonald GB, Sharma P, Mathews D, et al: Veno-occlusive disease of the liver after bone marrow transplantation: Diagnosis, incidence, and predisposing factors. *Hepatology* **4:**123–130, 1984.
48. McDonald GB, Shulman HM, Sullivan KM, et al: Intestinal and hepatic complications of human bone marrow transplantation. Part I. *Gastroenterology* **90:**460–477, 1986.
49. Marubbio AT, Danielson B: Hepatic veno-occlusive disease in a renal transplant patient receiving azathioprine. *Gastroenterology* **69:**739–743, 1975.
50. Eisenhauer T, Hartmann H, Rumpf KW, et al: Favorable outcome of hepatic veno-occlusive disease in a renal transplant patient receiving azathioprine, treated by portacaval shunt: Report of a case and review of the literature. *Digestion* **30:**185–190, 1984.
51. Weitz H, Gokel JM, Loeschka K, et al: Veno-occlusive disease of the liver in patients receiving immunosuppressive therapy. *Virchows Arch Pathol Anat* **395:**245–256, 1982.
52. Katzka DA, Saul SH, Jorkasky D, et al: Azathioprine and hepatic venocclusive disease in renal transplant patients. *Gastroenterology* **90:**446–454, 1986.
53. McLean C, Bras G, McLean AEM: Venous occlusions in the liver following dimethylnitrosamine. *Br J Exp Pathol* **3:**367–369, 1965.
54. Unigar H: Veno-occlusive disease of the liver and phlebectatic peliosis in the golden hamster exposed to dimethylnitrosamine. *Pathol Res Pract* **181:**180–187, 1986.
55. Setchell KDR, Gosselin SJ, Welsh MB, et al: Dietary estrogens as a probable cause of infertility and liver disease in captive cheetahs. *Gastroenterology* **93:**225–233, 1987.
56. Mellis C, Bale PM: Familial veno-occlusive disease with probable immune deficiency. *J Pediatr* **88:**236–242, 1976.

57. Goodman ZD, Ishak KG: Occlusive venous lesions in alcoholic liver disease: A study of 200 cases. *Gastroenterology* **83:**786–796, 1982.
58. Nakanuma Y, Ohta G, Doishita K: Quantitation and serial section observations of focal veno-occlusive lesions of the hepatic veins in liver cirrhosis. *Virchows Arch Pathol Anat* **405:**429–438, 1985.
59. Burt AD, MacSween RNM: Hepatic vein lesions in alcoholic liver disease: Retrospective biopsy and necropsy study. *J Clin Pathol* **39:**63–67, 1986.
60. Baert AL, Fevery J, Marchal G, et al: Early diagnosis of Budd–Chiari syndrome by computed tomography and ultrasonography: Report of five cases. *Gastroenterology* **84:**587–595, 1983.
61. Stark DD, Hahn PF, Trey C, et al: MRI of the Budd–Chiari syndrome. *AJR* **146:**1141–1148, 1986.
62. Murphy FB, Steinberg HV, Shires GT III, et al: The Budd–Chiari syndrome: A review. *AJR* **147:**9–15, 1986.
63. Friedman AC, Ramchandari P, Black M, et al: Magnetic resonance imaging diagnosis of Budd–Chiari syndrome. *Gastroenterology* **91:**1289–1295, 1986.
64. Vogelzang RL, Anschuetz SL, Gore RM: Budd–Chiari syndrome: CT observations. *Radiology* **163:**329–333, 1987.
65. Sanfey H, Boitnott JK, Cameron JL: Surgical management of patients with the Budd–Chiari syndrome. *World J Surg* **8:**706–715, 1984.
66. McDermott WV, Stone MD, Bothe A, et al: Budd–Chiari syndrome. Historical and clinical review with an analysis of surgical corrective procedures. *Am J Surg* **147:**463–467, 1984.
67. McCarthy PM, van Heerden JA, Adson MA, et al: The Budd–Chiari syndrome. Medical and surgical management of 30 patients. *Arch Surg* **120:**657–662, 1985.
68. Gupta S, Blumgart LH, Hodgson HJF: Budd–Chiari syndrome: Long-term survival and factors affecting mortality. *J Med* **60:**781–791, 1986.
69. Simson IW: Budd–Chiari syndrome and veno-occlusive disease, in Peters RL, Craig JR (eds): *Liver Pathology*. Churchill Livingstone, New York, 1986, pp. 299–314.
70. Nakamura T, Nakamura S, Aikawa T, et al: Obstruction of the inferior vena cava in the hepatic portion and the hepatic veins. *Angiology* **19:**479–498, 1968.
71. Simson IW: Membranous obstruction of the inferior vena cava and hepatocellular carcinoma in South Africa. *Gastroenterology* **82:**171–178, 1982.
72. Ishak KG, Sesterhenn IA, Goodman ZD, et al: Epithelioid hemangioendothelioma of the liver: A clinicopathologic and follow-up study of 32 cases. *Hum Pathol* **15:**839–852, 1984.
73. Taylor RW, Sylwesrtowicz T, Kossakowska AE, et al: Leiomyosarcoma of the inferior vena cava presenting as Budd–Chiara syndrome. *Liver* **7:**201–205, 1987.
74. Ishak KG: Malignant mesenchymal tumors of the liver, in Okuda K, Ishak KG (eds): *Neoplasms of the Liver*. Springer-Verlag, Tokyo, 1987, pp. 159–176.
75. Nakashima T, Kojiro M: *Hepatocellular Carcinoma*. Springer-Verlag, Tokyo, 1987.

30

Liver Disease of Pregnancy: Clinical Aspects

Rowen K. Zetterman and Rodney S. Markin

1. INTRODUCTION

The development of liver injury during pregnancy is unusual and occurs in less than 0.2% of cases. Jaundice develops in only 1 in 1500 pregnancies.[1] Liver injury can occur as a consequence of or coincident with pregnancy (Table I) developing in any trimester or even postpartum, depending on its etiology (Table II). The most common cause of liver injury in the pregnant patient is acute viral hepatitis accounting for up to 40% of cases. An enterically transmitted form of non-A, non-B (NANB) hepatitis has recently been observed that may cause an increased mortality rate in pregnant women. To date, it has only been observed in patients in or from developing countries. In some areas, such as Scandinavia or Chile, intrahepatic cholestasis of pregnancy occurs with high frequency and may account for 10–20% of jaundice during pregnancy. Other forms of liver injury are unusual during pregnancy.

2. NORMAL PREGNANCY

In the patient with uncomplicated pregnancy, other than occasional morning nausea, upper gastrointestinal (GI) symptoms should be absent. Physical examination may disclose spider angiomata over the upper body and palmar erythema in 50–60% of pregnant women. Occasionally, large numbers of small spider angiomata are seen. This may be confusing in a patient suspected of having prior chronic liver disease. Liver size during pregnancy is within the normal range. Hemodynamic changes also occur during pregnancy with an increase in blood volume of 30–40% during the third trimester.[2] While an associated increase in cardiac output with enhanced renal blood flow is observed, hepatic perfusion does not change.

Some laboratory tests may be altered during normal pregnancy. A gradual reduction in albumin, total protein, and blood urea nitrogen (BUN) in the latter months of pregnancy reflects the increased intravascular volume. Liver tests such as aminotransferases, bilirubin, and γ-glu-

Rowen K. Zetterman • Section of Digestive Diseases and Nutrition, Department of Internal Medicine, University of Nebraska Medical Center; Veterans Administration Medical Center, Omaha, Nebraska 68105. *Rodney S. Markin* • Department of Pathology and Microbiology, University of Nebraska Medical Center, Omaha, Nebraska 68105.

Table I. Liver Injury and Pregnancy

- Liver injury conincident with pregnancy
  - Acute viral hepatitis
  - Cholelithiasis/choledocholithiasis
  - Chronic liver diseases (e.g., primary biliary cirrhosis)
  - Disorders of bilirubin metabolism
  - Drug-induced liver injury (e.g., phenothiazines)
- Liver injury associated with pregnancy
  - Drug-induced liver injury (e.g., tetracycline)
  - Pyelonephritis/sepsis
- Liver injury as a consequence of pregnancy
  - Hyperemesis gravidarum
  - Intrahepatic cholestasis of pregnancy
  - Pre-eclampsia–eclampsia
  - Acute fatty liver of pregnancy
  - Budd–Chiari syndrome
  - Subcapsular hematoma/hepatic rupture

tamyltranspeptidase remain normal, while alkaline phosphatase, globulins, and fibrinogen levels increase.

Gallbladder function is also altered during pregnancy with increased gallbladder volume during fasting. Contractility is also impaired, and an increase in residual volume following eating is observed.[3] Gallbladder bile may also become more lithogenic.[4] No significant alteration of liver histology occurs during an uncomplicated pregnancy, with only slight Kupffer cell prominence described.[5]

3. HYPEREMESIS GRAVIDARUM

Although nausea and vomiting are common in early pregnancy, protracted vomiting associated with hyperemesis gravidarum is unusual. In those cases with dehydration and malnutrition of

Table II. Association of Duration of Pregnancy and Liver Injury

	Trimester			
	First	Second	Third	Postpartum
Hyperemesis gravidarum	X	—	—	—
Pre-eclampsia–eclampsia	—	—	X	X
Intrahepatic cholestasis of pregnancy	—	+/−	X	—
Acute fatty liver of pregnancy	—	—	X	X
Subcapsular hematoma/hepatic rupture	—	—	X	X
Budd–Chiari syndrome				X
Drug-induced liver injury	X	X	X	X
Pyelonephritis/sepsis	X	X	X	X
Disorders of bilirubin metabolism		X	X	X
Chronic liver disease		X	X	X
Cholelithiasis	X	X	X	X
Viral hepatitis	X	X	X	X

sufficient severity to require hospitalization, mild jaundice may be observed.[6] However, bilirubin elevations are usually <4 mg/dl, with transaminase elevations < 100 IU/liter. BSP clearance is reduced in patients with hyperemesis gravidarum when compared with those with uncomplicated pregnancy. Liver histology may be normal,[7] may demonstrate mild centrilobular cholestasis and focal hepatocellular necrosis,[8] or may show mild fatty metamorphosis.[7] Electron microscopy of the liver may exhibit changes typical of intrahepatic cholestasis.[8] It is likely that fatty metamorphosis of hyperemesis gravidarum is related to malnutrition and that the cholestasis and jaundice are due to dehydration and fasting. The differential diagnosis of vomiting and liver injury during pregnancy should include patients with intrahepatic cholestasis of pregnancy as early protracted vomiting may also be observed in this disorder.[9] Other etiologies to consider in the differential include acute viral hepatitis, drug-induced liver injury, cholecystitis/cholelithiasis, and pylonephritis (Table II). Treatment should be directed at controlling vomiting and correcting dehydration and malnutrition. There are no chronic hepatic sequelae of hyperemesis gravidarum though recurrent jaundice with recurrent hyperemesis gravidarum in subsequent pregnancies has been described.[8]

4. PRE-ECLAMPSIA–ECLAMPSIA

Pre-eclampsia is characterized by the development of pregnancy-induced hypertension, proteinuria, and peripheral edema. Coincident seizures or coma complete the definition of eclampsia. Pregnancy-induced hypertension is defined as a blood pressure of 140/90 mm Hg in a previously normotensive mother or by an increase in systolic blood pressure of 30 mm Hg and diastolic blood pressure of 15 mm Hg over prepregnancy levels.[10,11] Pre-eclampsia is common and affects approximately 5% of pregnancies. It occurs more frequently in primigravidas. Not all classic features need be present to establish a diagnosis of pre-eclampsia. Eclampsia can even occur in the absence of significant proteinuria or hypertension. This can also make the correct diagnosis difficult when associated with liver injury.

4.1. Clinical Features

Some patients with severe pre-eclampsia may develop hemolysis, abnormal liver tests, and thrombocytopenia. This syndrome has been called the HELLP syndrome becauses of *h*emolysis, *e*levated *l*iver tests, and *l*ow *p*latelet counts.[12–15] Women in whom this complication develops are usually multigravid and Caucasian. HELLP syndrome is said to occur in 4–12% of women with pre-eclampsia–eclampsia.[15]

Significant liver injury is uncommon in mild pre-eclampsia.[5,16] Liver biopsies reveal Kupffer cell hyperplasia, anisonucleosis, anisocytosis, and binucleate hepatocytes. With more severe pre-eclampsia, however, marked injury may occur. Fibrin is deposited in periportal sinusoids[17] and may be associated with focal hepatocyte necrosis. It is rarely noted in pre-eclampsia patient liver biopsies by routine stains.

HELLP syndrome is frequently associated with significant hepatic injury.[13–15,18] Although more common in subsequent pregnancies, it can occur in primigravidas as well. Most patients will have classic features of pre-eclampsia or eclampsia, although it can occur before all the manifestations of pre-eclampsia are recognized.[15,19,20]

Virtually all patients present with severe right upper quadrant (RUQ) or epigastric pain, fever, malaise, nausea, vomiting, and headache. Such symptoms should prompt further evaluation. Peptic ulcer disease, cholecystitis, and pancreatitis may also be considered. Physical findings include a slightly enlarged and tender liver. Laboratory abnormalities include anemia, thrombocytopenia, leukopenia, and abnormal peripheral blood smears with burr cells and schistocytes. Disseminated intravascular coagulation (DIC) may also occur in a small number of patients.[15] Elevations of liver enzymes will occur in all patients, with hyperbilirubinemia in approximately 50%.[13] Transaminases are frequently >500 IU/liter and may reach several thousand.[21] Lactate dehydrogenase levels are also increased in conjunction with hemolysis.[15]

Ultrasound or computed tomography (CT) of the liver and abdomen may aid in identifying the presence of significant liver injury.[15,22,23] An enlarged liver with areas of hemorrhage or infarction may be observed.

The histology of severe pre-eclampsia–eclampsia has recently been reviewed by Rolfes and Ishak.[24] In their series, most patients presented for reasons other than liver disease, with central nervous system (CNS) complications accounting for the majority of deaths. However, hepatic deaths also occurred associated with extensive infarction or subcapsular hematomas. Periportal fibrin deposition with hepatocellular necrosis is frequently seen. Necrosis may be focal, sublobular, or extensive. Infarction of up to 90% of the liver mass was described. Periportal hemorrhage was also observed, often in areas of heavy fibrin deposition. Other changes included cholestasis, mononuclear infiltration of the portal areas, cholangiolitis, and extramedullary hematopoiesis.

4.2. Intrahepatic Hemorrhage/Hepatic Rupture

Intrahepatic hemorrhage with subcapsular dissection of the hematoma or free rupture may develop either pre- or postpartum.[21,25–27] These patients often present with severe pre-eclampsia–eclampsia, RUQ pain, nausea, vomiting, and hepatic enlargement. With rupture, shock and abdominal distention may ensue. The diagnosis may be established by ultrasound or CT examination or by angiography.[28] The right lobe is principally involved. Paracentesis may also indicate fresh blood from hepatic rupture. For those with free rupture, prompt surgical intervention is usually mandated. Recently, transcatheter embolotherapy has also been successfully used.[29] If free rupture has not occurred, controversy exists as to the need for surgical intervention. Several recent reports have suggested that an expectant, conservative, nonoperative approach is appropriate.[30,31] Other causes of hepatic rupture during pregnancy should also be considered, including trauma, hepatic adenoma, ruptured splenic artery aneurysm, hepatocellular carcinoma, and rarely hemangioma or acute fatty liver of pregnancy. Both fetal and maternal mortality are increased with hepatic rupture.[25]

4.3. Pathogenesis

The pathogenesis of liver injury in severe pre-eclampsia–eclampsia is unclear. Fibrin deposition appears to develop first[17] and has been suggested to be the initiating event,[5,10] possibly as a consequence of a coagulopathy induced by release of tissue thromboplastin from the placenta. However, measurable DIC only occurs in 3% of severe pre-eclampsia cases,[15] suggesting that this mechanism is unlikely. Decreases in antithrombin III (AT III) levels during pre-eclampsia have also been observed in proportion to its severity.[32] Deficiencies of AT III are associated with thromboembolic phenomena and thrombosis of intrahepatic venous radicles with sinusoidal fibrin deposition has been suggested as well. Vasospasm also occurs during pre-eclampsia[11] and could account for injury to endothelial cells sufficient to cause ischemic liver cell necrosis.[24]

4.4. Prognosis

The prognosis for the mother and the fetus depends on early recognition of severe pre-eclampsia, even in the absence of classic signs, such as hypertension or proteinuria.[33] If fetal maturity permits, prompt delivery seems advisable as a fetal wastage of up to 30% can occur in severe cases.[34]

5. INTRAHEPATIC CHOLESTASIS OF PREGNANCY

Intrahepatic cholestasis of pregnancy (ICP)[35,36] is an unusual disorder characterized by pruritis and jaundice developing during the latter weeks of pregnancy that quickly resolves following delivery. Other than the discomfort of intense pruritis, the disease is usually of little consequence for the mother. It is the second most common cause of jaundice (after viral hepatitis) during pregnancy.[1]

The incidence of ICP is variable. In the United States, it is approximately 1 per 1000 pregnancies,[37,38] while in Scandinavia and Chile, it is 1–2%[39] and 10%,[37] respectively. It has not been reported in Asian women[37] and is extremely rare in blacks.[40]

5.1. Clinical Features

Intrahepatic cholestasis characteristically begins in the third trimester (70% of cases), although onset as early as 8–12 weeks has been observed.[41] It may recur or even initially occur in subsequent pregnancies or during use of oral contraceptives.[42,43]

Pruritis is the initial symptom and may be the only clue to the diagnosis. This has been termed pruritis gravidarum[44] and is now recognized as a nonicteric expression of ICP. Pruritis is typically more severe at night, usually involving the entire body, including the palms and soles. Within a few weeks, dark urine, light stools, and jaundice may appear. Hyperbilirubinemia is typically mild, although bilirubin of >30 mg/dl have been described.[45] Physical examination may show evidence of excoriations and icterus but otherwise should demonstrate no changes suggestive of chronic liver disease. Occasionally, the liver may be slightly enlarged. Once the patient delivers, the pruritis and jaundice usually resolves within 1–2 weeks. The patient may develop similar symptoms during subsequent pregnancies, although this is variable and can be more or less intense. Some patients will also develop symptoms during menstrual cycles, especially premenopausally,[46] and up to 50% will develop symptoms when using oral contraceptives.[46,47] Patients with familial benign recurrent intrahepatic cholestasis may also develop cholestasis during pregnancy.[48] However, they also demonstrate cholestasis during nonpregnant intervals. Patients with Dubin–Johnson syndrome may also become jaundiced during pregnancy.[49]

5.2. Laboratory Features

Laboratory features of cholestatis are usually present. The alkaline phosphatase may be increased, although it can remain within the range seen in uncomplicated pregnancy. γ-Glutamyltranspeptidase may also be elevated. Transaminases are usually modest and <200 IU/liter. Other laboratory findings can include hypercholesterolemia and hypertriglyceridemia. Serum bile acids[50] are also increased, and the presence of serum lipoprotein X[51] may be identified. Although serum bile acid levels may be increased, a direct correlation to the symptom of pruritis is difficult to ascribe. Because of a consequent decrease of intraluminal bile salts with cholestasis, fat malabsorption may also occur.[52] This probably accounts for vitamin K malabsorption and the consequent hypoprothrombinemia observed in ICP. It is important to recognize and correct hypoprothrombinemia predelivery to prevent postpartum hemmorrhage.

5.3. Pathology

The histology of ICP is typical of intrahepatic cholestasis with centrilobular bile plugs, with minimal inflammation and hepatocellular necrosis. (Figs. 1 and 2). Electron microscopy shows dilated bile canaliculi with loss of microvilli,[53,54] and hepatocyte mitochondria may be irregular and elongated. These changes disappear between pregnancies.

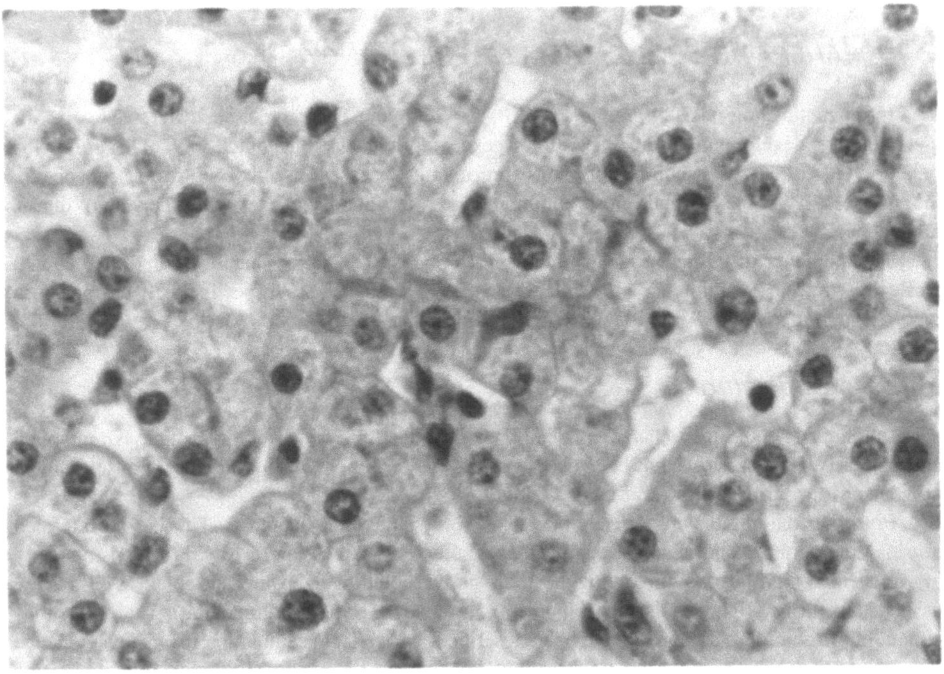

Figure 1. Intrahepatic cholestasis of pregnancy. Centrilobular region showing cholestasis without significant hepatocellular necrosis or inflammatory cell infiltrate. (H&E, ×80)

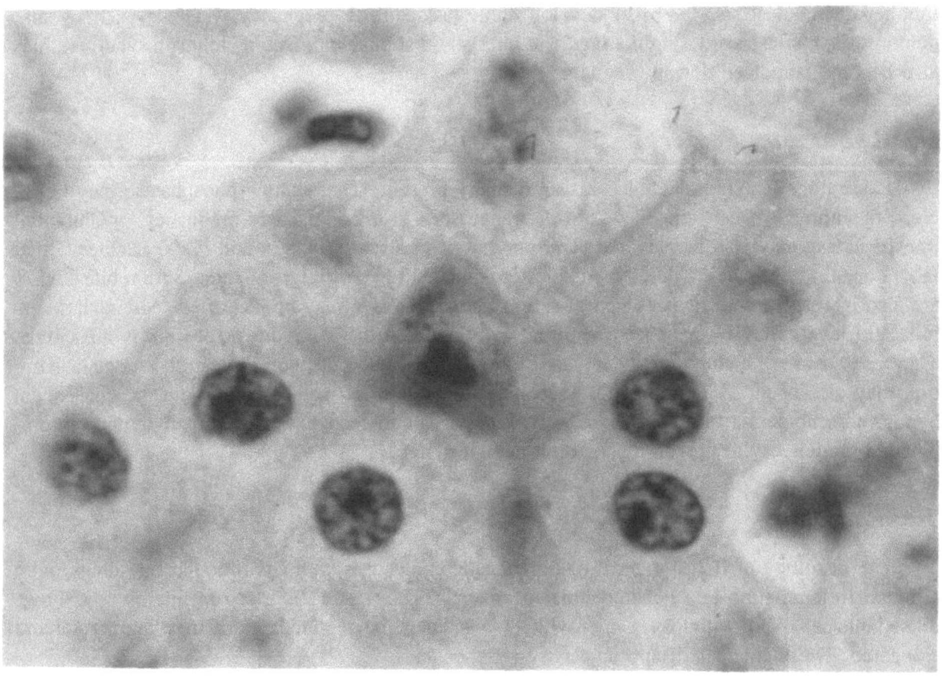

Figure 2. Bile staining of centrilobular hepatocytes with characteristic canalicular bile plug. (H&E, ×500)

5.4. Pathogenesis

The cause of ICP is unknown. Because of its relationship to the later stages of pregnancy and similar occurrence with oral contraceptive pills, it is assumed to be due to an abnormal sensitivity to estrogens. Challenge of affected subjects with ethinyl estradiol will also cause recurrence of symptoms.[55–57] What predisposes susceptible persons to this sensitivity is unknown. The increased frequency in certain geographic areas,[35–38] ethnic groups,[37,38] and families[1,3,5,36,46,51] has suggested a genetic basis for the disorder. Both men and women with a family history of ICP will develop altered BSP clearance following challenge with ethinyl estradiol.[57]

5.5. Prognosis and Treatment

The prognosis for the mother with ICP is excellent. Occasionally, the pruritis may be so intense that early delivery may be undertaken.[43] The outcome for the fetus may be more severe.[45,50,53,58] Premature labor is more frequent in those affected by ICP, and intrauterine fetal and neonatal deaths have been noted. The mechanism of fetal distress and premature labor is unknown but may be a consequence of elevated bile acid levels.[50] Placental abnormalities also occur[59] and may cause impaired transfer of oxygen and nutrients to the fetus.

During pregnancy, antihistamines (usually of minimal help) and cholestyramine may be administered to control pruritis. Phenobarbital may also improve pruritis,[60] although this effect is variable. It is also important to ensure that prothrombin levels are adequate before delivery and to administer vitamin K, if necessary.

Recently, it has been demonstrated that parenteral administration of *S*-adenosyl-1-methionine will reduce pruritis and decrease serum transaminases, bilirubin and total bile acids in patients with ICP.[61] Additional studies are required to assess its ability to alter the frequency of premature labor and adverse fetal outcome.

6. ACUTE FATTY LIVER OF PREGNANCY

Acute fatty liver of pregnancy (AFLP)[62] is an uncommon complication. Its recognized frequency is approximately one case per 13,328 deliveries.[63] However, many mild cases probably go unrecognized. Early reports and autopsy series have emphasized high maternal and fetal mortality rates,[64–66] although recent reports have indicated that the mortality rate is lower.[67,68] Whether this improvement is a consequence of earlier recognition with termination of pregnancy[69,70] or of improved supportive care[71] is unknown. It does not appear to be related to a change in disease severity.[71]

Acute fatty liver of pregnancy is more common in primigravidas but has occurred as late as the twelfth pregnancy[72] and is more likely to occur in twin gestations.[62,73,74] Furthermore, a male fetus is more likely present than a female.[73,75] Symptoms usually develop during the third trimester (or immediately postpartum), although onset as early as 24 weeks has been described.[76]

6.1. Clinical Features

Presenting features of AFLP are variable. It may follow an upper respiratory infection (URI)[73,77] or urinary tract infection (UTI).[62,73,78] Nausea and vomiting are common presenting complaints[75] and should not be ignored as nonspecific symptoms. Malaise, fatigue, and abdominal pain are also frequent. Abdominal discomfort may be epigastric, retrosternal, or RUQ. Jaundice may also develop. Pre-eclampsia may also occur in association with AFLP, with its additional symptoms and signs. Rarely, patients may present with seizures or signs of hepatic encephalopathy, including agitation, confusion, and somnolence. Because of associated coagulopathy, such problems as bleeding from puncture sites and GI and vaginal bleeding are also frequent.

At presentation, physical examination may not identify findings of significant liver injury. Low-grade fever may occur,[62] but associated infections are also frequent. Spider angiomata and palmar erythema are common accompaniments of uncomplicated pregnancy. Jaundice may or may not be present. Signs of pre-eclampsia, such as increased blood pressure and peripheral edema, may also be present.[68] The presence of a palpable tender liver or ascites should alert the clinician to AFLP. Although such findings may occur with any form of liver injury, the liver is not usually palpable during the third trimester of pregnancy, and ascites is abnormal. Overt signs of hepatic encephalopathy such as asterixis or agitation may also be noted.

6.2. Laboratory Features

Transaminases are usually modestly elevated. However, marked elevations have been described,[79] making the differentiation from other acute injuries such as viral hepatitis difficult. Alkaline phosphatase and γ-glutamyl-transpeptidase elevations also occur, indicating the presence of intrahepatic cholestasis. Bilirubin levels are generally increased at presentation. Hypoalbuminemia is also common.

Disseminated intravascular coagulation (DIC) may also develop in up to 60% of patients,[62,80,81] with thrombocytopenia and prolonged prothrombin and partial thromboplastin times. Antithrombin III levels may also be reduced.[62,82]

Other laboratory findings may include leukocytosis, hypoglycemia, and renal failure. The presence of nucleated red cells in the peripheral smear should also alert the clinician to AFLP. Pancreatitis can also develop.[77,83]

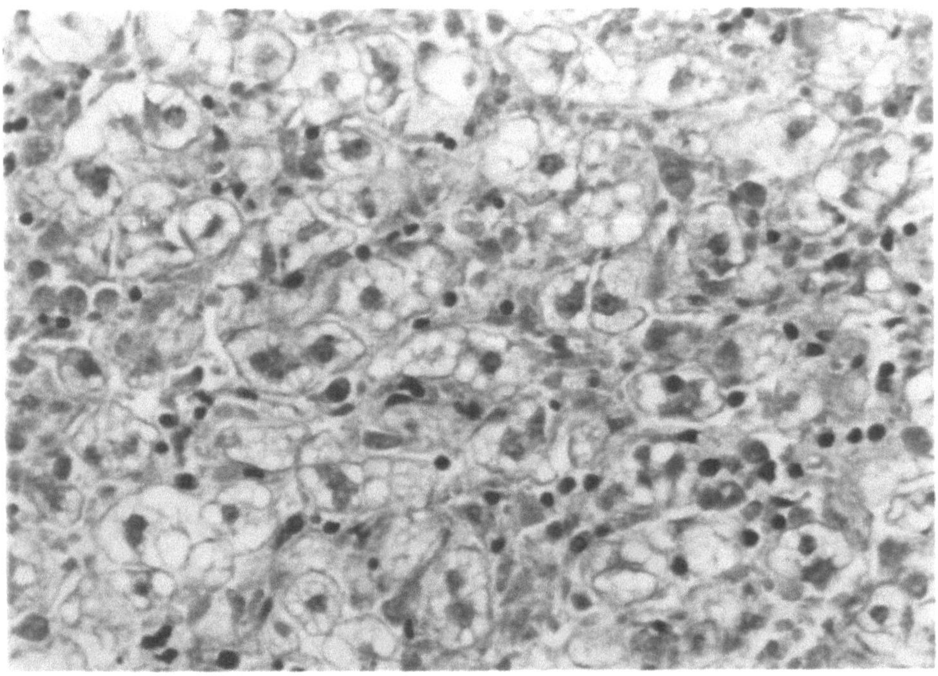

Figure 3. Typical section of acute fatty liver of pregnancy with microvesicular fatty change of hepatocytes. (H&E, ×80)

6.3. Pathology

The principal histologic lesion is microvesicular steatosis (Figs. 3 and 4). Microvesicular steatosis change has also been described in a variety of metabolic and toxic liver injuries (Table III). The accumulated fat within hepatocytes in AFLP is due to free fatty acids.[84]

The livers may become small and shrunken with loss of hepatocytes. Although hepatocellular necrosis may be observed as acidophilic bodies,[75] the majority of cell loss seems to be by hepatocytolosis of contiguous and single hepatocytes.[75,85] Additional features may include cholestasis, cholangiolitis, and extramedullary hematopoesis. Ballooning degeneration may also occur in centrilobular hepatocytes.

Electron microscopic examination of the liver[75,85,86] demonstrates free fat droplets, increased lysozomal fat, large pleomorphic mitochondria, and dilated smooth endoplasmic reticulum.

6.4. Pathogenesis

The mechanism for the development of AFLP is unknown. Initially, a strong relationship to tetracycline therapy was noted.[78,87–89] Although it has been suggested that AFLP may share a common pathogenesis with other microvesicular fatty liver diseases,[90] this seems unlikely. It does not have a definite relationship to preceding viral illness, as is typical of Reye syndrome. Furthermore, electron microscopic changes and enzyme studies of mitochondria in AFLP differ from those typically seen in Reye syndrome.[86] Inherited metabolic disorders also do not seem likely, as familial occurrence of AFLP is not reported, and survivors undergo subsequent pregnancies uneventfully.[62,74,91,92]

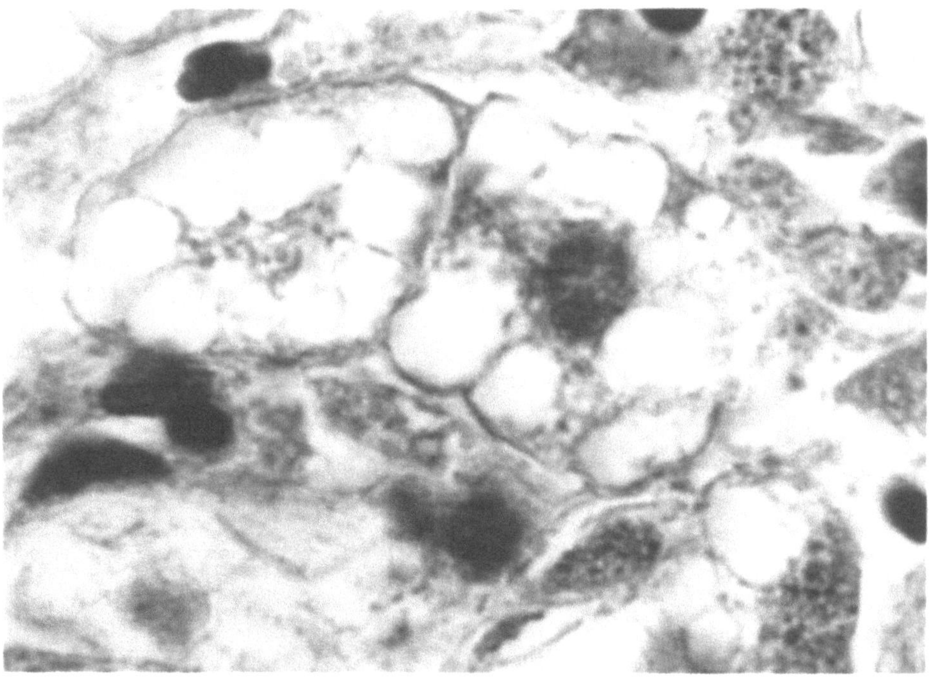

Figure 4. High-power magnification of acute fatty liver of pregnancy showing microvesicular fat accumulation without nuclear displacement. (H&E, ×500)

Table III. Microvesicular Fatty Liver[a]

Acute fatty liver of pregnancy
Reye syndrome
Jamaican vomiting disease
Valproic acid toxicity
Tetracycline toxicity
Alcoholic foamy degeneration
Labrea hepatitis
Yellow fever
Salicylate toxicity
Carnitine deficiency syndromes

[a]Adapted from Rolfes and Ishak[75] and Sherlock.[90]

6.5. Treatment

It is imperative to recognize AFLP promptly. The development of nausea, vomiting, and abdominal pain during the third trimester should alert the clinician to its possible occurrence. If clotting studies permit, the diagnosis can be confirmed by liver biopsy. A portion of the biopsy can be frozen, sectioned by cryostat, and stained by oil-red-O for fat. If clotting studies do not permit biopsy, increased echogenicity at ultrasound of the liver[93] or changes suggestive of fat accumulation on CT[94] may support the diagnosis. Clotting deficiencies and hypoglycemia should be controlled. Once the diagnosis is established, the pregnancy should be promptly terminated by cesarean section or by stimulated vaginal delivery.[69,70,95] Delay in delivery seems imprudent because of the potential for sudden deterioration. Furthermore, maternal liver dysfunction rapidly improves following delivery and steatosis is reported to disappear within 5 weeks of delivery.[96]

Complications of AFLP, such as pancreatitis, renal failure, and protein-losing enteropathy, may also occur despite improvement in liver function.[77,83]

Although intrahepatic hemorrhage with hepatic rupture is more common in toxemia of pregnancy, subcapsular hematoma[97] and hepatic rupture[98] have recently been described in AFLP. This complication should be considered if intervening hypotension, abdominal pain, or tenderness develops.

In addition, GI or vaginal hemorrhage and refractory hypoglycemia may occur postdelivery. Patients should receive fresh-frozen plasma and frequent antacids and should be observed for hypoglycemia.

Although patients who survive AFLP may not wish to go through subsequent pregnancies, there seems to be little reason to discourage them from having additional children. Subsequent pregnancies have been described [62,70,74,91,92,99–101] with no descriptions of recurrence.

REFERENCES

1. Haemmerli UP: Jaundice during pregnancy with special emphasis on recurrent jaundice during pregnancy and its differential diagnosis. *Acta Med Scand* **179**(suppl):1–111, 1966.
2. Pritchard JA: Changes in blood volume during pregnancy and delivery. *Anesthesia* **26**:393–397, 1965.
3. Everson GT, McKinley C, Lawson M, et al: Gallbladder function in the human female: Effect of the ovulatory cycle, pregnancy and contraceptive steroids. *Gastroenterology* **82**:711–719, 1982.
4. Kern FJ, Everson GT, DeMark B, et al: Biliary lipids, bile acids and gallbladder function in the human female: Effects of pregnancy and the ovulatory cycle. *J Clin Invest* **68**:1229–1242, 1981.
5. McKay DG, Merrill SJ, Weiner AE, et al: The pathologic anatomy of eclampsia, bilateral renal cortical

necrosis, pituitary necrosis, and other acute fatal complications of pregnancy, and its possible relationship to the generalized Schwartzman phenomenon. *Am J Obstet Gynecol* **66**:507–539, 1953.
6. Adams RH, Gordon J, Comes B: Hyperemesis gravidarum. I. Evidence of hepatic dysfunction. *Obstet Gynecol* **31**:659–664, 1968.
7. Sheeham HL: The pathology of hyperemesis and vomiting of late pregnancy. *J Obstet Gynecol Br Emp* **4b**:685–689, 1939.
8. Larrey D, Rueff B, Feldmann G, et al: Recurrent jaundice caused by recurrent hyperemesis gravidarum. *Gut* **25**:1414–1415, 1984.
9. Furhoff AK, Hellstrom K: Jaundice in pregnancy: A followup study of the series of women originally reported by L. Thorling. *Acta Med Scand* **193**:259–266, 1973.
10. Page EW: On the pathogenesis of pre-eclampsia and eclampsia. *J Obstet Gynaecol Commonw* **79**:883–894, 1972.
11. Worley RJ: Pathophysiology of pregnancy-induced hypertension. *Clin Obstet Gynecol* **27**:821–835, 1984.
12. Killam AP, Dillard SH, Patton RC, et al: Pregnancy-induced hypertension complicated by acute liver disease and disseminated intravascular coagulation. *Am J Obstet Gynecol* **123**:823–828, 1975.
13. Weistein L: Syndrome of hemolysis, elevated liver enzymes and low platelet count: A severe consequence of hypertension in pregnancy. *Am J Obstet Gynecol* **142**:159–167, 1982.
14. MacKenna J, Dover NL, Brame RG: Preeclampsia associated with hemolysis, elevated liver enzymes and low platelets—An obstetric emergency. *Obstet Gynecol* **62**:751–754, 1983.
15. Sibai BM, Taslimi MM, El-Nazer A, et al: Maternal–perinatal outcome associated with the syndrome of hemolysis, elevated liver enzymes and low platelets in severe preeclampsia-eclampsia. *Am J Obstet Gynecol* **155**:501–509, 1986.
16. Antia FP, Bharadwaj TP, Watsa MC, et al: Liver in normal pregnancy, preeclampsia and eclampsia. *Lancet* **2**:776–778, 1958.
17. Arias F, Mancilla-Jimenez R: Hepatic fibrinogen deposits in preeclampsia. *N Engl J Med* **295**:578–582, 1976.
18. Long RG, Scheuer PJ, Sherlock S: Pre-eclampsia presenting with deep jaundice. *J Clin Pathol* **30**:212–215, 1977.
19. Goodlin RC, Holdt D: Impending gestosis. *Obstet Gynecol* **58**:743–745, 1981.
20. Goodlin RC, Zetterman RK: When your pregnant patient develops jaundice. *Contemp Obstet Gynecol* **24**:27–44, 1984.
21. Manas KJ, Welsh JD, Rankin RA, et al: Hepatic hemorrhage without rupture in preeclampsia. *N Engl J Med* **312**:424–426, 1985.
22. Dammann HG, Hagemann J, Runge M, et al: In vivo diagnosis of massive hepatic infarction by computed tomography. *Dig Dis Sci* **27**:73–79, 1982.
23. Riely CA: The liver in preeclampsial/eclampsia: The tip of the iceberg. *Am J Gastroenterol* **81**:1218–1219, 1986.
24. Rolfes DB, Ishak KG: Liver disease in toxemia in pregnancy. *Am J Gastroenterol* **81**:1138–1144, 1986.
25. Biska, Waxman B: Rupture of the liver associated with pregnancy: A review of the literature and report of 2 cases. *Obstet Gynecol Surv* **31**:763–773, 1976.
26. Henny P, Lim AE, Brummelkamp WH, et al: A review of the importance of acute multidisciplinary treatment following spontaneous rupture of the liver capsule during pregnancy. *Surg Gyn Obstet* **156**:593–598, 1983.
27. Stalter KD, Sterling WA: Hepatic subcapsular hemorrhage associated with pregnancy. *Surgery* **98**:112–114, 1985.
28. Sommer DG, Greenway GD, Bookstein J, et al: Hepatic rupture with toxemia of pregnancy: Angiographic diagnosis. *AJR* **132**:455–456, 1979.
29. Loevinger EH, Vujic I, Lee WM, et al: Hepatic rupture associated with pregnancy: Treatment with transcatheter embolotherapy. *Obstet Gynecol* **65**:281–284, 1985.
30. Goodlin RC, Anderson JC, Hodgson PE: Conservative treatment of liver hematoma in the postpartum period. *J Reprod Med* **30**:368–370, 1985.
31. Woodhouse DR: Conservative management of spontaneous rupture of the liver in pregnancy. *Br J Obstet Gynaecol* **93**:1097–1099, 1986.
32. Weiner CP, Brandt J: Plasma antithrombin III activity: An aid in the diagnosis of preeclampsia–eclampsia. *Am J Obstet Gynecol* **142**:275–281, 1982.
33. Goodlin RC: Severe preeclampsia. Another great imitator. *Am J Obstet Gynecol* **125**:747–753, 1976.

34. Lin CC, Lindheimer MD, River P, et al: Fetal outcome in hypertensive disorders of pregnancy. *Am J Obstet Gynecol* **142**:255–260, 1982.
35. Svanborg A: A study of recurrent jaundice in pregnancy. *Acta Obstet Gynecol Scand* **33**:434–444, 1954.
36. Thorling L: Jaundice in pregnancy: A clinical study. *Acta Med Scand* **302** (suppl):1–123, 1955.
37. Reyes H, Gonzalez MC, Ribalta J, et al: Prevalence of intrahepatic cholestasis of pregnancy in Chile. *Ann Intern Med* **88**:487–493, 1978.
38. Reyes H: The enigm of intrahepatic cholestasis of pregnancy: Lessons from Chile. *Hepatology* **2**:87–96, 1982.
39. Forkman B, Ganrot PO, Genser G, et al: Plasma protein pattern in recurrent cholestasis of pregnancy. *Scand J Clin Lab Invest* **124** (suppl 29):89–99, 1972.
40. Wilson JAP: Intrahepatic cholestasis of pregnancy with marked elevation of transaminases in a black American. *Dig Dis Sci* **32**:665–668, 1987.
41. Furhoff AK, Hellstrom K: Jaundice in pregnancy. A follow-up study of the series of women originally reported by L. Thorling. *Acta Med Scand* **193**:259–266, 1973.
42. Drill VA: Benign cholestatic jaundice of pregnancy and benign cholestatic jaundice from oral contraceptives. *Am J Obstet Gynecol* **119**:165–174, 1974.
43. Berg B, Helm G, Petersohn L, et al: Cholestasis of pregnancy: Clinical and laboratory studies. *Acta Obstet Gynecol Scand* **65**:107–113, 1986.
44. Arfwedson H: Generalized pruritis in pregnancy: Symptom of liver dysfunction. *Obstet Gynecol* **7**:274–276, 1956.
45. Misra PS, Evanov FA, Wessely Z, et al: Idiopathic intrahepatic cholestasis of pregnancy. *Am J Gastroenterol* **73**:54–59, 1980.
46. Kreek MJ, Sleisenger MH, Jeffries GH: Recurrent cholestatic jaundice of pregnancy with demonstrated estrogen sensitivity. *Am J Med* **43**:795–803, 1967.
47. Orellano-Alcalde JM, Domingues JP: Jaundice and oral contraceptive drugs. *Lancet* **2**:1278–1280, 1966.
48. dePagler AGF, VanBerge Henegouwen GP, tenBokkel JA, et al: Familial benign recurrent intrahepatic cholestasis: Interrelation with intrahepatic cholestasis of pregnancy and from oral contraceptives. *Gastroenterology* **71**:202–207, 1976.
49. Cohen L, Lewis C, Arias IM: Pregnancy, oral contraceptives and chronic familial jaundice with predominately conjugated hyperbilirubinemia (Dubin–Johnson syndrome). *Gastroenterology* **62**:1182–1190, 1972.
50. Laatikainen T, Tulenheimo A: Maternal serum bile acid levels and fetal distress in cholestasis of pregnancy. *Int J Gynaecol Obstet* **22**:91–94, 1984.
51. Johnson P, Samsioe G, Gustafson A: Studies in cholestasis of pregnancy. I. Clinical aspects and liver function tests. *Acta Obstet Gynecol Scand* **54**:77–84, 1975.
52. Reyes H, Radrigan ME, Gonzalez MC, et al: Steatorrhea in patients with intrahepatic cholestasis of pregnancy. *Gastroenterology* **93**:584–590, 1987.
53. Eliakim M, Sadovsky E, Stein O, et al: Recurrent cholestatic jaundice of pregnancy. *Arch Intern Med* **117**:696–705, 1966.
54. Adlercreutz H, Svanborg A, Anberg A: Recurrent jaundice in pregnancy. I. A clinical and ultrastructural study. *Am J Med* **42**:335–347, 1967.
55. Holzbach RT, Sanders JH: Recurrent intrahepatic cholestasis of pregnancy. *JAMA* **193**:204–206, 1965.
56. Kreek MJ, Weser E, Sleisenger MH, et al: Idiopathic cholestasis of pregnancy: The response to challenge with synthetic estrogen, ethinyl estradiol. *N Engl J Med* **277**:1391–1395, 1965.
57. Reyes H, Ribalta J, Gonzalez MC, et al: Sulfobromophthalein clearance tests before and after ethinyl estradiol administration, in women and men with familial history of intrahepatic cholestasis of pregnancy. *Gastroenterology* **81**:226–231, 1981.
58. Reid R, Ivey KJ, Rencoret RH, et al: Fetal complications of obstetric cholestasis. *Br Med J* **1**:870–872, 1976.
59. Costoya AL, Leontic EA, Rosenberg HG, et al: Morphological study of placental terminal villi in intrahepatic cholestasis of pregnancy: Histochemistry, light and electron microscopy. *Placenta* **1**:361–368, 1980.
60. Espinoza J, Barnafi L, Schnaidt E: The effect of phenobarbital on intrahepatic cholestasis of pregnancy. *Am J Obstet Gynecol* **119**:234–238, 1974.
61. Frezza M, Pozzato G, Chiesa L, et al: Reversal of intrahepatic cholestasis of pregnancy in women after high dose S-adenosyl-l-methionine administration. *Hepatology* **4**:274–278, 1984.

62. Moore HC: Acute fatty liver of pregnancy. *J Obstet Gynecol Br Emp* **63:**189–198, 1956.
63. Pockros PJ, Peters RL, Reynolds TB: Idiopathic fatty liver of pregnancy: Findings in ten cases. *Medicine (Baltimore)* **63:**1–11, 1984.
64. Sheehan HL: The pathology of acute yellow atrophy and delayed chloroform poisoning. *J Obstet Gynecol Br Emp* **47:**49–62, 1940.
65. Ober WB, LeCompte PM: Acute fatty metamorphosis of the liver associated with pregnancy. *Am J Med* **19:**743–758, 1955.
66. Kahil MF, Fred HL, Brown H, et al: Acute fatty liver of pregnancy. *Arch Intern Med* **113:**63–69, 1964.
67. Bernuau J, Degott C, Nouel O, et al: Non-fatal acute fatty liver of pregnancy. *Gut* **24:**340–344, 1983.
68. Riely CA, Latham PS, Romero R, et al: Acute fatty liver of pregnancy: A reassessment based on observations in nine patients. *Ann Intern Med* **106:**703–706, 1987.
69. Hou SH, Levin S, Ahola S, et al: Acute fatty liver of pregnancy: Survival with early cesarean section. *Dig Dis Sci* **29:**449–452, 1984.
70. Ebert EC, Sun EA, Wright SH, et al: Does early diagnosis and delivery in acute fatty liver of pregnancy lead to improvement in maternal and infant survival? *Dig Dis Sci* **29:**453–455, 1984.
71. Pockros PJ, Reynolds TB: Acute fatty liver of pregnancy. *Dig Dis Sci* **30:**601–602, 1985.
72. Haemmerli UP: Jaundice during pregnancy with special emphasis on recurrent jaundice during pregnancy and its differential diagnosis. *Acta Med Scand* **444** (suppl):1–111, 1966.
73. Hague WM, Fenton DW, Duncan SLB, et al: Acute fatty liver of pregnancy. *J R Soc Med* **76:**652–659, 1983.
74. Burroughs AK, Seong NH, Dojcinov DM, et al: Idiopathic acute fatty liver of pregnancy in 12 patients. *Q J Med* **204:**481–497, 1982.
75. Rolfes DB, Ishak KG: Acute fatty liver of pregnancy: A clinicopathologic study of 35 cases. *Hepatology* **5:**1149–1158, 1985.
76. Sun E, Decker J, Wright S, et al: Acute fatty liver of pregnancy: Criteria for early diagnosis and management. *Gastroenterology* **80:**1296, 1981.
77. Hatfield AK, Stein JH, Greenberger NJ, et al: Idiopathic acute fatty liver of pregnancy: Death from extrahepatic manifestations. *Dig Dis* **17:**167–178, 1972.
78. Kunelis CT, Peters RL, Edmondson HA: Fatty liver of pregnancy and its relationship to tetracycline therapy. *Am J Med* **38:**359–377, 1965.
79. Brown MS, Reddy KR, Hensley GT, et al: The initial presentation of fatty liver of pregnancy mimicking acute viral hepatitis. *Am J Gastroenterol* **82:**554–557, 1987.
80. Holzbach RT: Acute fatty liver of pregnancy with disseminated intravascular coagulation. *Obstet Gynecol* **43:**740–744, 1974.
81. Cano RI, Delman MR, Pitchumoni CS, et al: Acute fatty liver of pregnancy complicated by disseminated intravascular coagulation. *JAMA* **231:**159–161, 1975.
82. Laursen B, Frost L, Mortensen JZ, et al: Acute fatty liver of pregnancy with complicating disseminated, intravascular coagulation. *Acta Obstet Gynecol Scand* **62:**403–407, 1983.
83. Riely CA: Acute hepatic failure at term. *Postgrad Med* **68:**118–127, 1980.
84. Eisele JW, Barker EA, Smuckler EA: Lipid content in the liver of fatty metamorphosis of pregnancy. *Am J Pathol* **81:**545–560, 1975.
85. Malatjalian DA, Bradley BWD: Acute fatty liver of pregnancy: Light and electron microscopic studies. *Gastroenterology* **84:**1384, 1983.
86. Weber FL, Snodgrass PJ, Powell DE, et al: Abnormalities of hepatic mitochondrial urea-cycle enzyme activities and hepatic ultrastructure in acute fatty liver of pregnancy. *J Lab Clin Med* **94:**27–41, 1979.
87. Schultz JC, Adamson JS, Workman WW, et al: Fatal liver disease after intravenous administration of tetracycline in high dosage. *N Engl J Med* **269:**999–1004, 1963.
88. Schiffer MA: Fatty liver associated with administration of tetracycline in pregnant and nonpregnant women. *Am J Obstet Gynecol* **96:**326–332, 1966.
89. Wenk RG, Gebhardt FC, Bhagavan BS, et al: Tetracycline-associated fatty liver of pregnancy, including possible pregnancy risk after chronic dermatologic use of tetracycline. *J Reprod Med* **26:**135–141, 1981.
90. Sherlock S: Acute fatty liver of pregnancy and the microvesicular fat diseases. *Gut* **24:**265–269, 1983.
91. Breen KJ, Perkins KW, Mistilis SP, et al: Idiopathic acute fatty liver of pregnancy. *Gut* **11:**822–825, 1970.
92. Davies MH, Wilkinson SP, Hanid MA, et al: Acute liver disease with encephalopathy and renal failure in late pregnancy and the early puerperiun. *Br J Obstet Gynecol* **87:**1005–1014, 1980.

93. Campillo B, Bernuau J, Witz M-O, et al: Ultrasonography in acute fatty liver of pregnancy. *Ann Intern Med* **105**:383–384, 1986.
94. McKee CM, Weir PE, Foster JH, et al: Acute fatty liver of pregnancy and diagnosis by computed tomography. *Br Med J* **292**:291–292, 1986.
95. Riely CA: Acute fatty liver of pregnancy—1984. *Dig Dis Sci* **29**:456–457, 1984.
96. Duma RJ, Dowling EA, Alexander HC, et al: Acute fatty liver of pregnancy: Report of a surviving patient studied with serial liver biopsies. *Ann Intern Med* **63**:851–858, 1965.
97. Rohs LS: Subcapsular hematoma in fatty liver of pregnancy. *J Forensic Sci* **31**:1509–1513, 1986.
98. Minuk GY, Lui RC, Kelly JK: Rupture of the liver associated with acute fatty liver of pregnancy. *Am J. Gastroenterol* **82**:457–460, 1987.
99. Sakamoto S, Tsuji Y, Koga S, et al: Idiopathic fatty liver of pregnancy with a subsequent uncomplicated pregnancy and a progressive increase in serum cholinesterase activity in the third trimester. *Hepatogastroenterology* **33**:9–10, 1986.
100. MacKenna J, Pupkin M, Grenshaw C, et al: Acute fatty metamorphosis of the liver: A report of two patients who survived. *Am J. Obstet Gynecol* **127**:400–404, 1977.
101. Jenkins WJ, Darling MR: Idiopathic acute fatty liver of pregnancy: Subsequent uncomplicated pregnancy. *J Obstet Gynecol* **1**:100–101, 1980.

31

Liver Disease of Pregnancy: Pathology

Donald B. Rolfes

1. INTRODUCTION

Liver disease is not common in pregnancy. Jaundice is the most frequent clinical manifestation and is present in only one of every 1500 pregnancies.[1] The disorders that affect the liver during this period can be divided into two groups: those that simply occur simultaneously with gestation but that are etiologically unrelated to it, and those that develop only within the context of pregnancy. The former is responsible for two thirds of the cases of liver dysfunction during gestation. Acute viral hepatitis is reputed to be the most common cause of jaundice during pregnancy; however, the entire spectrum of liver disease can occur in the gravid patient. As a general rule, the course of these diseases remains unaffected by gestation. Acute viral hepatitis is no more severe in the pregnant patient, provided she is well nourished, than in the nonpregnant patient.[2] Special consideration is given to these entities in other general references on the topic.[3,4] This chapter examines those diseases that develop exclusively during pregnancy. These include acute fatty liver of pregnancy, liver disease in toxemia of pregnancy, intrahepatic cholestasis of pregnancy and liver disease in hyperemesis gravidarum.

2. THE LIVER DURING NORMAL PREGNANCY

The morphology of the liver is normal during gestation. There are no consistent or distinctive features to characterize a liver of pregnancy. Histologic changes do not accompany the mild increases in total and direct serum bilirubin that can be detected in 20% of pregnant women and that reflect physiologic cholestasis related to increased circulating estrogens.

3. ACUTE FATTY LIVER OF PREGNANCY

Acute fatty liver of pregnancy (AFLP) is a disease of the third trimester that occurs anywhere from the thirtieth to the fortieth week of gestation. Both primigravidas and multiparas are affected. An increased incidence is observed with twin gestations and in pregnancies with male offspring.

Donald B. Rolfes • Department of Pathology, Holy Cross Hospital, Silver Spring, Maryland 20910.

The illness typically has a rapid clinical course which lasts 3 weeks. It begins with a prodrome of malaise, nausea, and vomiting. The patient subsequently becomes jaundiced and shortly afterward develops hepatic encephalopathy. Liver-function tests reflect a predominantly cholestatic disorder with serum bilirubin of 10–15 mg% and moderate alkaline phosphatase elevations. The serum transaminases are modestly elevated, usually below 300 IU/liter and almost always less than 500 IU/liter. Hypoglycemia, a correctable manifestation of the liver failure, and hyperuricemia are commonly observed. Extrahepatic complications frequently accompany AFLP and include azotemia and renal failure, disseminated intravascular coagulation (DIC), peptic ulceration with gastrointestinal (GI) bleeding, and acute pancreatitis. Signs and symptoms of mild toxemia, i.e., hypertension and proteinuria, develop in 20–40% of cases.[5] Their presence should not discourage the physician from considering a diagnosis of AFLP.

This is the most serious of the pregnancy-associated liver diseases. A review of cases reported in the literature up to 1980 found maternal and fetal mortalities of 75% and 85%, respectively.[6] Recent series, with one exception,[7] have shown a dramatic improvement in the prognosis associated with this disorder. Maternal mortality rates in them have ranged from 8 to 33% while fetal deaths occurred in 14–66% of cases.[5,8–12] The explanation for this changing outlook is twofold.[13–15] One is prompt termination of the pregnancy upon diagnosis of this disorder, as well as better supportive care for the hepatic encephalopathy and extrahepatic complications which develop. The other is the recognition that milder cases exist. Older series were based largely on autopsies while more recent studies are clinical reviews and better document the natural course of this disease. It is now evident that some mothers do not develop hepatic encephalopathy, while others manifest early stages of it but do not inevitably progress to coma. In fact, AFLP should be considered in the differential diagnosis of any woman in the third trimester of pregnancy with evidence of liver dysfunction, including those who are anicteric.[7] It has been suggested that the newer imaging techniques, such as computed tomography (CT), ultrasonography, and magnetic resonance imaging (MRI), could be helpful in early diagnosis.[16] A case of AFLP diagnosed by CT has been reported.[17]

Thirteen women are now known to have had normal pregnancies following one complicated by AFLP, and there are no reports of recurrences.[5,9,10,18–21] Therefore, an attitude of guarded optimism can be expressed to patients who wish to become pregnant again.

Affected livers are grossly yellow and often small, a reflection of substantial loss of parenchyma. Microvesicular steatosis is the most characteristic microscopic feature. This is also observed with tetracycline toxicity,[22–24] Reye syndrome,[25] alcoholic foamy degeneration,[26] valproic acid injury,[27] salicylate intoxication,[28] cholesterol ester storage disease,[29] and Wolman disease.[30] The clinical setting should readily distinguish these conditions from AFLP.

Fatty change may involve the liver in a panacinar distribution or zonally, affecting both acinar zones 2 and 3 or may be restricted to the latter. Some reports propose periportal sparing of hepatocytes as a feature distinguishing AFLP from tetracycline toxicity,[7] but this criterion is unreliable. There is no direct correlation between the degree of fatty change and prognosis. The amount of fat observed in the liver probably depends on when in the course of the illness the biopsy was performed. In women who survive, there is rapid mobilization of the lipid, which recedes toward the terminal hepatic venule. Fatty metamorphosis, which is only suspected in occasional zone 3 hepatocytes, is characteristic of biopsies 3 weeks after the onset of jaundice.[8] It may be undectable after 1 month of convalescence.[12,31] A normal hepatic architecture is reconstituted and scarring or other chronic sequelae do not develop.

In most instances, the small fat droplets produce discrete vacuoles in the hepatocyte and the fatty change is readily recognized by light microscopy (Fig. 1A). However, liver cells containing fine fat droplets (less than 1 μm in diameter) do not exhibit distinct vacuolation, but have an appearance of diffuse cytoplasmic ballooning[12,32] (Fig. 1B). These represent a continuum of changes due to increasing enlargement and confluence of lipid droplets. Ballooning is the earliest morphologic expression in which minute fat droplets less than one μm in diameter are present, but are not appreciated by light microscopy.

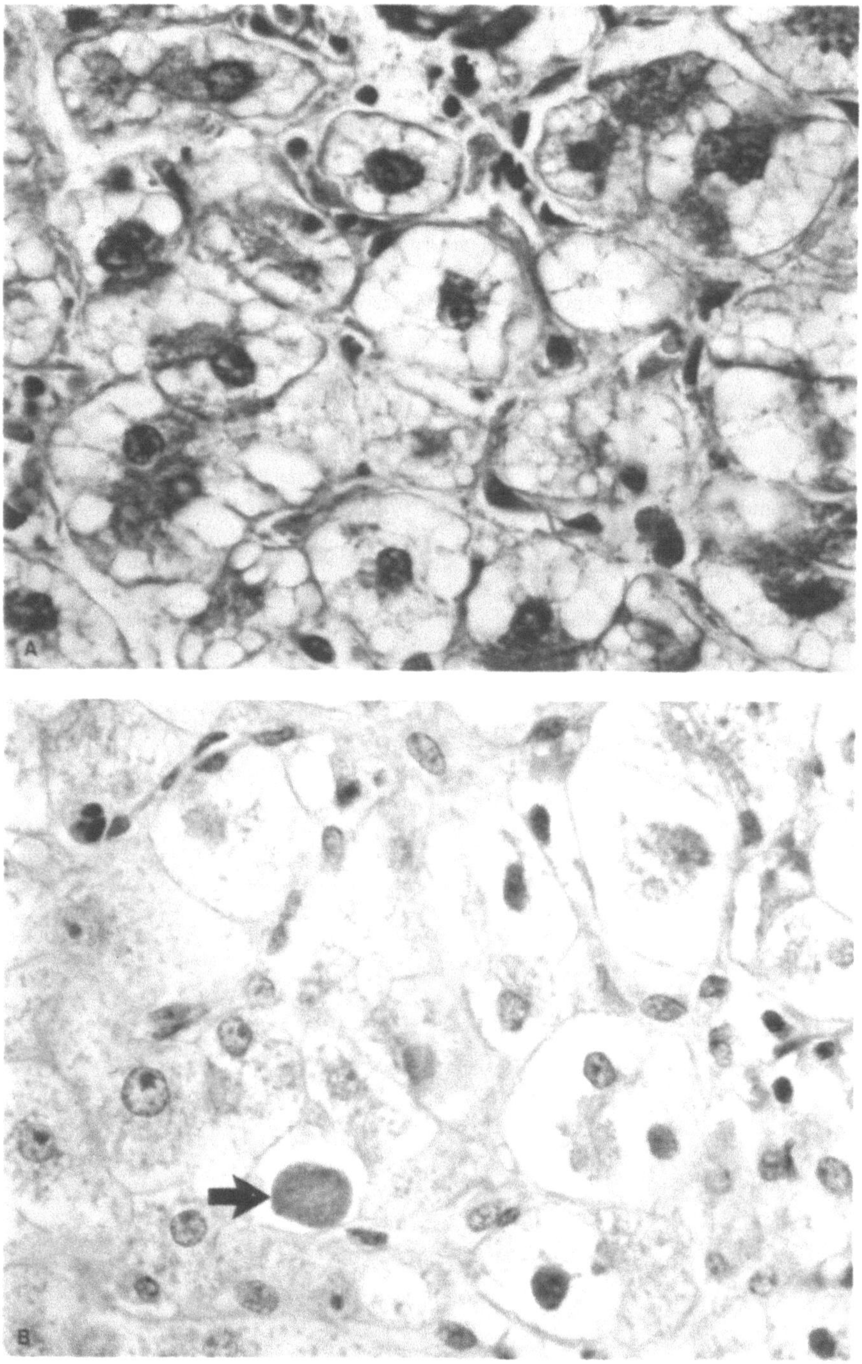

Figure 1. Liver cells undergoing microvesicular fatty change may show distinct varying sized microvesicles (A) or diffuse cytoplasmic ballooning (B). An acidophil body is present (arrowhead). (H&E, ×630)

In some biopsies, ballooning is pronounced and the presence of the lipid is masked. This mimics the hydropic swelling of liver cells in acute viral hepatitis, and it is particularly confusing when accompanied by a lymphoplasmacytic infiltrate and acidophil bodies which are present in 10–20% of the cases.[12] In such instances, the differentiation of AFLP from acute viral hepatitis may be impossible by routine light microscopy (Fig. 2). Unfortunately, this is most often why the biopsy has been performed in cases that are clinically confusing. Termination of pregnancy has not been shown to improve the outcome in acute viral hepatitis, and the additional stress placed on the liver, particularly if a general anesthetic is used for cesarean section, may cause further harm. Therefore, if acute fatty liver is in the differential diagnosis, a small piece of the specimen should not be processed but kept fresh frozen for the potential need to demonstrate the lipid with an oil-red-O stain. While acute viral hepatitis may, on occasion, lead to mild fatty change, its degree does not approach that seen in acute fatty liver of pregnancy, nor is it zonal in distribution.

Microvesicular steatosis is commonly accompanied by other changes. Intrahepatic cholestasis is an almost regular finding, including bile in canaliculi and hepatocytes as well as acute cholangiolitis. Liver cell necrosis occurs and is predominantly due to hepatocytolysis, the histologic expression of which is subtle. Single and small groups of hepatocytes disappear leaving behind hyperplastic aggregates of Kupffer cells, which have phagocytosed and degraded the cellular debris. Finally, extramedullary hematopoiesis including erythroid islands, myeloid groups, and megakaryocytes may be present in the sinusoids.

Speculation on the pathogenesis of AFLP has included the role of mitochondrial injury and the free fatty acid content of the liver. Hepatic mitochondrial enlargement, pleomorphism, and crystalline inclusions are regular ultrastructural findings,[9,33] and megamitochondria may be ob-

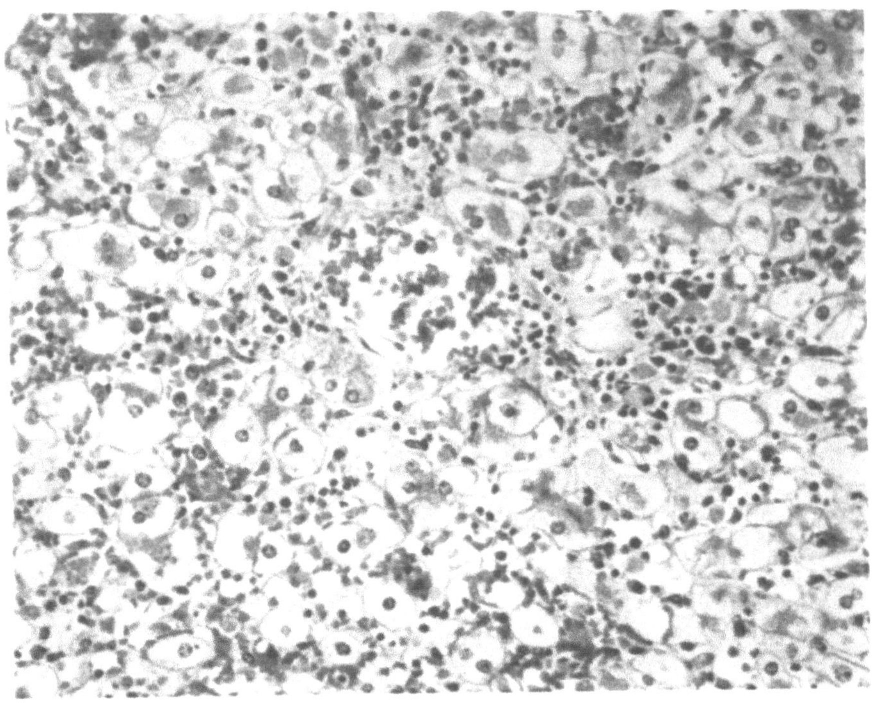

Figure 2. Acute fatty liver of pregnancy may on occasion mimic acute viral hepatitis. Liver cells surrounding a terminal hepatic vesicle are diffusely swollen without discrete vacuoles. A moderate lymphocytic infiltrate is present and hemorrhage is evident in areas of hepatocytolysis. (H&E, ×250)

served by light microsopy.[12] A deficiency of mitochondrial urea cycle enzyme activity has also been demonstrated in several patients.[33] However, unlike the specific mitochondrial changes associated with Reye syndrome, these morphologic alterations can be observed in a wide variety of circumstances and, along with the urea cycle enzyme deficiencies, are not invariably present.[34] They probably represent secondary degenerative or adaptive phenomena to an altered metabolic environment.

Lipid that accumulates in the liver in alcoholism, obesity, and diabetes is mainly neutral tryglyceride.[35,36] In these disorders, fatty change is the result of liver cell injury—and not its cause. Biochemical analysis of fatal cases of AFLP, however, have shown the fat to be predominantly in the form of free fatty acids.[35] These are toxic to both cells and tissue. In AFLP, then, the lipid accumulation may significantly contribute to hepatocellular dysfunction.

4. LIVER DISEASE IN TOXEMIA OF PREGNANCY

Pre-eclampsia is characterized by pregnancy-induced or aggravated hypertension in association with proteinuria and peripheral edema. Convulsions and coma may follow and this stage is termed eclampsia. These complications develop in 5% of pregnancies, occur in the second half of gestation, usually in the third trimester, and principally affect primigravidas.

The liver is not primarily involved in early toxemia, but it is a target organ damaged in severe pre-eclampsia and eclampsia. Hepatic involvement usually manifests as upper abdominal pain, nausea, and vomiting and occasionally jaundice. Laboratory evaluation reflects hepatocellular dysfunction with predominant elevation of the serum transaminases, which can be in the hepatitic range. Bilirubin increases are typically mild, usually below 6 mg%, and largely related to an accompanying microangiopathic hemolytic anemia. Occasionally, deep jaundice develops and in these instances hepatocellular dysfunction also likely contributes to the hyperbilirubinemia.[37] Liver disease most often occurs in women with advanced toxemia due to poor prenatal care. It is usually accompanied by other manifestations of severe disease including a high diastolic blood pressure (>110 mm Hg), high levels of proteinuria (persistently >2+), oliguria, elevated serum creatinine, cerebral and visual disturbances, thrombocytopenia, and fetal growth retardation. Within this clinical context, the cause of the liver disease is usually recognized. Some women with pre-eclampsia present principally with clinical manifestations of hepatic dysfunction and have laboratory evidence of *h*emolytic anemia, *e*levated *l*iver *e*nzymes, and *l*ow *p*latelets,[38–44] an atypical presentation of advanced toxemia termed the HELLP syndrome.[45] Affected patients often have only mild elevations of the blood pressure and proteinuria. Hepatic symptoms within this context may be mistaken for acute viral hepatitis, cholecystitis, gastroenteritis, pancreatitis, or other abdominal emergencies.

Macroscopically, the liver in toxemia shows diffuse, fine or blotchy hemorrhages over the capsular and the cut surface (Fig. 3). Histopathologically, periportal regions reveal variable combinations of fibrin deposition, hemorrhage, and hepatocellular necrosis[32,46] (Fig. 4). Periportal fibrin deposition may occur. This is precipitated within the sinusoids from the immediate periportal areas to the mid-portions of the acinus. Intact liver cell plates initially persist between thin fibrin strands, but the entrapped hepatocytes undergo ballooning and lysis as well as acidophilic degeneration and necrosis, with progressive accumulation of fibrin. Dense wide bands of fibrin eventually replace all adjacent liver cells. Portal tract capillary thrombi are often observed. Less frequently, hepatic arterial thrombi and occlusion of intrahepatic portal veins are observed. In some cases, primary hemorrhage occurs. Red cells dissect through the portal connective tissue and the walls of hepatic arteries and replace the surrounding hepatocytes, forming blood lakes. These hemorrhages may be restricted to the immediate periportal zones or may extend peripherally, in some instances becoming confluent with similar areas of hemorrhage eminating from other portal tracts. Finally, in some instances, evidence of both fibrin deposition and hemorrhage is present. Dense deposits of

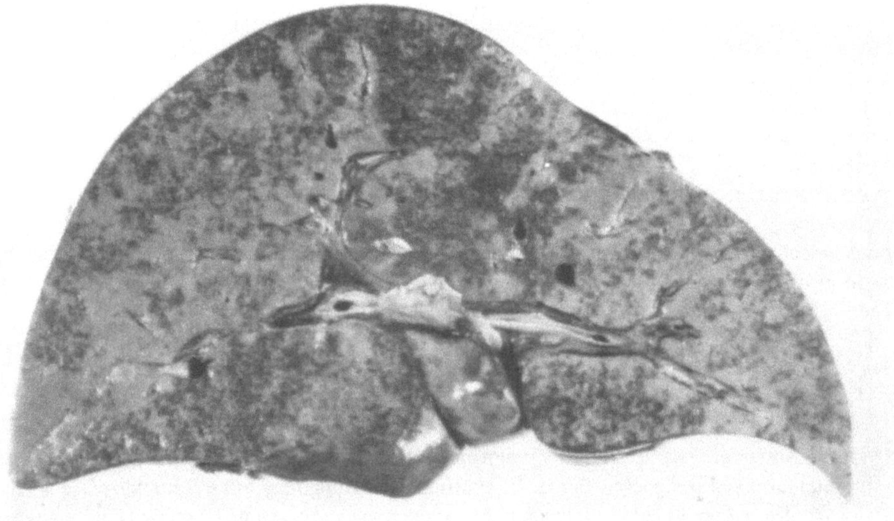

Figure 3. Hepatic involvement in toxemia gives the liver a mottled appearance due to diffuse fine areas of hemorrhage and necrosis.

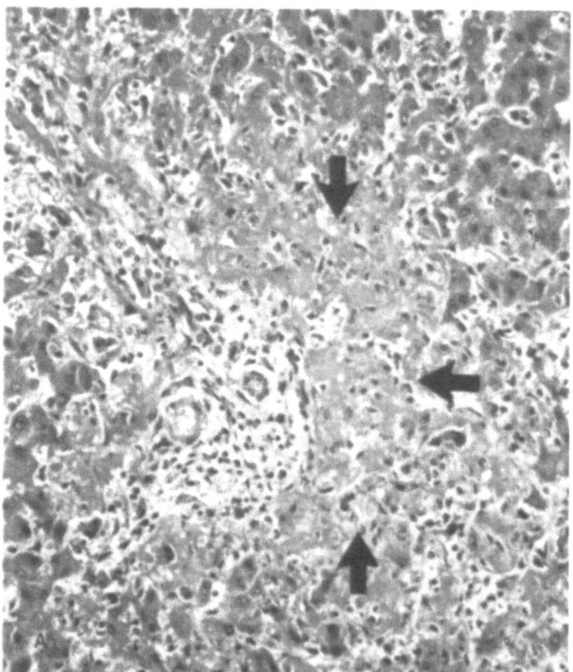

Figure 4. In toxemic liver disease periportal fibrin deposition and/or hemorrhage develop. Pure fibrin deposition (arrowheads) is seen in sinusoids and replacing liver cells in the acinus (A). Red cells flood the portal connective tissue and adjacent acinus (B).

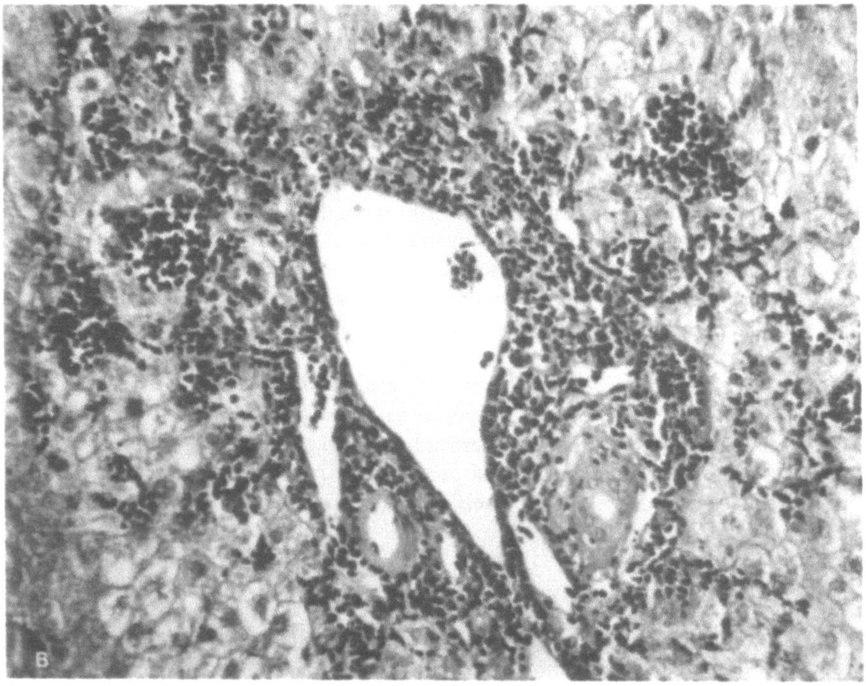

Figure 4. (*Continued*)

fibrin develop in the immediate periportal regions, while more peripherally the acinus is effaced by hemorrhage.

These characteristic periportal lesions are detected at autopsy in more than 75% of women dying with eclampsia.[47] They are observed less often in needle-biopsy specimens from living patients due to sampling artifact and the presence of generally milder disease.[48–52] They are seen in only 25% of such specimens from women with eclampsia and rarely in women with pre-eclampsia. Reconstitution of a normal liver architecture occurs in patients who survive.

Opinions have differed on the sequence and cause of the changes seen in the liver in toxemia. Most have considered periportal sinusoidal fibrin deposition as primary and have attributed it to disseminated intravascular coagulation (DIC).[50,53] However, only a few patients with eclampsia have such coagulation abnormalities.[52,54–59] Some investigators have suggested that liver cell necrosis or hemorrhage is the primary events, but these views are not supported by histologic observations.

Segmental vasospasm creating alternating regions of constriction and dilation along the systemic arterial tree is important in the pathogenesis of toxemia.[44,57,59] It has been proposed that this may produce a vasculopathy, which could explain the changes observed in the liver.[32,52,56] Vasospasm could injure endothelial cells and expose collagen, resulting in a localized consumptive coagulopathy with platelet adherence and aggregation, as well as fibrin precipitation. Hemorrhage could develop secondary to periportal liver cell necrosis resulting from the sinusoidal occlusion. Alternatively, the increased pressure in the dilated regions could lead to mural arterial hemorrhage and tears and could rupture vascular anastomoses (i.e., to sinusoids and hepatic portal veins). An exaggeration of these phenomena at the level of the small hepatic arteries could result in fibrin deposition, hemorrhage, or both, developing within and surrounding the portal tracts.

Central nervous system (CNS) catastrophies are the usual cause of death in toxemia; however, liver involvement may also be responsible. Extensive periportal lesions may lead to liver failure, and two rare complications, rupture and infarction, often prove fatal.

Eighty percent of women with spontaneous hepatic hemorrhage in pregnancy are toxemic.[4,60] These women are often multigravid and they present late in the third trimester or the early postpartum period. Sudden right upper quadrant pain, an abdominal mass and rapidly progressive shock is the characteristic feature. Rupture of the liver is preceded by an hepatic hematoma (Fig. 5). This detaches, elevates, and eventually tears the capsule resulting in exsanguinating hemorrhage. Even the intact hepatic hematoma is potentially fatal. However, these may be managed conservatively with blood product replacement and close monitoring, as long as the patient remains hemodynamically stable.[61] When abdominal bleeding begins, surgery to control hemostasis is usually quoted as the patient's only chance for survival.[62] Even with such treatment, maternal and fetal mortality are high, each approximately 60%. Transcatheter embolotherapy has recently been used in the management of this problem.[63]

Hepatic infarction may occur in toxemia. This can involve localized areas in the liver or as much as 50–90% of the parenchyma. Intense arterial vasospasm may be responsible in some instances. Women with massive hepatic infarction have often had profound episodes of shock. The poor perfusion of the liver during these periods, superimposed on the obstruction to sinusoidal blood flow created by the fibrin deposition, probably accounts for the severe ischemia that leads to such widespread necrosis.

5. INTRAHEPATIC CHOLESTASIS OF PREGNANCY

Intrahepatic cholestasis of pregnancy is second only to viral hepatitis, as a cause of jaundice during gestation, and accounts for 20% of cases. It can occur at any time during the first to the third trimester. It begins with a prodrome of pruritus, and in some instances no further symptoms will develop, a forme fruste referred to as pruritus gravidarum. In most cases, the pruritus is followed in 2 weeks by the onset of mild jaundice, often with dark urine and light stools. Both pruritus and jaundice persist for the duration of the pregnancy. Laboratory studies typically reveal mild elevation

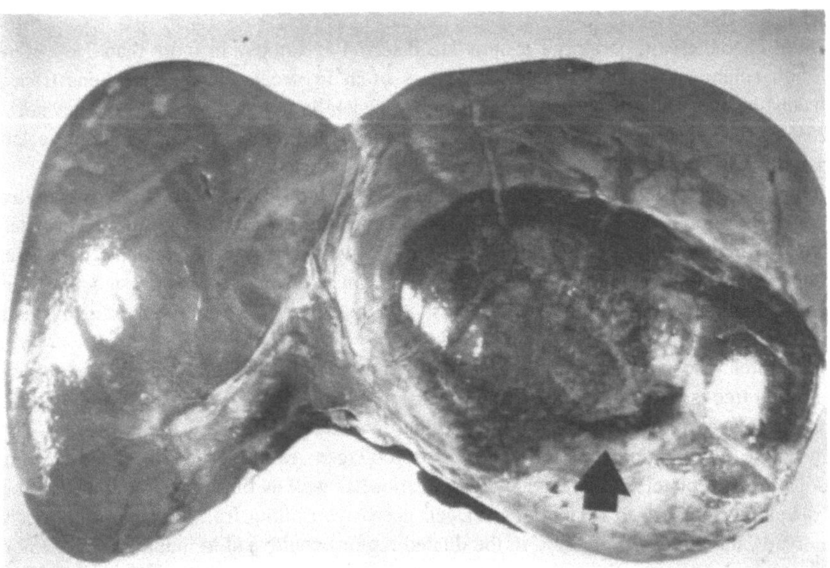

Figure 5. A subcapsular hematoma (arrowhead) precedes hepatic rupture in toxemia of pregnancy. Persistent hepatic hemorrhage will produce a capsular tear and massive peritoneal bleeding.

of the serum bilirubin (<5 mg%, predominantly direct reacting) and alkaline phosphatase activity. Serum bile acids are increased 10–100 times, accounting for the pruritus. The serum aminotransferase values may be increased but are usually less than 250 IU/liter.

This disorder is benign for the mother, and all signs and symptoms resolve, usually within 2 weeks following delivery. Mild pruritis during pregnancy may respond to the use of antihistamines, and more severe symptoms sometimes improve with cholestyramine. Preliminary trials with *S*-adenosyl-L-methionine have been encouraging.[64] A subsequent risk of developing cholelithiasis and gallbladder disease is observed in these women.[65,66] The fetus, however, is at risk in these pregnancies. Fetal distress, fetal death, and premature deliveries can occur. A role for maternal bile salts which cross the placenta has been postulated.[67,68] The overall fetal perinatal mortality is four times that of controls and close perinatal monitoring is necessary.

The histopathology is characterized by acinar cholestasis (Fig. 6). Bile is seen in canaliculi and hepatocytes, predominantly in zone 3. These changes are often subtle. Inflammation and necrosis are typically not observed, and portal tracts are not affected. Intrahepatic cholestasis of pregnancy is due to maternal hypersensitivity to the cholestatic effects of estrogens. Symptoms frequently recur in subsequent pregnancies and during the administration of oral contraceptives or synthetic estrogens.[69] This tendency seems to be inherited, since close family members are affected. Genetic transmission is also implicated because of the variable expression in certain ethnic and geographically isolated groups. Intrahepatic cholestasis of pregnancy occurs with a very high incidence in Chile, where it develops in 10% of pregnant women and is also common in Scandinavian countries.[70]

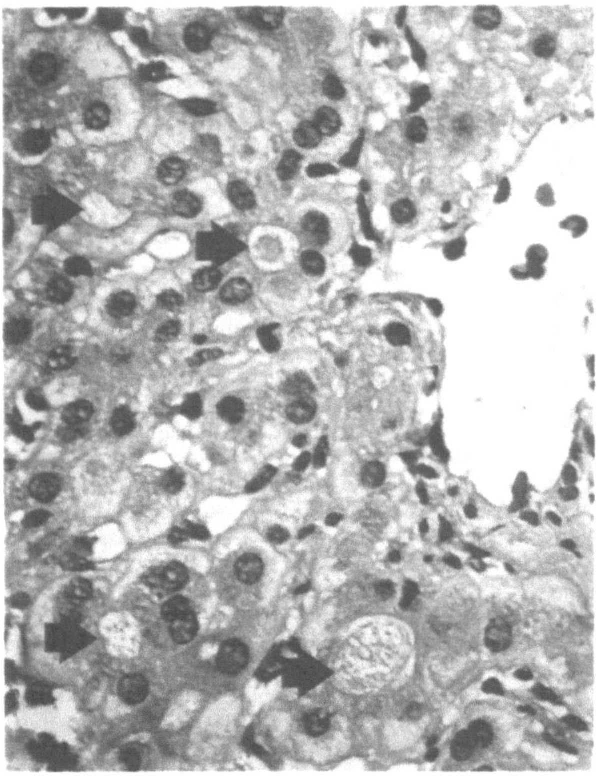

Figure 6. Intrahepatic cholestasis of pregnancy produces canalicular bile plugs (arrowheads) which are most pronounced in acinar zone 3 adjacent to the terminal hepatic venule. (H&E, ×555)

6. LIVER DISEASE IN HYPEREMESIS GRAVIDARUM

Nausea and vomiting are common accompaniments of pregnancy and, when severe, can be associated with liver dysfunction.[71] Such patients are usually diagnosed inhospital after being admitted for dehydration and malnutrition. Occasionally, jaundice develops, but asymptomatic abnormalities of liver-function tests are observed more frequently. The level of bilirubin is usually <4 mg%, the aminotransferases may be increased up to 200 IU/liter, and the alkaline phosphatase activity may be mildly raised. Liver biopsies are only rarely performed on these patients. They usually show a normal parenchyma, or mild fatty change, but a recent report recorded cholestasis and scarce necrotic hepatocytes.[72] Liver dysfunction responds to the control of vomiting and the correction of dehydration and malnutrition.

REFERENCES

1. Haemmerli UP: Jaundice during pregnancy with special emphasis on recurrent jaundice during pregnancy and its differential diagnosis. *Acta Med Scand* **179:**1–111, 1966.
2. Snydman DR: Hepatitis in pregnancy. *N Engl J Med* **313:**1398–1401, 1985.
3. Krejs GJ: Jaundice during pregnancy. *Semin Liver Dis* **3:**73–82, 1983.
4. Steven MM: Pregnancy and liver disease. *Gut* **22:**592–614, 1981.
5. Pockros PJ, Peters RL, Reynolds TB: Idiopathic fatty liver of pregnancy: Findings in ten cases. *Medicine (Baltimore)* **63:**11, 1984.
6. Varner M, Rinderknecht NK: Acute fatty metamorphosis of pregnancy. A maternal mortality and literature review. *J Reprod Med* **24:**177–180, 1980.
7. Hague WM, Duncan SLB, Slater DN, et al: Acute fatty liver of pregnancy. *J R Soc Med* **76:**652–661, 1983.
8. Bernuau J, Degott C, Nouel O, et al: Non-fatal acute fatty liver of pregnancy. *Gut* **24:**340–344, 1983.
9. Burroughs AK, Seong NH, Dojcinov DM, et al: Idiopathic acute fatty liver of pregnancy in 12 patients. *Q J Med* **204:**481–497, 1982.
10. Davies MH, Wilkinson SP, Hanid MA, et al: Acute liver failure with encephalopathy and renal failure in late pregnancy and the early puerperium, a study of 14 patients. *Br J Obstet Gynecol* **87:**1005–1014, 1980.
11. Riely CA: Acute hepatic failure at term. *Postgrad Med* **68:**118–127, 1980.
12. Rolfes DB, Ishak KG: Acute fatty liver of pregnancy: A clinicopathologic study of 35 cases. *Hepatology* **5:**1149–1158, 1985.
13. Kaplan MM: Acute fatty liver of pregnancy. *N Engl J Med* **313:**367–370, 1985.
14. Riely CA: Acute fatty liver of pregnancy—1984. (Editorial.) *Dig Dis Sci* **29:**456–457, 1984.
15. Sherlock S: Acute fatty liver of pregnancy and the microvesicular fat diseases. *Gut* **24:**265–269, 1983.
16. Bova JG, Schenker S: Acute fatty liver of pregnancy. *N Engl J Med* **313:**1608, 1985.
17. McKee CM, Weir PE, Foster JH, et al: Acute fatty liver of pregnancy and diagnosis by computed tomography. *Br Med J* **292:**291–292, 1986.
18. Breen KJ, Perkins KW, Schenker S, et al: Uncomplicated subsequent pregnancy after idiopathic fatty liver of pregnancy. *Obstet Gynecol* **40:**813–815, 1972.
19. Ebert EC, Sun EA, Wright SH, et al: Does early diagnosis and delivery in acute fatty liver of pregnancy lead to improvement in maternal and infant survival? *Dig Dis Sci* **29:**453–455, 1984.
20. Jenkins WJ, Darling MR: Idiopathic acute fatty liver of pregnancy: Subsequent uncomplicated pregnancy. *J Obstet Gynecol* **1:**100–101, 1980.
21. Mackenna J, Pupkin M, Crenshaw C, et al: Acute fatty metamorphosis of the liver. A report of two patients who survived. *Am J Obstet Gynecol* **127:**400–404, 1977.
22. Kunelis CT, Peters RL, Edmondson HA: Fatty liver of pregnancy and its relationship to tetracycline therapy. *Am J Med* **38:**359–377, 1965.
23. Peters RL, Edmondson HA, Mikkelsen WP, et al: Tetracycline-induced fatty liver in non-pregnant patients. *Am J Surg* **113:**622–632, 1967.
24. Robinson MJ, Rywlin AM: Tetracycline associated fatty liver in the male. *Dig Dis* **15:**857–862, 1970.
25. Bove KE, McAdams AJ, Partin JC, et al: The hepatic lesion in Reye's syndrome. *Gastroenterology* **69:**685–697, 1975.

26. Uchida T, Kao H, Quispe-Sjogren M, et al: Alcoholic foamy degeneration—A pattern of acute alcoholic injury of the liver. *Gastroenterology* **84**:683–692, 1983.
27. Zimmerman HJ, Ishak KG: Valproate-induced hepatic injury: Analyses of 23 fatal cases. *Hepatology* **2**:591–597, 1982.
28. Starko KM, Mullick FG: Hepatic and cerebral findings in children with fatal salicylate intoxication: Further evidence for a causal relation between salicylate and Reye's syndrome. *Lancet* **1**:326–329, 1983.
29. Dincsoy HP, Rolfes DB, McGraw CA, et al: Cholesterol ester storage disease and mesenteric lipodystrophy. *Am J Clin Pathol* **81**:263–269, 1984.
30. Miller R, Bialer MG, Rogers JF, et al: Wolman's disease. Report of a case with multiple studies. *Arch Pathol Lab Med* **106**:41–45, 1982.
31. Duma RJ, Dowling EA, Alexander HC, et al: Acute fatty liver of pregnancy. Report of a surviving patient studied with serial liver biopsies. *Ann Intern Med* **63**:851–858, 1965.
32. Rolfes DB, Ishak KG: Liver disease in pregnancy. *Histopathology* **10**:555–570, 1986.
33. Weber FL, Snodgrass PJ, Powell DE, et al: Abnormalities of hepatic mitochondrial urea cycle enzyme activities and hepatic ultrastructure in acute fatty liver of pregnancy. *J Lab Clin Med* **94**:27–41, 1979.
34. Maier J, Daugherty CC, Hug G, et al: Hepatic mitochondrial enzymes and ultrastructural abnormalities in acute fatty liver of pregnancy. *Gastroenterology* **82**:1123, 1982 (abst).
35. Eisele JW, Barker EA, Smuckler EA: Lipid content in the liver of fatty metamorphosis of pregnancy. *Am J Pathol* **81**:545–560, 1975.
36. Hoyumpa AM, Greene HL, Dunn GD, et al: Fatty liver: Biochemical and clinical considerations. *Dig Dis* **20**:1142–1170, 1975.
37. Long RG, Scheuer PJ, Sherlock S: Pre-eclampsia presenting with deep jaundice. *J Clin Pathol* **30**:212–215, 1977.
38. Goodlin RC: Severe preeclampsia: Another great imitator. *Am J Obstet Gynecol* **125**:747–753, 1976.
39. Goodlin RC, Holdt D: Impending gestosis. *Obstet Gynecol* **58**:743–745, 1981.
40. Killam AP, Dillard SH, Patton RC, et al: Pregnancy-induced hypertension complicated by acute liver disease and disseminated intravascular coagulation. Five case reports. *Am J Obstet Gynecol* **123**:823–828, 1975.
41. Lindheimer MD, Katz AI: Hypertension in pregnancy. *N Engl J Med* **313**:675–680, 1985.
42. Mackenna J, Doven NL, Brame RG: Preeclampsia associated with hemolysis, elevated liver enzymes and low platelets—An obstetric emergency? *Obstet Gynecol* **62**:751–754, 1983.
43. Ogle ME, Sanders AB: Preeclampsia. *Ann Emerg Med* **13**:368–370, 1984.
44. Worley RJ: Pathophysiology of pregnancy-induced hypertension. *Clin Obstet Gynecol* **27**:821–835, 1984.
45. Weinstein L: Syndrome of hemolysis, elevated liver enzymes and low platelet count: A severe consequence of hypertension in pregnancy. *Am J Obstet Gynecol* **142**:159–167, 1982.
46. Rolfes DB, Ishak KG: Liver disease in toxemia of pregnancy. *Am J Gastroenterol* **81**:1138–1144, 1986.
47. McKay DG: Clinical significance of the pathology of toxemia of pregnancy. *Circulation* **30**(suppl 2):66–75, 1964.
48. Ingerslev M, Teilum G: Biopsy studies on the liver in pregnancy. III. Liver biopsy in albuminuria of pregnancy, eclampism and eclampsia. *Acta Obstet Gynecol Scand* **25**:361–367, 1945.
49. Sheehan HL: *Toxemias of Pregnancy, Human and Veterinary.* Blakiston, Philadelphia, 1950.
50. McKay DG, Merrill SJ, Weiner AE, et al: The pathologic anatomy of eclampsia, bilateral renal cortical necrosis, pituitary necrosis and other fatal complications of pregnancy and its possible relationship to the generalized Schwartzman reaction. *Am J Obstet Gynecol* **66**:507–539, 1953.
51. Anita FP, Bharadway TP, Watsa MC, et al: Liver in normal pregnancy, pre-eclampsia and eclampsia. *Lancet* **2**:776–778, 1958.
52. Arias I, Mancilla-Jimenez R: Hepatic fibrinogen deposits in preeclampsia. *N Engl J Med* **295**:578–582, 1976.
53. Page EW: On the pathogenesis of pre-eclampsia and eclampsia. *J Obstet Gynaecol Br Commonw* **79**:883–894, 1972.
54. Naish P, Clark AD, Winston RML, et al: Serum and urine fibrinogen derivatives in normal pregnancy and preeclampsia. *Obstet Gynecol* **42**:861–867, 1973.
55. Condie RG: A serial study of coagulation factors XII, XI and X in plasma in normal pregnancy and in pregnancy complicated by pre-eclampsia. *Br J Obstet Gynecol* **83**:636–639, 1976.

56. Pritchard JA, Cunningham FG, Mason RA, et al: Coagulation changes in preeclampsia: Their frequency and pathogenesis. *Am J Obstet Gynecol* **124:**855–864, 1976.
57. Gant NF, Worley RJ: *Hypertension in Pregnancy: Concepts and Management.* Appleton and Lange, East Norwalk, Connecticut, 1980.
58. Sibai BM, Anderson GD, McCubbin JH: Eclampsia. II. Clinical significance of laboratory findings. *Obstet Gynecol* **59:**153–157, 1982.
59. DeVoe SJ, O'Shaughnessy R: Clinical manifestations and diagnosis of pregnancy-induced hypertension. *Clin Obstet Gynecol* **27:**836–853, 1984.
60. Bis KA, Waxman B: Rupture of the liver associated with pregnancy: A review of the literature and report of two cases. *Obstet Gynecol Surv* **31:**763–773, 1976.
61. Manas KJ, Welsh JD, Rankin RA, et al: Hepatic hemorrhage without rupture in preeclampsia. *N Engl J Med* **312:**424–426, 1985.
62. Stalter KD, Sterling WA: Hepatic subcapsular hemorrhage associated with pregnancy. *Surgery* **98:**112–113, 1985.
63. Loevinger EH, Vujic I, Lee WM, et al: Hepatic rupture associated with pregnancy: Treatment with transcatheter embolotherapy. *Obstet Gynecol* **65:**281–284, 1985.
64. Frezza M, Pozzato G, Chiesa L, et al: Reversal of intrahepatic cholestasis of pregnancy in women after high dose S-adenosyl-L-methionine administration. *Hepatology* **4:**274–278, 1984.
65. Samsioe G, Suendsen P, Johnson P, et al: Studies in cholestasis of pregnancy. *Acta Obstet Gynecol Scand* **54:**417–423, 1975.
66. Misra PS, Evanov FA, Wessely Z, et al: Idiopathic intrahepatic cholestasis of pregnancy. Report of an unusual case and review of the recent literature. *Am J Gastroenterol* **73:**54–59, 1980.
67. Laatikainen TJ: Fetal bile acids in pregnancies complicated by maternal intrahepatic cholestasis. *Am J Obstet Gynecol* **122:**852–856, 1975.
68. Laatikainen TJ, Tulenheimo A: Maternal serum bile acid levels and fetal distress in cholestasis of pregnancy. *Int J Gynecol Obstet* **22:**91–94, 1984.
69. Kreek MJ, Weser E, Sleisenger MH, et al: Idiopathic cholestasis of pregnancy. The response to challenge with the synthetic estrogen, ethinyl estradiol. *N Engl J Med* **277:**1391–1395, 1967.
70. Reyes H: The enigma of intrahepatic cholestasis of pregnancy: Lessons from Chile. *Hepatology* **2:**87–95, 1982.
71. Adams RH, Gordon J, Combes B: Hyperemesis gravidarum. Evidence of hepatic dysfunction. *Obstet Gynecol* **31:**659–664, 1968.
72. Larrey D, Rueff B, Feldmann G, et al: Recurrent jaundice caused by recurrent hyperemesis gravidarum. *Gut* **25:**1414–1415, 1984.

32

Hepatocellular Carcinoma: Clinical Aspects

Chao H. Chan

1. INTRODUCTION

Hepatocellular carcinoma is one of the most common malignancies worldwide. The incidence is particularly high in Africa and Asia.[1–8] Accurate figures on the incidence of hepatocellular carcinoma are not available due to the inclusion of gallbladder carcinoma and cholangiocarcinoma as primary liver and biliary tract cancer.[7,9]

The incidence of hepatocellular carcinoma has been reported to be as high as 98.2 per 100,000 males per year for Mozambique and a low of 1.9 for Yugoslavia[7] (Table I). Hepatocellular carcinoma is a relatively uncommon tumor in the United States. The incidence at the Los Angeles County Hospital, based on autopsies, suggest that the occurrence of this tumor is rising.[10] At the University of Arkansas and Veterans Administration Medical Centers, Little Rock, Arkansas, the incidence of hepatocellular carcinoma seen from January 1, 1980 to December 31, 1985 was 2.2% and 2.1% of autopsies, respectively. This figure is comparable with the 2.06% for the whole of Japan[11] and is much higher than those reported from the Los Angeles County Hospital (Table II). The cause of this rise in incidence in the United States is unclear.

2. ETIOLOGIC FACTORS

2.1. Hepatitis B Viral Infection

Worldwide, the frequency of hepatocellular carcinoma parallels the hepatitis B carrier rate (Table III). Countries with a high liver cancer rate also have high HBsAg carrier rate in the general population.[12] In a prospective study conducted in Taiwan, Beasley[13] noted a 390-fold increase risk of liver cancer rate in those government employees who were HBsAg positive than in those who were HBsAg negative on entry into the study. In the Peoples Republic of China, 33–60% of hepatoma patients were HBsAg positive, in contrast to the HBsAg-positive rate of 20% in the general population[14] (Table III). Using recombinant DNA technique and gel electrophoresis,

Chao H. Chan • Gastroenterology Division, University of Arkansas for Medical Sciences; John L. McClellan Memorial Veterans Administration Medical Center, Little Rock, Arkansas 72205.

Table I. Incidence of Primary Liver Cancer

Country	Incidence (per 100,000 males per year)
Mozambique	98.2
China	17.0
South Africa	14.2
Japan	4.6
Denmark	3.4
England and Wales	3.0
United States	
Hawaii	7.2
Other states	2.7
Chile	2.6
Columbia	2.0
Yugoslavia	1.9

Table II. Incidence of Hepatocellular Carcinoma: Autopsy Studies

Source	Percent autopsies
Kurume University (Japan)	3.17
Tokyo Medical University (Japan)	1.36
Whole of Japan (1958–1967)	2.06
Los Angeles County Hospital	
1958–1963	0.21
1954–1963	0.31
1963–1973	0.96
Arkansas	
University of Arkansas 1980–1985	2.2
Veterans Administration Medical Center 1980–1985	2.1

Table III. Frequency of Positive HBsAg in Hepatocellular Carcinoma Patients

Country	Percent positive
United States	3–6
Japan	34–93
Taiwan	44
Singapore	55
Africa	45–88
China	33–60

Shafritz et al.[15] were able to demonstrate the integration of hepatitis B viral DNA into the genome of nontumorous and/or tumor tissues in patients with hepatocellular carcinoma. This integration can be demonstrated in some patients who were seronegative for HBsAg but positive for antibody to HBsAg.[15]

Brechot et al.[16] recently reported a high frequency of positive serum hepatitis B viral DNA (9.5%) and positive liver tissue hepatitis B viral DNA (59%) in 134 patients with chronic liver disease with negative serum tests for HBsAG. In the 20 patients with hepatocellular carcinoma included in this series, HBV DNA hybridizable sequences were detected in the liver tissue of 17 patients. In 12 of these 17 patients, both tumor and nontumorous tissue was available. In nine patients, HBV DNA was detected in both samples. In the other three patients, HBV DNA was only noted in the tumor-bearing tissue. These strong epidemiologic and HBV DNA studies strongly suggest an important pathogenetic role of hepatitis B virus in the development of hepatocellular carcinoma. In the United States, however, the prevalence of hepatitis B virus (HBV) markers in hepatocellular carcinoma patients is relatively low, suggesting that other cocarcinogens or promoters may play an important role in the pathogenesis of liver cancer.[17,18]

2.2. Toxins

A large number of toxins have been implicated in carcinogenesis. They include aflatoxin, nitrosamines, butter yellow, and *Senecio* alkaloids. In liver carcinogenesis, the most important is aflatoxin,[19] produced by the mold, *Aspergillus flavus*. In experimental studies, aflatoxin can induce hepatocellular carcinoma in the monkey, guinea pig, mouse, and rainbow trout.[20] In humans, aflatoxin contamination of food has been positively correlated with the development of hepatocellular carcinoma (Table IV). For instance, Kenyans living in low altitude have twice the incidence of primary liver cancer than those living in higher altitudes, probably due to the higher aflatoxin intake from contaminated food. Similar observations were also noted in Thailand.[21]

2.2.1. Drinking Water and Liver Cancer

At the 1986 Shanghai International Symposium on Liver Cancer and Hepatitis, Yu[22] reported the association of drinking water and hepatoma in Quidong County. The mortality rate of hepatocellular carcinoma in the population that drank pond water was 140 per 10^5—3.5 times higher than that of river water drinkers (40 per 10^5) and seven times higher than that of well-water drinkers (20 per 10^5). Serologic studies of hepatitis B markers showed a comparable HBsAG-positive (11%, 8.9%, 12.6%) and anti-HBs-positive (50.5%, 49.8%, 49.3%) rate, respectively, for pond, river, and well-

Table IV. Aflatoxin Intake and Hepatocellular Carcinoma

Country	Aflatoxin intake (ng/kg per day)	Incidence of hepatocellular Ca (per 100,000/year)
Mozambique	222.4	13
Thailand[a]	45.6	6
Thailand[b]	5.0	2
Kenya[a]	10.0	4
Kenya[b]	3.5	1.2

[a]Low altitude.
[b]High altitude.

water drinkers. Yu concluded that the difference in hepatocellular carcinoma rate could not be accounted for by the HBV infection. Further study of aflatoxin intake and analysis of water content of DDT and BHC (Table V) as a marker of chemical or toxin contamination suggested that pond and river water have higher chemical contaminants than does well water. These contaminants may serve as a promoter or cocarcinogen in the development of liver cancer in Quidong County. Yu quoted an Environmental Protection Agency (EPA) study that reportedly showed the presence of 2221 contaminants in drinking water, including 22 carcinogens, 42 suspected carcinogens, 27 cocarcinogens, 56 mutagens, and 15 suspect mutagens.[23] Initial epidemiologic analysis of the Arkansas hepatocellular carcinoma cases suggests clustering of patients along certain parts of the Arkansas River. Further investigation into toxin contamination is planned.

2.3. Cirrhosis and Liver Cancer

Hepatocellular carcinoma is superimposed on cirrhosis in varying frequency.[10,24,25] In the United States, 80–90% of hepatocellular carcinoma was superimposed on cirrhosis,[10,26] whereas in Africa and India, cirrhosis may not be as prevalent (30–40%).[26] Hepatocellular carcinoma has developed in cirrhosis associated with hemochromatosis,[24,25] α_1-antitrypsin deficiency,[27] alcoholic cryptogenic primary biliary cirrhosis, and chronic active hepatitis (CAH).[24] One notable exception is Wilson disease, which is seldom associated with the development of liver cancer.[28]

2.4. Alcohol

Hardell et al.[29] reported a fourfold increased risk of hepatocellular carcinoma in alcoholics in North America and Europe. Similar associations have been noted by others.[30–32] By contrast, Ugarte and Donoso[33] reported a low incidence of hepatocellular carcinoma despite a very high alcohol consumption and cirrhosis in Chile. Since most of the positive association of hepatocellular carcinoma and alcoholics was in cirrhotics, the etiologic role of alcohol per se is difficult to document. A high prevalence of HBV marker in the alcoholic cirrhotic[34] and the demonstration of integrated HBV DNA in liver and tumor tissue of alcoholic cirrhotics with hepatocellular carcinoma[35] cast further doubt that alcohol per se plays a primary role in the development of hepatocellular carcinoma.

2.5. Miscellaneous Factors

Oral and anabolic steroids have rarely been reported to cause hepatocellular carcinoma as well.[36,37] Association of hepatocellular carcinoma and non-A, non-B (NANB) hepatitis infection is uncertain. Although some cases of NANB post-transfusion hepatitis have reportedly developed into hepatocellular carcinoma.[38,39]

Table V. Drinking Water Source, Chemical Contamination, and Hepatocellular Carcinoma: Quidong County, China

Source of water	Approximate mortality rate/100,000	Aflatoxin B intake (ng/kg per day)	Contaminant DDT (ppb)	Contaminant BHC (ppb)
Pond	140	2.51	0.0153	0.4786
River	40	7.28	0.0206	0.3934
Well, shallow	20	3.51	0.0033	0.0552

Hepatocellular carcinoma seemed to evolve by exposure to an initiating factor, which may be HBV infection, leading to integration of HBV viral DNA into host cells. This was accompanied by a simultaneous or subsequent exposure to a promoter or promoters, which may be toxin, alcohol, cirrhosis, androgen, and so forth. The initiating and promoter factors combined results in formation of hepatocellular carcinoma.

3. CLINICAL FEATURES

3.1. Age and Sex

In the United States, primary liver cancer is a disease of the elderly (65–80 years); in Asia, it is prevalent in the middle aged (45–65 years), while in Africa it was noted primarily in the young adult (under 40 years). Hepatocellular carcinoma is predominantly a male disease with a male-to-female ratio of 4 : 1–9 : 1. In the United States, however, the male-to-female ratio may be lower (2 : 1–4 : 1).[40–44]

3.2. Clinical Symptoms

The most frequent presenting symptom in the Arkansas series[40] is abdominal pain (69%). Weight loss/anorexia (60%) and weakness (35%) are other common symptoms. Jaundice, however, was the presenting symptom in only 18% of our patients.[40] A cirrhotic patient who presents with sudden deterioration with increasing ascites, hepatic encephalopathy, or unexplained fever should alert one to the possibility of hepatocellular carcinoma.

3.3. Physical Signs

The most common physical finding is hepatomegaly, noted in 80–90% of all patients (Table VI); tender hepatomegaly was found in approximately one half of the patients. Hepatic bruits, although noted in 6–25% of some series,[26,43] were seldom noted in our Arkansas patients.

3.3.1. Systemic Syndromes Associated with Liver Cancer

A panoramic variety of paraneoplastic and systemic syndromes associated with hepatocellular carcinoma such as erythrocytosis, hypercalcemia, hypoglycemia, hypercholesteronemia, abnormal globulin, abnormal isoferritin, aberrant alkaline phosphatase, dysfibrinogenemia, cryofibrinogenemia, carcinoid syndrome, porphyria cutanea tarda, cystathioninemia, and precocious puberty have been summarized in the literature[10,26,45] but are seldom seen in most North American series.[40,41]

Table VI. Physical Signs

Sign	Arkansas (%)	Literature (%)
Hepatomegaly	73	80–95
Tenderness	48	15–60
Splenomegaly	6	20–45
Fever	9	10–50
Jaundice	20	10–40

3.4. Laboratory Findings

Anemia is the most common hematologic abnormality noted (60–75%). Erythrocytosis noted in 2–10% of patients in the literature was not seen in our Arkansas series.[40] Leukocytosis (30%) and prolonged prothrombin time (70%) were also quite common. Routine liver tests such as serum bilirubin, aspartate aminotransferase (SGOT), alanine aminotransferase (SGPT), alkaline phosphatase, and lactic dehydrogenase (LDH), were frequently abnormal (Table VII). Serum bilirubin level, however, is only moderately increased (mean 3.4 mg%). SGOT values were in the 100–200 range, with SGOT/SGPT of two to four, similar to those observed in alcoholic liver diseases. Serum alkaline phosphatase and LDH levels were usually two- to fourfold elevated.[40]

4. DIAGNOSIS

The diagnosis of hepatocellular carcinoma depends on a high index of suspicion. A cirrhotic patient with unexplained deterioration or the development of right upper quadrant (RUQ) pain in an HBsAg carrier should alert one to the possibility of hepatocellular carcinoma. However, as pointed out by Chlebowski et al.,[41] most hepatoma patients (67%) in their series have no prior diagnosis of liver disease despite the presence of cirrhosis in 63% and positive HBsAg in 52% of their patients. Elevated levels of α-fetoprotein (AFP) and des-r-carboxyprothrombin noted in 40–85% of hepatocellular carcinoma patients are good collaborative tests.[46,47] Definitive diagnosis, however, requires liver biopsy performed percutaneously or under ultrasound or CT guidance. Selective arteriographic studies may be necessary to determine vascular anatomy and extent of hepatic involvement, especially when hepatic resection is contemplated.[48] Recently, radioimmunoassay (RIA) techniques using monoclonal antibody tagged with AFP or ferritin have been proposed as a new method of detection and diagnosis.[49] Others suggest the use of iodized oil as an aid in the detection of hepatocellular carcinoma.[50]

5. PROGNOSIS AND SURVIVAL

Okuda et al.[51] recently published their analysis of 600 consecutive hepatoma patients seen in Japan. These investigators staged their patients based on four factors: presence of ascites, tumor size more than 50% of liver mass, albumin <3 g%, or bilirubin >3 mg%. Stage I included patients with none of the factors present; stage II, with one or two factors present; and stage III, with three or four factors present. Using this staging system, survival of hepatocellular carcinoma patients depends on the stage of disease and on whether the treatment is surgical or nonsurgical. The 5-year survival for

Table VII. Liver Tests in 112 Patients in Arkansas[a]

Liver tests[b]	LRVA	UAMS	Other
Total bilirubin mg% (<1.2 mg%)	3.4 ± 3.8	2.9 ± 4.7	4.5 ± 7.9
SGOT (<45 μm)	137 ± 132	124 ± 94	259 ± 501
SGPT (<45 μm)	72 ± 94	54 ± 25	62 ± 36
LDH (<190 μm)	401 ± 480	429 ± 375	475 ± 75
Alk pH (<115 μm)	390 ± 308	318 ± 286	488 ± 62

[a]LRVA, Little Rock Veterans Administration Hospital; UAMS, University of Arkansas Hospital; Other, other Arkansas hospitals.
[b]Values in parentheses represent normal values.

the whole series was 34% for the surgically treated group, and only 5% for nonsurgically treated patients. The median survival for stage I patients was 32.4 months in the surgical group but only 8.1 months in the nonsurgical group. For stage II patients, the surgically treated group had a median survival of 7.4 months, compared with 2.1 months for the nonsurgically treated group. For stage III patients, nonsurgically treated patients had a median survival of only 0.7 months. There were no stage III surgically treated patients. Early detection and surgical resection seem to be the key to prolonged survival.

6. PREVENTION AND SCREENING

The most effective preventive measure is mass vaccination of the susceptible population with hepatitis B vaccine.[52,53] Currently, massive efforts to vaccinate all newborns are being conducted in the People's Republic of China. The Chinese are conducting trials aimed at screening of high-risk persons such as HBsAg carriers and patients with history of post-transfusion hepatitis who are over 45 years of age. Screening tests consist of periodic (every 3–6 months) serum AFP and ultrasonography every 6 months. Tang claimed that such screening may permit the detection of small hepatocellular carcinoma at an early stage, which can be surgically resected successfully.[49] Similar screening of a high-risk Alaskan population has also been reported by Hayward et al.[54] to be beneficial. Several recent studies emphasized screening[55–57] and detection of small hepatocellular carcinoma.[58–60] Despite these claims in the literature, there were no randomized control trials documenting their effectiveness.

7. TREATMENT

Early detection and hepatic resection remain the most effective mode for cure for hepatocellular carcinoma.[49,58] Hepatic artery ligation or embolization,[49,61] radiation,[61] and chemotherapy either systemic or via hepatic artery infusion,[61,62] although reported to be beneficial, were not substantiated by well-controlled studies. The lack of regional and distant metastasis in 25% of our Arkansas autopsy cases,[40] despite large tumor mass, raised the possibility of transplantation in these patients. Hepatic transplantation has yielded satisfactory results in the series of Cuervas-Mons et al.,[63] especially in young patients with fibrolamellar hepatocellular carcinoma.

REFERENCES

1. Anthony PP: Primary carcinoma of the liver: A study of 282 cases in Ugandan Africans. *J Pathol* **110**:37–48, 1973.
2. Berman C: Primary carcinoma in the Bantu races of South Africa. *S Afr J Med Sci* **5**:54–72, 1960.
3. Geddes EW, Falkson G: Malignant hepatoma in the Bantu. *Cancer* **25**:1271–1278, 1970.
4. Steiner PE: Cancer of the liver and cirrhosis in Trans-Saharan Africa and the United States of America. *Cancer* **13**:1085–1166, 1960.
5. Tull JC: Primary carcinoma of the liver: A study of one hundred and thirty-four cases. *J Pathol* **35**:557–562, 1932.
6. Vogel CL, Anthony PP, Mody N, et al: Hepatitis-associated antigen in Ugandan patients with hepatocellular carcinoma. *Lancet* **2**:621–624, 1970.
7. Doll R, Payne P, Waterhouse J: *Cancer Incidence in Five Continents*. International Union Against Cancer and Springer-Verlag, Heidelberg, 1966.
8. Beasley RP, Hwang LY, Lin CC, et al: Hepatocellular carcinoma and hepatitis B virus. *Lancet* **2**:1129–1132, 1981.
9. American Cancer Society: *Cancer Facts and Figures*, American Cancer Society, New York, 1985.

10. Edmondson HA, Craig JR: Neoplasm of the liver, in Schiff L, Schiff E (eds): *Disease of the Liver*, 6th ed. JB Lippincott, Philadelphia, 1987, pp. 1109–1158.
11. Okuda K, Peters RL (eds): *Hepatocellular Carcinoma*. Wiley, New York, 1976.
12. Lutwick LI: Relationship between aflatoxins and hepatitis B virus and hepatocellular carcinoma. *Lancet* **1**:755–757, 1979.
13. Beasley RP: Hepatitis B virus as the etiologic agent in hepatocellular carcinoma—Epidemiologic considerations. *Hepatology* **2**:21s–26s, 1982.
14. Kang LY: Epidemiology and prevention of viral hepatitis in China, in *Proceedings of the 1986 Shanghai International Symposium on Liver Cancer and Hepatitis* pp. 230–259.
15. Shafritz DA, Shouval D, Sherman HI, et al: Integration of hepatitis B virus DNA into the genome of liver cells in chronic liver disease and hepatocellular carcinoma. *N Engl J Med* **305**:1067–1073, 1981.
16. Brechot C, Degos F, Lugassy C, et al: Hepatitis B virus DNA in patients with chronic liver disease and negative tests for hepatitis B surface antigen. *N Engl J Med* **312**:270–276, 1985.
17. Omata M, Ashcavai M, Liew CT, et al: Hepatocellular carcinoma in the U.S.A. Etiologic considerations. *Gastroenterology* **76**:279–287, 1979.
18. Tabor E, Gerety RJ, Vogel CL, et al: Hepatitis B virus infection and primary hepatocellular carcinoma. *J Natl Cancer Inst* **58**:1197–1200, 1977.
19. Enwonwu CO: The role of dietary aflatoxin in the genesis of hepatocellular cancer in developing countries. *Lancet* **2**:956–958, 1984.
20. Busby WF, Wogan GN: Food-borne mycotoxins and alimentary mycotoxicoses, in Riemann H, Bryan FL (eds): *Food-borne Infections and Intoxications*. Academic, Orlando, Florida, 1979, pp. 519–610.
21. Linsell CA, Peers FG: Aflatoxin and liver cell cancer. *Trans R Soc Trop Med Hyg* **71**:471–473, 1977.
22. Yu SZ: Drinking water and primary liver cancer, in *Proceedings of the 1986 Shanghai International Symposium on Liver Cancer and Hepatitis*. pp. 260–278.
23. Report to Congress: *Preliminary Assessment of Suspected Carcinogens in Drinking Water*. U.S. Environmental Protection Agency, Washington, D.C., 1975.
24. Zaman SN, Melia WM, Johnson RD, et al: Risk factors in development of hepatocellular carcinoma in cirrhosis: Prospective study of 613 patients. *Lancet* **1**:1357–1360, 1985.
25. Bradbear RA, Bain C, Siskind V, et al: Cohort study of internal malignancy in genetic hemochromatosis and other chronic nonalcoholic liver diseases. *J Natl Cancer Inst* **75**:81–84, 1985.
26. Chan CH: Primary carcinoma of the liver. *Med Clin North Am* **50**:989–994, 1975.
27. Berg NO, Eriksson S: Liver disease in adults with alpha-l-antitrypsin deficiency. *N Engl J Med* **287**:1264–1267, 1972.
28. Wilkinson ML, Portmann B, Williams R: Wilson's disease and hepatocellular carcinoma: possible protective role of copper. *Gut* **24**:767–771, 1983.
29. Hardell L, Bengtsson NO, Jonsson U, et al: Etiologic aspects of primary liver cancer with special regard to alcohol, organic solvents and acute intermittent porphyria—An epidemiological investigation. *Br J Cancer* **50**:389–397, 1984.
30. Faivre J, Milan C, Bugnon P, Legoux JL, et al: Primary liver cancer in Cote d' Or (Burgundy). Results of three years systematic registration in a well-defined French population. *Biomedicine* **31**:150–152, 1979.
31. Lee F: Cirrhosis and hepatoma in alcoholics. *Gut* **7**:77–85, 1966.
32. Leevy C, Gellene R, Ning M: Primary liver cancer in cirrhosis of the alcoholic. *Ann NY Acad Sci* **114**:1026–1040, 1964.
33. Ugarte G, Donoso S: Primary hepatic tumors in Chile, in Remmer H, Bolt HM, Bannasch P, et al (eds): *Primary Liver Tumors*, MTP Press, Lancaster, 1978, pp. 165–169.
34. Bassendine MF, Seta L, Salmerons J, et al: Incidence of hepatitis B virus infection in alcoholic liver disease. HBsAg negative chronic active liver disease and primary liver cell cancer in Britain. *Liver* **3**:65–70, 1983.
35. Brechot C, Nalpas B, Courouce AM, et al: Evidence that hepatitis B virus has a role in liver cell carcinoma in alcoholic liver disease. *N Engl J Med* **306**:1384–1387, 1982.
36. Neuberger J, Portmann B, Nunnerley HB, et al: Oral contraceptive associated liver tumours: Occurrence of malignancy and difficulties in diagnosis. *Lancet* **1**:273–276, 1980.
37. Shar SR, Kew MC: Oral contraceptives and hepatocellular carcinoma. *Cancer* **49**:407–410, 1982.
38. Kiyosawa K, Akahane Y, Nagata A, et al: Hepatocellular carcinoma after non-A, non-B post-transfusion hepatitis. *Am J Gastroenterol* **79**:777–781, 1984.
39. Resnick RH, Stone K, Antonioli D: Primary hepatocellular carcinoma following non-A, non-B post-transfusion hepatitis. *Dig Dis Sci* **28**:908–911, 1983.

40. Chan CH, Slaton D, Morrison D, et al: Hepatocellular carcinoma in Arkansas, clinical and epidemiologic features in 112 patients. (in preparation)
41. Chlebowski RT, Tong M, Weissman J, et al: Hepatocellular carcinoma: Diagnostic and prognostic features in North American patients. *Cancer* **53**:2701–2706, 1984.
42. Inouye AA, Whelan TJ Jr: Primary liver carcinoma: A review of 205 cases in Hawaii. *Am J Surg* **138**:53–61, 1979.
43. Ihde DC, Sherlock P, Winawer SJ, et al: Clinical manifestations of hepatoma: A review of 6 year's experience at a cancer hospital. *Am J Med* **56**:83–91, 1974.
44. Kew MC: Clinical, pathologic and etiologic heterogeneity in hepatocellular carcinoma: Evidence from southern Africa. *Hepatology* **1**:366–369, 1981.
45. Margolis S, Homcy C: Systemic manifestations of hepatoma. *Medicine (Baltimore)* **51**:381–391, 1972.
46. Soulier JP, Gozin D, Lefrere JJ: A new method to assay des-r-carboxyprothrombin. *Gastroenterology* **91**:1258–1262, 1986.
47. Liebman HA, Furie BC, Tong MJ, et al: Des-gamma-carboxy (abnormal) prothrombin as a serum marker of primary hepatocellular carcinoma. *N Engl J Med* **310**:1427–1431, 1984.
48. Williamson BWA, Blumgart LH, McKellar NJ: Management of tumors of the liver, combined use of arteriography and venography in the assessment of resectability, especially in hilar tumors. *Am J Surg* **139**:210–215, 1980.
49. Proceedings of the *1986 Shanghai International Symposium on Liver Cancer and Hepatitis*. pp. 1–171.
50. Ohishi H, Uchida H, Yoshimura H, et al: Hepatocellular carcinoma detected by iodized oil. *Radiology* **154**:25–29, 1985.
51. Okuda K, Obata H, Nakajima Y, et al: Prognosis of primary hepatocellular carcinoma. *Hepatology* **4**:3s–6s, 1984.
52. Lee SD, Lo KJ, Wu JC, et al: Prevention of maternal-infant hepatitis B virus transmission by immunization: The role of serum hepatitis B virus DNA. *Hepatology* **6**:369–373, 1986.
53. Blumberg BS, London WT: Hepatitis B virus and the prevention of primary cancer of the liver. *J Natl Cancer Inst* **71**:267–273, 1985.
54. Heyward WL, Lanier AP, McMahon BJ, et al: Early detection of primary hepatocellular carcinoma. *JAMA* **254**:3052–3054, 1985.
55. Kobayashi K, Sugimoto T, Makino H, et al: Screening methods for early detection of hepatocellular carcinoma. *Hepatology* **5**:1100–1105, 1985.
56. Liaw YF, Tai DI, Chu CM, et al: Early detection of hepatocellular carcinoma in patients with type B hepatitis. *Gastroenterology* **90**:263–267, 1986.
57. Ebara M, Ohto M, Shinagawa T, et al: Natural history of minute hepatocellular carcinoma smaller than three centimeters complicating cirrhosis. *Gastroenterology* **90**:289–298, 1986.
58. Tang Z-Y (ed): *Subclinical Hepatocellular Carcinoma*. China Academic Publishers, Beijing-Springer-Verlag, Berlin, 1985.
59. Sheu JC, Sung JL, Chen DS, et al: Early detection of hepatocellular carcinoma by real-time ultrasonography. *Cancer* **56**:660–666, 1985.
60. Sheu JC, Sung JL, Chen DS: Growth rate of asymptomatic hepatocellular carcinoma and its clinical implications. *Gastroenterology* **89**:259–266, 1985.
61. Cady B, Macdonald JS, Gunderson LL: Cancer of the hepatobiliary system, in Devita VT Jr, Hellman S, Rosenberg SA (eds): *Cancer, Principles and Practice of Oncology*, 2nd ed. JB Lippincott, Philadelphia, 1985, pp. 747–753.
62. Lighdsdale CJ, Daly J: Management of primary and metastatic cancer of the liver, in Devita VT Jr, Hellman S, Rosenberg SA (eds): *Cancer, Principles and Practice of Oncology*, 2nd ed. JB Lippincott, Philadelphia, 1985, pp. 1159–1170.
63. Cuervas-Mons V, Martinez AJ, Dekker A, et al: Adult liver transplantation: An analysis of early causes of death on 40 consecutive cases. *Hepatology* **6**:495–501, 1986.

33

Hepatocellular Carcinoma: Pathology

Donald B. Rolfes

1. USUAL HEPATOCELLULAR CARCINOMA

Hepatocellular carcinoma is the most common primary malignancy of the liver. This neoplasm is relatively rare in the United States but is the most common fatal malignancy in many parts of the world. Hepatocellular carcinoma usually develops in the cirrhotic liver of older adults. Hepatitis B infection is present in 85% of cases worldwide, although alcoholism is the most common associated disease in developed countries of the Western world.[1]

Grossly, these tumors are typically widely disseminated in a cirrhotic liver, replacing regenerating nodules, or they are multicentric at the time of diagnosis (Fig. 1). Vascular invasion is common with both the portal and hepatic veins being involved, as well as the inferior vena cava. As a consequence, these neoplasms are usually unresectable and have a grim prognosis, with survival measured in months. A variant that may have prognostic significance is the encapsulated hepatocellular carcinoma.[2] These tumors tend to be solitary and to grow slowly, forming a thick fibrous capsule. Consequently, they are more often resectable than other types of hepatocellular carcinoma.

Microscopically, the cells of most hepatocellular carcinomas resemble normal liver cells to a variable degree. They have distinct cell membranes and oncocytic finely granular cytoplasm. Bile canaliculi can usually be demonstrated between the cells. Bile pigment may be present in tumor cells or in dilated bile canaliculi and is the most helpful feature establishing the diagnosis. A variety of cellular products reflecting normal and pathologic liver cell function can often be demonstrated. These include glycogen, Mallory bodies, α_1-antitrypsin, and α-fetoprotein (AFP).

Several histologic growth patterns are found in hepatocellular carcinoma.[3] Since the cytologic features can be so variable, recognizing one of these patterns may be very helpful in arriving at a diagnosis. The most frequent is the trabecular pattern (Fig. 2). The trabeculae are separated by sinusoid-like vascular spaces with little or no supporting connective tissue. The trabeculae may be only a few cells thick (microtrabecula), or more than 20 cells thick (macrotrabecula). Sometimes the centers of the trabeculae contain a dilated canaliculus, producing a pseudoglandular pattern. Solid or "cobblestone" patterns are produced when trabeculae grow together, forming sheets of tumor cells. Occasional carcinomas develop large vascular lakes within the tumor, mimicking peliosis hepatis and producing the pelioid type of hepatocellular carcinoma.

These various histologic patterns are not thought to have any particular prognostic significance.

Donald B. Rolfes • Department of Pathology, Holy Cross Hospital, Silver Spring, Maryland 20910.

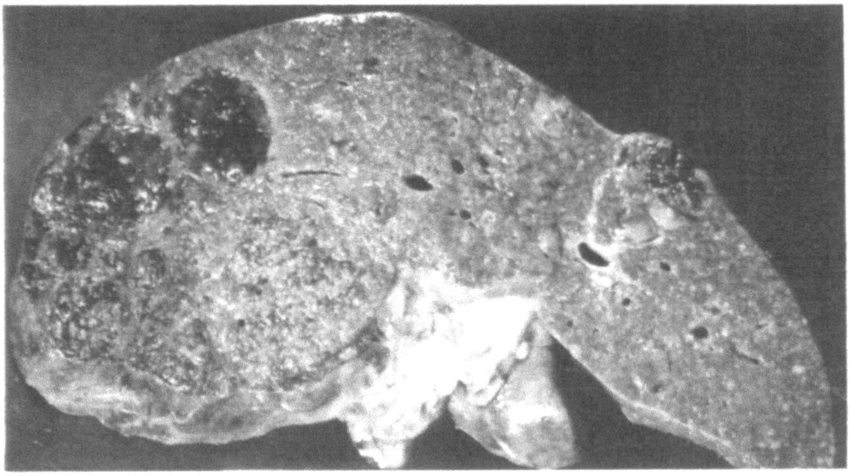

Figure 1. Widespread hemorrhagic nodules of hepatocellular carcinoma present in a cirrhotic liver.

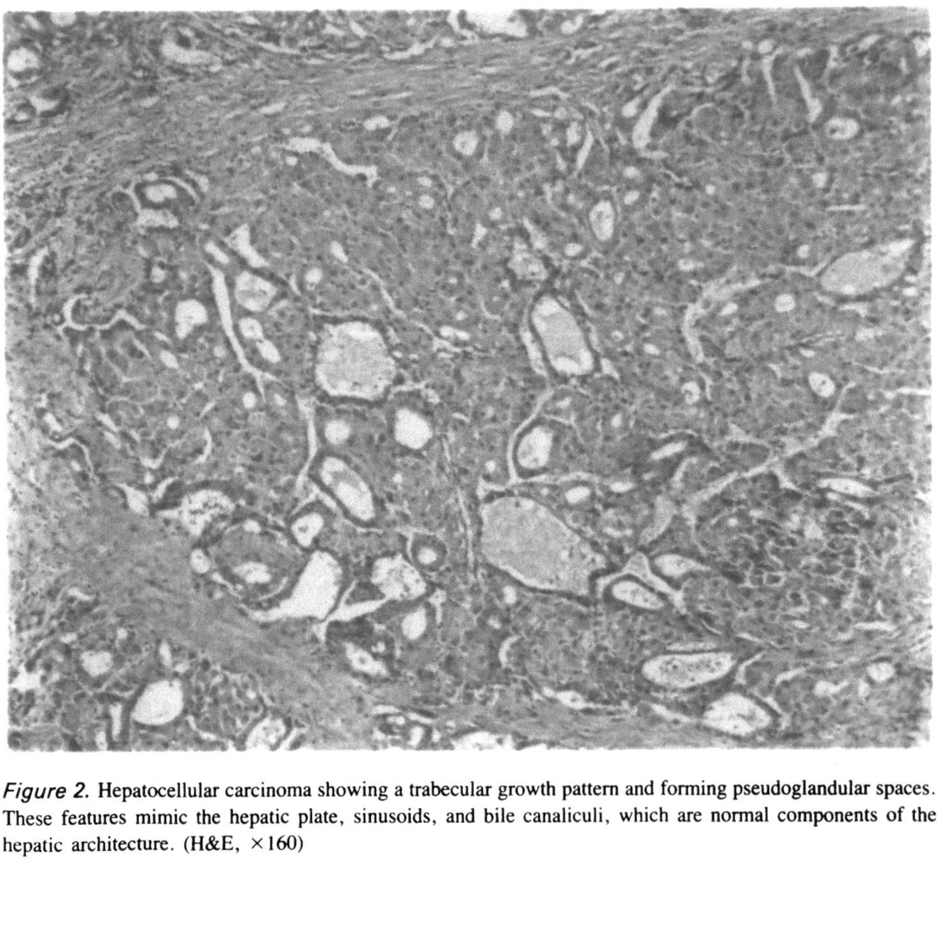

Figure 2. Hepatocellular carcinoma showing a trabecular growth pattern and forming pseudoglandular spaces. These features mimic the hepatic plate, sinusoids, and bile canaliculi, which are normal components of the hepatic architecture. (H&E, ×160)

However, a histologic variant that appears to have a somewhat better prognosis is the clear cell type of hepatocellular carcinoma. The clear cell appearance is caused by large amounts of fat and/or glycogen in the tumor cells and can sometimes be difficult to distinguish histologically fror :lear cell carcinomas of the kidney. The overall prognosis, however, is still quite poor.[4]

2. FIBROLAMELLAR CARCINOMA OF THE LIVER

Fibrolamellar carcinoma (FLC) is a variant of hepatocellular carcinoma; its separation as a distinct entity is justified by clinicopathologic features that sharply contrast with those commonly observed (Table I). The existence of this neoplasm was confirmed almost simultaneously by Berman et al.[5] and Craig et al.[6] in 1980. While this neoplasm constitutes only 1–2% of all hepatocellular carcinomas, 40% of those seen in children and young adults are of this type.[7] At diagnosis, the tumor is frequently localized in the liver, surgically resectable, and potentially curable. Its recognition is consequently critical.

2.1. Clinical Aspects

Fibrolamellar carcinoma usually develops in patients 5–35 years of age. It is seen with equal incidence in males and females. No association with oral contraceptive use has been found.[8] Presenting symptoms are nonspecific and include abdominal pain, malaise, and weight loss. An abdominal mass is palpable in two thirds of patients.

Liver-function tests reveal nonspecific mild elevations of the serum transaminases, alkaline phosphatase, and bilirubin. Increase in the serum AFP, which is seen in 85% of ordinary hepatocellular carcinomas, is observed in fewer than 10% of cases. Other potential tumor markers have been identified, including increased serum vitamin B_{12}-binding capacity and vitamin B_{12} levels,[9] neurotensin,[10,11] and carcinoembryonic antigen (CEA).[12] The former are due to an abnormal transcobalamin-1 protein, which is either synthesized by the tumor or represents circulating transcobalamin-1 that has been chemically modified by it.

The most helpful clue radiographically is the presence of calcification within the tumor, an otherwise uncommon finding in untreated hepatocellular carcinoma.[13,14] This may be detected on

Table I. Comparison of Clinicopathologic Features of Fibrolamellar Carcinoma with Usual Hepatocellular Carcinoma

Factor	FLC	HCC
Age group	5–35 years	50–70 years
Sex distribution	Males = females	Males predominate (3.5 : 1)
Non-neoplastic liver	Normal	Cirrhotic (75%)
Serum HBsAg	Absent	Present (60%)
Serum α-fetoprotein	Normal	Elevated (85%)
Histopathology		
Fibrosis	Prominent	Absent
Cytology	Abundant eosinophilic, cytoplasm	Variable
Extent of disease in liver at diagnosis	Localized	Widely disseminated
Surgical resectability	50–75%	10–20%
Mean survival from time of diagnosis	32–68 months	<6 months

plain films of the abdomen or by computed tomography (CT) (Fig. 3). These neoplasms produce a defect on sulfur colloid liver–spleen scintigram, are echogenic by ultrasound, and hypodense by unenhanced computed tomography. The latter two imaging modalities may detect a central scar, manifested by areas of increased echogenicity and lower density within the neoplasm, respectively, which can create confusion with focal nodular hyperplasia. Angiograms show a highly vascularized tumor whose arterial phase is characterized by abnormal vessels arranged in a septate fashion. Early arteriovenous shunting to the hepatic portal vein, if present, is a good clue to the presence of FLC.[15]

2.2. Pathology of Fibrolamellar Carcinoma

Fibrolamellar carcinoma usually occurs in a noncirrhotic otherwise normal-appearing liver. Two thirds of reported cases have been located in the left lobe. Grossly, the tumor is usually a sharply circumscribed solitary mass with a scalloped border (Fig. 4). Occasionally, smaller adjacent satellite nodules are present. Fibrous septa course through the tumor, in some instances radiating from a central scar mimicking the appearance of focal nodular hyperplasia. The distribution of metastases is similiar to that of ordinary hepatocellular carcinoma, with a tendency for abdominal lymph node, peritoneal, and pulmonary spread.

The distinctive histologic characteristics of this tumor include both stromal and cytologic components. Fibrosis, which is typically inconspicuous in hepatocellular carcinoma, is abundant in FLC (Fig. 5). Collagen and fibroblast are arranged in parallel lamellae about nests, pseudoglands, cords, and sheets of neoplastic cells. This desmoplastic response is also apparent in metastases, although it is often less pronounced. The neoplastic cells have an abundant deeply eosinophilic cytoplasm (Fig. 6). Most have a centrally placed vesicular nucleus with a single prominent nucleolus. Mitotic figures are rare. Cytoplasmic pale bodies (Fig. 7) and eosinophilic globules (Fig. 6), both of which represent various secretory products of the cells, are common. The latter are usually positive with periodic acid-Schiff (PAS) staining following diastase pretreatment and often represent accumulation of α_1-antitrypsin.[16,17] Fibrinogen is often present in the pale bodies,[18] which are PAS negative. Copper and copper-binding protein can frequently be detected with special stains (Rhodanine, Shikata orcein) and are distinctive features of this neoplasm.[12,17,19] Bile production is common, and mucin may be present.[20]

Ultrastructural descriptions have accompanied many reports of this tumor.[6,7,16,18,21–25] The outstanding feature has been the presence of abundant mitochondria, which fill the cytoplasm and account for its eosinophilic appearance by light microscopy.

2.3. Treatment and Prognosis

The outlook for patients with ordinary hepatocellular carcinoma is dismal, with a mean survival of 6 months. By contrast, the average survival of patients with FLC has been 32–68 months. This improved prognosis is due to multiple factors, which include the tumor's greater resectability and indolent growth. A more aggressive approach by surgeons, influenced by the young age of these patients and the lack of complicating cirrhosis, probably also plays a role in the more favorable prognosis.

Complete surgical resection is the basis for treatment of this tumor and can be accomplished in 50–75% of cases.[6,26,27] A simple lobectomy is the procedure of choice, but with very large tumors, right or left trisegmentectomy may be required.[28] Successfully treated patients have an excellent chance for long-term survival and the potential for cure. Cumulative figures from four large series,[5,7,26,29] involving 37 patients, show 24% alive and disease-free greater than 5 years following complete resection, 19% healthy 2–5 years following surgery, and another 19% well less than 2 years following the procedure; 38% had developed recurrences or died of their disease. Further heroic efforts are probably justified for those patients with more advanced disease. When primary resection of the tumor is not possible, hepatic transplantation has been employed.[29] Resection of

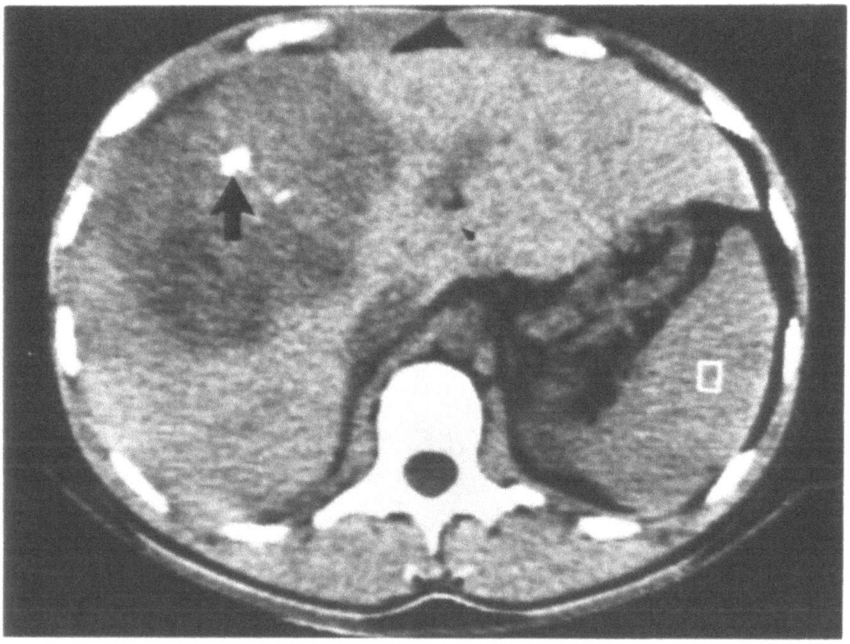

Figure 3. Unenhanced computerized axial tomography shows a well-defined hypodense mass with lobulated borders in the anterior segment of the right lobe of the liver. A central area of calcification is apparent (arrowhead).

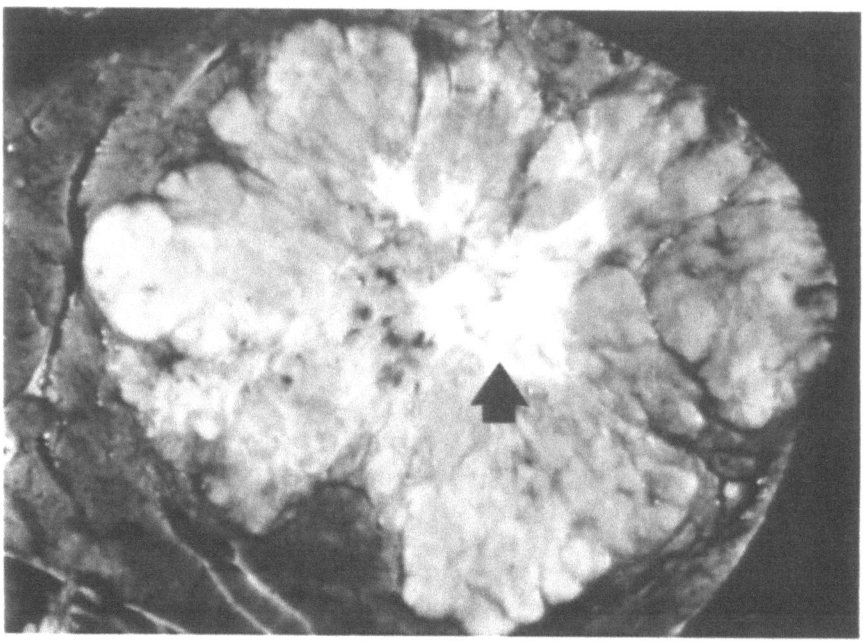

Figure 4. Surgical resection of fibrolamellar carcinoma is frequently possible because the tumor is often localized and sharply circumscribed at diagnosis. Fibrous septa course through the neoplasm giving it a multinodular appearance and radiate from a central scar (arrowhead) mimicking focal nodular hyperplasia.

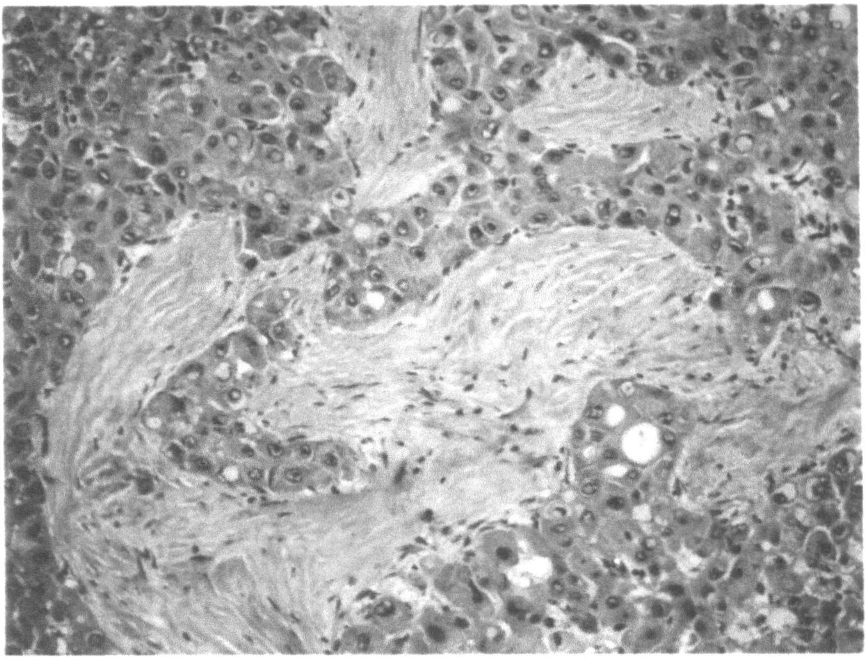

Figure 5. In fibrolamellar carcinoma, parallel lamellae of collagen and fibroblasts surround nests and anastomosing cords of tumor cells (H&E, ×160)

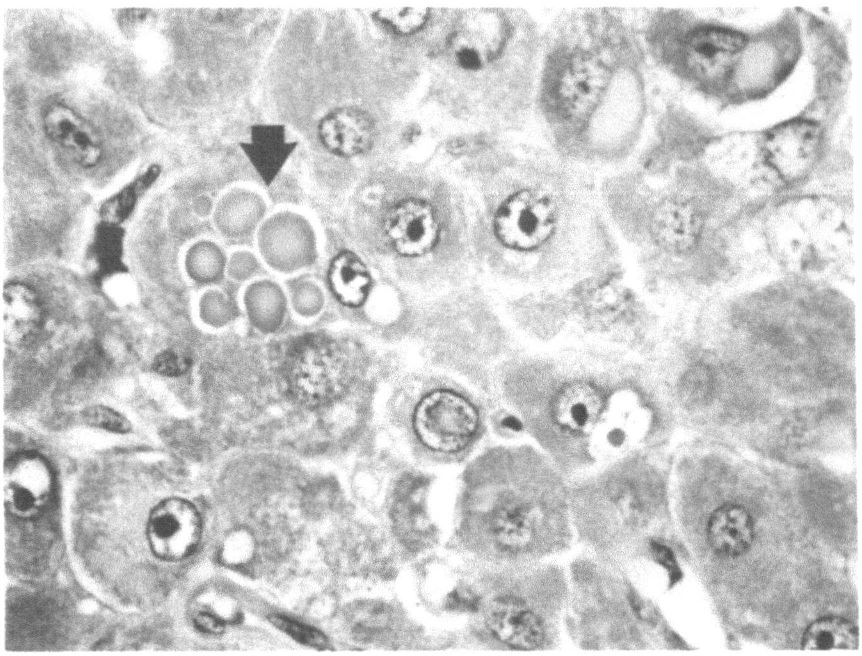

Figure 6. Neoplastic hepatocytes are characterized by abundant finely granular and deeply eosinophilic cytoplasm. Nuclei have a vesicular chromatin distribution and prominent nucleoli. Eosinophilic globules (arrowhead) are frequently observed. (H&E, ×630)

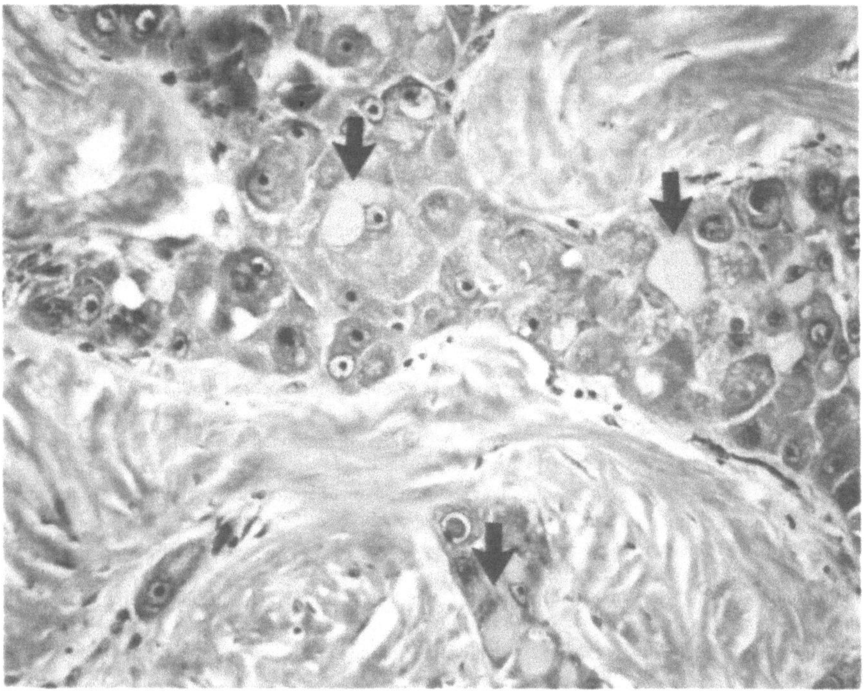

Figure 7. Pale cytoplasmic inclusions (arrowheads) are characteristically present in fibrolamellar carcinoma. (H&E, ×250)

recurrences in the liver and extrahepatic metastases may be beneficial and, in some instances, curative.[5,26]

Even patients with nonresectable tumors and distant metastases have prolonged survival, indicating that this tumor is intrinsically less malignant than HCC. In one study, such patients survived an average of 24 months.[30] Various chemotherapeutic regimens have been used within this context,[12,29,30] with partial responses observed in occasional patients, but they have had no demonstrable impact on overall survival. There are no reports of radiotherapy being successfully employed.

REFERENCES

1. Kew MC, Popper H: Relationship between hepatocellular carcinoma and cirrhosis. *Semin Liver Dis* **4:**136–146, 1984.
2. Okuda K, Musha H, Nakajima Y: Clinicopathologic features of encapsulated hepatocellular carcinoma: A study of 26 cases. *Cancer* **40:**1240–1245, 1977.
3. Anthony PP: Tumours and tumour-like lesions of the liver and biliary tract, in MacSween NM, Anthony PP, Scheuer PJ (eds): *Pathology of the Liver,* 2nd ed. Churchill Livingstone, Edinburgh, 1987, pp. 574–645.
4. Lai CL, Lew PC, Lam KC, et al: Histologic prognositic indicators in hepatocellular carcinoma. *Cancer* **44:**1677–1683, 1979.
5. Berman MM, Libbey NP, Foster JH: Hepatocellular carcinoma. Polygonal cell type with fibrous stroma—An atypical variant with a favorable prognosis. *Cancer* **46:**1448–1455, 1980.
6. Craig JR, Peters RL, Edmondson HA, et al: Fibrolamellar carcinoma of the liver: A tumor of adolescents and young adults with distinctive clinicopathologic features. *Cancer* **46:**372–379, 1980.

7. Farhi DC, Shikes RH, Murari PJ, et al: Hepatocellular carcinoma in young people. *Cancer* **52:**1516–1525, 1983.
8. Goodman ZD, Ishak KG: Hepatocellular carcinoma in women: Probable lack of etiologic association with oral contraceptive steroids. *Hepatology* **2:**440–444, 1982.
9. Paradinas FJ, Melia WM, Wilkinson ML, et al: High serum vitamin B12 binding capacity as a marker of the fibrolamellar variant of hepatocellular carcinoma. *Br Med J* **285:**840–842, 1982.
10. Collier NA, Bloom SR, Hodgson JHF, et al: Neurotensin secretion by fibrolamellar carcinoma of the liver. *Lancet* **1:**538–540, 1984.
11. Wood JR, Melia WM, Wood SM, et al: Neurotensin and hepatocellular carcinoma. (Letter to the editor.) *Lancet* **1:**687, 1984.
12. Teitelbaum DH, Tuttle S, Carey LC, et al: Fibrolamellar carcinoma of the liver. Review of three cases and the presentation of a characteristic set of tumor markers defining this tumor. *Ann Surg* **202:**36–41, 1985.
13. Friedman AC, Lichtenstein JE, Goodman ZD, et al: Fibrolamellar hepatocellular carcinoma. *Radiology* **157:**583–587, 1985.
14. Francis IR, Agha FP, Thompson NW, et al: Fibrolamellar hepatocarcinoma: Clinical, radiologic and pathologic features. *Gastrointest Rad* **11:**67–72, 1986.
15. Wong LK, Link DP, Frey CF, et al: Fibrolamellar hepatocarcinoma: Radiology, management and pathology. *AJR* **139:**172–175, 1982.
16. Caballero T, Aneiros J, Lopez-Caballero J, et al: Fibrolamellar hepatocellular carcinoma. An immunohistochemical and ultrastructural study. *Histopathology* **9:**445–456, 1985.
17. Lefkowitch JH, Muschel R, Price JB, et al: Copper and copper-binding protein in fibrolamellar liver cell carcinoma. *Cancer* **51:**97–100, 1983.
18. Stromeyer FW, Ishak KG, Gerber MA, et al: Ground glass cells in hepatocellular carcinoma. *Am J Clin Pathol* **74:**254–258, 1980.
19. Sheahan DG: Fibrolamellar carcinoma of the liver: An immunohistochemical study. *Lab Invest* **54:**57, 1986 (abst).
20. Goodman ZD, Ishak KG, Langloss JM, et al: Combined hepatocellular-cholangiocellular carcinoma. A histologic and immunohistologic study. *Cancer* **55:**124–135, 1985.
21. Vecchio FM, Fabrino A, Ghirlanda G, et al: Fibrolamellar carcinoma of the liver: The malignant counterpart of focal nodular hyperplasia with oncocytic change. *Am J Clin Pathol* **81:**521–526, 1984.
22. An T, Ghatak N, Kastner R, et al: Hyaline globules and intracellular lumina in a hepatocellular carcinoma. *Am J Clin Pathol* **79:**392–396, 1983.
23. Baithum SI, Pollock DJ: Oncocytic hepatocellular tumor. *Histopathology* **7:**107–112, 1983.
24. Farhi DC, Shikes RH, Silverberg SG: Ultrastructure of fibrolamellar oncocytic hepatoma. *Cancer* **50:**702–709, 1982.
25. Mierau GW, Orsini EN: Case for diagnosis. *Ultrastruct Pathol* **5:**273–279, 1983.
26. Nagorney DM, Adson MA, Weiland LH, et al: Fibrolamellar hepatoma. *Am J Surg* **149:**113–119, 1985.
27. Lack EE, Neave C, Vawter GF: Hepatocellular carcinoma. Review of 32 cases in childhood and adolescence. *Cancer* **52:**1510–1515, 1983.
28. Craig JR, Van Thiel DH: Fibrolamellar carcinoma, in Ishak KG (ed): *Hepatopathology 1985. Syllabus of the Postgraduate Course of the American Association for the Study of Liver Disease, Chicago, 3–4, Nov. 1985.* Slack, Thorofare, New Jersey, pp. 361–371.
29. Starzl TE, Iwatsuki S, Shaw BW, et al: Treatment of fibrolamellar hepatoma with partial or total hepatectomy and transplantation of the liver. *Surg Gynecol Obstet* **162:**145–148, 1986.
30. Ihde DC, Matthews MJ, Makuch RN, et al: Prognostic factors in patients with hepatocellular carcinoma receiving systemic chemotherapy. Identification of two groups of patients with prospects for prolonged survival. *Am J Med* **78:**399–406, 1985.

Index

MIX
Papier aus verantwortungsvollen Quellen
Paper from responsible sources
FSC® C105338

If you have any concerns about our products,
you can contact us on
ProductSafety@springernature.com

In case Publisher is established outside the EU,
the EU authorized representative is:
Springer Nature Customer Service Center GmbH
Europaplatz 3, 69115 Heidelberg, Germany

Printed by Libri Plureos GmbH
in Hamburg, Germany